The Art and Science of Cardiac Physical Examination

with Heart Sounds, Jugular and Precordial Pulsations on CD

2nd Edition

Includes 12-Lead ECG Interpretation

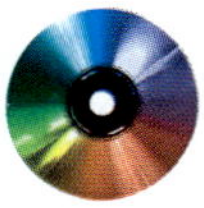

***System requirements*:**

- **Operating System—Windows Vista or above**
- **Recommended Web Browser—Google Chrome & Mozilla Firefox**
- **Essential plugins—Java & Flash player**
  - Facing problems in viewing content—it may be your system does not have Java enabled.
  - If Videos do not show up—it may be the system requires Flash player or need to manage Flash setting. To learn more about Flash setting click on the link in the help section.
  - You can test Java and Flash by using the links from the help section of the CD/DVD.

Accompanying CD/DVD Rom is playable only in Computer and not in DVD player.

CD/DVD has Autorun function—it may take few seconds to load on your computer. If it does not works for you then follow the steps below to access the contents manually:

- Click on My Computer
- Select the CD/DVD drive and click open/explore—this will show list of files in the CD/DVD
- Find and double click file—"launch.html"

For more information about troubleshoot of Autorun click on:
http://support.microsoft.com/kb/330135.

The Art and Science of Cardiac Physical Examination

with Heart Sounds, Jugular and Precordial Pulsations on CD

Includes 12-Lead ECG Interpretation

Narasimhan Ranganathan MBBS FRCP(C) FACP FACC FAHA
Associate Professor in Medicine
University of Toronto, Ontario, Canada
Senior Cardiology Consultant
St. Joseph's Health Centre
Toronto, Ontario, Canada

Vahe Sivaciyan BSc MD FRCP(C)
Assistant Professor in Medicine
University of Toronto, Ontario, Canada
Staff Cardiologist, St. Joseph's Health Centre
Toronto, Ontario, Canada

Franklin B Saksena MD CM FACP FRCP(C) FACC FAHA
Associate Professor in Medicine
Northwestern University School of Medicine
Chicago, Illinois, USA

Foreword

Sriram Rajagopal MD DM

JAYPEE *The Health Sciences Publisher*

New Delhi | London | Philadelphia | Panama

Jaypee Brothers Medical Publishers (P) Ltd

Headquarters
Jaypee Brothers Medical Publishers (P) Ltd.
4838/24, Ansari Road, Daryaganj
New Delhi 110 002, India
Phone: +91-11-43574357
Fax: +91-11-43574314
E-mail: jaypee@jaypeebrothers.com

Overseas Offices
J.P. Medical Ltd.
83, Victoria Street, London
SW1H 0HW (UK)
Phone: +44-20 3170 8910
Fax: +44(0)20 3008 6180
E-mail: info@jpmedpub.com

Jaypee Medical Inc.
The Bourse
111 South Independence Mall East
Suite 835
Philadelphia, PA 19106, USA
Phone: +1 267-519-9789
E-mail: jpmed.us@gmail.com

Jaypee Brothers Medical Publishers (P) Ltd.
Bhotahity, Kathmandu, Nepal
Phone: +977-9741283608
E-mail: kathmandu@jaypeebrothers.com

Jaypee-Highlights Medical Publishers Inc.
City of Knowledge, Bld. 237, Clayton
Panama City, Panama
Phone: +1 507-301-0496
Fax: +1 507-301-0499
E-mail: cservice@jphmedical.com

Jaypee Brothers Medical Publishers (P) Ltd.
17/1-B, Babar Road, Block-B, Shaymali
Mohammadpur, Dhaka-1207
Bangladesh
Mobile: +08801912003485
E-mail: jaypeedhaka@gmail.com

Website: www.jaypeebrothers.com
Website: www.jaypeedigital.com

Inquiries for bulk sales may be solicited at: jaypee@jaypeebrothers.com

The Art and Science of Cardiac Physical Examination

Second Edition: **2016**

ISBN: 978-93-5152-777-0

Printed at: Sanat Printers

Dedication

Narasimhan Ranganathan, Vahe Sivaciyan and Franklin B Saksena wish to dedicate this book to their respective wives, Saroja, Ayda and Kathleen. For without their support, this book would not have been possible.

Foreword

I feel privileged to be asked to write a foreword to this book *The Art and Science of Cardiac Physical Examination.*

The authors are very experienced and senior clinicians, and have more than three decades of rigorous, scientific research into clinical signs and their mechanisms. They have made seminal contributions to the literature in this field, particularly in the area of the jugular venous pulse. Further, they are deeply committed to teaching and communicating the knowledge and insights that they have acquired over the years.

The past few decades have seen considerable changes in the science and practice of cardiology. The plethora of new discoveries, new imaging modalities and newer modes of treatment has tended to overshadow the importance of sound clinical examination. Indeed, there is a widespread feeling that both the time and the importance accorded to the formal teaching of clinical skills in many contemporary cardiology training programs are inadequate. The authors' effort in bringing out this excellent book (and companion CD) serves as an effective and timely step to correct this trend.

The treatment of the subject matter is comprehensive, with each of the main chapters starting with a detailed review of the normal physiology underlying a clinical phenomenon as well as the pathophysiology in different abnormal states, providing a clear understanding of the basis of the clinical sign. The chapters on the arterial pulse and jugular venous pulse are particularly illuminative in this respect. The correct technique of elicitation of the finding is then lucidly outlined, often with unique methods to demonstrate phenomena and insightful tips to improve bedside skills. Finally, the interpretation and integration of the information obtained is rightly emphasized, so that the finding can be placed in the context of the larger clinical picture in a cogent and meaningful manner. The summary at the end of each chapter provides a concise and rapid review to enhance learning. The chapters are extensively referenced providing rich material for further learning. The creative and original methods described in the chapter entitled "Elements of Auscultation" serve to beautifully unify the "Art" and "Science" aspects of auscultation. A separate chapter on "Pathophysiologic Basis of Symptoms and Signs in Cardiac Disease" serves to reiterate concepts described elsewhere in the book in the particular context of specific conditions.

The novel use of audiovisual aids in the companion CD further remarkably enhances the value of this book as a learning resource. Examples from years of clinical observation have been carefully documented and painstakingly converted to video and audio clips that provide an unprecedented level of realism. The readers are provided with a "clinical experience" where they can literally see and hear the findings and can verify their skills of observation and interpretation in a "real-life" setting. This edition introduces two new chapters on electrocardiography, now widely regarded as part of the clinical evaluation. The first of these chapters provides extensive coverage of the principles of electrocardiography and interpretation, while the second chapter on "Integration of ECG into the Cardiac Diagnosis" provides a succinct account of the correlation of ECG findings in a wide range of cardiac disorders with the pathophysiology of these conditions. The section on self-assessment is also a valuable educational aid and serves to reinforce the message on the integration of information from different sources.

This book is bound to be of immense value to any individual interested in clinical cardiology, from the fresh medical student (who will benefit from a sound and lucid introduction to the subject) to the senior and experienced clinician (who will gain new understanding and insight). The companion CD is well-suited to serve as an important tool for both individual and group teaching. The authors are to be commended for their extraordinary effort in distilling decades of clinical experience into this extremely valuable contribution to the important field of clinical cardiology.

Sriram Rajagopal MD DM
Chief Cardiologist
Southern Railway Headquarters Hospital
Chennai, Tamil Nadu, India

Preface to the 2nd Edition

The first edition of our book was the result of our long-lasting interest in promoting the usefulness and value of proper cardiac physical examination in the assessment of cardiac patients. It is a culmination of our long-lasting experience in teaching and training physicians and students of cardiology. We have offered a course annually of the same title in Toronto over the last 35 years. Modern technological advances both invasive and non-invasive have contributed significantly to our knowledge and understanding of cardiac physical signs and their pathophysiologic correlates. Both students and the teachers alike become impressed by these technological tools to the extent of neglecting the age-old art as well as the substantial body of science behind the cardiac physical examination. These technological advances are here to stay. However, some have even gone to the extent of suggesting that a "physician should have an all purpose tool in his or her pocket that would be more in keeping with the 21st century than the stethoscope, a 200-year-old technology whose time should be over".[1] One must never forget that any tool or instrument is only as good as the person using it. The information that can be derived from the proper assessment of the jugular contours, the precordial pulsations, the arterial pulses as well as cardiac auscultation can never be considered waste in terms of the assessment of a cardiac patient, in our opinion. It is not only cost effective and satisfying and can never be counterproductive to the patient's needs. In addition, it could be lifesaving under certain circumstances (such as in remote locations, during power failure and times of disaster). Neglect of these basic skills, expected of physicians and cardiologists to be, will not augur well for the future generation of the physicians and patients alike.

The positive features of our book include among other things innovative and proven effective teaching methods with the use of recordings of not only heart sounds and murmurs but also the actual video-recordings of both normal and abnormal jugular pulsations as well the precordial pulsations together with arterial flow signals and/or the heart sounds for timing of the events in relation to the cardiac cycle. We were pleased and not totally surprised however, when we discovered that our book was translated into Chinese, a few years ago.[2] It suggests also that not all physicians share the opinion of some who would like to name the stethoscope as "archaic instrument" and lock it up in their office chest. In addition, it indicates a need to reach out to more medical schools and the institutions in many developed and developing nations. We are hoping that it would achieve that goal with our current publishers of this new and improved second edition.

In addition to the 'The Art and Science of Cardiac Physical Examination', we have also been interested in teaching 12-lead ECG interpretation to physicians and trainees for many years offering annual courses. ECG is often considered an integral part of the office assessment of a cardiac patient and almost considered to be an extension of cardiac physical assessment. Most physicians either have or have access to an ECG machine in their offices. ECG is also indispensable in the assessment of patients presenting with acute symptoms of chest pain and or dyspnea. Therefore, when we were faced with the opportunity of providing a second edition, we wanted to make the book even more comprehensive. In addition to updating new and relevant information in several of the previous chapters of the first edition, we have included three new chapters. These consist of the following: a complete chapter consisting of six different sections which cover fully the 12-lead Electrocardiogram Interpretation, a second chapter showing how to integrate the ECG into Cardiac Diagnosis and a third and final chapter for Self-Assessment at the end with several interesting clinical cases from our own practice. In addition, we have added a self-assessment section in the companion CD with several new clinical examples. We believe that these self-assessment sections would serve as a good review as well as being useful for reinforcement purposes both in self-teaching and/or group learning sessions.

Before we end this preface, we would like to take the opportunity to reminisce and thank for the friendship and the association we have had both during the formative years of becoming a cardiologist as well as in the later years of career as a practicing cardiologist and as a teacher. During the years of training, I (the senior author) had the opportunity to work with some of the well-known cardiologists including Dr George E Burch and Dr John Phillips of the reputed Tulane University medical school as well as Dr E Douglas Wigle and Dr Malcolm Silver (Cardiac Pathologist) of the University of Toronto. However, the longest association of teaching both cardiac physical examination and 12-lead ECG interpretation was with Dr Jules Constant from the State University of Buffalo, New York, USA. We in fact used to invite him over to teach along with us in Toronto almost annually for many years in our annual cardiac physical examination course. I have also taken part in teaching along with him in 'the 12-lead ECG interpretation courses' which he used to organize in the month of February in the warmer southern climate. He had a fine sense of empathy for the beginners, which was admirable. One's own teaching technique also becomes more refined watching other masters perform. In fact, Dr. Constant was still alive at the time of the release of our first edition of the book. We wish to list the names of these individuals here in order not only to recognize their contribution in the field of cardiology but also to express our gratitude.

Finally, we present this book again with a firm belief that it will be an invaluable asset and it will serve as useful aid in stimulating and learning as well as in teaching clinical cardiology.

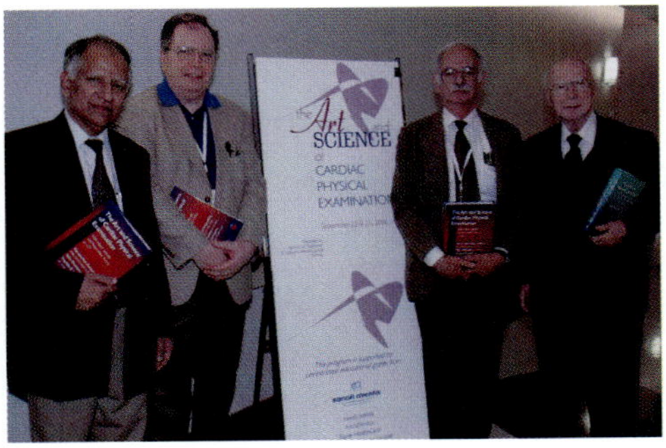

REFERENCES

1. Mehta M, Jacobson T, Peters D, et al. Handheld Ultrasound Versus Physical Examination in Patients Referred for Transthoracic Echocardiography for a Suspected Cardiac Condition. JACC Cardiovasc Imaging. 2014 Oct;7(10):983-90.
2. Translation from the English language Edition of The Art and Science of Cardiac Physical Examination, by Narasimhan ranganathan, Vahe Sivaciyan and Franklin B. Saksena. Beijing, China: www.sciencep.com; 2009.

Narasimhan Ranganathan MBBS FRCP(C) FACP FACC FAHA
Associate Professor in Medicine
University of Toronto, Ontario, Canada
Senior Cardiology Consultant
St. Joseph's Health Centre
Toronto, Ontario, Canada

Vahe Sivaciyan BSc MD FRCP(C)
Assistant Professor in Medicine
University of Toronto, Ontario, Canada
Staff Cardiologist, St. Joseph's Health Centre
Toronto, Ontario, Canada

Preface to the 1st Edition

It has been our experience that teaching of the physical examination of the heart in medical schools has been deteriorating since the advent of the modern diagnostic tools such as the 2-dimensional echocardiography and nuclear imaging. At best it has been sketchy and too superficial for the student to appreciate the pathophysiologic correlates. Both the invasive and the non-invasive modern technological advances have contributed substantially to our knowledge and understanding of the cardiac physical signs and their pathophysiological correlates. However, both the students and the teachers alike appear to be mesmerized by these technologic advances to the neglect of the age-old art as well as the substantial body of science of the cardiac physical examination. It is also sad to see that reputed journals also give low priority to articles related to the clinical examination.

Our experience is substantiated by a nationwide survey of the teaching and practice of cardiac auscultation during internal medicine and cardiology training which concluded that there was in fact low emphasis on this and perhaps also on other bedside diagnostic skills.[1] The state of the problem is well-reflected in the concerns expressed in previous publications.[2-4] including the editorial in the American Journal of Medicine 2001;110:233-5, entitled "Cardiac auscultation and teaching rounds: how can cardiac auscultation be resuscitated?" as well as in the rebuttal, "Selections from current literature. Horton hears a Who but no murmurs—does it matter?".[5] The latter goes to the extent of suggesting that auscultation be performed only when cardiac symptoms are encountered in patients. This appears to be based on an exaggerated concern for the waste of time and resources. Implicit in this statement if one chooses to agree with it, will be the acknowledgment of one's failure as a physician caring for patients.

On the contrary, we not only share the opinion of others that cardiac auscultation is a cost effective diagnostic skill[6] and we would like to go one step further and suggest that all aspects of cardiac physical examination are very cost-effective and rewarding in many ways. A properly obtained detailed and complete history of the patient's problems and a thorough physical examination are never counterproductive to the interests of the patient.

Modern technological advances are here to stay and they should be adjunct to the clinical examination of the patient but should not be allowed to replace them. Let us not forget that many of these tools do add to the rising costs of healthcare all over the world. A well carried out physical examination of the heart often provides the critical information necessary to choose the right investigative tool and to avoid the unnecessary ones. Even if one ignores the cost factor, a physician caring for a patient under conditions where these techniques may not be accessible (at nights and on the weekends in some institutions, remote locations, during power failure and during times of natural or other disasters) should be able to assess and diagnose cardiac function and probable underlying pathology using the fives senses, a stethoscope and a sphygmomanometer.

Mackenzie integrated the jugular venous pulse as part of the cardiovascular physical examination.[7] Wood further went on to show that the precise analysis of the jugular venous pulse waveforms and the measurement of the venous pressure with reference to the sternal angle is possible at the bedside.[8] Interpretation of the jugular venous pulse contour and the assessment of the pressure yet remains an occult art practiced only by experienced clinicians. Poor, ill-defined and vague terms such as jugular venous distension are commonly used and written about even in reputed journals when cardiac physical findings are mentioned.

One of the satisfying features of medicine aside from contributing to the clinical improvement of an ailing patient, is the intellectual excitement and satisfaction of arriving at the right conclusion through proper reasoning based on clues derived from the clinical examination of the patient. In addition, not surprisingly some of the physical signs have also been shown in this day and age of 'Evidence based Medicine', to be of prognostic importance. For instance elevated jugular venous pressure and the third heart sound in patients with symptomatic heart failure had been shown to have independent prognostic information.[9] We believe that a proper understanding of the pathophysiologic correlates of the various signs and symptoms would help in developing skills of logical thinking required of a good clinician at work. It is all the more important if one were to plan to study the validity or the worthiness of the detection of an abnormal sound or sign in relationship to other cardiac measurements.[10] Improper understanding would only result in testing of wrong hypotheses and misleading conclusion.

The purpose of this book is to arm the student of cardiology with the proper techniques and understanding of the art and science of the cardiac physical examination, to dispel myths and confusion and to help develop skills required of any astute clinician.

This book is a culmination of our efforts resulting from our long-standing experience of teaching and training physicians and trainees and students of cardiology. In fact an annual course entitled by the same name as our book has been organized and offered by us at our institution in Toronto over 25 years. They have been always well received and extremely appreciated for the teaching methods and the content by the attendees. Audio recordings of heart sounds and murmurs, as well as video recordings of jugular and precordial pulsations with simultaneously recorded sounds and flow signals for timing from actual patients collected over many years of clinical practice have been utilized in this course. Video display of the actual sounds and murmurs provides a real-time playback effect and enhances the group teaching and learning experience using multiple listening devices with infrared transmission of sounds. The teaching material and methods have been developed and refined over many years, stimulated by enthusiastic and inquisitive students and trainees and aided by our own research and studies particularly with reference to the jugular venous flows and pulsations as well as with regard to the precordial pulsations.

The organization of the material presented in this book warrants some elaboration. We believe that the information is presented in a fashion integrating the science with concepts useful for logical integration into clinical applications. The teaching method adopted is somewhat unique and we believe totally original in some sections. This would be evident in chapters on Jugular Venous Pulse, the Precordial pulsations as well as the Arterial Pulse. The approach to the interpretation of the jugular venous pulsations presented here brings to the forefront the proper method of integration of the art with the science at the bedside. We believe that it is different in many ways from other books dealing with cardiac examination.

Every important topic has a summary of salient and practical points from the point of view of clinical assessment. This would serve for quick review as well as act as pointers needing reinforcement. Many illustrations of sounds and murmurs used in the text are derived from digital display of actual audio recordings from patients The pathophysiology of some of the important clinical cardiac conditions are shown in flow diagrams as well as in tabular format permitting logical review and reinforcement. The references given at the end of the chapters are specially chosen to provide a variety of pertinent as well as the classic papers.

A special chapter deals with local and systemic manifestations of cardiovascular disease authored by our colleague and friend Dr Franklin B Saksena (Senior Attending Physician, Division of Adult Cardiology, John Stroger, Jr. Hospital of Cook County and Assistant Professor of Medicine, Northwestern University, Chicago, Attending Physician, Swedish Covenant Hospital, Attending Physician, Saint Mary of Nazareth Hospital). It provides several useful illustrations as well as a major list of references.

The audio and the video recordings of sounds and murmurs, the jugular and the precordial pulsations from actual patients with a variety of clinical cardiac problems are also available in a companion CD which will have all the videofiles playable through the Windows Media player on any new modern computer. These video recordings made from actual patients are meant to further enhance individual learning as well as group teaching of students and trainees in cardiology. They will provide a real time play back effect of heart sounds and murmurs displayed on an oscilloscopic screen. Another unique feature in the videofiles includes the presentation of simultaneous recordings of the 2-dimensional echocardiographic images together with the audiorecordings of the heart murmurs from a few patients with specific cardiac lesions.

We present this book with a firm belief that it will be an invaluable asset and hope it will serve as a very useful tool in learning and teaching clinical cardiology.

REFERENCES

1. Mangione S, Nieman LZ, Gracely E, et al. The teaching and practice of cardiac auscultation during internal medicine and cardiology training. A nationwide survey. Ann Intern Med 1993;119:47-54.
2. Schneiderman H. Cardiac auscultation and teaching rounds: how can cardiac auscultation be resuscitated? Am J Med 2001;110:233-5.
3. Lok CE, Morgan CD, Ranganathan N. The accuracy and interobserver agreement in detecting the 'gallop sounds' by cardiac auscultation. Chest 1998; 114:1283-8.
4. Tavel ME. Cardiac auscultation. A glorious past—but does it have a future? Circulation 1996;93:1250-3.
5. Kopes-Kerr CP. Selections from current literature. Horton hears a Who but no murmurs—does it matter? Fam Pract 2002;19:422-5.
6. Shaver. J. A. Cardiac auscultation: a cost-effective diagnostic skill. Curr Probl Cardiol 1995;7:441-530.
7. Mackenzie J. The study of the Pulse. London: Pentland, 1902.
8. Wood P. Diseases of the Heart and Circulation. Philadelphia,: JB Lippincott Vo, 1956.
9. Drazner MH, Rame JE, Stevenson LW, et al. Prognostic importance of elevated jugular venous pressure and a third heart sound in patients with heart failure. N Engl J Med 2001;345:574-81.
10. Marcus GM, Gerber IL, McKeown BH, et al. Association between phonocardiographic third and fourth heart sounds and objective measures of left ventricular function. Jama 2005;293:2238-44.

Narasimhan Ranganathan MBBS FRCP(C) FACP FACC FAHA
Associate Professor in Medicine
University of Toronto, Ontario, Canada
Senior Cardiology Consultant
St. Joseph's Health Centre
Toronto, Ontario, Canada

Vahe Sivaciyan BSc MD FRCP(C)
Assistant Professor in Medicine
University of Toronto, Ontario, Canada
Staff Cardiologist, St. Joseph's Health Centre
Toronto, Ontario, Canada

Acknowledgments to the 2nd Edition

First of all, I would like to express my sincere thanks to all my colleagues at both the St. Michael's Hospital as well as the St. Joseph's Health Centre who have been supportive of my teaching endeavors during the years of my hospital practice. In addition we wish to express our sincere gratitude to all of our patients who had volunteered their time in this regards for the purposes of cardiac teaching. This second edition however, could not be successfully completed without the help of Mr. Roger Harris. He was also quite helpful in the preparation of the first edition of the book as mentioned in the previous acknowledgments. We wish to express and record here our profound thanks and acknowledgments for the invaluable assistance of Mr. Roger Harris in the production of not only the newer illustrations but also in the preparation of the companion CD and its content files for the second edition. Mr. Roger Harris is currently the retired chief of the audiovisual department of the St. Joseph's Health Centre in Toronto. We had numerous audio recordings from actual clinical patients to choose from. But our desire to provide them in a similar format as the previous CD with real time playback effect had some tremendous obstacles to overcome. Video recordings of the oscilloscopic tracings of the phono signals and adjusting them for asynchrony between the video and the audio signals due to playback and recording involving different devices was the most difficult and time consuming of these. Luckily for us, the efforts of Mr. Roger Harris were not only very fruitful and victorious but also timely. Thus we are really indebted to him and therefore sincerely express our thanks to Roger for his invaluable assistance.

We wish to express our sincere gratitude and thanks to Dr. Sriram Rajagopal, Chief of Cardiology, at the Southern Railway Headquarters Hospital, Chennai, a premier tertiary cardiac care centre in India with recognized postgraduate training program in Cardiology, for writing the Foreword to this second edition.

Finally, we would also like to thank Mr. Jitendar P Vij (Group Chairman), Mr. Ankit Vij (Group President), Ms Chetna Malhotra Vohra (Associate Director), Ms Angima Shree (Development Editor) and Production team of Jaypee Brothers Medical Publishers (P) Ltd., New Delhi, India.

Narasimhan Ranganathan

Acknowledgments to the 1st Edition

I wish to express on behalf of all the authors our sincere thanks and gratitude to many individuals who had helped either directly or indirectly our efforts in teaching of bedside clinical cardiology over the years and thereby had made the publication of this work possible. First our thanks go to all the patients who had kindly volunteered their time for the purpose of medical education and teaching. I wish to express also my sincere thanks to all my colleagues in the Cardiology division of the St. Michael's Hospital, University of Toronto with whom I had worked between the years of 1970 through 1988, my colleagues at the St. Joseph's Health Centre from 1989 up to the present as well as the administration of the St. Joseph's Health Centre for their support of our educational programs and endeavours. A special thanks is also due to Mr John Cooper and his family whose kind donation towards the Cardiology service at St. Joseph's Health Centre allowed the acquisition of a computer with a fast processor and modern video editing capabilities, which eventually helped in the conversion of old technology to modern technology. We would like to express our thanks also to Professor Emeritus Rashmi Desai from the Department of Physics at the University of Toronto and his colleague Dr Katrin Rohlf from the Department of Chemistry, University of Toronto for their input and comments.

Our profound gratitude and sincerest thanks however, we owe to Mr. Roger Harris, who is the head of the Audio-Visual department at St. Joseph's Health Centre, without whose ingenuity and dedicated and continued assistance, the publication of this book and the companion video CD would not be possible. Most of the audio recordings were originally made on a four channel Cambridge magnetic disc recorder of the 1960s. In fact we originally used to play these discs even during our annual continuing medical education courses, using a storage oscilloscope with the help of a television camera connected to large monitors for instant display of the waveforms. In 1989, I had the good fortune of associating with Mr Roger Harris after I joined St. Joseph's Health Centre. With his assistance and advice, the audio recordings were initially converted to video recordings. When reliable video editing programs with good and acceptable synchrony between the audio and the video tracks became available, Roger helped to digitise and archive these video recordings. In addition it is through his efforts we have made the successful transition to current technology with display capability through the Windows Media player on any modern computer. Furthermore, his assistance has been invaluable for the production of all of the illustrations in the text as well as the production of the companion Video CD. Therefore his dedication and contributions are gratefully acknowledged and very much appreciated.

Finally, we also wish to express our sincere gratitude and appreciation to Mr Balu Srinivasan for his timely and dedicated professional assistance in the preparation of the final design and format of the companion Video CD.

Narasimhan Ranganathan

Contents

CD Content List

Heart Sounds, Jugular and Precordial Pulsations

Chapter 1 Approach to the Physical Examination of the Cardiac Patient

Snapshot

- Reasons for which Cardiac Assessment is Sought
- Cardiac Symptoms and their Appraisal
- Generation of Working List of Possible Diagnoses
- The Approach to a Focused Physical Examination
- Practical Points to a Focused Cardiac Physical Examination

Performance of a proper cardiac physical examination and the interpretation of the findings require a good understanding of both the physiology of the cardiovascular system and the pathophysiology involved in the abnormal states caused by various cardiac lesions and disorders. The development of good bedside skills not only requires dedication on the part of the student of cardiology but also require the instruction methods be sound and based on both science and logic. The clinician instructor and the student clinician then come to appreciate that the whole process involves the integration of the science with the art of the physical examination.

While each of the various aspects of the cardiac physical examination is dealt with in a detailed manner in the subsequent chapters, the very first chapter is devoted to the general approach to the physical examination of the cardiac patient.

In this chapter the following points are discussed:

1. The various reasons for which a cardiac assessment might be sought.
2. The appraisal of the various cardiac symptoms and their proper interpretation in order that an intelligent list of the various possible etiologic causes of the problem can be generated.
3. The generation of the possible etiologic causes of the symptoms of the patient.
4. The physical examination that is focused to derive pertinent information helpful in the differential diagnosis and thereby enables one to plan the subsequent investigation and management.
5. The material is illustrated by two different patient histories. In the first case, the discussion of the physical findings is somewhat general, and in the second case, it is more specific. We believe that both clinical cases can be treated as material for self-testing by the interested student or the trainee, both before and after studying the remainder of the book.

REASONS FOR WHICH CARDIAC ASSESSMENT IS SOUGHT

The patient for cardiovascular assessment may present generally as a result of one of the following reasons:

1. *For confirmation and assessment of a suspected cardiac lesion or disease.*
2. *Because of the presence of abnormal cardiac findings on physical examination (such as a heart murmur), and/or one of the laboratory tests (such as an abnormal ECG, chest X-Ray or echocardiogram).*
3. *Because of symptoms pertaining to other systems or regions of the body that, however, might have a cardiac source.*
4. *Because of the presence of cardiac symptoms (such as dyspnea, chest pain and syncope).*

In the patient with a suspected cardiac lesion or disease, one needs to have a clear mental picture of associated symptoms and signs and risk factors if any. The examiner then should analyze the patient's history, symptoms and signs from this perspective. For instance, if the patient is sent with a diagnosis of atrial septal defect, the mental picture of this lesion should be one of a precordial pulsation dominated by the right ventricle, inconspicuous left ventricle and fixed splitting of the second heart sound. If that patient were to have a large area hyperdynamic left ventricular apical impulse, then either the diagnosis is incorrect or the lesion is complicated by an additional condition such as mitral regurgitation, which may be significant.

If the patient were referred because of an abnormal finding on physical examination such as a heart murmur, the examiner in addition to confirming the finding also needs to establish the cause and the severity of the lesion. In patients with abnormal laboratory test results, the abnormality must be identified and confirmed. One needs to have a clear knowledge of the associated lesions and causes for proper evaluation of such instances. For instance a patient referred for cardiomegaly on the chest X-ray should have the X-ray reviewed to rule out apparent cardiomegaly from causes such as scoliosis or poor technique. Physical examination and, in some cases, a two-dimensional echocardiogram may be essential to determine the actual chamber dimensions and wall thickness. Sometime a markedly hypertrophied ventricle with reduced internal dimensions may cause an increased cardiothoracic ratio on the chest radiograph.

In patients with abnormal electrocardiograms (ECGs), the identification of the abnormality often can give directions to diagnosis. For instance, the presence of left ventricular hypertrophy and strain pattern should indicate the presence of left ventricular outflow obstruction, hypertrophic cardiomyopathy or hypertensive heart disease. If the ECG were to show an infarct, besides ischemic heart disease, one needs to consider other conditions that can cause infarct patterns on the ECG, such as hypertrophic cardiomyopathy or pre-excitation as seen in Wolff-Parkinson-White syndrome.

Patients may sometimes present with clinical symptoms and signs pertaining to other systems or regions of the body that may actually have resulted from a cardiac source. These include symptoms consistent with systemic arterial embolism that could vary depending on the territory or region involved. They are often of sudden onset and result in ischemic symptoms related to arterial occlusion that could be either transient and/or of prolonged duration. When the source of the systemic embolism arises from the heart, the most common region that will be affected is the brain. This, of course, will cause stroke and/or transient cerebral ischemic symptoms. The cardiac sources that need to be considered include infective endocarditis with vegetations on the valve, formation of a left ventricular mural thrombus over an area of akinetic myocardium as a result of a recent and large myocardial infarction. The most common cause is often the onset of atrial fibrillation that will predispose to formation of thrombus in the left atrial appendage due to loss of atrial contraction and the resultant tendency for blood to sludge in the left atrium. The atrial fibrillation can occur in patients with pre-existing valvular disease most commonly mitral disease. However, atrial fibrillation unrelated to valvular disease is becoming the most common arrhythmia especially in the elderly patients and often the cause in a substantial portion of patients who present with stroke and/or transient cerebral ischemia.[1–3] Rarely the thrombus may in fact be of systemic venous origin such as due to a deep venous thrombosis in the lower extremities and/or the pelvic veins and embolize not only to the lungs but also end up in the arterial system. In order for this to occur, one will have to have a communication between the right and the left side of the heart. Patients who present with such a *paradoxical embolism* may often have a patent foramen ovale and/or a small atrial septal defect that had been undetected previously. Such communications are usually associated with small left-to-right shunts, since the left atrial pressure is normally higher than the right atrial pressure, and the right ventricle offers less resistance to filling than the left ventricle. However, when sudden venous embolism occurs into the right heart and to the lungs, it can cause elevation of right ventricular and right atrial pressure. This can set the stage for transient reversal of flow across the atrial septum and result in paradoxical embolism. This may have to be considered especially when transient cerebral ischemia or stroke occurs in relatively younger patients with no significant risk factors for stroke or obvious cause such as valvular disease and/or atrial fibrillation. However, one will have to resort to two-dimensional echocardiographic (either transthoracic or transesophageal) study for confirmation, since cardiac physical examination may not necessarily reveal anything abnormal due to very small left-to-right shunt at rest.[4]

However, most of the patients seen for cardiac assessments are referred primarily on account of their predominant cardiac symptoms. Often a clear evaluation of the symptoms and their severity could lend itself to ***an analytical approach*** to diagnosis.

CARDIAC SYMPTOMS AND THEIR APPRAISAL

Symptoms could be grouped to identify underlying pathology:

1. ***Definite orthopnea and/or nocturnal dyspnea*** should point to the presence of ***high left atrial pressure*** and therefore help in generating possible list of causes to look for in the examination.
2. ***Triad of dyspnea, chest pain and exertional presyncope or syncope*** should indicate ***fixed cardiac output lesions*** (where cardiac output fails to increase adequately during exercise) such as due to outflow tract obstruction (e.g. aortic stenosis).
3. *Low output symptoms of fatigue, lassitude and light-headedness* could be caused by *severe inflow obstructive lesions, severe cardiomyopathy of ischemic or non-ischemic etiology, constrictive pericarditis, cardiac tamponade or severe pulmonary hypertension.*
4. ***Syncope and presyncope*** in addition to outflow obstructive lesions *may also be caused by significant brady- or tachyarrhythmias, hypotension of sudden onset brought by postural change, vagal reaction or of neurogenic origin.*

While symptoms and signs of ***peripheral edema and ascites*** may be caused by ***congestive heart failure,*** may also be due to other causes such as ***severe tricuspid regurgitation and constrictive pericarditis.*** They may also be due to other non-cardiac causes related to low-serum albumin of hepatic, gastrointestinal or renal causes as well as venous obstruction. Only when the pitting edema is of cardiac origin, significant elevation in the jugular venous pressure would be expected.

In the assessment of patients with symptoms described as ***dizziness,*** one ***needs to distinguish*** as far as possible ***presyncopal*** feeling (weakness or a drained feeling as though one is about to faint) from ***vertiginous*** sensation that often is not cardiac in origin and often is related to the peripheral or central vestibular system. Vertiginous feeling should be considered if a sensation of spinning or imbalance is experienced with or without nausea.

Chest pain, which is often a common reason for cardiac referral, needs to be properly assessed with regard to character, location, duration, frequency, provoking and relieving factors as well as the associated presence or absence of coronary risk factors (history of smoking, gender, age, diabetes, hyperlipidemia, hypertension, obesity, family history). Careful analysis should allow the chest pain to be defined as ***one of the three following categories:***

1. ***Typical angina*** (central chest discomfort often described as tightness, heaviness, squeezing or burning sensation or sensation of oppression or weight on the chest with or without typical radiation to the arms, shoulders, back, neck and/or jaw with or without accompanying dyspnea, related often to activity and relieved usually within a few minutes of rest or after nitroglycerine).

2. ***Atypical angina*** (meaning that the chest discomfort has some features of angina and yet other features not so typical—e.g. left anterior or central chest tightness related to physical exertion but requiring a long period of rest for relief such as having to lie down for extended period of time).
3. ***Non-cardiac chest pain*** such as those related to musculoskeletal, pleuritic, esophageal and others.

Exertional angina although commonly associated with ***ischemic*** (coronary) ***heart disease*** could also be caused by conditions that increase the myocardial oxygen demands *such as aortic stenosis, aortic regurgitation and severe uncontrolled hypertension.* Systemic factors, which could aggravate the problem, would also need to be considered such as anemia and hyperthyroidism. Classical ***anginal discomfort occurring unprovoked at rest*** but nevertheless responding to nitroglycerine should elicit consideration of coronary ***vasospasm (Prinzmetal's or variant angina)*** as well as *possible unstable coronary syndrome. Prolonged (>20 minutes in duration) and/or severe central chest discomfort or tightness with or without radiation* should raise suspicion of ***acute coronary syndromes and their mimickers.*** Among the latter conditions ***acute pericarditis and dissection of the aorta*** deserve special mention. The discomfort of acute ***pericarditis*** gets aggravated in the supine position and ***relief*** in the intensity of the discomfort is often experienced with patient sitting ***upright and leaning forward.*** The discomfort caused by ***dissection of aorta*** may be described as ***sudden tearing sensation or crushing*** feeling often with ***wide radiation particularly to the back*** sometimes to the neck and arms and occasionally to the abdomen. It may also be intermittent. Sometimes patients with acute myocardial *infarction* particularly that of ***the inferior wall*** might have discomfort primarily in the ***epigastrium*** accompanied by symptoms of nausea or vomiting. Acute infarct could of course occur without any discomfort and sometimes with minimal symptoms such as some numbness in the arm or hand. It requires often a high index of suspicion, given appropriate clinical markers to identify all of them accurately.

Angina occasionally may present as ***exertional belching.*** Occasionally, exertional ***dyspnea*** and even nocturnal dyspnea in addition to being symptoms indicative of elevated left atrial pressure may represent ***anginal equivalent symptoms*** with discomfort being totally absent.

If the ***angina is atypical,*** one should ***consider not only coronary artery disease*** but also other conditions such as *mitral valve prolapse syndrome, hypertrophic cardiomyopathy, unrecognized uncontrolled systemic hypertension, pulmonary hypertension and hyperthyroidism.*

The assessment also requires one to define the degree of severity of the cardiac symptomatic disability. This requires one to classify the severity of the cardiac symptoms such as dyspnea or angina using one of the accepted classification systems like that of the *New York Heart Association (NYHA) Classification of dyspnea or heart failure symptoms into classes I, II, III and IV.*[5]

Class I is defined as symptoms on severe exertion, while ***Class IV*** implies symptoms at rest. ***Class III*** implies symptoms on light or less than ordinary exertion and ***Class II*** implies symptoms on moderate level of exertion or ordinary exertion. The ordinary exertion that the patient could normally do without symptoms would also depend both on the age of the patient as well as on the mental attitude or wishes. For instance, even between two patients of similar age, one could be satisfied with walking comfortably while the other might insist on playing tennis, considering this to be a normal activity for him. *The Canadian Cardiovascular Society classification has a class 0 that simply means asymptomatic. It often is used for defining severity of anginal symptoms.*[6]

GENERATION OF WORKING LIST OF POSSIBLE DIAGNOSES

A. *In the evaluation of the cardiac patient, an analytical approach to a full and complete cardiac history should point to a working list of possible diagnoses. One can enumerate possibilities, which could produce all, or most of the predominant symptoms of the patient.*

B. *The enumeration should draw from broad categories of both congenital and acquired cardiac disorders.* The categories can be similar to what is shown in Tables 1.1 and 1.2.

Congenital: This is a simplified scheme useful for the purposes of thinking about possible congenital cardiac lesions in the adults. For more complete list, one can refer to a pediatric cardiology textbook.

In addition, one should ***also consider possible precipitating factors, which*** could be causative in the presence of pre-existing cardiac disorders, which are otherwise asymptomatic. Such precipitating factors may include some extracardiac factors. These will include:

- ***Infection such as pneumonia***
- ***Anemia***
- ***Hyperthyroidism***
- ***Pulmonary thromboembolism***
- ***Hypoxemia secondary to pulmonary and ventilatory disorders such as sleep apnea***
- ***Salt and fluid overload secondary to renal insufficiency***
- ***Iatrogenic causes (e.g. use of non-steroidal anti-inflammatory drugs or cox-2 inhibitors)***

The next step involves a careful examination and definition of the arterial pulses, the jugular pulsations, the precordial pulsations, as well as the peripheral and systemic signs. Each and all of these need to be evaluated in relation to the possibilities listed from the history. When this is done properly, often a

Table 1.1: Categories of congenital heart defects.

Acyanotic forms without a shunt:		
Outflow Obstruction	• Pulmonary Stenosis, Aortic, Stenosis, Coarctation of Aorta	
Inflow Obstruction	• Mitral Stenosis	
Regurgitant Lesions	• Mitral	• Congenitally corrected transposition, anomalous origin of the left coronary artery from the pulmonary artery
	• Tricuspid	• Ebstein's Anomaly
	• Aortic	• Bicuspid Aortic valve
Acyanotic forms with left to right shunts:		
Atrial Level	• Atrial Septal Defect Primum/Secundum	
Ventricular Level	• Ventricular Septal Defect	
Aortic Level	• Persistent Ductus Arteriosus, Aorto-Pulmonary Window	
Other Communications	• Coronary A-V Fistulae, Ruptured Sinus of Valsalva Aneurysm	
Cyanotic forms:		
Eisenmenger Syndrome	• Reversed shunt with pulmonary hypertension due to pulmonary vascular disease	
Tetralogy/Tetralogy type Lesions	• Decreased Pulmonary Flow	
Mixed Chamber Defects	• Single atrium, Single Ventricle Truncus Arteriosus	
Others:		
Conduction system disorders	• Congenital A-V Block, Accessory pathways	

clear and definitive diagnosis can be established or arrived at even before auscultation is performed. Auscultation, which is often the last step in the physical examination of the cardiac patient, may sometimes become the confirmatory step in this process. Only mild lesions are diagnosed only on the basis of auscultation alone (e.g. mitral valve prolapse, hypertrophic obstructive cardiomyopathy and others).

THE APPROACH TO A FOCUSED PHYSICAL EXAMINATION

Clinical Exercise

This approach can be *illustrated by discussing two different patients* each presenting with specific cardiac symptoms. One could use the following sections

Table 1.2: Categories of acquired cardiac disorders.

1. *Valvular disease*:
   - Stenotic lesions
   - Regurgitant lesions
2. Infective endocarditis
3. Ischemic heart disease
4. Hypertensive heart disease
5. *Myocardial diseases*:
   - Cardiomyopathies
   - Hypertrophic, restrictive and dilated,
   - Myocarditis
6. *Pericardial diseases*:
   - Acute pericarditis
   - Pericardial effusion with or without cardiac compression (tamponade)
   - Chronic constrictive pericarditis
7. *Cardiac tumors* (Atrial myxoma)
8. *Conduction system disorders*:
   - Tachyarrhythmia
   - Bradyarrhythmia
9. Pulmonary hypertension

that deal with two patients both as pre- and post-tests, namely before and after studying the remaining chapters in the book.

Case A. A 70-year-old woman previously healthy presents with sudden onset of dyspnea and orthopnea with radiologic signs of pulmonary edema.

The symptom complex with radiologic evidence of pulmonary congestion obviously indicates a pathologic process associated with *high left atrial pressure if high altitude and acute pulmonary injury are not involved.* The latter two can be easily solved by the relevant history surrounding the onset. One can then develop a list of all possible lesions both congenital and acquired, which can cause this problem. Then evidence in the history both in favor and against each listed condition should be considered.

Congenital

The only congenital lesion that could possibly be considered is bicuspid aortic valve with stenosis and/or regurgitation. But the age of the patient is somewhat against this.

Acquired

- Valvular lesions
- Mitral stenosis or obstruction

Patient with mitral stenosis may present with acute pulmonary edema due to the sudden onset of atrial fibrillation. Rapid ventricular rate such as that accompanying uncontrolled atrial fibrillation might be the precipitating cause of acute pulmonary edema in a patient with significant mitral stenosis that the patient otherwise is able to tolerate. The rapid heart rate by shortening the diastolic filling time impedes emptying of the left atrium in mitral stenosis, thereby raising the left atrial pressure acutely. But this type of presentation in rheumatic mitral disease is more likely to be seen in the fourth and the fifth decades. However, mitral obstruction due to ***atrial myxoma*** could occur in the age group of this patient and therefore cannot be excluded. Occasionally, patient with prosthetic mitral valve with previous history of mitral valve replacement could present in pulmonary edema because of an acute thrombus formation on the prosthetic valve obstructing inflow and preventing proper prosthetic valve function.

Mitral Regurgitation

Chronic mitral regurgitation: Chronic mitral regurgitation does not usually present with pulmonary edema unless its severity is suddenly markedly increased. This can happen *with rupture of chordae tendineae (spontaneous or due to infective endocarditis)* or may be due to other additional problems, which also affect the mitral valve function (such as due to ischemic papillary muscle dysfunction with or without avulsion of chordae or severe uncontrolled hypertension).

Acute severe mitral regurgitation: This is likely to present with acute pulmonary edema and may be caused by ***spontaneous rupture of chordae tendineae,*** for instance, in a patient with previously unrecognized myxomatous degeneration of the mitral leaflets, sometimes due to ***avulsion of chordae, due to papillary muscle infarction*** in a patient with acute coronary syndrome and ***rarely due to papillary muscle rupture*** with acute myocardial infarction. None of these could be excluded or considered low on the list based primarily on the history.

Aortic Stenosis

While this lesion on an acquired basis (calcific or degenerative) is more common in men, can nevertheless present with acute left ventricular failure, and usually some preceding history of the presence of a heart murmur and the classical triad of symptoms, namely dyspnea, angina and exertional presyncope or syncope, should be looked for. However, absence of any of these does not exclude this condition from consideration.

Aortic Regurgitation

Chronic aortic regurgitation: This can arise from valvular lesions (bicuspid valve, rheumatic involvement, trauma, endocarditis and others) or aortic root dilatation (Marfan's syndrome, syphilitic aortitis, spondylitis and others). The compensated state may last for a long time, and when the left ventricular failure sets in, it can be quite dramatic and associated with pulmonary edema. Therefore, this needs to be seriously considered.

Acute severe aortic regurgitation: Acute severe aortic regurgitation (often caused by ***endocarditis*** on a native valve or a prosthetic aortic valve with virulent pathogens such as staphylococci) obviously can present with acute pulmonary edema. Sometimes the symptom complex and some of the physical signs ***may be mimicked by ruptured sinus of Valsalva aneurysm, which*** also needs to be considered.

Ischemic Heart Disease

Acute myocardial infarction of course is by far the most common cause of sudden de novo acute pulmonary edema and therefore needs to be on the top of the list of all the causes of acute pulmonary edema. While the presence of chest discomfort or pain at onset and/or the presence of coexisting coronary risk factors raise the suspicion to high levels, neither the absence of chest discomfort nor the absence of significant coronary risk factors exclude it from consideration. The diagnosis of course would require either electrocardiographic and/or enzymatic determination of cardiac markers such as an elevated troponin level or creatine kinase MB fraction.

Hypertensive Heart Disease

Acute uncontrolled or poorly controlled hypertension can present sometimes with acute pulmonary edema. It can be seen, for instance, in younger females when complicating glomerulonephritis or pregnancy. However, these conditions need not be present. The systolic left ventricular function could be normal and yet ***due to significant diastolic dysfunction,*** the left ventricular diastolic filling pressures could be severely elevated causing the symptoms. This is particularly not uncommon in the elderly female. Occasionally, ***chronic renal failure might coexist*** in these patients aggravating the fluid and volume overload. The renal failure could itself be caused by hypertensive nephrosclerosis and/or diabetic nephropathy. Thus, this is an important entity to consider.

Cardiomyopathies

Acute dyspnea and pulmonary edema could occur in patients with *hypertrophic obstructive cardiomyopathy with significant resting aortic outflow tract gradient.* Similar symptomatology could occasionally occur in patients with ***dilated cardiomyopathy*** (of various etiologies including, idiopathic, viral, alcoholic and others). They are, therefore, not excluded on the basis of the history alone. Restrictive cardiomyopathy with etiologies like those caused by infiltrative processes such as amyloid or myxedema is not likely to present with such dramatic onset.

Conduction System Disorders

These by themselves will not be implicated for this presentation; however, conduction system involvement by electrocardiographic findings as part of the underlying cardiac disease may be detected; for instance, the presence of left bundle branch block on the ECG may be noted in a patient with idiopathic dilated or restrictive cardiomyopathy or in calcific aortic stenosis (Lev's disease).

Pericardial Diseases

Pericardial diseases of acute or chronic origin are not expected to cause acute symptoms of high left atrial pressure. While acute dyspnea may be caused by pericardial effusion that is causing significant cardiac compression, it is unlikely to produce radiologic signs of pulmonary edema. Unilateral left-sided constriction from chronic constrictive pericarditis is extremely rare and unlikely to present acutely.

Cardiac Tumors

Primary cardiac tumors such as a myxoma because of its location and mobility due to attachment by a stalk to the underlying endocardial wall could cause obstructive symptoms. If the myxoma is left atrial in location, then it can cause acute symptoms of high left atrial pressure due to mitral obstruction.

Pulmonary Hypertension

All lesions listed above that cause significant elevations in the left atrial pressure and symptoms thereof will more than likely raise the pulmonary arterial pressures and cause pulmonary hypertension. However, in this instance the symptoms primarily stem from the high left atrial pressure. However, in chronic pulmonary hypertension when significant, the right ventricle gets the brunt of the problem and will raise the systemic venous pressures with or without secondary tricuspid regurgitation and will eventually lead to diminished right ventricular output. The former will cause systemic venous congestion and peripheral edema, the latter would only diminish the left ventricular output and cause low cardiac output symptoms but not pulmonary congestion. Therefore, this pathophysiologic process is not under consideration here.

In view of the acute onset of symptoms presumably unprovoked, some of the likely precipitating and/or aggravating factors also need to be considered in the evaluation process since these may be really operative when there is pre-existing left ventricular dysfunction that is otherwise tolerated and asymptomatic.

Precipitating or Aggravating Factors

Rapid ventricular rate: Rapid heart rate due to uncontrolled atrial fibrillation or similar supraventricular tachyarrhythmia such as uncontrolled atrial flutter, atrial tachycardia and occasionally even ventricular tachycardia could precipitate onset of acute pulmonary edema ***in patients with pre-existing left ventricular dysfunction*** of varied etiologies *(ischemic heart disease with prior myocardial infarction, uncontrolled hypertensive heart disease, hypertrophic or dilated cardiomyopathies) all of which might have been otherwise asymptomatic.*

Acute Infection such as Pneumonia: This needs to be considered in the elderly since both systolic and/or diastolic left ventricular dysfunction of varied and/or multiple etiologies (ischemic, hypertensive and non-ischemic cardiomyopathies) are common in the elderly particularly in the very old (in the eighties and above). In these individuals, systemic infection and particularly pulmonary infection might throw them into left ventricular failure ***due to additional hypoxemia,*** which can further depress cardiac function.

Acute Pulmonary Embolism: This will not be expected to cause left ventricular dysfunction directly and therefore will not present as acute left ventricular failure when the left ventricular function is normal. *However, when the underlying left ventricular function is already previously compromised by other pre-existing cardiac disease, then it can aggravate the same leading to pulmonary edema.* The mechanisms involve hypoxia, tachycardia or atrial tachyarrhythmia, which it may produce, and increased reflex vasoconstriction (could be mediated by catecholamines, serotonin and others), which can raise the afterload.

It is of utmost importance that the patient in acute pulmonary edema be treated for the same with appropriate measures, which should include oxygenation, intravenous diuretics, morphine as well as ventilatory support when considered essential. It is even appropriate to look, at the ECG quickly for signs of an acute myocardial infarction given the fact that it is often the most leading cause of acute pulmonary edema. The discussion here is not meant to be about management of the patient rather as to how one goes about considering the various possible etiologies, since it is important for the complete management of the patient.

2. *Discuss the physical findings noted on the cardiac examination, and synthesize further to narrow down the possibilities to arrive at the proper diagnosis.*

Presyncopal symptoms on exertion would point to transient abrupt fall in cardiac output. The first comment that one can make regarding this particular patient is that *the exertion that caused the presyncopal symptom in this relatively young man who has been "previously well", however, appears to be quite minimal. Therefore, the symptoms may or may not be related to the exertion.* Therefore, while generating possible conditions that could have caused the symptoms, *one cannot totally limit these to lesions associated with exertional syncope (namely fixed output lesions such as due to severe outflow obstruction) alone. Abrupt onset of any tachyarrhythmia supraventricular or ventricular if it were rapid (rate > 160) and sufficiently long in duration (at least >30 seconds) could cause a fall in cardiac output and therefore cause symptoms. Similarly, any significant bradycardia (pauses > 4.0 seconds or rates < 35) can be associated with a fall in cardiac output, which may be symptomatic.*

The ability to generate such a list requires some background knowledge of various disorders and their typical presenting features. But one can certainly think of them in general categories and add individual disorders appropriate to the level of the experience and knowledge of the physician. This likely would vary whether the individual is a beginner or student or he/she is a cardiac fellow.

The list of ***possible etiologies*** would include the following.

Congenital

- Obstructive outflow lesions*:* Significant aortic/pulmonary stenosis
- Inflow obstruction: Unlikely but cannot exclude atrial myxoma
- ***Severe Pulmonary hypertension*** secondary to Eisenmenger's syndrome*:* With reversed intracardiac shunt from pulmonary vascular disease
- ***Disorders associated with significant tendency for tachyarrhythmias:***
    - Ebstein's anomaly of the tricuspid valve
    - Arrhythmogenic right ventricle
    - Conduction System Disorders with tendency for tachyarrhythmias
- ***With tendency for bradyarrhythmias:*** Congenital AV block

Acquired

Left ventricular outflow obstruction:

- Valvular aortic stenosis (unlikely at this age unless congenital in origin)
- Hypertrophic obstructive cardiomyopathy
- Inflow obstruction such as due to atrial myxoma (mitral stenosis unlikely)

Regurgitant valvular lesions: By themselves they are not expected to cause such symptoms. Occasionally, however, ventricular tachyarrhythmias may be seen in patients with advanced mitral regurgitation. Rarely severe ventricular tachyarrhythmias might also occur in patients with mitral valve prolapse syndrome with redundant myxomatous degeneration of the valves.

Ischemic heart disease:

- Ischemia with ventricular arrhythmia (patient relatively young but cannot be excluded).
- Coronary vasospasm with ventricular tachyarrhythmia or bradycardia or AV block depending on the coronary artery involved.

Cardiomyopathies: Ventricular tachyarrhythmias, in the presence of underlying non-obstructive or obstructive hypertrophic cardiomyopathy, dilated cardiomyopathy or bradyarrhythmias in the presence of restrictive cardiomyopathy.

Pericardial diseases: Unlikely to be associated with the symptoms of presyncope unless there is severe pericardial effusion, then invariably other symptoms such as lassitude, fatigue and dyspnea would be present.

Conduction system disorders:

- With tendency for tachyarrhythmia
- Pre-excitation syndromes (Wolff-Parkinson-White syndrome, Lown-Ganong-Levine syndrome)
- Long QT syndrome
- Re-entrant tachycardia in the absence of pre-excitation
- Paroxysmal atrial tachycardia
- *Severe pulmonary hypertension:* Secondary to severe pulmonary disease, ventilatory disorders such as sleep apnea and others
- *Primary pulmonary hypertension:* More common in females
- *Acute Pulmonary Embolism:* Can cause drop in cardiac output suddenly and may also induce arrhythmias. Not very typical but cannot be excluded

Others

Vasovagal reaction: Usually occurs secondary to anxiety, acute pain somatic or visceral, and distension of viscus organ and rarely secondary to ischemia. Usually associated with sweating, nausea and/or vomiting.

Cardiac Examination Findings in Patient B

- ***Patient slightly tachypneic 5'7"; weighing 185 lb; BP 125/80; heart rate 95/min; respirations 25/min.***
- ***Arterial pulse: Normal volume or amplitude pulse with normal upstroke in the carotids. All pulses palpable and symmetrical***
- ***Jugular venous pulse: Jugular venous pressure 8 cm above the sternal angle at 45°. The contour showed x′ = y; the venous pressure tended to rise on inspiration.***

- ***Precordial pulsations: Apical impulse normal with medial retraction. Right ventricular impulse palpable on deep inspiration by subxiphoid palpation.***
- ***Auscultation: S2 palpable at the II LICS. S2 splitting appeared to be somewhat wide but appeared to vary normally on inspiration. S3 and S4 were both heard at the lower left sternal area and over the xiphoid area and appeared to increase slightly on inspiration. No significant murmurs. Chest was clear.***

Interpretations of the Physical Findings of Patient B

1. Mild tachypnea and increased respiratory rate should raise suspicion about possible hypoxemia.
2. The arterial pulse upstroke being normal rules out significant left-sided obstruction. It also is not suggestive of hypertrophic cardiomyopathy, where the arterial pulse upstroke is often brisk. The normal pulse volume or amplitude and the normal pressure indicate adequate stroke volume and tend to rule out any significant cardiac compression.
3. The elevated jugular venous pressure indicates rise in the diastolic pressures in the right ventricle. The abnormal contour of ***x′ descent = y descent*** can occur both with and without significant pulmonary hypertension. The preservation of x' indicates preserved right ventricular systolic function. The prominent ***y descent*** would indicate increased ***v wave*** pressure head in the right atrium, which is usually caused by raised right ventricular diastolic pressures ***(the pre a wave pressure).*** This contour in the absence of pulmonary hypertension can occur in pericardial effusion with some cardiac compression. However, the preserved ***y descent*** excludes cardiac tamponade since early diastolic emptying of the right atrium must be free and unrestricted. The same $x' = y$ contour in the presence of pulmonary hypertension, however, would indicate significant pulmonary hypertension severe enough to alter the diastolic function of the right ventricle.
4. Both the palpable S2 in the second left interspace and right ventricular impulse subxiphoid would indicate the presence of pulmonary hypertension. This will be the evidence to conclude that the jugular venous pulse contour abnormalities arise from significant degree of pulmonary hypertension.
5. The apical impulse with medial retraction suggests a left ventricular impulse. It has been described as normal indicating presumably normal and perhaps no more than mild left ventricular dysfunction. Therefore, the left ventricular dysfunction is not the cause of the pulmonary hypertension.
6. The widely split S2 moving physiologically may indicate some right ventricular dysfunction due to pulmonary hypertension, since pulmonary

hypertension per se by increasing the pulmonary impedance would make the P2 to occur earlier and cause a narrower split S2. Other possibility is an electrical delay such as a coexisting right bundle branch block.

7. The presence of S3 and S4 heard over the lower left sternal border and xiphoid area; both of which being described as slightly increasing on inspiration suggest right-sided events compatible with right ventricular diastolic dysfunction and acute decompensation of the right ventricle.

Synthesis

1. *So far the predominant right-sided signs all point to the presence of significant pulmonary hypertension with right ventricular diastolic dysfunction. Since the patient is described previously well and the history being rather of sudden and recent onset, acute cause of pulmonary hypertension such as acute pulmonary embolism must be considered to be present unless proven otherwise.*
2. *Such a conclusion is also suggested by the presence of mild tachycardia and mild tachypnea.*
3. *Such an analysis should lead to immediate application of appropriate measures of management including treatment and diagnostic investigations.*

PRACTICAL POINTS TO A FOCUSED CARDIAC PHYSICAL EXAMINATION

1. *Proper evaluation of the cardiac symptoms and their severity would ultimately require defining the appropriate causal cardiac disorder. Therefore, it helps to group symptoms to identify underlying pathology.*
2. *Definite orthopnea and/or nocturnal dyspnea should point to the presence of high left atrial pressure. Triad of dyspnea, chest pain and exertional presyncope or syncope should indicate fixed cardiac output lesions. Fatigue, lassitude and light-headedness may be due to low output. Significant brady- or tachyarrhythmias or hypotension of sudden onset may also cause syncope and presyncope in addition to outflow obstructive lesions. Peripheral edema and ascites represent congestive symptoms due to high right atrial pressure.*
3. *Proper evaluation of cardiac symptoms includes generation of a working list of possible etiologies drawn from a broad range of cardiac disorders and lesions.*
4. *While a complete and a thorough cardiac examination is performed, each finding both normal and abnormal should be analyzed with regard to their significance in relation to the etiologic causes under consideration of the particular patient problem. This automatically becomes a sound tool or method for arriving at proper conclusions with regard to both the diagnosis and the management.*

REFERENCES

1. Go AS, Hylek EM, Phillips KA, et al. Prevalence of diagnosed atrial fibrillation in adults: national implications for rhythm management and stroke prevention: the AnTicoagulation and Risk Factors in Atrial Fibrillation (ATRIA) Study. JAMA. 2001 May ;285(18):2370-5.
2. Albers GW, Dalen JE, Laupacis A, et al. Antithrombotic therapy in atrial fibrillation. Chest. [Review]. 2001;119(1 Suppl): 194S-206S.
3. January CT, Wann LS, Alpert JS, et al. 2014 AHA/ACC/HRS Guideline for the Management of Patients With Atrial Fibrillation: Executive Summary: A Report of the American College of Cardiology/American Heart Association Task Force on Practice Guidelines and the Heart Rhythm Society. Circulation. 2014.
4. Windecker S, Stortecky S, Meier B. Paradoxical embolism. J Am Coll Cardiol. [Review]. 2014;64(4):403-15.
5. The Criteria Committee for the New York Heart Association: Nomenclature and Criteria for Diagnosis of Diseases of the Heart and Great Vessels, Ninth Edition, Little Brown and Company. Boston, Mass, 1994.
6. Hemingway H, Fitzpatrick NK, Gnani S, et al. Prospective validity of measuring angina severity with Canadian Cardiovascular Society class: the ACRE study. Can J Cardiol. 2004;20(3):305-9.

Chapter

2 Arterial Pulse

Snapshot

- Physiology of the Arterial Pulse
- Assessment of the Arterial Pulse
- Practical Points in the Clinical Assessment of the Arterial Pulse

PHYSIOLOGY OF THE ARTERIAL PULSE

Although the arterial pulse, which is considered a fundamental clinical sign of life itself from time immemorial had been the subject of study by many physiologists as well as clinicians in the past,[1-28] it received less attention by the clinicians for many years after the discovery of the sphygmomanometer.[29] However, there has been a renewed interest in this field in recent years, since new techniques such as applanation tonometry are now being applied for its study.[30-33] However, the physiology of the arterial pulse is quite complicated and the subject is often given only cursory description even in the most popular textbooks in cardiology. Also, the retained terminology and nomenclature do not help to clarify the issues.[21,34] Most detailed review of the complicated physiology of both the normal and the abnormal arterial pulse can be found in some of the excellent papers of O'Rourke and his coworkers.[21,35-38] However, the subject has remained somewhat elusive even to most interested clinicians. Therefore, in this chapter, attempt will be made to simplify some of the concepts for the sake of understanding.

The purpose of the arterial system is to deliver oxygenated blood to the tissues but more importantly to convert intermittent cardiac output into a continuous capillary flow. This is primarily achieved by its structural organization.[6] The central vessels namely the aorta up to the iliac bifurcation and its main branches namely the carotid and the innominate arteries are very elastic and act in part as a reservoir in addition to being conduits. The vessels at the level of the radial and femoral arteries are more muscular, whereas the iliac, the sub-clavian and the axillary vessels are intermediate or transitional in structure. When an artery is put into stretch the readily extensible fibers of the vessel wall govern its behavior. More elastic is the vessel, the greater is the volume accommodated for a small rise in pressure.

It is well known that the recording obtained with a pulse transducer placed externally over the carotid artery has a contour and shape very similar to a pressure curve obtained through a catheter placed internally in the carotid artery and recorded with a strain gauge manometer system (Figs. 2.1A and B). While the former records displacement of the vessel

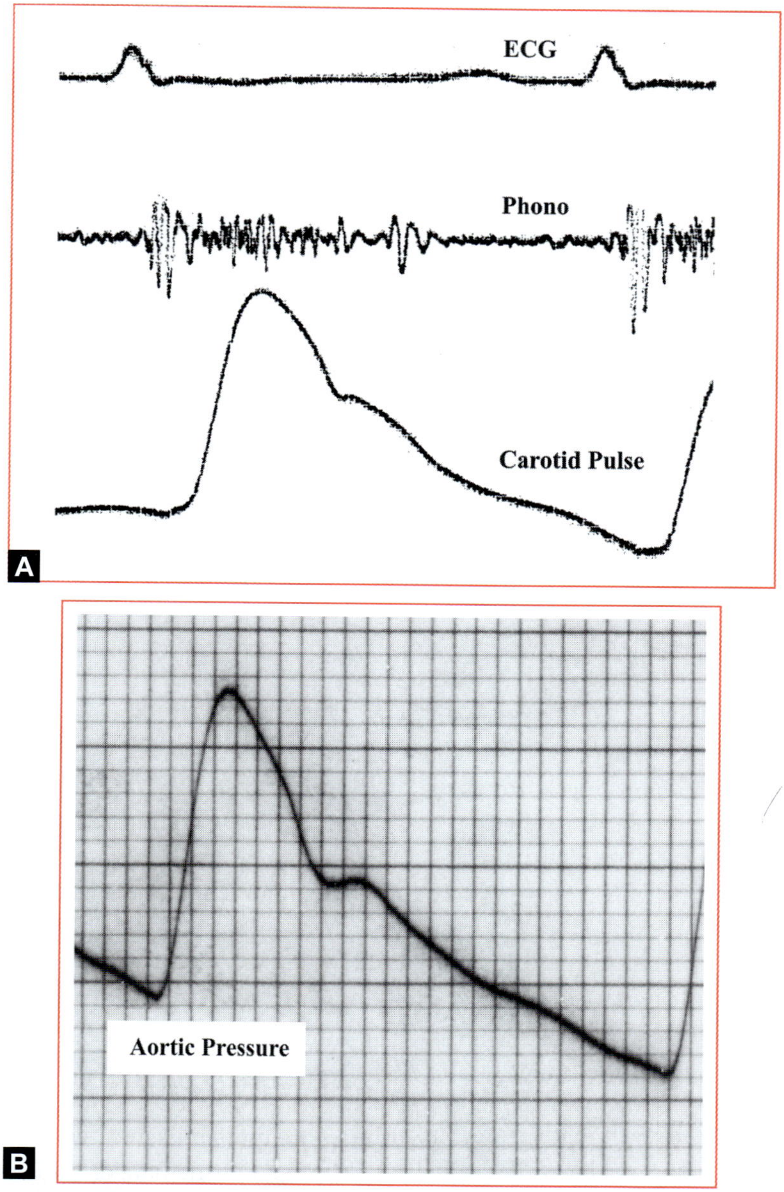

Figs. 2.1A and B: (A) Simultaneous recordings of ECG, phonocardiogram and the carotid pulse. (B) Intra-aortic pressure recording in the same patient. Note the similarity of the carotid pulse tracing and the aortic pressure recording. (ECG: Electrocardiogram).

transmitted to the skin through overlying soft tissues, the latter is a true recording of the internal pressure changes. The displacement in the externally recorded tracing is due to changes in the wall tension of the vessel similar to the recording of an apical impulse reflecting the change in left ventricular wall tension. *The wall tension is governed by the principles of Laplace relationship. The tension is directly proportional to the pressure and the radius and inversely related to the thickness of the vessel wall.* Since ejection of the major portion of the stroke volume takes place in the early and mid-systole, the cause of major change in tension in early and mid-systole is due to changes in both volume and pressure. During the later part of systole and during diastole, however, the pre-dominant effect must be primarily due to changes in pressure although volume may also be playing a part. The dominance of the pressure pulse effect on the tension of the vessel wall for the greater part of the cardiac cycle is the main reason for the similarity of the externally recorded carotid pulse tracing and the internally recorded pressure curve.

The contraction of the left ventricle imparts its contractile energy on the blood mass it contains, developing and raising the pressure to overcome the diastolic pressure in the aorta in order to open the aortic valve and eject the blood into the aorta. As the ventricle ejects the blood mass into the aorta with each systole, it creates a pulsatile pressure as well as a pulsatile flow. By appropriate recording techniques applied in and/or over an artery, one can show the pulsatile nature of the pressure wave, the pulsatile nature of the flow wave as well as the dimensional changes in the artery as the pressure wave travels.[36]

What is actually felt when an artery is palpated by the finger, is not only the force exerted by the amplitude of the pressure wave but also the change in the diameter. For instance the pressure pulse of both arteriosclerosis and hypertension in the elderly as well as that caused by significant aortic regurgitation will look similar when recorded. It will show a rapid rise in systole and a steep fall in diastole with an increased pulse pressure (the difference between the systolic and the diastolic pressure). However, the arterial pulse in these two different situations will feel different to the palpating fingers. The difference is essentially in the diameter change. The pulse of aortic regurgitation is associated with a significant change in diameter, whereas it is usually not the case in arteriosclerosis. The diameter change due to the high volume of the pulse in aortic regurgitation can be further exaggerated by elevating the arm, which helps to reduce the diastolic pressure in the brachial and the radial artery.

Since pressure and radius are two important factors, which affect wall tension as shown by Laplace relationship, it is probably reasonable to consider both of them together. What is actually felt when the arterial pulse is palpated can therefore be restated as the effect caused by a change in the wall tension of the artery.

Laplace's Law

Tension = P (pressure) × r (radius) for a thin walled cylindrical shell.

If the wall has a thickness, then the circumferential wall stress is given by **Lame's equation**, as follows:

$$\text{Tension} \propto \frac{\text{P (pressure)} \times \text{r (radius)}}{\text{2h (wall thickness)}}$$

Amplitude of the pulse will depend not only on the amplitude of the pressure wave but also on the change in dimensions between diastole and systole (or simply the amount of change in wall tension).

The Volume Effect

According to Laplace's Law, the volume has a direct effect on the wall tension since it relates to the radius. The actual volume of blood received by each segment of the artery and its effect on the change in wall tension, on that segment, depends also on the vessel involved. The proximal elastic vessels (aorta and its main branches) receive almost all of the stroke volume of the left ventricle. The elastic nature of these vessels allows greater displacement and change in their radius. However as one goes more peripherally, total cross-sectional area increases. Therefore, each vessel receives only a fraction of the stroke volume. In addition, the vessels are more muscular and less distensible. For similar rise in pressure, the change in vessel diameter is less. The corollary of this is that to achieve similar diameter change in the peripheral vessels, the pressure developed must be higher.

Pressure in the Vessel

The pressure pulse generated by the contraction of the left ventricle is transmitted to the most peripheral artery almost immediately and yet the blood that leaves the left ventricle takes several cardiac cycles to reach the same distance. *Thus, it must be emphasized that pressure pulse wave transmission is different and not to be confused with actual blood flow transmission in the artery. The analogy that can be given is the transmission of the jolt produced by an engine of the train to a series of coaches while shunting the coaches on the track as opposed to the actual movement of the respective coaches produced by the push given by the engine. This is the classic analogy given by Bramwell.*[6]

The mechanics of flow dictate that it is the pressure gradient not the pressure that causes the flow in the arteries. There is very little drop in the mean pressure in the large arteries. Almost all of the resistance to flow is found in the precapillary arterioles. This is where most of the drop in mean pressure also occurs in the arterial system.[11,12,35] The shape of the pressure pulse changes, as it propagates through to the periphery. Although the mean pressure decreases slightly, the pulse pressure (systolic pressure minus the diastolic pressure) increases distally so that the peak pressure actually increases as the wave propagates.[11,37] The higher peak systolic pressure achieved in the less distensible and more muscular peripheral vessels helps to accommodate the volume received by the distal vessels.

Reflection

Experimental studies have clearly shown that pressure pulse wave generated artificially by a pump connected to a system of fluid-filled closed tubes or branching tubes with changing caliber gets reflected. The reflective sites appear to be branching points.[11,12] This implies that the incident pressure pulse ***(not flow)*** produced by the contracting left ventricle gets reflected back. *It is reflection of the pressure pulse that gives the pulse wave its characteristic contour (Fig. 2.2).* The pressure and the velocity waveforms vary markedly at different sites in the arteries. The peak velocity generally occurs before the peak in pressure at all sites.[17] As one moves to the periphery the pulsatile pressure fluctuations increase while the oscillations of flow diminish as a result of damping. The peripheral pressure fluctuations often become amplified to the extent of exceeding the central aortic systolic pressure. This is further evidence that the pressure waves get reflected peripherally.[17,37]

Since the pressure pulse normally travels very fast (meters per second), the recorded arterial pressure wave at any site in the arterial system is usually the result of the combination of the incident pressure wave produced by the contracting left ventricle and the reflected wave from the periphery.[37,38]

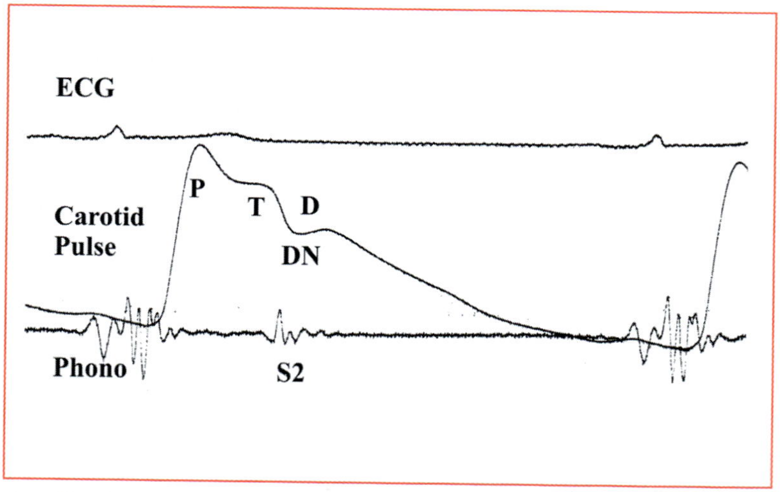

Fig. 2.2: Simultaneous recordings of ECG, carotid pulse tracing and the phonocardiogram. The carotid pulse shows the percussion wave (P), the tidal wave (T) and the dicrotic wave (D) that follows the dicrotic notch (DN). (ECG: Electrocardiogram).

Pulse Wave Contour

When one records the arterial pulse wave with a transducer, one may be able to identify three distinct components in its contour:

1. *The percussion wave that is the initial systolic portion of the pressure pulse.*
2. *The tidal wave that is the later systolic portion of the pressure pulse.*
3. *The dicrotic wave that is the wave following the dicrotic notch (roughly corresponding to the timing of the second heart sound) and therefore diastolic.*

Factors that Affect the Magnitude of the Initial Systolic Wave

Although this portion of the arterial pulse may also be influenced and modified by reflected waves from the periphery, *the rate of rise and the amplitude of the incident pressure wave of the arterial pulse are still dependent on the ejection of blood into the aorta by the contracting left ventricle.* Thus, the characteristics of the proximal arterial system and the effect of the left ventricular pump become pertinent (Table 2.1 and Fig. 2.3).

Table 2.1: Determinants of arterial pressure pulse and contour

Components	*Determining factors*
1. Incident pressure wave	• Compliance of aorta • Stroke volume • Velocity of ejection • Left ventricular pump – Preload – Afterload – Contractility – Pattern of ejection – Impedance to ejection
2. Pulse wave velocity	• Mean arterial pressure • Arterial stiffness/compliance • Vasomotor tone
3. Intensity of reflection	• Peripheral resistance (arteriolar tone)
Increased	• Vasoconstriction
Decreased	• Vasodilatation
4. Effects of wave reflection	• Distance from reflecting sites • Pulse wave velocity • Timing of arrival in cardiac cycle • Duration of ejection
Diastolic wave	• Compliant arteries • Slow transmission • Shortened duration of ejection
Late systolic wave	• Stiff arteries • Rapid transmission • Long duration of ejection

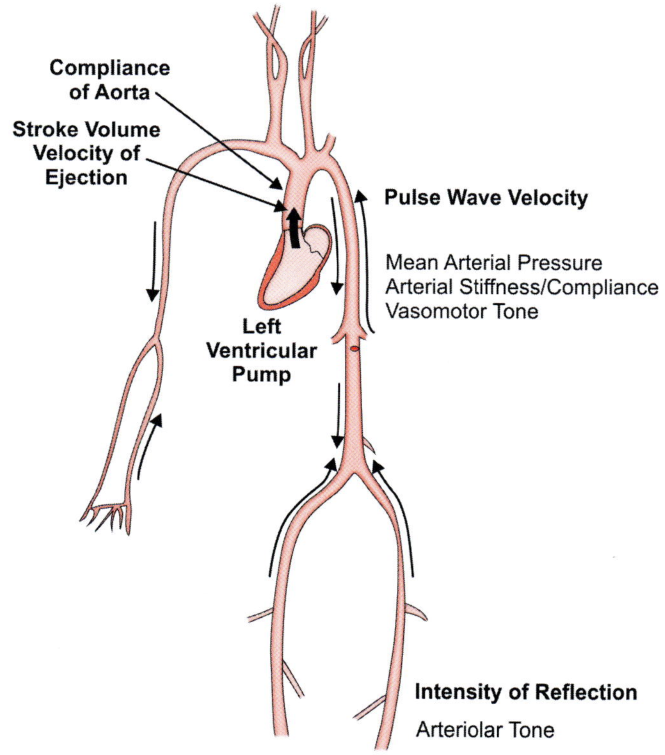

Fig. 2.3: Diagrammatic representation of factors involved in the arterial pressure pulse wave contour, including the incident pressure wave, pulse wave velocity, transmission and reflection.

Characteristics of the Proximal Arterial System

Ejection of blood into the aorta by the contracting left ventricle during systole leads to the rise in aortic pressure from the diastolic level at the time of the aortic valve opening to the peak in systole. The rise in aortic pressure from its diastolic to the systolic peak is determined by the compliance of the aorta as well as the stroke volume. The aorta is very compliant due to its greater content of elastin compared to the smooth muscle and the collagen in its walls. Since the walls of the aorta are compliant, it expands to accommodate the blood volume. The increase in pressure for any given stroke volume will be determined by the compliance of the aorta. Increasing age leads to changes in the structural components of the walls of the aorta leading to a reduced compliance.[39] When the aorta is rigid and stiff the pressure will rise steeply to an increased peak systolic pressure giving rise to an increased pulse pressure.

In some elderly patients, the decreased compliance of the proximal vessels could be severe enough to hide the slowly rising percussion wave of the aortic stenosis due to marked increase in pressure despite small increase in volume.[36]

In addition, the pressure rise will be steeper and faster if the stroke volume is delivered to the aorta with a faster rate of ejection as would be expected with increased contractility.

The Left Ventricular Pump

The left ventricular output is dependent on the filling pressures (preload), the intrinsic myocardial function and the afterload against which it pumps (determined by the vascular properties of the arterial system that affect its compliance, the peripheral resistance and the peak systolic pressure). When the ventricle begins to contract at the end of diastole, the intraventricular pressure rises as more and more myocardial fibers begin to shorten. When the left ventricular pressure exceeds the left atrial pressure, closing the mitral valve, the isovolumic phase of contraction begins. During this phase, the rate of pressure development is rapid. The rate of change of pressure ($d\boldsymbol{P}/d\boldsymbol{t}$) during this phase usually is reflective of the contractile state of the left ventricle. It is increased when the left ventricle is hypercontractile and is usually depressed when the ventricular function is diminished. When the left ventricular pressure exceeds the aortic diastolic pressure the aortic valve opens and the ejection phase of systole begins. Recordings of pressures in the left ventricle and the aorta obtained by special microtip sensors show that the left ventricular pressure exceeds that of the aorta in the early part of systole.[40-42] This pressure gradient is termed the impulse gradient since it is generated by the ventricular contraction. The aortic flow velocity reaches a peak very soon after the onset of systole. During the later half of systole, the rate of myocardial fiber shortening slows and the left ventricular pressure begins to fall. When the left ventricular pressure falls below that in the aorta, the gradient reverses and this is associated with the deceleration of aortic outflow. The initial rapid rise in the aortic outflow velocity to its peak is caused by early and abrupt acceleration of blood flow out of the left ventricle. This acceleration is achieved as a result of the force generated by the ventricular contraction. The peak aortic flow velocity achieved is dependent on the magnitude of the force ***(F)*** multiplied by the time ***(t)*** during which it acts. The physical term "impulse" describes ***(F)*** × ***(t)***.

The kinetic energy imparted by the ventricular contraction to the blood mass it ejects can be viewed as the total momentum gained by the blood mass. The force of contraction and the peak rate of pressure development ($d\boldsymbol{P}/d\boldsymbol{t}$) by determining the rate of acceleration of flow should influence the rate of rise of the incident pressure. Both the mass ***(m)*** of blood ejected namely the stroke volume and the velocity ***(v)*** of ejection would be expected to affect the amplitude of the incident pressure wave. The stroke volume and the velocity of ejection together represent the ***momentum of ejection (mv).*** The effect of the maximum momentum achieved during ejection as well as the rate of change in momentum on the rate of rise and the amplitude of the pressure pulse can be explained by an analogy. This is best understood by observing a strength testing game in carnivals where a person hits a platform on the ground with a large wooden hammer displacing a metal weight vertically. The aim is usually to raise the weight high enough to ring a bell at the top of the column to show strength and win a prize. The force with which the platform is struck results in the ***launching momentum.*** The harder the platform is struck, the faster and higher the weight will rise.

Momentum of Ejection (mv)

Mass (Stroke Volume)

In conditions with large stroke output, momentum of ejection will be augmented causing increased amplitude of the pressure wave. The stroke volume will be increased in hyperdynamic and hypervolemic states such as anemia, hyperthyroidism, Paget's disease, and pregnancy. Large stroke volumes can also occur in the absence of the above, in certain cardiovascular conditions such as aortic regurgitation and persistent ductus arteriosus (Fig. 2.4). In addition, bradycardia as seen with chronic complete atrioventricular (AV) block, by virtue of increased diastolic filling of the ventricle can also produce increased stroke volume.

Diminished stroke volume will therefore be expected to cause decreased momentum of ejection and decreased amplitude of the pressure pulse. This will occur in conditions with significant obstruction to either left ventricular outflow or inflow. Severe aortic stenosis often with some left ventricular dysfunction and severe mitral stenosis are examples of such states. Cardiac failure with poor pump function will also result in severe reduction in stroke

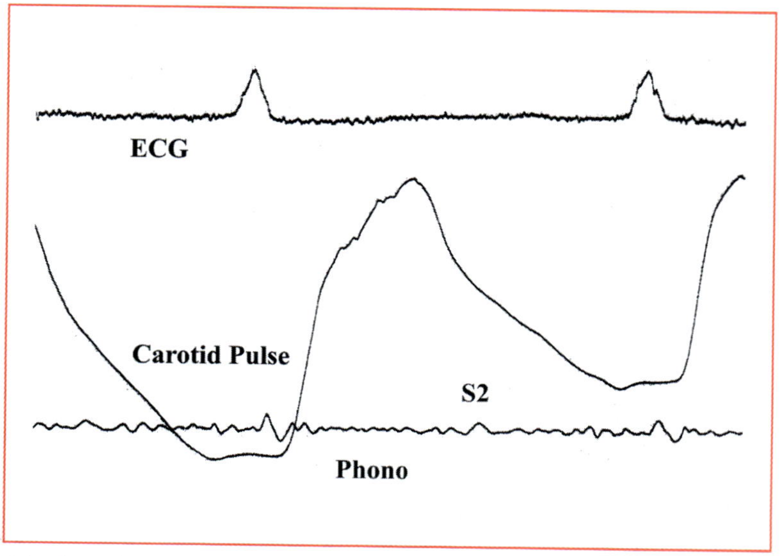

Fig. 2.4: Carotid pulse recording in a patient with aortic regurgitation. Note the wide pulse excursion.

volume. Severe reduction in filling of the left ventricle as seen in patients with cardiac tamponade also will have similar effect on the stroke volume and therefore on the momentum of ejection.

Velocity of Ejection

The velocity of ejection will be determined by the strength with which the left ventricle contracts, as well as by the impedance to ventricular ejection.

Contractility

Increased velocity of ejection, in the absence of outflow obstruction, will likely lead to larger amplitude of the pressure pulse in the aorta, since more volume will be delivered over a shorter duration. The rapid velocity also implies a stronger contractile force and increased dP/dt, and therefore will be expected to cause a faster rate of rise of the pressure pulse or rapid upstroke of the pulse.

In the absence of obstruction to the left ventricular outflow, the velocity of ejection is mainly determined by the pump function of the left ventricle as well as the preload and the afterload. In conditions with large stroke volume due to Starling effect, the ejection velocity would also be increased unless significant left ventricular dysfunction coexists.

In mitral regurgitation, there is increased contractility due to Starling effect of the increased filling of the left ventricle (from both the normal pulmonary venous return and the volume of blood that went backward into the left atrium due to the regurgitation), resulting in faster ejection. However, there is no increased stroke volume received by the aorta, since the left ventricle has two outlets during systole namely the aorta and the left atrium. The amplitude of the pressure pulse is expected to be normal but the rate of rise may be rapid.[43]

In hypertrophic cardiomyopathy, the ventricle is hypercontractile and ejects the blood very fast. This leads to a very rapid rise of the arterial pulse. In addition, in this condition, the pattern of ejection is such that the flow into the aorta often may be biphasic with a smaller secondary peak in late systole, which may partly contribute to a secondary late systolic pressure rise in the aorta.[44] This is more pronounced in the patients who have a dynamic obstruction to the outflow when during the middle of systole the anterior leaflet of the mitral valve gets pulled from its closed position and moves anteriorly toward the interventricular septum ***(systolic anterior motion or SAM).*** While there is still controversy as to the cause of the ***SAM,***[45] it has been attributed to a Venturi effect caused by the rapid outflow velocity. This septal mitral contact obstructs ejection and the aortic flow ceases. In late systole when the intraventricular pressure begins to fall, the anterior mitral leaflet moves away from the septum, the obstruction subsides and the ejection resumes. This will then give rise to a second peak in the pulse in late systole, which however will be smaller than the first peak.

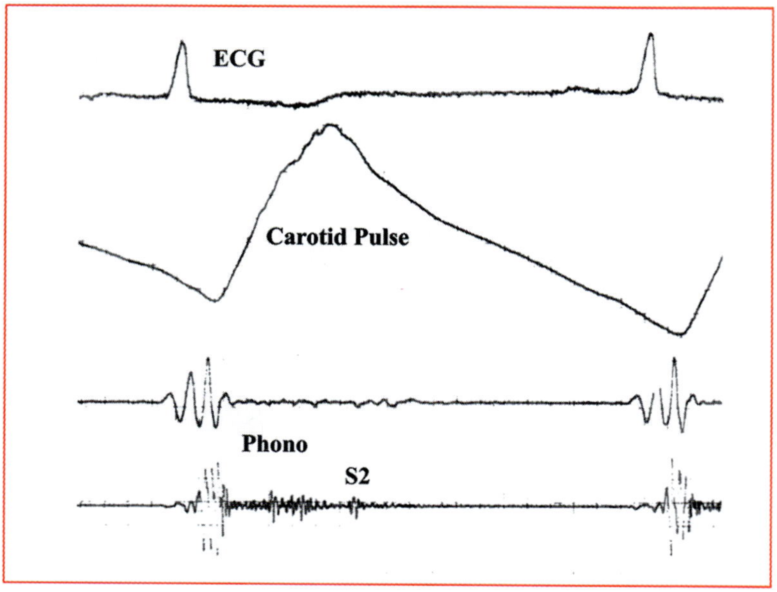

Fig. 2.5: Carotid pulse tracing in a patient with aortic stenosis. The delayed or slow upstroke with peak of the pulse at the end of systole, almost at the timing of the second heart sound (S2).

In aortic stenosis, although the ejection velocity is significantly increased due to the obstruction, the accompanying volume increment is low. Therefore, the increase in radius and the tension in the aortic wall will be expected to be slow. In addition, the increased velocity of the aortic jet through the stenotic valve, by a Venturi effect, will cause a decrease in the lateral pressure,[26,46] *thereby contributing to a slower rate of pressure rise in the aorta, giving rise to a delayed upstroke and a shoulder in the ascending limb of the pressure wave called the anacrotic shoulder (Fig. 2.5).*

Impedance to Ejection

In addition to the factors affecting the afterload, impedance to ejection includes the vascular properties of the arterial system and the peripheral resistance. The load that the ventricle needs to handle during contraction is usually termed the afterload. This is sometimes considered synonymous with the intraventricular systolic pressure. In fact afterload is more closely related to the left ventricular wall tension or stress. According to Laplace relationship, the tension is directly proportional to the pressure and the radius and is inversely related to the thickness. Thus when the left ventricle faces a chronic pressure load (e.g. hypertension or aortic stenosis) or volume load (e.g. mitral or aortic regurgitation), eventually its walls will undergo hypertrophy. This will then tend to normalize or reduce the wall stress or tension. Since wall tension is an important determinant of myocardial oxygen consumption, increased afterload would be disadvantageous to the ventricular myocardial fiber shortening.

The vascular properties of the arterial system especially the aorta are also important since they determine the yield or the compliance. The peripheral resistance is due to the combined resistance to flow of all the vessels in the arterial system. This is pre-dominantly determined by the precapillary arteriolar tone (commonly referred to as the resistance vessels). The level of the sympathetic activation generally determines this vasomotor tone. In addition, the arteries in general will offer variable resistance to flow depending on the bulk of the smooth muscle, the relative content of collagen and elastin in their walls as well as the tone of the smooth muscle in the media.[39] The tone of the smooth muscle is in turn locally mediated by the endothelial function. It is well known that the normal endothelium produces nitric oxide, which causes smooth muscle relaxation.[47] The basal diastolic tension in the arteries is related to the tone of the vessels and the peripheral runoff. *The change in wall tension caused by the pressure wave amplitude as felt by palpation is to a certain extent dependent on the basal diastolic tension in the vessel before ejection.*

Low Peripheral Resistance

Low peripheral resistance may result from:

a. *Peripheral vasodilatation due* to withdrawal of the sympathetic tone as seen in patients with aortic regurgitation (large stroke volume turning off the renin angiotensin system leading to precapillary vasodilatation), due to certain drugs and due to septic or anaphylactic shocks.
b. Development of arteriovenous communications congenital (arteriovenous malformations), iatrogenic (arteriovenous fistulae) or due to pathologic processes in various systemic organs (cirrhosis of the liver, chronic renal disease, chronic pulmonary disease, Paget's disease, and Beriberi).

Conditions with low peripheral resistance and vasodilatation will lead to increased amplitude of the pulse since the diastolic pressure and the diastolic tension in the vessels in these states is low and therefore the effect of change in tension is better appreciated. Conditions that are associated with increased stroke output (mass augmenting momentum of ejection) with low peripheral resistance (e.g. persistent ductus or arteriovenous communications, aortic regurgitation) cause increased velocity of ejection. Both these factors lead to a large amount of change in tension leading to greater amplitude of the pulses (bounding pulses).

High Peripheral Resistance

...pathetic tone causing

of the proximal vessels making them less distensible as well as causing increased basal diastolic tension in the arteries. Therefore, the change in tension during systole is less. The increased resistance to ejection will decrease ejection velocity and to some degree the volume.

In severe hypertension, the basal tension being high in diastole, the change in tension during systole may be poorly felt since much of the change in tension is due to pressure rise alone. It is not uncommon to find constricted and poorly felt peripheral arterial pulses in the context of significantly elevated intra-arterial pressures in some patients receiving inotropic and vasoactive agents. However in some very elderly patients with stiffened arteries due to arteriosclerosis (medial degeneration and sclerosis of the media), the arterial pressure rise might be quite steep and large with large amplitude pulses due to very marked increase in the pulse pressure.[15,35,37,38] *The diastolic pressure and tension in these elderly patients' vessels are not usually increased.*

Transmission or Velocity of Propagation of the Pulse Wave

As mentioned earlier, the velocity of pulse transmission is generally very rapid. The velocity of pulse transmission is not to be confused with the velocity of ejection or blood flow. The latter can be easily measured by Doppler and is only about 0.3 m/s at the radial, whereas at the level of the femoral, the pulse wave transmission velocity is almost close to 10 m/s. It gets faster as one moves more peripherally since the peripheral vessels are more muscular and therefore stiffer. *The pulse wave velocity is normally faster in the elderly due to the stiffness of the vessels.*[4] *Vasoconstriction and the increased tone of the vessel walls also make the arterial system stiffer and allow faster propagation. The elasticity of the arterial segments is also influenced by the distending pressure.*[39] As distending pressure increases, the vessel becomes more tense. This is due to greater recruitment of the inelastic collagen fibers and consequently a reduction in elasticity and conversely an increase in stiffness.[27,48] *The mean arterial pressure determines the background level of distending pressure in the arterial system. Thus when the mean arterial pressure rises, the arteries become more tense and allows the pulse wave to travel faster.*[39] *Pressure pulse wave travels slowly when the mean arterial pressure is lower.*[36,37,39]

The concept can also be demonstrated by plucking the middle of a string, which is held steady and firm at either end. The oscillations produced by the transmission of the wave and its reflection will be grossly visible when the string is held loose. When it is held tight, the transmission is fast and the oscillations become a blur and when the frequencies reach audible range, one can hear a tone as well. The tightness, with which the string is held, is analogous to the stiffness of the vessels in the arterial system.

In severe left ventricular failure, with very low cardiac

and lead to a low amplitude arterial pulse and if the mean arterial pressure is low, this will tend to slow pulse wave velocity. In aortic stenosis, the velocity of ejection is increased; however, the rate of change in momentum is very slow due to less mass or volume being ejected per unit time. In addition, the increased velocity of ejection caused by the pressure gradient across the aortic valve gives rise to a Venturi effect causing a decrease in lateral pressure in the aorta.[26,46] This results in a slowly rising low volume pulse with lower mean arterial pressure, which may also be transmitted slowly to the periphery. In severe aortic stenosis, one may actually feel an appreciable delay between the upstroke of the brachial arterial pulse and that of the radial arterial pulse ***(brachioradial delay)*** in the same arm. This is a rare sign,[49] which has also been observed by us in some patients with severe degree of aortic stenosis with low output. It is conceivable that the delay may also be due to other factors including more compliant arteries, which will also make the wave travel slower.[50,51]

Reflection

Wave of propagation would eventually die out in a completely open system. The arterial system is far from being a completely open system. Although the total collective cross-sectional area increases peripherally, because of change in caliber and branching, reflection of the incident pressure wave occurs from these sites. Complete occlusion of a vessel or a branch will result in complete and fast reflection. Under normal conditions close to 80% of the incident wave gets reflected from the periphery. The main reflection site for the proximal segment of the arterial system may be the aortoiliac bifurcation.[22] For the more peripheral muscular portion of the arterial system, reflecting sites are at the level of the arterioles. *Increase in peripheral resistance or vasoconstriction will increase the intensity of wave reflection (reflection coefficient).[37,38] On the other hand, the effect of lowering the peripheral resistance and vasodilatation will cause a decrease in wave reflection. This can be demonstrated pharmacologically by the intra-arterial injection of nitroglycerine or acetylcholine[25,52] as observed by the changes in the arterial pressure pulse waveform.*

The arterial pulse waveforms have been studied by breaking it down into its component harmonics much like a musical wave. The majority of the energy of the pulse is contained in its first five harmonics. Vascular impedance studies relating corresponding harmonic component of pressure and flow waves have allowed quantitative analysis and have given better insights into arterial pressure and flow mechanics.[11,14,15]

The peripheral circulation has been considered to provide two discrete components of the reflecting sites, one representing the resultant of all reflecting sites from the upper body and the other one representing the resultant of all reflecting sites from the trunk and the lower extremities. This has been described as an ***asymmetric T tube in shape model.***[36,38,53]

The Effects of Wave Reflection on the Pressure and the Flow Waveforms

1. *The effect of wave reflection is related to the time of arrival of the reflected wave during the cardiac cycle. The latter will depend not only on the pulse wave velocity but also on the distance from the individual reflecting sites. Reflected waves from the upper limbs arrive earlier at the ascending aorta compared to those that arrive from the lower body. Reflected waves from the most peripheral reflecting sites will arrive earlier at the larger peripheral arteries before they will arrive at the central aorta.*
2. *When the reflected wave is in the same direction, as the incident wave it will facilitate flow, whereas when it has an opposite direction to the incident wave it will diminish flow. Therefore, the upper and lower body reflections will have different effects on the ascending and the descending aortic flow. Reflected waves from the lower body arriving in the upper arm vessels show the effect of facilitation of forward flow altering its contour from that seen in the ascending aorta.*
3. *Reflected pressure wave always adds to the pressure waveform.*
4. *The recorded arterial pressure waveform will depend on the incident wave, the intensity of wave reflection from the peripheral sites, the timing of reflection during the cardiac cycle where the two meet and merge.*[36,37]
   Reflection added to the incident central aortic pressure wave contributes to the shape of the central aortic pressure. In general, it tends to augment the central aortic pressure. In the peripheral more muscular arteries such as at the level of the femoral or the radial artery, the reflection from the distal sites arrive in such a way as to fuse with the peak of the incident pressure wave giving rise to an elevated systolic pressure and a larger pulse pressure compared to the central aortic pressure wave. Such amplification of the pressure pulse peripherally is more marked in the lower extremities than in the upper extremities. The peripheral amplification in the arterial pressure appears to be somewhat related to the frequency component. In fact, transfer of pressure wave to the periphery has been studied by relating the degree of amplification of the peripheral pressure compared to the aortic pressure to the individual harmonic frequency component of the pressure pulse. The amplification appears to be least in the lower frequencies peaking relatively at higher frequencies.[36,37] This must be taken in relation to the fact that most of the energy of the arterial pressure pulse is actually in the first five harmonics.

When the arteries are relatively compliant and the pulse wave velocity is relatively slow (as in young adults), reflected waves return to the central aorta in diastole augmenting diastolic pressure and therefore coronary blood flow, which occurs pre-dominantly during diastole. *In these normal young individuals, reflected wave from the periphery causes a secondary wave or hump in diastole (dicrotic wave) to the central aortic pressure* (Fig. 2.6A). When arteries are stiffer and the pulse wave velocity is higher as with increasing age, reflected waves arrive earlier and augment the central aortic systolic pressure, causing a second late systolic peak to the waveform (tidal wave) that is higher than the first peak[22] (Fig. 2.6B). It adds also to the duration of the pressure pulse. This would in effect increase the left ventricular workload and compromise the coronary perfusion.[54,55]

5. *The duration of ejection (ejection time) also plays an important role as to how the central aortic pressure contour will become modified by the reflected wave from the periphery.*[17,19,35] *When the ejection duration is increased, the reflected wave from the periphery will arrive at the central aorta during late systole and thus cause a secondary wave in late systole (Fig. 2.6B). When the ejection time is shortened, the reflected wave will arrive after the incisura on the aortic pressure curve (dicrotic notch on the carotid pulse), which corresponds, to the aortic valve closure. This will obviously give rise to a diastolic wave (dicrotic wave) (Fig. 2.8A). The importance of the effect of ejection time or duration of ejection has been demonstrated in humans during Valsalva maneuver. During this maneuver, one tries to exhale forcefully against a closed glottis. During the strain phase, there is increased intrathoracic and intra-abdominal pressures. This will lead to decrease in venous return. This is accompanied by decreased stroke volume and falling blood pressure, which causes reflex tachycardia secondary to sympathetic stimulation. All of these lead to a shortened duration of ejection. And when the straining phase ends, there is a sudden surge of all the damped venous return from the splanchnic and the peripheral veins. This will in turn increase the stroke output, which will be ejected into an arterial system that is constricted by the marked sympathetic stimulation that occurred during the strain phase. Ejection of a larger stroke volume into constricted arterial system would lead to a sudden rise in the arterial pressure (blood pressure overshoot). This, in turn, will cause reflex bradycardia due to baroreceptor stimulation. The ejection time will, therefore, be increased during the poststrain phase. The pattern with late systolic peak has been observed in the beats with longer duration of ejection and the pattern with the diastolic (dicrotic) wave when the duration of ejection is short and the arterial pressure is low*[8,17,23,36,37] *(Table 2.1).*

Intensity of Reflection

Intensity of reflection is related to the degree of arteriolar tone. Vasoconstriction will intensify reflection and vasodilatation will abolish the same. Vasodilatation associated with exercise will be expected to cause less amplification of pressure in the active limb, whereas in the inactive limb the amplification

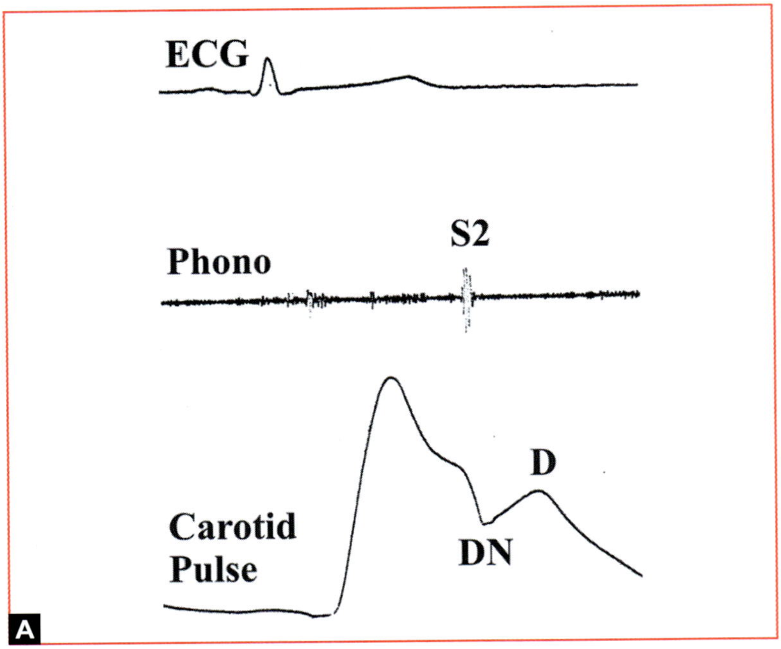

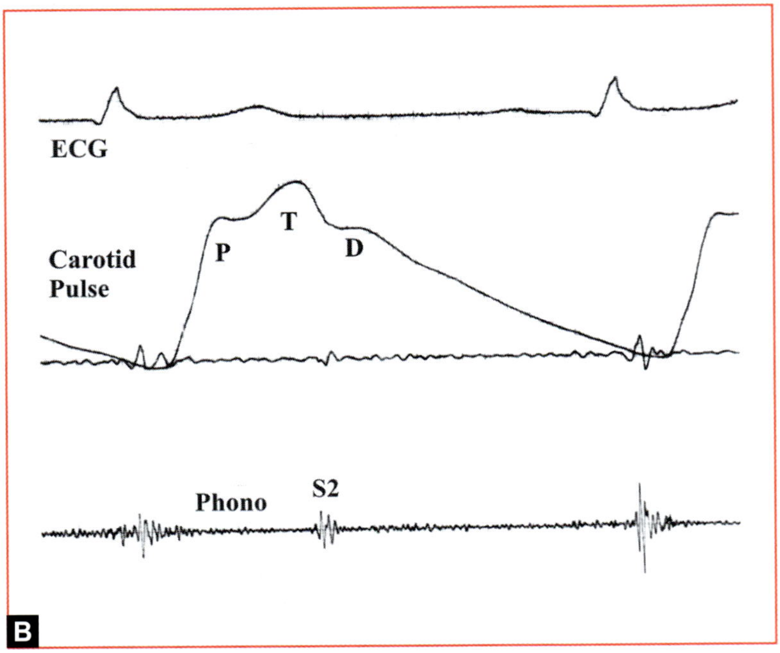

Figs. 2.6A and B: (A). Simultaneous recordings of ECG, phonocardiogram and carotid pulse recording. Note the prominent diastolic (dicrotic D) wave that comes after the dicrotic notch that occurs at the time of S2 and aortic valve closure marking the end of systole. (B) Simultaneous recordings of ECG, phonocardiogram and carotid pulse recording. Note the percussion (P) and the tidal (T) wave in the carotid pulse tracing. The late systolic (tidal wave) peak is higher than the initial systolic wave. (ECG: Electrocardiogram).

may in fact be greater. The amplification of brachial pressures caused by leg exercise can be abolished by reactive hyperemia of the arm.[56] Intra-arterial injection of nitroglycerine or acetylcholine in a single vascular bed can be shown to abolish secondary diastolic waves (which are usually caused by reflection) in the arterial pressure wave.[25,37]

In summary, multiple factors determine pressure pulse wave reflection and its effects, including vasomotor tone, vascular properties, mean arterial pressure, left ventricular ejection time (LVET) and the pattern of left ventricular ejection[37] (see Table 2.1 and Fig. 2.3).

Clinical Implications of Pressure Pulse Wave Reflection

The multiple factors, which determine wave reflection and its effects discussed above, are of clinical relevance in the assessment of the arterial pulse:

1. Wave reflection is the primary reason for the alteration of the incident pressure wave centrally in the aorta contributing to the change in its contour and duration as stated above. If the reflected waves arrive in diastole and cause diastolic pressure rise it helps in the coronary perfusion, whereas if it arrives in systole and augments the late systolic pressure, then it will add to the increased left ventricular workload, thereby increasing the systolic left ventricular wall tension, which is one of the major determinants of myocardial oxygen consumption.[37,38]
2. If the left ventricular function is relatively good, then the contracting left ventricular pump despite the increased demand of myocardial oxygen may sustain the increased pressure load in late systole. However in situations where the left ventricular systolic function is severely compromised, as in late stages of myocardial dysfunction of any etiology, then the left ventricle will be unable to sustain the late systolic augmentation of the pressure. In fact, the reflected pressure wave will impede forward flow from the left ventricle causing it to diminish its output. This will in turn abbreviate the LVET or duration. Such patients are usually in cardiac failure with poor left ventricular function and decreased stroke output. This will not be an issue in patients with cardiac failure purely on the basis of diastolic dysfunction where the congestive symptoms are related to decreased compliance and stiffness of the ventricular myocardium resulting in elevated ventricular diastolic filling pressures. They will have normal LVET.[37]
3. *When the initial (percussion) and the late systolic (tidal) portion of the arterial pressure pulse are well separated, one may feel a bifid or bisferiens pulse, e.g. bisferiens pulse of combined aortic stenosis and aortic regurgitation.*[21,35,36] In this situation, aortic stenosis causes slower rate of change in momentum of ejection leading to slower rate of pressure rise as discussed previously. However when the bisferiens pulse is felt, usually the coexisting aortic regurgitation is usually significant. The high stroke volume

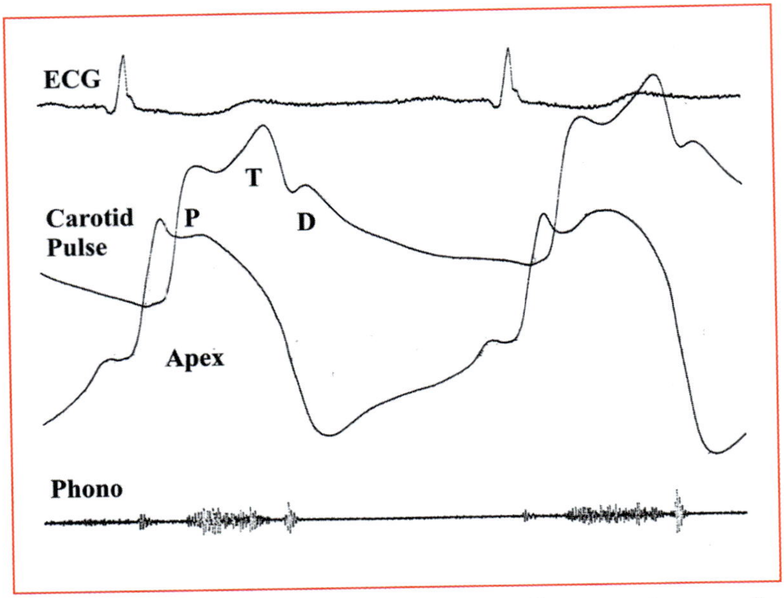

Fig. 2.7: Simultaneous ECG, carotid pulse, phonocardiogram and apexcardiogram from a patient with aortic stenosis and aortic regurgitation. Carotid pulse shows a well separated initial systolic (percussion—P) and late systolic (tidal—T) waves that were palpable as a bisferiens pulse.

accompanying the aortic regurgitation will cause a large amplitude pressure pulse wave. The increased velocity of turbulent flow at peak systole due to the obstruction, however, will cause a decrease in lateral pressure in the aorta due to the Venturi effect similar to that seen in isolated aortic stenosis (Fig. 2.7) leading to a drop in pressure rise during the middle of systole, thereby separating the initial from the late systolic peak.[38,46] In this instance, however, the late systolic peak will be greater than the initial one. In aortic valve disease, the ejection duration is prolonged and this may have some effect on the harmonic components of the arterial pressure pulse wave since the left ventricular pump ejects its stroke volume over a longer period of systole. The pressure pulse has been noted to have pre-dominance of lower frequencies.[19]

4. *When the dicrotic (diastolic) wave becomes large and palpable it may mimic the bisferiens pulse. This is usually produced under circumstances of low momentum of ejection (usually due to low stroke volume), e.g. severe left ventricular failure, cardiac tamponade and cardiomyopathy (Figs. 2.8A and B). In these states, there may be increased sympathetic stimulation and activation of the renin-angiotensin system. Sympathetic stimulation will cause vasoconstriction. This will be accompanied by increased intensity of reflection. The pulse wave velocity could be normal or low. The activation of renin-angiotensin system by making the vessels stiffer will favor increased pulse wave velocity. However, the poor left*

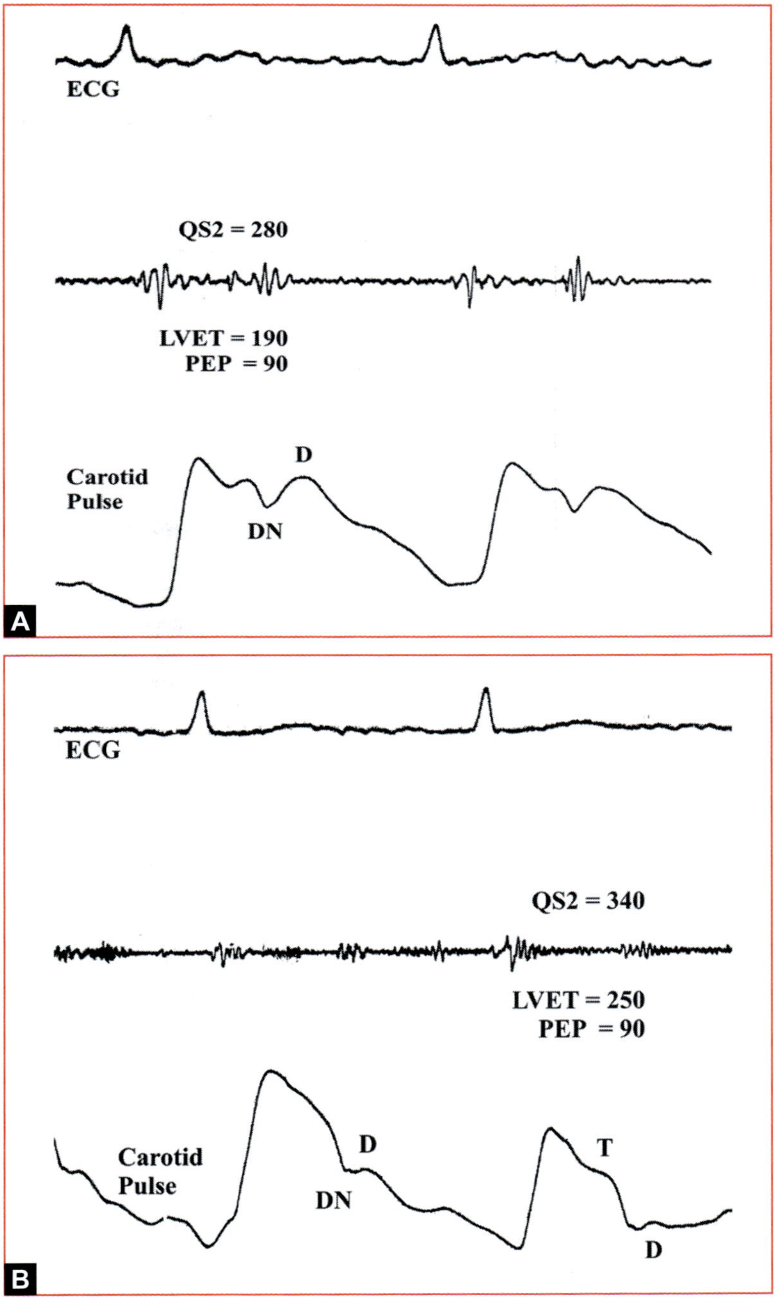

Figs. 2.8A and B: (A). Carotid pulse in a patient with cardiac tamponade. Note the prominent dicrotic wave D. If palpable, it could give rise to a bifid pulse. DN, dicrotic notch. Systolic time intervals QS2 (total duration of electromechanical systole), LVET (left ventricular ejection time) and the PEP (pre-ejection period) are given in milliseconds. (B) Same patient as in (A), after pericardiocentesis. Note the change in the dicrotic wave D. It is much smaller. The improvement in the stroke output following the relief of tamponade is evidenced by the increase in LVET.

ventricular function and output will cause a poor momentum of ejection, resulting in decreased rise in the mean arterial pressure. The low mean arterial pressure will make the pulse wave travel slower. The ejection time may be shortened due to the low stroke volume. Intense vasoconstriction will be associated with good intensity of reflection. Thus, the reflected wave will arrive in the central aorta after the aortic valve closure, i.e. after the incisura in diastole.

5. *The three conditions, which govern reflection in severe cardiac failure, are also present in low output states such as shock and cardiac tamponade.[21,37] They are as follows:*
   a. *The low arterial pressure that favors slow wave travel*
   b. *Intense vasoconstriction that intensifies wave reflection*
   c. *Shortened LVET, which makes the reflection to arrive in diastole (dicrotic wave) after aortic valve closure.*

The importance of low stroke volume and shortened ejection duration has also been demonstrated by the fact that the dicrotic wave gets exaggerated, in beats following shorter diastoles, during strain phase of Valsalva maneuver[8,20,37] (which is breathing against the closed glottis) and during amyl nitrite inhalation. Amyl nitrite is a rapidly acting arterial dilator. It is fairly quickly inactivated in the lungs and the effect is primarily on the arterial system that causes rapid onset of arterial dilatation with fall in blood pressure. The brisk sympathetic stimulation secondary to the hypotension produces reflex sinus tachycardia and decreased stroke output initially and decreased ejection time. The reflex sympathetic stimulation leads to vasoconstriction, which favors reflection. All the three conditions are thus met to cause prominent dicrotic waves. The sympathetic stimulation also leads to venoconstriction causing increased venous return. The increased venous return results in increased cardiac output (stroke volume × the heart rate per minute) (Fig. 2.9).

Compliant arterial system (as in the younger patients, post-aortic valve replacement in patients with aortic regurgitation) with associated slow pulse wave velocity can cause reflected wave to travel slowly enough to augment diastolic portion of the arterial pressure wave, thereby causing a prominent dicrotic wave.

Arterial Pulse Contour in Hypertrophic Cardiomyopathy

In hypertrophic cardiomyopathy obstructive or non-obstructive, the left ventricular contractility is markedly increased. The pattern of ejection is such that the aortic outflow tends to be biphasic in systole unlike the normal monophasic outflow.[44] This is particularly marked in patients with obstruction to the outflow caused by the sudden systolic anterior motion of the anterior mitral leaflet toward the interventricular septum during the middle of systole presumably caused by the Venturi effect of the rapid outflow velocity. The latter mechanism has been questioned by some and the SAM

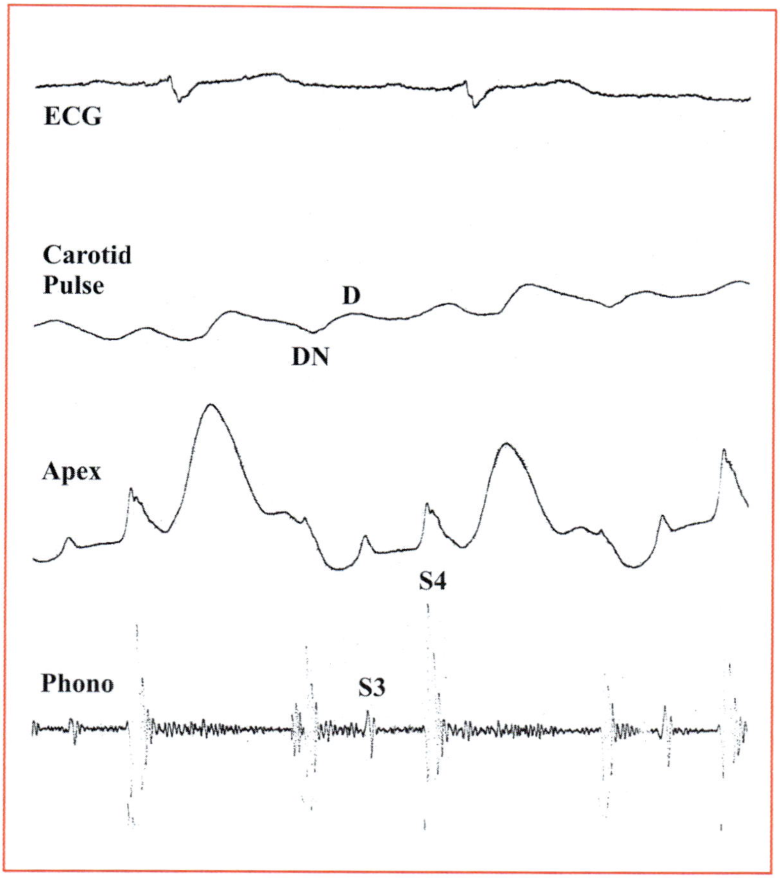

Fig. 2.9: Prominent dicrotic wave (D) following amyl nitrite inhalation in a patient with hypertrophic cardiomyopathy. Amyl nitrite causes rapid onset of arterial dilatation with fall in blood pressure. The brisk secondary sympathetic stimulation produces increased vasoconstriction and tachycardia with shortening of ejection time. Venoconstriction with increased venous return will eventually increase the cardiac output. While the cardiac output is increased, the stroke volume may actually fall due to the tachycardia. The exaggerated diastolic inflow in the presence of the hypertrophic cardiomyopathy brings out the third (S3) and the fourth (S4) heart sounds. Apexcardiogram (apex) reflects these events with exaggerated rapid filling wave and atrial kick.

has been attributed to pushing or pulling of the mitral valve by the anatomic distortion aggravated by vigorous contraction in these patients with marked hypertrophy of the left ventricular walls associated with small cavity.[45] In any event, the flow ceases in mid-systole and resumes in late systole. The biphasic outflow, therefore, generates a bifid contour of the pressure wave in the aorta. The late systolic pressure may also be augmented by reflected wave from the periphery. The initial part of ejection being rapid and strong is associated with a faster and greater momentum of ejection resulting in a sharply rising and peaked initial systolic (percussion) wave, which has larger amplitude than the late systolic (tidal) wave (Figs. 2.10 and 2.11).

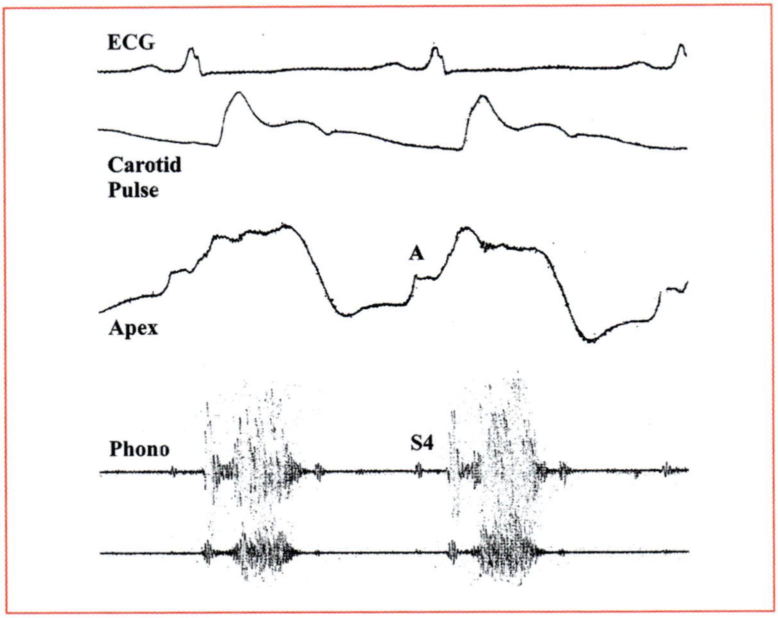

Fig. 2.10: Simultaneous recordings of the ECG, the carotid pulse, the Phonocardiogram and the Apexcardiogram from a patient with hypertrophic obstructive cardiomyopathy. Carotid pulse shows a rapid rate of rise of the percussion wave. (ECG: Electrocardiogram).

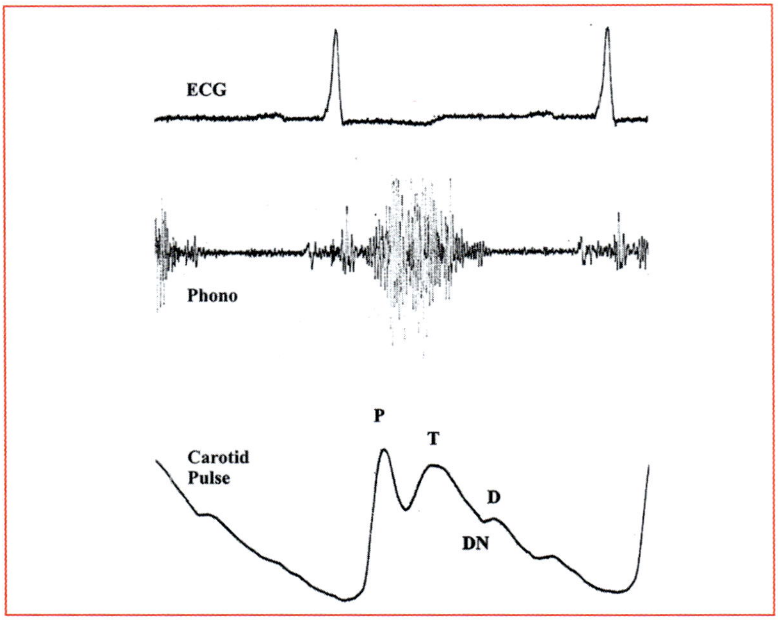

Fig. 2.11: Bisferiens carotid pulse in a patient with hypertrophic obstructive cardiomyopathy. The initial systolic or percussion (P) and the late systolic tidal (T) waves can be felt separately. The initial systolic wave is more prominent than the late systolic tidal wave.

ASSESSMENT OF THE ARTERIAL PULSE

The essential elements of examination of the arterial pulse should be geared toward the assessment of the volume, the upstroke and the pulse contour abnormalities. In addition to these essential points, the observer would also be able to assess heart rate, rhythm and arterial wall characteristics. *The assessment of the arterial pulse will be discussed under the following headings:*

1. *Rates, Rhythm and Pulse Deficit*
2. *Symmetry and Radiofemoral Delay*
3. *Vessel Wall Characteristics*
4. *Amplitude*
5. *Upstroke*
6. *Contour Abnormalities*
7. *Bruits*
8. *Pulsus Alternans*
9. *The Peripheral Signs of Aortic Regurgitation*

Rate, Rhythm and Pulse Deficit

The heart rate per minute can be quickly ascertained in most instances by counting the peripheral arterial pulse from any site for at least 15 seconds. When the pulse rhythm is irregular, the presence of an arrhythmia is suggested. In such instances, the pulse rate may not reflect correctly the heart rate. *Simultaneous cardiac auscultation and palpation of the peripheral arterial pulse will reveal a faster rate at the apex of the heart than suggested by the peripheral pulse. This difference is termed the pulse deficit. Simultaneous auscultation may also allow in determining the possible cause of the irregularity.* A pause in the peripheral pulse due to an extrasystole or premature beat can be correctly distinguished from that caused by a dropped beat such as seen in second degree sinoatrial or atrioventricular block. An exaggerated pulse deficit is most often present in atrial fibrillation especially when the ventricular rate is not well controlled. The R-R intervals in atrial fibrillation are usually variable. This leads to varying lengths of diastole. The ventricular filling following short diastole is poor leading to low stroke volume and ejection velocity resulting in poor ejection momentum and therefore poor pulse, which cannot be felt. Similar effect can also be caused by premature beats.

Symmetry and Radiofemoral Delay

All peripheral pulses should be palpated including the temporal arteries in the head, the carotids in the neck, the brachial, the radial and the ulnar in the upper extremities, the abdominal aorta, the femoral, the popliteal, the posterior tibial and the dorsalis pedis in the lower extremities. The presence of the pulse at all these sites must be ascertained. Comparison of the similar pulse at opposite sides of the body should be made. An absence of the pulse at any site and also the presence of significant discrepancy between the two sides usually indicate a proximal blockage in the vessel with the absent or weaker pulse.

The temporal artery is usually felt for the presence of tenderness commonly seen in temporal arteritis. *The carotid pulse being most central and closer to the aorta should be preferentially used for the assessment of the pulse volume, upstroke as well as detection of contour abnormalities*. It may be occasionally anatomically difficult to palpate in some patients with short and thick necks. It is usually located somewhat medially to the sternomastoid muscles.

The brachial pulse is located medially in the antecubital fossa. The brachial arterial pulse is commonly used for measurement of blood pressure in the arms. It should also be felt for the proper placement of the stethoscope for blood pressure measurement. The radial and the ulnar pulses are felt laterally and medially, respectively, on the anterior aspect of the wrist. One of these could be congenitally absent. Both these arteries are usually connected in the hand through the anastomotic arches. In some patients, these connections may be inadequate. Radial artery often is used for intra-arterial blood pressure monitoring in critically ill patients and such instrumentation may lead to occlusion of the vessel. This is usually tolerated by most because of the anastomotic connections in the hand, which continues to be perfused through the ulnar artery. In patients with poor anastomotic connections such iatrogenic blockage may lead to gangrene of the hand. *The adequacy of the anastomosis in the hand must be determined* prior to any such instrumentation. This is usually determined ***by the radial compression test (Allen's test).*** Both the radial and the ulnar arteries should be blocked by direct compression of the vessels against the underlying wrist bones. The patient is asked to make a tight fist thus emptying the hand of the venous blood. This should leave the hand pale until the radial artery is released from the compression. This should result in immediate hyperemia of the hand, resulting in the disappearance of the pallor and return of the normal pink appearance. The test should be repeated a second time with release of the ulnar artery. Similar result should be obtained to indicate intact anastomosis.

The abdominal aorta may or may not be palpable in the adult depending on the degree of obesity. In obese individuals, the mere palpability may be an indication of the presence of an aneurysm. *Palpability of a wide area of pulsation over the region of the abdominal aorta particularly when the pulsation is expansile would indicate the presence of an abdominal aortic aneurysm.* Expansile pulsation can be easily checked by palpating with two index fingers of each hand placed on either side of the pulsating aorta approximately one to two inches apart. If the fingers are further separated by each pulsation as opposed to being lifted up without separation, then the pulsation can beconsidered expansile.

The femoral arteries should be palpated in each groin below the inguinal ligament. Diminished or absent femoral pulses indicating proximal blockage is often seen in peripheral vascular disease. Normally the femoral and the radial pulses occur simultaneously. *When the femoral pulse lags behind the radial (radiofemoral delay), occlusion of the aorta either due to coarctation or atherosclerosis is indicated.*

The differential effects of the anatomic variations in coarctation of aorta may be diagnosable at the bedside by the careful comparison of the brachial pulses between the two arms. If both the brachial pulses and the carotids are strong with delayed or diminished femoral pulses, it will indicate the coarctation to be distal to the left sub-clavian artery. However, when the left brachial arterial pulse is weak or diminished compared to the right, it will indicate the coarctation to be proximal to the left sub-clavian artery. If the right sub-clavian has an anomalous origin from the aorta distal to the coarctation, then the right brachial pulse will be diminished or poor.

Popliteal pulses are felt by applying pressure over the popliteal fossa with both hands encircling the knee with the thumbs on the patella and the finger tips held over the popliteal fossa with the knees very slightly bent to relax the muscles. *The normal popliteal pulse is often difficult to feel especially in heavy patients. Popliteal pulses may be more easily felt in patients with significant aortic regurgitation and in other causes of wide pulse pressure.*

The dorsalis pedis and the posterior tibial can have marked anatomic variations, resulting in the occasionally absence of one or the other without proximal occlusive disease. Other signs of occlusive disease, causing absence of these pulses in the feet should be looked for (temperature of the foot, color, skin perfusion assessment by blanching, presence or absence of hair on the dorsum of the toes).

Vessel Wall Characteristics

The readily accessible arteries such as the brachials and the radials can be rolled between the finger and the bone to get a feel for the thickness and the stiffness of the walls. A calcified vessel will feel hard and not easily compressible. Vessels affected by medial sclerosis would feel thicker and stiffer and less pliable.

Amplitude

The amplitude of the pulse is assessed by determining the displacement felt by the palpating fingers. The displacement is dependent on the change in tension between diastole and systole developed in the arterial wall palpated. The tension is increased according to Laplace's law as the radius and the pressure increase. The radius is increased with large stroke volumes. Patients with low output and low stroke volume will have a "thready" or weak pulse due to poor displacement and reduced level of tension developed. Such a low amplitude pulse (low volume pulse) is known as ***pulsus parvus.*** The peak systolic arterial pressure also contributes to the tension developed on the vessel wall. Thus, the presence of a marked increase in pulse pressure could also result in increased amplitude of the pulse.

The amplitude of the arterial pulse should be assessed in general using the carotid pulse. Carotid pulse amplitude may be low in the presence of significant obstructive lesions such as severe aortic and mitral stenoses. Large stroke volumes as seen in aortic regurgitation would result in exaggerated pulse displacement of the carotids, which may be even visible from a distance (Corrigan's pulse). The large amplitude pulsation may be felt also in more peripheral vessels as well and reflects the increased change in wall tension secondary to increased stroke volumes. The low basal tension due to the low diastolic pressure, low peripheral resistance and vasodilatation is also associated with increase in the pulse pressure (*see* Figs. 2.4 and 2.7).

In the presence of a large stroke volume associated with low diastolic pressure as in aortic regurgitation or its mimickers (aortic sinus rupture or communication with another low pressure cardiac chamber such as the right atrium, aortopulmonary window, and persistent ducts arteriosus), the arterial pulse feels strong and bounding with large volume of expansion. Therefore, the amplitude is often casually referred to as the volume of the pulse. *In patients with significant hypertension, in the presence of severe vasoconstriction, the peripheral pulses may even be difficult to palpate due to the decreased change in radius and wall tension.*

In patients with combined aortic stenosis and regurgitation where both are significant, the amplitude of the carotid pulsation often would reflect the aortic stenosis whereas the aortic regurgitation will show its effects on the amplitude more peripherally such as in the popliteal arteries. The augmented systolic pressures due to reflection in these more muscular and peripheral vessels together with the low diastolic pressure secondary to vasodilatation and retrograde flow into the left ventricle would cause wide change in tension between diastole and systole causing more prominent pulsation.

Upstroke

The arterial pulse upstroke is best judged at the carotid. This is a palpatory assessment of the rate of rise of the pulse from its onset to the peak. The normal rate of rise of the carotid arterial pulse is usually sharp and rapid and indicates unobstructed ejection by a healthy ventricle. This in essence rules out significant fixed type of aortic stenosis. The normally rising carotid pulse transmits a sharp tapping sensation to the palpating finger. When the upstroke is delayed due to significant aortic stenosis, the rise is slow and gives more sustained gentle type of pushing sensation reflecting the gradual rise. In fact, the sensation in some patients may be jagged and simulates a "thrill" or "shudder". In normals, most of the stroke volume is ejected during the first third of systole causing a rapid rise in the aortic pressure, giving rise to a rapid upstroke. In aortic stenosis, this rapid ejection cannot occur. In fact, it takes all of systole to eject the same volume. The decreased mass or volume ejected per unit time leads to considerable decrease in ejection momentum despite increased velocity of ejection. In addition, the increased velocity of flow caused by the significant pressure gradient between the left ventricle and the aorta caused by the stenosis produces a Venturi effect on the lateral walls of the aorta. This has the effect of significantly reducing the net pressure rise in the aorta. *Thus, the rate of rise of the arterial pressure pulse is slow in aortic stenosis. The net effects on the arterial pulse in valvular aortic stenosis are diminished amplitude (small), slow ascending limb (parvus) and a late and poorly defined peak (tardus).* When the stenosis is very severe and accompanied by failing ventricle, the upstroke and the pulse may be poorly felt if felt at all *(pulsus tardus et parvus, meaning late, slow and small). When the carotid pulse amplitude is judged to be very low, one will have extreme difficulty in assessing the rate of rise accurately.*

The decreased momentum of ejection particularly in severe cases with decreased stroke volume will result in a low mean arterial pressure. This may be accompanied by slow pulse wave velocity, which in rare instances may actually be felt as an appreciable delay between the brachial and the radial artery pulses (brachioradial delay). In the normals, simultaneous palpation of the brachial and the radial arterial pulse of the same side will not show any delay at the onset of the pulses over the two vessels. If in fact one feels an appreciable delay between the two pulses then this would indicate a slow transmission of the pulse wave. This is ***a rare sign, which may be present in severe aortic stenosis.***[49]

In aortic stenosis, the peripheral amplification of pressures is diminished but may be still present. This must be taken into account in assessing the gradient of pressure between the left ventricle and a peripheral artery especially in children.

In the elderly patients with stiffened arteries, even significant aortic stenosis may fail to be detected by the assessment of the upstroke. *When the compliance of the aorta is decreased as seen in the elderly, even the small volume that gets ejected in the early systole will cause a significant rise in pressure thus increasing the tension in the carotids quickly enough to hide the expected effect of the stenosis on the pulse.*

In some elderly patients with stiff vessels with rapid pulse wave velocity and reflection, there may be a hump or shoulder felt in the upstroke (anacrotic shoulder). This may mimic a delayed upstroke. These patients may be falsely diagnosed as having aortic stenosis especially when the findings are associated with aortic sclerosis and ejection murmurs.

Therefore in the elderly, interpretation of carotid pulse upstroke should take these factors into account. The reason for this effect is the rapid transmission of the incident and the reflected pulse waves.

Very rapid or a "brisk" upstroke of carotid pulse when felt in association with a large amplitude pulse suggests a hyperdynamic state such as due to aortic regurgitation or aortic regurgitation mimickers (aortic sinus rupture or communication with another low pressure cardiac chamber such as the right atrium, aortopulmonary window, persistent ductus arteriosus). When the upstroke is brisk and the pulse amplitude is normal or low, hypertrophic cardiomyopathy with or without sub-valvular muscular dynamic mid-systolic obstruction must be considered (see Fig. 2.10). In severe mitral regurgitation also the upstroke may tend to be brisk due to a Starling effect on the left ventricle secondary to the volume overload. However, the amplitude will tend to be normal.[43]

In supravalvular aortic stenosis, the right brachial pulse and the carotid may be stronger than the left brachial. This will be reflected in an increased pulse pressure in the right arm than the left. It has been attributed to a ***Coanda effect*** (the tendency of a jet of fluid when properly directed, to get attached to a convex surface instead of moving in a straight line).[43] The obstruction in the supravalvular aortic stenosis is such that the high velocity jet is directed toward the right innominate artery and gets carried by this Coanda effect. *It probably means that the direct impact pressure at the center of the jet is received by the right innominate artery. There may be actually a Venturi effect of lowered lateral pressure in the aorta distal to the stenosis transmitted to the left sub-clavian and the left brachial artery.*

Contour Abnormalities

The normal arterial pulse has a single impulse with each cardiac systole. Occasionally in certain abnormal states, the pulse may be felt as a double impulse. This abnormality of the contour of the impulse is termed "pulsus bisferiens" or simply bifid pulse. ***Bifid pulse contours may be felt and recorded in arterial pulse tracings.***

The conditions that may exhibit bifid pulse contours are as follows:

a. Hypertrophic cardiomyopathy with obstruction
b. Severe aortic regurgitation with some aortic stenosis

The mechanisms are different in these two conditions and have been dealt with previously. The arterial pulse will tend to have an increased volume and amplitude in combined aortic stenosis and regurgitation than in hypertrophic cardiomyopathy. The effect of aortic regurgitation on the amplitude will be particularly evident in the periphery, while the aortic stenosis effect may be more appreciable in the carotid. The bisferiens of aortic stenosis and regurgitation also gets altered in peripheral arteries where they may not be recognizable as such. It is always best detected in the carotids and the bisferiens is usually such that the late peak is always higher than the initial peak. This is different in the hypertrophic cardiomyopathy where the initial peak is often brisk and higher that the late peak.

Dicrotic wave when exaggerated ***may become palpable and cause*** a bisferiens effect on the pulse. *The difference lies in the appreciation of the fact that the second impulse is diastolic and will occur after the second heart sound as judged by simultaneous auscultation and palpation. The exaggerated dicrotic wave is usually associated with low momentum of ejection due to low stroke volume as in severe heart failure, cardiomyopathy and cardiac tamponade. In these instances, the pulse amplitude will be expected to be low. The mechanisms and factors favoring the development of prominent dicrotic waves have been discussed previously.*

Bruits

Bruits are audible noise often systolic, caused by turbulence in flow usually due to partial obstruction of the lumen of the arteries and very occasionally due to high flow. These are often heard over large arteries and detected by auscultation with a stethoscope. Routine assessment of the arterial pulse must, therefore, include auscultation over all large peripheral arteries such as the carotid, sub-clavians, vertebrals, abdominal aorta, the renals, the iliacs and the femorals. Often a systolic murmur originating from the aortic valve and occasionally from the mitral valve may radiate to the carotids. This can be differentiated by noting ***the location of maximal loudness of the bruit-murmur.*** The carotid bruit is maximally loud as expected over the carotids as opposed to a radiating murmur, which should be maximally loud over the precordium. In high flow states, continuous bruit lasting throughout systole and diastole may be heard over the intercostal vessels. This could occur in situations that lead to development of collateral flow such as seen in patients with aortic coarctation. Peripheral arteriovenous shunts (congenital or acquired AV fistulae) may also produce continuous bruits over the vessels involved.

Pulsus Alternans

When the pulse amplitude changes beat-by-beat alternating between higher and lower pulse amplitude as a result of alternating stroke volume, the resulting pulse is termed pulsus alternans. The alternating weaker and stronger pulses can be both felt and recorded. In such patients when the intra-arterial pressures are monitored, similar changes in both systolic and pulse pressures are noted. It can be detected by palpation and can be confirmed by blood pressure recording. Korotkoff sounds will be seen to double in rate once the cuff pressure is lowered and the lower systolic peaks of the weaker beats are detected. Pulsus alternans if detected clinically, it usually indicates severe degree of myocardial dysfunction and left ventricular failure.

Pulsus alternans is, however, a normal phenomenon in as much as it can be induced after a premature beat. The effect of alternans in normal subjects can only be demonstrated by measurements of the systolic time intervals (Fig. 2.12). The ***systolic time intervals*** consist of the following:

1. The duration of the total electromechanical systole is measured by the interval "QS2" between the onset of the QRS in the electrocardiogram (ECG) and the end of systole as depicted by the onset of the second heart sound (S2) on the simultaneously recorded phonocardiogram.
2. The LVET is measured from the onset of the upstroke of the simultaneously recorded carotid artery pulse tracing to the dicrotic notch.
3. The third interval, which is derived from these two measurements, is the pre-ejection period (PEP). This is obtained by sub-tracting the LVET from the QS2.

The stronger beat has better stroke output and therefore has longer LVET. The increased contractility of the stronger beat is reflected in shorter PEP. The weaker beat has the opposite namely a longer PEP. The effect of the alternans after an extrasystole in normal subjects lasts for two beats. As left ventricular function deteriorates the alternans effect is more pronounced and tends to persist for a longer period. When the left ventricular function is severely depressed the alternans becomes more pronounced and may become clinically noticeable and palpable in the arterial pulse (Figs. 2.13A and B). This

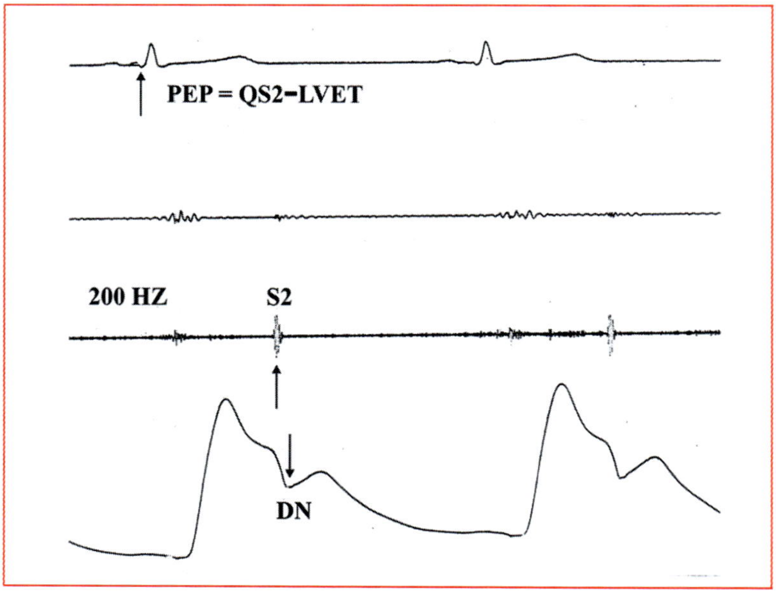

Fig. 2.12: Simultaneous recordings of ECG, phonocardiogram and carotid pulse tracings, showing measurement of systolic time intervals. QS2, total electromechanical systole; LVET, left ventricular ejection time; PEP, pre-ejection period. All intervals are in milliseconds. (ECG: Electrocardiogram).

may sometimes last for long periods of time such as several hours or days. Pulsus alternans is often initiated by an extrasystole. Although the mechanism is not fully elucidated, it is perhaps related in some ways to the phenomenon of post-extrasystolic potentiation.[57,58]

It is well known that the beat following an extrasystole is associated with increased contractility and stroke volume. This post-extrasystolic potentiation is partially related to the compensatory pause, which follows the extrasystole providing increased time for diastolic filling, which in turn through the

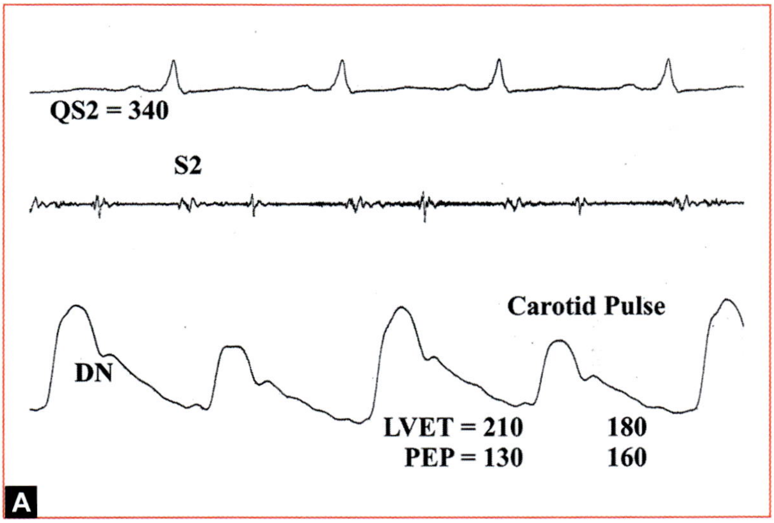

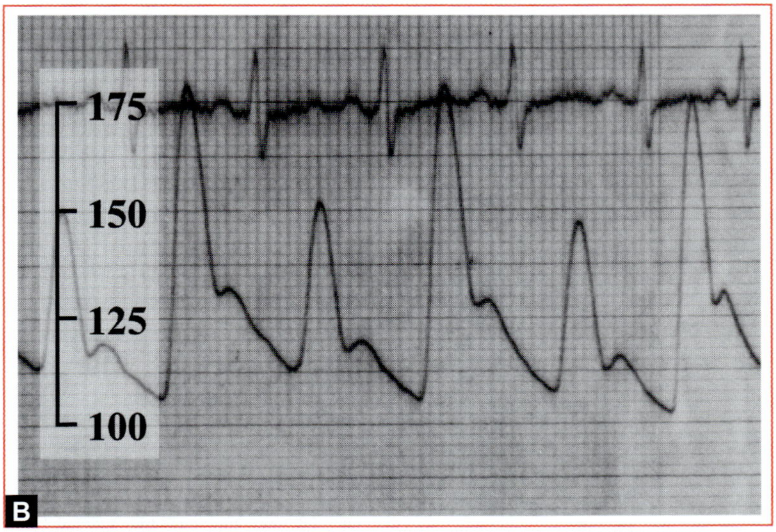

Figs. 2.13A and B: (A) Carotid pulse recording from a patient with cardiomyopathy showing pulsus alternans. (B) In the same patient, intra-aortic pressures showing alternating levels of increased and decreased systolic pressures and pulse pressures.

Starling effect would help increase the contractility and stroke volume. The long pause will also allow more time for peripheral runoff and drop in diastolic pressure. This will, in turn, help the post-premature beat by decreasing the afterload. However, the post-extrasystolic potentiation can be demonstrated even when there is no compensatory pause, thereby keeping both the filling and the afterload constant by pacing studies. In this instance, the increased contractility is probably due to increased levels of intracellular calcium availability for the actin–myosin interaction. The premature depolarization caused by an extrasystole is thought to release more intracellular calcium from the sarcoplasmic reticulum (SR) before all the calcium released during the previous beat could be taken back up by SR. The increased calcium is, therefore, available for the post-premature beat, thereby increasing its contractile force by more actin–myosin interaction. The calcium uptake and release may actually fluctuate alternatingly from beat-to-beat reaching probably the steady state in the normals after a couple of beats. However in the severely diseased myocytes of patients with severe cardiomyopathy or end-stage heart failure, the steady state may not be reached for prolonged periods of time.[59] This becomes manifest as alternating strong and weak contractions of pulsus alternans.

The Peripheral Signs of Aortic Regurgitation

1. Quincke's sign
2. Corrigan's pulse
3. Water-hammer pulse
4. Pistol-shot sounds
5. Duroziez's sign
6. de-Musset's sign
7. Hill's sign

Most of these peripheral signs of aortic regurgitation[60] are related to the large stroke volume, increased ejection velocity and momentum together with decreased peripheral resistance, and widened pulse pressure with low diastolic pressure secondary to retrograde flow into the left ventricle and peripheral vasodilatation. *Some of these signs may, therefore, be present in aortic regurgitation mimickers (aortic sinus rupture or communication with another low pressure cardiac chamber such as the right atrium, aortopulmonary window, and persistent ductus arteriosus) as well as other conditions fulfilling the same pathophysiologic requirements (Paget's disease, arteriovenous communications, severe anemia).*

Quincke's sign: This sign refers to the capillary pulsation as detected in the nail bed. This sign is elicited by applying slight pressure at the tip of the fingernail enough to cause blanching of the distal nail bed while shining the penlight through the pulp of the fingertip. The observer should look for movement of the proximal edge of the blanched area. This sign is not diagnostic of aortic regurgitation and can occur in many other states with increased pulse pressure and may even be detected in normal young individuals.

Corrigan's pulse: This term already explained refers to the visible large amplitude carotid pulsation.

Water-hammer pulse: This term refers to a toy, which consists of a sealed tube of vacuum partially filled with water so that when it is turned upside down the water falls with a palpable slap. The peripheral arterial pulse such as the radial, in patients with aortic regurgitation and other similar states as mentioned above, is usually peaked and with rapid rise which is poorly sustained followed by a rapid fall. When the radial artery is palpated with the palm of the hand while the arm is held raised, which helps to lower the diastolic pressure further in the arm palpated, the sharp slapping quality may be exaggerated.

Pistol-shot sounds: The phenomenon responsible for water-hammer effect upon auscultation over large vessels such as the femorals produces loud slapping sounds, which mimic literally pistol shots. These are short loud sounds. The mechanism has not been clearly established, but it has been thought to be due to shock waves generated when the flow velocities exceed pressure velocities locally.[35] It is also conceivable that they may be associated with actual reflection at these sites.

Duroziez's sign: This is also termed "the intermittent femoral double murmur of Duroziez".[60] It is elicited by compressing the femoral artery by applying gradual pressure over the stethoscope, which is placed over the femoral artery. At a certain moment of pressure, a double murmur will be heard. The second method is to listen over the femoral artery while applying pressure with the finger in succession first 2 cm upstream (meaning proximal to) and then 2 cm downstream (meaning distal to) of the stethoscope. The upstream pressure will produce a systolic murmur and the downstream pressure will produce a diastolic murmur. The mechanism involved is the turbulent flow caused by the partial obstruction. The turbulence gives rise to bruit, and its presence in relation to the site of obstruction should suggest direction of flow. The systolic bruit is easy to understand, since flow is toward the periphery during systole; one would expect the bruit to be distal to site of obstruction. Since diastolic bruit is heard proximal to the obstruction, the turbulent flow must also be proximal to the obstruction indicating retrograde flow. Retrograde flow in some major arteries including the coronaries during diastole has been documented by angiography in aortic regurgitation.

Duroziez's sign may be falsely positive in other high output states such as thyrotoxicosis, severe anemia, fever, persistent ductus and arteriovenous fistula. In high output states, the diastolic component of the bruit may be due to forward flow. The specificity of the sign can be increased by eliciting the sign slightly differently by applying the partial compression of the femoral artery with the proximal or the distal edge of the stethoscope while listening for the loudest diastolic component. In retrograde flow states (such as aortic regurgitation and persistent ductus arteriosus) as opposed to high output states, the diastolic components are louder when the distal edge of the stethoscope is pressed.

de-Musset's head bobbing sign: This sign is best elicited by watching the patient's upper body and head while seated at the edge of the examining table. The upper body and head will be seen to move back and forth rhythmically with each systole. This is the result of the exaggerated ballistographic effect of the large stroke volume and wide pulse pressure together with low peripheral resistance. Ballistocardiography, an old physiologic method,[61] involves recording of the reaction of the whole body to the action of ejection of blood into the aorta (Newton's third law of motion). The recoil of the aorta itself may play a part in contributing to the movement. Special instrument and bed are required to detect these in the normal subjects with normal stroke volume. However, it becomes so exaggerated in aortic regurgitation that it becomes visible and detectable clinically.

Hill's sign: This sign is elicited by measurement of the systolic blood pressure in the arm and the leg simultaneously or in very quick succession.[3,62] *It must be emphasized that the Hill's sign refers to systolic blood pressure differential as obtained by indirect blood pressure measurements using the traditional cuff. The pressure is obtained in the usual way at the arm over the brachial artery. The pressure in the leg can be elicited over the popliteal artery or at the ankle by palpation of the posterior tibial artery. Intra-arterial pressure recordings at the femoral level are not the way to look for this difference accurately. The reason for this is that the femoral artery is probably not peripheral enough to show this exaggerated effect.*

Normally, the peripheral pressures are usually amplified due to the muscular nature of these vessels allowing rapid transmission of the pulse wave in both directions resulting in summation of the reflected with the peak of the incident wave. This peripheral amplification is usually more pronounced in the leg than in the arm. In normal subjects, this difference in peak pressure between the arm and the leg is in the order of 15–20 mm Hg. This difference may be markedly exaggerated in patients with significant aortic regurgitation (Figs. 2.14A and B).

A difference of 20–40 mm Hg in the peak pressure can easily be seen in other conditions with wide pulse pressures (e.g. thyrotoxicosis, anemia, fever or Paget's disease). The difference of between 40 and 60 mm Hg is

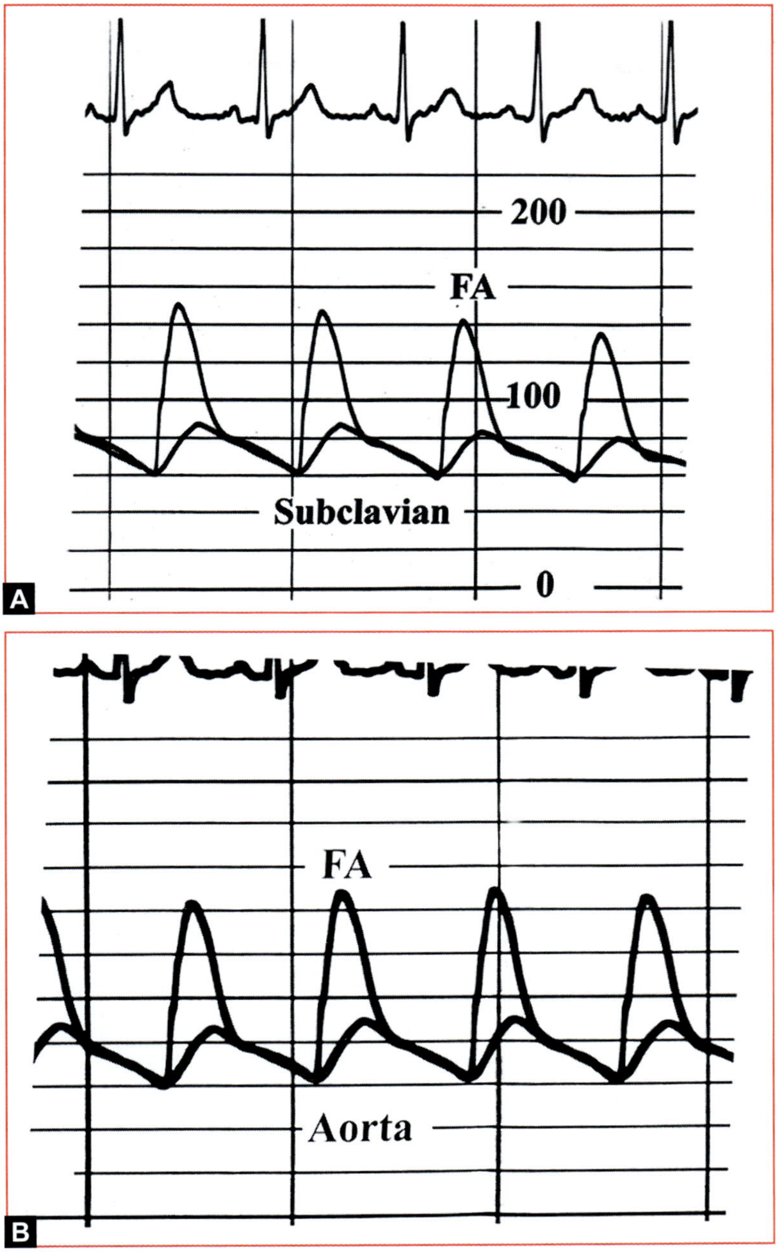

Figs. 2.14A and B: (A) Simultaneous intra-arterial pressure recordings through catheters placed in the femoral artery (FA) and the sub-clavian artery in a patient with aortic regurgitation. Note the significant difference in the systolic pressures. (B) The catheter is withdrawn from the sub-clavian artery to the central aorta and simultaneous recording of aortic, and femoral arterial pressures are shown. Note that there is no significant difference of systolic pressures between the central aorta and the sub-clavian artery. However, there is about a 60 mm difference in pressures between the FA and the central aorta.

associated with moderate degree of aortic regurgitation, whereas that in excess of 60 mm Hg is usually indicative of moderately severe aortic regurgitation. Therefore, Hill's sign is somewhat related to the degree of aortic regurgitation and, therefore, useful in following the patients with aortic regurgitation.

The blood pressure differential between the arm and the leg is probably multifactorial in origin even in the normal subjects:

1. The reflecting sites in the lower extremities are probably more than in the arm.
2. The vessels of the lower extremities are probably more muscular.
3. It is known that the age-related change in the compliance of the arteries is less in the upper limb vessels than in the lower limb vessels.[36,37]
4. The upper arm vessels tend to arise anatomically at approximately 90° angle from the aortic arch. The diameter of these vessels being smaller than the aorta, the relative rapid flow in the aortic arch may cause a Venturi effect of relative suction on these cephalobrachial vessels. This may tend to reduce the net effect of peripheral amplification of pressures caused by reflection. This effect of suction can be demonstrated in the side arm of a tap by running water through it when the side arm is of a smaller diameter and at right angles to the direction of water flow.

   This concept derives support from the fact that when direct impact pressure gets transmitted preferentially to the orifice of the innominate artery as it happens in supravalvular aortic stenosis, the pressure is actually higher in the right arm supplied by that vessel.[43] Presumably here, the Venturi effect of reduction in lateral pressure does not apply, since the direct impact pressure of the jet gets directed preferentially toward the orifice due to the anatomic nature of the stenosis.
5. In aortic regurgitation, the increased momentum of ejection will produce larger amplitude incident pressure wave. The increased momentum of ejection as well as the increased duration of ejection may in fact alter the harmonic components of the wave. It has been shown that peripheral amplification is less with lower frequencies than with higher frequencies of the pressure pulse wave. It has been suggested, therefore, that peripheral amplification is generally less in aortic regurgitation.[36,38] While these may be valid, it is known that in Echo Doppler measurements of pure aortic regurgitation, the aortic outflow velocity is quite variable. Sometimes it can be quite high without the presence of any stenosis. In patients with aortic regurgitation and high velocities of flow in the aortic arch, one can expect exaggerated result from the Venturi effect. This may explain variations seen in the sensitivity of the Hill's sign in patients with aortic regurgitation. In patients who have a positive Hill's sign, it becomes useful in their long-term follow-up.

PRACTICAL POINTS IN THE CLINICAL ASSESSMENT OF THE ARTERIAL PULSE

In the clinical assessment of the arterial pulse, it is worth remembering the following points:

1. *The three features of the arterial pulse that should be diligently sought for are the amplitude, the upstroke and the pulse contour abnormalities.*
2. *The other features include the determination of rate, rhythm, pulse deficit, symmetry, radiofemoral delay, bruits and specifically looking for the peripheral signs of aortic regurgitation when indicated.*
3. *The palpation of the carotid arterial pulsation is necessary to determine the pulse upstroke and for the detection of abnormal contours. The amplitude may be judged by palpation of the carotid as well as the more peripheral vessels.*
4. *The amplitude of the pulse is assessed by determining the displacement felt by the palpating fingers. The displacement is dependent on the change in tension in the artery between diastole and systole. The amplitude of the pulse must be judged as to whether it is normal, low or increased.*
5. *The low amplitude (the low volume) pulse usually indicates low momentum of ejection due to decreased stroke volume and low pulse pressure as seen in significant obstructive lesions of the outflow or the inflow tracts (severe aortic or mitral stenoses), poor ventricular pump function as in severe cardiomyopathy or heart failure and severe reductions in left ventricular filling as in cardiac tamponade or significant loss in the blood volume or the extracellular fluid volume.*
6. *In severe systemic hypertension with excessive vasoconstriction, the peripheral pulse amplitude may be poor due to decreased change in radius and wall tension.*
7. *If the pulse amplitude is considered increased or exaggerated ("bounding pulses") then conditions associated with large stroke volume and low peripheral resistance must be considered. These include aortic regurgitation and aortic regurgitation mimickers (aortic sinus with a communication to a low pressure chamber such as the right atrium, aortopulmonary window and persistent ductus arteriosus).*
8. *The pulse amplitude will also be exaggerated in conditions associated with vasodilatation and low peripheral resistance since in these states (e.g. septic states, drugs causing vasodilatation, arteriovenous communications congenital or iatrogenic or due to pathologic processes in systemic organs as in cirrhosis of the liver, chronic renal disease, chronic pulmonary disease, Paget's disease and Beriberi) the diastolic pressure in the vessel is low and therefore the change in tension is better appreciated.*

9. *In patients with combined aortic stenosis and regurgitation where both are significant, the amplitude of the carotid pulsation often would reflect the aortic stenosis, whereas the aortic regurgitation will show its effects on the amplitude more peripherally such as in the popliteal arteries.*
10. *In the elderly with decreased compliance of the large arteries, ejection of normal stroke volume may cause significant systolic hypertension. The pulse amplitude will be high due to rapid pulse wave velocity caused by the increased stiffness and reduced compliance of the arteries, resulting in increased augmentation of central systolic and pulse pressure due to reflection. In fact even the presence of aortic stenosis may be masked in such patients.*
11. *The upstroke of the pulse is best assessed over the carotid artery. The normal rate of rise is felt as a sharp tap by the palpating finger. The delayed upstroke is felt as a gentle sustained push. In some, the sensation may be jagged simulating a "thrill" or "shudder". A normally rising carotid pulse rules out significant fixed aortic stenosis. The delayed carotid upstroke, on the other hand, is indicative of fixed left ventricular outflow obstructive lesions. Rare exceptions are of course the elderly patients. Delayed upstroke may be masked in the elderly with stiff aorta where the pressure rise may be steep due to the decreased compliance of aorta. The elderly may also have a hump on the upstroke due to an exaggerated anacrotic shoulder mimicking a delayed upstroke without the presence of any significant aortic stenosis. When the amplitude of the pulse is low as in low stroke output, then the rate of the rise of the pulse is often difficult to judge.*
12. *When the upstroke of the pulse is thought to be brisk or rapid and if the pulse amplitude is normal or low then conditions associated with rapid left ventricular ejection such as hypertrophic cardiomyopathy with or without sub-valvular dynamic muscular obstruction must be considered. If the upstroke is brisk and the pulse amplitude is normal, then rapid ejection with normal stroke volume as in significant mitral regurgitation must be considered.*
13. *Bifid pulse contours or pulsus bisferiens must lead one to consider hypertrophic cardiomyopathy with possible obstruction as well as combined aortic regurgitation and stenosis where the aortic regurgitation is more dominant and hemodynamically significant than the aortic stenosis. In hypertrophic cardiomyopathy with obstruction, amplitude of the pulse is low while the upstroke will be brisk and the initial peak will be brisk and taller than the late peak. In combined aortic stenosis and regurgitation with bisferiens, the amplitude will be large and the upstroke will be relatively normal. The second peak will be larger than the first peak.*
14. *Exaggerated dicrotic wave may occasionally be the cause of a bifid pulse contour. The second impulse in this instance will occur in diastole as timed by auscultation. The exaggerated dicrotic wave is usually associated*

with low momentum of ejection usually due to low stroke volume as in severe heart failure, cardiomyopathy and cardiac tamponade. In these instances, the pulse amplitude will be expected to be low.

REFERENCES

1. Mahomed F. The physiology and clinical use of the sphygmograph. Medical Times and Gazette, London. 1872;1:62-65.
2. Mackenzie J. The study of the pulse. Arterial, venous and hepatic and of the movements of the heart. Edinburgh: Pentland; 1902.
3. Hill L, Rowlands RA. Systolic blood pressure. (1) in change of posture, (2) in cases of aortic regurgitation. Heart. 1911;3:219-32.
4. Bramwell JC, Hill AV. Velocity of transmission of the pulse wave and elasticity of arteries. Lancet. 1922;1:891-2.
5. Wiggers CJ. The Pressure Pulses in the Cardiovascular System. New York: Longmans Green and Co; 1928.
6. Bramwell JC. The arterial pulse in health and disease. Lancet. 1937;2:239-47.
7. Kroeker EJ, Wood EH. Comparison of simultaneously recorded central and peripheral arterial pressure pulses during rest, exercise and titlted position in man. Circulation Res. 1955;3:623-32.
8. Kroeker EJ, Wood EH. Beat to beat alterations in relationship of simultaneously recorded central and peripheral arterial pressure pulses during Valsalva maneuver and prolonged expiration in man. J Appl Physiol. 1956;8:483-94.
9. Remington JW, Wood EH. Formation of peripheral pulse contour in Man. J Appl Physiol. 1956;9:433-42.
10. Wood P. Diseases of the Heart and Circulation. Philadelphia: JB Lippincott Co; 1956. pp. 26-32.
11. McDonald DA. Blood Flow in Arteries. London: Edward Arnold Publishers Ltd; 1960.
12. Attinger EO (Ed). Pulsatile Blood Flow. Proceedings of the first International Symposium on Pulsatile Blood Flow. New York: McGraw Hill Book Company; 1963.
13. Ikram H, Nixon PGF, Fox JA. The Hemodynamic implications of bisferiens pulse. Br Heart J. 1964;26:452-9.
14. O'Rourke MF, Taylor MG. Input impedance of the systemic circulation. Circ Res. 1967;20:365-80.
15. O'Rourke MF, Blazek JV, Morreels CL, Jr, et al. Pressure wave transmission along the human aorta: changes with age and in arterial degenerative disease. Circulation Res. 1968;23:567-79.
16. Barner HB, Willman VL, Kaiser GC. Dicrotic pulse after open heart operation. Circulation. 1970;42:993-7.
17. Mills CJ, Gabe IT, Gault JH, et al. Pressure-flow relationships and vascular impedance in man. Cardiovasc Res. 1970;4:405-17.
18. Mills CJ, Gabe IT, Gault JH, et al. Blood velocity and pressure waveforms in the major arteries in man. Clin Sci. 1970;38:10P.
19. O'Rourke MF. Influence of ventricular ejection on the relationship between central aortic and brachial pressure pulse in man. Cardiovasc Res. 1970;4: 291-300.
20. Meadows WR, Draur RA, Osadjan CE. Dicrotism in heart disease. Correlations with cardiomyopathy, pericardial tamponade, youth, tachycardia, and normotension. Am Heart J. 1971;82:596-608.

21. O'Rourke MF. The arterial pulse in health and disease. Am Heart J. 1971;82: 687-702.
22. Murgo JP, Westerhof N, Giolma JP, et al. Aortic input impedance in normal man: relationship to pressure wave forms. Circulation. 1980;62:105-16.
23. Murgo JP, Westerhof N, Giolma JP, Altobelli SA. Manipulation of ascending aortic pressure and flow wave reflections with the Valsalva maneuver: relationship to input impedance. Circulation. 1981;63:122-32.
24. Murgo JP, Westerhof N, Giolma JP, et al. Effects of exercise on aortic input impedance and pressure wave forms in normal humans. Circ Res. 1981; 48:334-43.
25. Hamilton WF. The patterns of the arterial pressure pulse. Am J Physiol. 1944; 141:235-41.
26. Dow P. The development of anacrotic tardus pulse of aortic stenosis. Am J Physiol. 1941;131:432-6.
27. Roach MR, Burton AC. The reason for the shape of the distensibility curves of arteries. Can J Biochem Physiol. 1957;35:681-90.
28. O'Rourke MF. Pressure and flow waves in systemic arteries and the anatomical design of the arterial system. J Appl Physiol. 1967;23:139-49.
29. Ruskin A. Classics in arterial hypertension. Springfield: Thomas; 1956.
30. Drzewiecki GM, Melbin J, Noordergraaf A. Arterial tonometry: review and analysis. J Biomech. 1983;16:141-52.
31. Kelly RP, Hayward C, Ganis J, et al. Non-invasive registration of arterial pressure waveform using high-fidelity applanation tonometry. J Vasc Med Biol. 1989;1: 142-9.
32. Karamanoglu M, O'Rourke MF, Avolio AP, Kelly RP. An analysis of the relationship between central aortic and peripheral upper limb pressure waves in man. Eur Heart J. 1993;14:160-7.
33. Chen CH, Nevo E, Fetics B, et al. Estimation of central aortic pressure waveform by mathematical transformation of radial tonometry pressure. Validation of generalized transfer function. Circulation. 1997;95:1827-36.
34. Glossary of cardiologic terms related to physical diagnosis. IV. Arterial pulses. Am J Cardiol. 1971;27:708-9.
35. O'Rourke MF. Arterial Function in Health and Disease. Edinburgh: Churchill Livingstone; 1982.
36. O'Rourke MF, Kelly R, Avolio A. The Arterial Pulse. Philadelphia, PA: Lea & Febiger; 1992.
37. Nichols WW, O'Rourke MF. McDonald's Blood Flow in Arteries. London: Edward Arnold; 1998.
38. Vlachopoulos C, O'Rourke M. Genesis of the normal and abnormal arterial pulse. Curr Probl Cardiol. 2000;25:303-67.
39. Oliver JJ, Webb DJ. Non-invasive assessment of arterial stiffness and risk of atherosclerotic events. Arterioscler Thromb Vasc Biol. 2003;23:554-66.
40. Rushmer RF. Origins of pulsatile flow: the ventricular impulse generators. In: Attinger EO (Ed). Pulsatile Blood Flow. New York: McGraw Hill Book Company; 1963. pp.221-34.
41. Noble MI. The contribution of blood momentum to left ventricular ejection in the dog. Circ Res. 1968;23:663-70.
42. Murgo JP, Altobelli SA, Dorethy JF, et al. Normal ventricular ejection dynamics in man during rest and exercise. In: Leon DF, Sharer JA (Eds). Physiologic Principles of Heart Sounds and Murmurs, Vol. 92. New York: American Heart Association; 1975.

43. Perloff JK. The physiologic mechanisms of cardiac and vascular physical signs. J Am Coll Cardiol. 1983;1:184-98.
44. Murgo JP, Alter BR, Dorethy JF, et al. Dynamics of left ventricular ejection in obstructive and non-obstructive hypertrophic cardiomyopathy. J Clin Invest. 1980;66:1369-82.
45. Sherrid MV, Gunsburg DZ, Moldenhauer S, et al. Systolic anterior motion begins at low left ventricular outflow tract velocity in obstructive hypertrophic cardiomyopathy. J Am Coll Cardiol. 2000;36:1344-54.
46. O'Rourke MF. Impact pressure, lateral pressure, and impedance in the proximal aorta and pulmonary artery. J Appl Physiol. 1968;25:533-41.
47. Kinlay S, Creager MA, Fukumoto M, et al. Endothelium-derived nitric oxide regulates arterial elasticity in human arteries in vivo. Hypertension. 2001;38: 1049-53.
48. Bank AJ, Wang H, Holte JE, et al. Contribution of collagen, elastin, and smooth muscle to in vivo human brachial artery wall stress and elastic modulus. Circulation. 1996;94:3263-70.
49. Leach RM, McBrien DJ. Brachioradial delay: a new clinical indicator of the severity of aortic stenosis. Lancet. 1990;335:1199-201.
50. Caro CG, Parker KH. Brachioradial delay and severity of aortic stenosis. Lancet. 1990;335:1535.
51. O'Rourke MF, Avolio AP, Karamanoglu M, et al. Brachioradial delay. Lancet. 1990;336:1377-8.
52. O'Rourke MF, Taylor MG. Vascular impedance of the femoral bed. Circ Res. 1966;18:126-39.
53. O'Rourke MF, Avolio AP. Pressure and flow waves in systemic arteries and the anatomical design of the arterial system. J Appl Physiol. 1967;23:139-49.
54. Bogren HG, Mohiaddin RH, Klipstein RK, et al. The function of the aorta in ischemic heart disease: a magnetic resonance and angiographic study of aortic compliance and blood flow patterns. Am Heart J. 1989;118:234-47.
55. Ohtsuka S, Kakihana M, Watanabe H, et al. Chronically decreased aortic distensibility causes deterioration of coronary perfusion during increased left ventricular contraction. J Am Coll Cardiol. 1994;24:1406-14.
56. Rowell LB, Brengelmann GL, Blackmon JR, et al. Disparities between aortic and peripheral pulse pressures induced by upright exercise and vasomotor changes in man. Circulation. 1968;37:954-64.
57. Ranganathan N, Sivaciyan V, Chisholm R. Effects of post-extrasystolic potentiation on systolic time intervals. Am J Cardiol. 1978;41:14-22.
58. Voss A, Baier V, Schumann A, et al. Post-extrasystolic regulation patterns of blood pressure and heart rate in patients with idiopathic dilated cardiomyopathy. J Physiol. 2002;538:271-8.
59. Eisner DA, Diaz ME, Li Y, et al. Stability and instability of regulation of intracellular calcium. Exp Physiol. 2005;90:3-12.
60. Sapira JD. Quincke, de Musset, Duroziez, and Hill: some aortic regurgitations. South Med J. 1981;74:459-67.
61. Eblen-Zajjur A. A simple ballistocardiographic system for a medical cardiovascular physiology course. Adv Physiol Educ. 2003;27:224-9.
62. Frank MJ, Casanegra P, Migliori AJ, et al. The clinical evaluation of aortic regurgitation. With special reference to a neglected sign: the popliteal-brachial pressure gradient. Arch Intern Med. 1965;116:357-65.

Chapter

3 Blood Pressure and its Measurement

Snapshot

- Physiology of Blood Flow and Blood Pressure
- Physiology of BP Measurement
- Points to Remember when Making the BP Measurement
- Factors which Affect Blood Pressure Readings
- Interpretation of Blood Pressure Measurements
- Use of BP Measurement in Special Clinical Situations

PHYSIOLOGY OF BLOOD FLOW AND BLOOD PRESSURE

The purpose of the arterial system is to provide oxygenated blood to the tissues by converting the intermittent cardiac output into a continuous capillary flow, and this is achieved by the structural organization of the arterial system.

The blood flow in a vessel is basically determined by two factors:

1. *The pressure difference between the two ends of the vessel that provides the driving force for the flow*
2. *The impediment to flow, which is essentially the vascular resistance*

This can be expressed by the following formula:

$Q = \Delta P/R$,

where Q is the flow, ΔP is the pressure difference and R is the resistance.

The pressure head in the aorta and the large arteries is provided by the pumping action of the left ventricle ejecting blood with each systole. The arterial pressure peaks in systole and tends to fall during diastole.

Briefly the peak systolic pressure achieved is determined by (*see* Chapter 2 on Arterial Pulse):

1. The momentum of ejection (the stroke volume, the velocity of ejection that in turn are related to the contractility of the ventricle and the afterload)
2. The distensibility of the proximal arterial system
3. The timing and amplitude of the reflected pressure wave

When the arterial system is stiff as in the elderly, for the same amount of stroke output, the peak systolic pressure achieved will be higher. The poor distensibility causes a greater peak pressure (Laplace relationship).

In addition, a stiff arterial system results in faster transmission and reflection of the pressure wave, thereby adding to the peak pressure. The narrow and peaked pressure seen in the more peripheral muscular arteries is the effect of such reflection. The level to which the arterial pressure will fall during diastole is primarily dependent on the state of the peripheral resistance, which controls the runoff. Conditions with low peripheral resistance and vasodilatation will cause the diastolic pressure to fall to low levels.

The ***mean arterial pressure*** is the average of all the pressures obtained over an entire duration of a cardiac cycle. Since diastole is longer than systole, the mean pressure is estimated as the sum of 60% of the diastolic pressure and 40% of the systolic pressure. More accurate measurement will be by integrating the area under a recorded pressure curve. The ***pulse pressure,*** which is the difference between the systolic and the diastolic pressure, reflects not only the stroke volume but also the state of the peripheral resistance. Conditions associated with a large stroke volume and low peripheral resistance will be expected to give rise to a large pulse pressure and this will be reflected in the amplitude of the arterial pulse by palpation.

While the control of the cardiac output is usually determined by local tissue flow under physiologic states, the control of the arterial pressure is independent of these and is regulated through a complex system that involves nervous reflexes and neurohumoral mechanisms for short-term needs (such as "flight", "fright" and "fight" type reactions or in situations like those following acute loss of blood volume) and neuroendocrine, renin–angiotensin–aldosterone system and renal mechanisms for long-term adaptation. These control systems in the normal as well as their alterations in hypertension and in heart failure are well discussed in standard texts in physiology and medicine. In this chapter, our focus will be mainly in relation to the measurement of blood pressure (BP) by the sphygmomanometer and its use in special clinical situations.

PHYSIOLOGY OF BP MEASUREMENT

The indirect measurement of BP by the sphygmomanometer involves the application of a controlled lateral pressure by an inflatable cuff to occlude the artery by compression, thereby stopping the flow. The detection of the resumption of flow during slow deflation allows the determination of the pressure. The cuff is normally applied to the arm over the brachial artery. When the cuff pressure exceeds the systolic pressure, the brachial artery is fully occluded and the flow ceases. When the cuff is deflated to pressures just below the systolic peak, the flow begins to resume with each cardiac systole. The jet of blood coming through the partially occluded vessel is associated with tapping type sounds, which can be recognized using the stethoscope placed over the brachial artery just distal to the cuff. These sounds termed the Korotkoff sounds help in identifying the systolic and the diastolic pressures in the artery. As the cuff is being deflated, the pressure when the Korotkoff sounds first appear is noted. This corresponds to the systolic pressure. The disappearance of the Korotkoff sounds with further deflation will correspond to the diastolic pressure. Korotkoff sounds generally become muffled first when the cuff is being deflated before they totally disappear. It is always advisable to take the diastolic pressure to the level at which the sounds disappear, since it is less likely to introduce errors.[1]

The Mechanism of Origin of the Korotkoff Sounds

The exact mechanism of origin of Korotkoff sounds is not completely established. They have been thought to be due to turbulence of flow coming through the partially occluded artery. This is thought to be supported by the following.

They become muffled ***(phase IV)*** and eventually disappear ***(phase V)*** generally when the flow resumes in diastole, i.e. when the cuff is deflated below the diastolic pressure allowing the artery to be open throughout the cardiac cycle. In addition, before they become muffled and completely disappear, they may sound like a short bruit (initially as soft bruit in ***phase II*** and louder bruit as in ***phase III).***

However, they do not always sound like murmurs and often sound as sharp sounds. The possibility of Water hammer theory had been previously suggested (not to be confused with the water hammer pulse in aortic regurgitation) to explain the presence of distinct sounds.[2] The sounds are thought to be produced by the deceleration of high velocity jet of flow coming through the vessel, as it opens up from an occluded state, against the stationary column of blood distal to the occlusion. The intensity of the sounds, however, may vary being loud and persistent to low diastolic pressures or throughout diastole in certain situations as in aortic regurgitation in children and in pregnancy. In aortic regurgitation, the stroke volume tends to be large with increased velocity of ejection. Children generally have hyperkinetic circulation, and pregnant women tend to have a high cardiac output with increased sympathetic tone. On the other hand, the Korotkoff sounds tend to be poor in low output states.

When an oversized cuff is used it may lead to underestimation of the systolic BP. It has been shown that the state of the distal vasculature in the limb where the BP is being measured affects the intensity of the Korotkoff sounds. Vasodilatation makes the sounds louder, and vasoconstriction softer.[3,4] When the peripheral resistance in the arm distal to the cuff was changed by interventions such as heating, cooling and by induction of reactive hyperemia, the amplitude of the Korotkoff sounds appeared to change. Thus, these effects may lead to either over or under estimation of both systolic and diastolic pressures.[5] In fact, when the Korotkoff sounds are poorly heard, they are best augmented by raising the arm (decreasing venous distension) and having the patient open and close their fist on the side where the pressure is being measured a few times.[6,7] This is thought to increase the forearm flow.

Others have proposed that the pressure pulse wave itself may be the source of the Korotkoff sounds. The sounds may be attributed to "shock waves" where the flow velocity of blood in the narrowed segment may exceed the pulse wave propagation velocity and give rise to vibrations in the audible frequency range. This would be analogous to the sonic boom heard when the speed of a jet plane reaches and surpasses the speed of sound.

It is also possible that the Korotkoff sounds are related to energy (vibrations) that results from sudden termination of the pressure pulse wave at the site of the inflated cuff, which leads to partial occlusion of the vessel, causing this to become a terminating site favoring reflection. Between the systolic peak and the diastolic pressures during which time the Korotkoff sounds are present there is a considerable degree of termination and reflection together with beginning onward transmission of the pressure pulse wave. Once the cuff pressure is lowered below the diastolic pressure there is no more termination or reflection at the site of the cuff application and the pressure pulse is further transmitted along the artery. Therefore, there is no sound to be heard. This may be supported by the fact that when an oversized cuff is used it may lead to underestimation of the systolic BP. In conditions where the Korotkoff sounds are loud and last longer to low levels of diastolic pressure such as aortic regurgitation, there is a more rapid and higher launching momentum to the pressure pulse wave because of the large stroke volume which is ejected with a rapid velocity. Thus, there may be more energy for dissipation at the termination sites. In significant aortic regurgitation, one often feels "pistol shots" over the femoral arteries, which are also often sites of reflection because of bifurcation. On the other hand, this mechanism does not explain why the Korotkoff sounds are heard distal to the cuff and not proximal to it.

Tavel et al. had previously shown using invasive pressure measurements that the Korotkoff sounds correspond to the steepened portion of the anacrotic limb of the pressure pulse.[8] More recently, Drzewiecki et al. have proposed an alternate origin for the production of the Korotkoff sounds. They relate it to the distortion of the pressure pulse under the cuff in the narrowed segment, and a change in both pressure and flow distal to the cuff resulting in a nonlinear pattern of pressure-flow relationship. This results in a steeper pulse slope distal to the cuff with higher frequency harmonic content of this steeper pulse slope reaching the audible frequency range. This interesting theory was proposed based on a mathematical model representing the structures involved, which was able to predict the range of features of the Korotkoff sounds previously reported.[9] However, it does not satisfactorily explain as to why in some people the Korotkoff sounds persist even when the cuff is fully deflated.

It is clear from the short description above that the origin of the Korotkoff sounds is far from being completely established.

POINTS TO REMEMBER WHEN MAKING THE BP MEASUREMENT

The following points are worth noting when taking BP measurements:[10–12]

1. First, determine roughly the systolic pressure by palpation of the radial artery pulse, as the cuff is gradually being deflated so that ***an auscultatory gap*** *(during which Korotkoff sounds may disappear altogether and reappear again when the cuff is being deflated further) if present will not be missed. This sometime occurs in some hypertensive patients.*[13] *The auscultatory gap may also be due to venous congestion and decreased velocity of blood flow in the extremity where the BP is being measured.*[6] The systolic pressure estimated by the palpation of the distal radial artery (while compressing the proximal brachial artery) is usually 10 mmHg lower than the systolic pressure as assessed by the auscultatory method. Some studies have shown that assessment of central aortic pressure by measurement of the brachial BP by cuff method underestimates the systolic pressure by 5–20 mm Hg and overestimates the diastolic pressure by 12–20 mm Hg. This has been related to interobserver variability. Specially, for the diastolic pressure some may take phase IV and others phase V as the true pressure. This discrepancy is even more exaggerated during vasoconstriction.[14–16]
2. Keep the position of the antecubital fossa at the level of the heart to avoid the hydrostatic effect of gravity on the column of blood in the arm.
3. Deflate the cuff slowly. The recommended deflation rate is usually 3 mm Hg/s. This rate should actually vary according to the patient's heart rate (relatively slow deflation rate during bradycardias and relatively faster deflation rate during tachycardias).
4. Avoid venous congestion that tends to muffle Korotkoff sounds, by raising the arm and by inflating the cuff faster.[6]
5. When the BP is first determined in a new patient it should be measured in both arms. If a difference is noted then the higher reading of the two must be considered as the patient's BP. Slight variation between the two arms is common. The normal difference should not exceed 15 mm Hg. The difference may be due to the fact that the innominate on the right side and the subclavian on the left side may arise from the aorta at different angles. The relative suction due to a Venturi effect of the flow through the aortic arch between the two arms may be different for this reason. When the difference is abnormally high then it will be indicative of obstruction on the side with the lower reading. Conditions such as coarctation of aorta (one proximal to the origin of the left subclavian), atherosclerotic or embolic obstruction (rare in the upper extremities), and aortic dissection

are some of the conditions that may have to be considered depending on the clinical situation. In coarctation of aorta proximal to the left subclavian, the right arm pressure will be naturally higher than the left. In supravalvular aortic stenosis, the direction of the jet of flow tends to be directly directed into the innominate artery. This often results in the direct impact pressure of the central jet being transmitted to the right arm, thus making the right arm pressure higher than the left due to a Coanda effect.[17]

6. When Korotkoff sounds persist, take the point where they become muffled as the level of the diastolic pressure.
7. When Korotkoff sounds are poor, have the patient exercise their hand as pointed out earlier, thereby augmenting the intensity of the Korotkoff sounds.[7]
8. Always have a cuff of proper size for the arm especially for very obese individuals. The width of the bladder in the cuff should be roughly 40% of the arm circumference. In most patients (normal size), a 5-inch wide cuff would be the appropriate choice. Too wide a cuff may lead to erroneous recognition of the onset of the Korotkoff sounds for the site of auscultation may be too distal to the site of actual occlusion of the artery. This may make the Korotkoff sounds to be too soft in intensity to be heard and may result in underestimation of the pressure. A narrow cuff will allow overdistension of the bladder of the cuff before actual occlusion of the brachial artery can occur. Some of the pressures applied may be spent in distending the bladder rather than compressing the artery. This will lead to an overestimation of the systolic and even the diastolic pressures. Larger size cuff (8 inches wide) is needed in obese patients where the arm circumference is >35 cm.[18,19] The bladder of the cuff should cover at least 50% of the circumference of the limb where the BP is being measured.
9. Support the arm so that patient's arm muscles are relaxed. If not, isometric contraction may occur that will raise the peripheral resistance, thereby raising the diastolic pressure. This would also adversely influence the BP reading by muffling the Korotkoff sounds, thereby raising the diastolic pressure and most likely lowering the systolic pressure.
10. Avoid aneroid manometers, which can have problems in calibration. If an aneroid manometer is used it is recommended that it be calibrated, against a mercury manometer, yearly in fact probably more frequently.[20]
11. Local changes in the limb are known to affect BP readings. If the patient has washed his/her hand with cold or hot water just before getting the BP measured, the reading obtained may be higher or lower, respectively, and may not correctly reflect the central aortic pressure. When BP is taken more than once, they should be done at least 5 minutes apart to avoid reactive hyperemic vasodilatation during the second measurement. This lowers the recorded BP locally leading to false estimation of central aortic pressure.[5]

FACTORS WHICH AFFECT BLOOD PRESSURE READINGS

1. Anxiety, stress and/or pain. Sometimes the mere fact of having the BP taken by a physician can excite a nervous and anxious patient to cause significant rise in the BP of the patient. (The so-called white coat syndrome.)[21,22]
2. Exercise such as climbing a couple of flights of stairs, and even mild activity involving bending or stooping in the elderly could raise the pressures. It should be noted that the transfer of energy of pulse pressure wave to the periphery is greater at low frequencies (<2.5 Hz) in patients at rest because of slower heart rates and longer ejection time. With exercise and the associated faster heart rates and shorter ejection time, the energy transfer occurs at higher frequencies (>2.5 Hz). Since higher frequencies are amplified more, the systolic brachial pressure will be measured to be elevated and may not necessarily reflect the true central aortic systolic pressure.[23–25]
3. Exposure to cold by causing sympathetic vasoconstriction will raise the pressures.
4. Postprandial state will tend to lower the pressure. In addition to increased vagal tone necessary for increased peristalsis, the lower pressure is likely related to vasodilatation in the mesenteric vessels diverting more blood to the gut for the purpose of proper digestion. This probably also relates to the increase in angina or postprandial decrease in exercise tolerance in patients with exertional angina. The increased demand of blood supply to the gut, increasing the work load of the heart coupled with the decreased diastolic pressure (coronary perfusion pressure), leads to mismatch between the oxygen demand and the coronary blood supply resulting in angina.
5. Alcohol acutely will lower the pressure while chronic alcohol consumption raises the pressures.
6. Both chronic and acute cigarette smoking tend to cause elevated pressures.
7. Illicit drugs such as cocaine use may cause significant elevations in BP.
8. Excessive use of liquorice can lead to sustained hypertension.
9. Distension of viscus organ such as the urinary bladder, gall bladder and bowels can cause severe increase in pressures.
10. Significant drop in BP may be noted on postural change from a supine to erect position ***(postural hypotension)*** in patients with hypovolemia, following use of certain antihypertensive drugs and in patients with diabetes with autonomic dysfunction. This is more common in type I diabetics.
11. Since pregnant uterus can compress the inferior vena cava in the supine position and cause decreased venous return, thereby lowering the BP, it is always advisable to measure the BP in a pregnant woman in the sitting position.

INTERPRETATION OF BLOOD PRESSURE MEASUREMENTS

The following important points need to be kept in mind in the interpretation of BP recordings:

1. Diagnosis of hypertension requires demonstration of sustained elevations of BPs under normal resting conditions. *The normal upper level of BP for adults regardless of age is 140/80. In fact, some newer studies suggest that mortality and cardiac events are less frequent in those with BPs <125/75. This, in fact, may become the normal for the future. In fact, in diabetics present recommendations suggest the BP to be controlled to 130/80, and if renal disease or microalbuminuria is also present the pressure should be 120/70 or lower. It appears that lower is better as long as the patient does not suffer any symptoms or adverse effects of hypotension and remains asymptomatic. Documentation of sustained elevations of BPs, therefore, requires more than one observation. Sometimes self-recorded pressures at home and/or recordings using an ambulatory monitoring system may have to be resorted to particularly in nervous and anxious individuals. In addition, one may also have to look for evidence of end-organ damage such as the presence of retinal changes, electrocardiographic and/or echocardiographic evidence of left ventricular hypertrophy.*
2. *While one cannot make a diagnosis of hypertension in a patient with one isolated elevation in BP, significance of such elevations nevertheless should be interpreted in relation to the clinical problem. For instance, an elderly patient who has exertional angina or dyspnea, with a resting BP of 130/80 mm Hg may have been noted to have a BP reading of 180/90 soon after undressing himself, untying his shoe laces and getting on the examining couch. Although one may not label this patient as hypertensive on the basis of that one recording of high pressures, it nevertheless points to the fact that the elevations in BP in this patient was not only inappropriate to the level of exercise and most likely are the contributing factor to the exertional symptoms. The lowering of the pressure with the use of medications such as angiotensin converting enzyme inhibitor and/or a β-blocker will be the right management strategy for such a patient.*
3. In the young patients due to peripheral amplification secondary to reflected waves in the more muscular stiffer vessels in the extremities, the systolic BP obtained may not correctly reflect the systolic central aortic pressure and may in fact be 50% higher. In these patients, the diastolic pressure may more accurately reflect the diastolic pressure in the central aorta.

   In the elderly because of arteriosclerosis and stiffened aorta and arteries in general, the pressure pulse wave travels faster. The wave reflection, therefore, tends to arrive early in the central vessels, augmenting the systolic pressure. In these patients, no peripheral amplification is noted and the brachial systolic pressure more accurately reflects the central aortic systolic pressure.[26–30]

In atherosclerosis, there may be significant differences between the upper and the lower limb pressures. Because atherosclerosis tends to involve the lower extremities more, one may actually find in these patients decreased pulse amplitude together with lower BP in the lower limbs compared to the arms. This is in contrast to the usual findings in the young and/or normal patients, where the pressures in the legs are in fact 10–20 mm Hg higher than the brachial pressures.

4. In some patients, without any evidence of hypertensive end-organ damage, significantly elevated systolic BPs may be obtained in doctors' offices. These high office BP readings at times are associated with normal BP readings throughout the day when 24 hours ambulatory BP monitoring is carried out. Not so surprisingly the first and the last readings (normally readings taken in the laboratory in the presence of the technician) during these recordings also show significant BP elevations. This is known as "white coat syndrome" and is likely related to anxiety reaction on the part of the patient. Generally, this condition is felt to be relatively benign, although there always is a concern that they may become hypertensive in the future.

White coat hypertension has been defined and classified[31,32] into three groups:

1. ***White coat hypertension:*** Abnormal office systolic BP >150 mm Hg and daytime average systolic BP <140 mm Hg. (Patients are not on antihypertensive therapy).
2. ***White coat syndrome—normotensive:*** Patients' BPs controlled on antihypertensives. Their daytime average systolic BP < 140 mm Hg and office BP reading of > 150 mm Hg.
3. ***White coat syndrome—hypertensive:*** Patients may be on or off antihypertensive medications with daytime average systolic BP of > 140 mm Hg and office systolic BP measurement of > 150 mm Hg which is at least 15 mm Hg higher than the average daytime systolic BP.

"White coat hypertension/syndrome" may not be as benign as it once was thought to be.[33] There appears to be higher incidence of increased mean albumin levels in the urine of some of these patients. Some show increased albumin/creatinine ratios > 30%.

USE OF BP MEASUREMENT IN SPECIAL CLINICAL SITUATIONS

Determination of Pulsus Paradoxus

Effects of Respiration on the BP in the Normal Subjects

The effects of respiration on the level of BP in the normal must be understood in relation to the changes in the respiratory variations of the intrathoracic pressures as well as the venous return. On inspiration, there is generally a lower systolic pressure compared to the end of expiration. The intrathoracic pressure falls on inspiration, which helps to augment venous return to the heart. The inspiratory expansion of the lungs by increasing its pulmonary venous capacity accommodates for the extravolume of blood returned to the right side on inspiration and the consequent increase in right ventricular output. The increased venous return on inspiration is, therefore, not immediately available to the left heart. In fact, the return to the left heart may slightly decrease on inspiration, the expanded lungs holding the extravolume for at least a few cardiac cycles. By that time the expiratory phase usually occurs. The intrathoracic pressure on expiration becomes relatively more positive. The aorta being an intrathoracic structure, these changes in the intrathoracic pressures will also affect the aortic pressure. There is generally a fall in the systolic BP with normal inspiration and the magnitude of this fall is about 5–10 mm. This is due to both the fall in the intrathoracic pressure and the effect of the expanded lungs holding the extra venous return, thereby diminishing the return to the left heart and therefore its output. The opposite occurs on expiration, the intrathoracic pressure rises and the lungs contract in volume by exhaling air. This aids in increased pulmonary venous inflow to the left side increasing the stroke output. The net effect leads to an increased arterial pressure on expiration. In the normal, the expansion of the right ventricle on inspiration does not usually result in shift of the interventricular septum to the left, since the normal pericardium does not limit physiologic changes in ventricular volumes.[34]

In the normal, the effect of this ***inspiratory fall*** in the systolic BP is not detectable by palpation of the arterial pulse. However, the magnitude of the inspiratory fall in the BP can be easily assessed by the BP cuff at the bedside. *When the cuff is being slowly deflated to detect the onset of the Korotkoff sounds, careful observation will reveal that initially the Korotkoff sounds are audible only at the end of expiration. With each inspiration they will be seen to become inaudible. The level of the BP at the end of expiration when the Korotkoff sounds begin to be heard must first be noted. With further cuff deflation however, it will be observed that the Korotkoff sounds are audible throughout both inspiration and expiration. The level at which this begins to happen must be noted next. The difference between the two systolic levels namely the number of mm Hg to which the cuff was needed to be deflated (when Korotkoff sounds no longer remain inaudible on inspiration) gives the magnitude of the inspiratory fall in the BP.*

Pulsus Paradoxus in Cardiac Tamponade

In cardiac tamponade, there is an exaggeration of the normal inspiratory fall in the systolic BP leading to a truly definable ***"pulsus paradoxus".*** The fall in the stroke volume of the heart and consequently the systolic BP despite the increased venous return to the heart caused by inspiration is the paradox that has led to this term. In fact in significant cardiac tamponade, the palpation of the arterial pulse may reveal that its amplitude is less or the pulse may not even be felt on inspiration. This, of course, is not the case in the normal. The mechanism of this exaggerated fall in the BP on inspiration is attributable to the compressive effect of the fluid in the pericardial space, which is under a high pressure. In cardiac tamponade, all the four chambers of the heart are as if they were boxed in this tight pericardial space. In the absence of pre-existing cardiac disease, the pressures in the right and the left atria, the intrapericardial pressures as well as the right and left ventricular diastolic pressures are all elevated to the same level. In extreme cases of tamponade, the thinner walled structures like the right ventricle get compressed more completely than the thicker walled left ventricle. When inspiration increases the venous return to the right heart as in the normal, the expansion of the right ventricle within this enclosed tight pericardial space will of necessity push the interventricular septum to the left side, thereby further diminishing the left heart filling and its compliance. This will lead to decreased left ventricular output. The septal bulge on inspiration to the left side can in fact be demonstrated in echocardiograms of patients with tamponade.

Since the pericardium is attached to the diaphragm, the descent of the diaphragm with inspiration may also pull on the pericardium, thereby altering its global shape to a more spindle shape. This physically can lead to further rise in the intrapericardial pressure. The effects of the inspiratory fall in the intrathoracic pressures as well as the effects of the inspiratory expansion of the lungs and pulmonary venous pooling leading to diminished left heart filling that were mentioned above in the normal are also still operative in patients with cardiac tamponade. The net effect of these changes on the left heart filling as well as the intrathoracic pressures will cause a greater fall in the left ventricular stroke output and the BP on inspiration. The opposite changes occur on expiration leading to a higher arterial pressure on expiration. The effect of the inspiratory pulmonary venous pooling is particularly more dramatic when the left ventricular stroke output is already diminished due to the tamponade.

The BP cuff is used in the same manner as mentioned above to determine the magnitude of fall in mmHg due to the pulsus paradoxus. The pulsus paradoxus by BP measurement must exceed 15 mm Hg to be considered significant.

In the presence of significant elevations of the left ventricular diastolic pressures due to pre-existing cardiac disease, cardiac tamponade does not cause pulsus paradoxus. The raised diastolic pressures offer greater resistance to the compressive effects of the intrapericardial pressures. Cardiac tamponade also does not lead to pulsus paradoxus in two other conditions, namely aortic regurgitation and atrial septal defect. In the former, the extrasource of left ventricular filling due to the aortic regurgitation keeps the left ventricular volumes from falling, thereby preventing the respiratory fluctuations in left heart filling. Similarly in atrial septal defect, the left-to-right shunt accommodates for respiratory changes in venous return, thereby preventing a fall in left heart filling during inspiration.[35–43]

Conditions Other than Cardiac Tamponade with Pulsus Paradoxus

Constrictive pericarditis: In constrictive pericarditis, pulsus paradoxus is much less common than in cardiac tamponade. It is more common in the effusive subacute type constriction than in the chronic cases. Pulsus paradoxus is absent in the chronic cases due to poor transmission of the intrathoracic pressures to the cardiac chambers due to the thickened and fibrosed and sometimes calcified pericardium. When pulsus paradoxus is seen, it is probably due to a combination of two factors, namely the septal shift to the left and the increased pulmonary venous pooling on inspiration. The diaphragmatic pull on the pericardium on inspiration is also unlikely to be operative on a thickened and scarred pericardium.[38]

Bronchial asthma and chronic obstructive pulmonary disease: The exaggerated swings in the intrathoracic pressures may be directly transmitted to the aorta, affecting the systolic and the diastolic pressures with very little change in the stroke volume or the pulse pressure. In the presence of significant airways obstruction, there is marked increase in the intrathoracic pressures during expiration caused by the intercostal muscles to overcome the airways obstruction. This elevated intrathoracic pressure is directly transmitted to the aorta raising the expiratory pressure in the aorta. Thus, there is an ***expiratory gain*** in BP rather than the usual inspiratory fall in the normal. However, the net effect on the BP is the same.

Hypovolemic shock and acute pulmonary embolism: In some patients with hypovolemic shock, pulsus paradoxus may be noted.[44] This is due to an exaggerated effect of the inspiratory pulmonary venous pooling on the already diminished stroke volume. The change in the percentage of the stroke volume is higher compared to the normal individuals with normal cardiac output.

Similarly, the reduced capacity of the pulmonary arterial bed due to embolic obstruction in the presence of the normal pulmonary venous bed may also lead to an accentuated effect of the inspiratory pulmonary venous pooling on the left ventricular stroke volume.[45]

Blood Pressure Response to the Valsalva Maneuver

The ***Valsalva maneuver*** is basically a forced expiration against a closed glottis. This maneuver is used in our daily life when we try to bear down or strain. One way of producing this maneuver is to ask a patient simply to hold the breath and strain as if to imitate straining on the toilet. One can produce this also by asking a supine patient to push actively their abdominal wall against the palm of the examiner's hand placed on the patient's abdomen so as to offer some pressure without causing pain. A more controlled way of doing the maneuver will be to have the patient blow into a hollow tube connected to an aneroid manometer to raise the pressure to about 40 mm Hg and sustain it at that level for about 20–30 seconds.

The arterial pressure response in the normal during the Valsalva maneuver:

Four phases are recognized with continuous arterial pressure recordings. Initially, the effort of strain raises the intrathoracic pressures, which is directly transmitted to the aorta causing an initial rise in the arterial pressure. During the ***first phase,*** the rising intrathoracic pressure contracts the pulmonary venous bed to its lowest volume thus helping the left ventricular output to increase. With the continued strain, the venous return drops due to damping of venous circulation from the abdominal viscera and the periphery. This leads to a significant drop in the stroke output, which is accompanied by a fall in the systolic and diastolic BPs as well as the pulse pressure ***(the second phase).*** The decreased stroke output stimulates the sympathetic system to cause a reflex increase in the heart rate at this time. Upon release of the strain, there is a sudden drop in the intrathoracic pressures, which again affects directly the aortic pressures and, therefore, the arterial pressure. The ***third phase*** is quite momentary and is only appreciated by continuous recordings of arterial pressure. This is almost immediately followed by a sudden surge of venous return from the splanchnic bed and the periphery augmented by the fall in the intrathoracic pressure. This leads to a significant increase in the right and the left ventricular stroke output. ***During the fourth phase,*** the increased stroke volume ejected into an arterial system, which has been primed by a significant sympathetic stimulation during the earlier strain phase, causes an ***overshoot of the arterial pressure*** over and above the control level. The increased stroke volume effect is reflected in the increase in the pulse pressure as well. The rise in the arterial pressure also causes a reflex slowing of the heart rate through the baroreceptor stimulation (Fig. 3.1).

The arterial pressure response to the Valsalva maneuver in patients with Heart failure:

The response of patients with heart failure can be described as *a* ***square wave response*** as seen on a continuous recording of the arterial pressures (Fig. 3.2). The initial rise in the intrathoracic pressure during the strain and the immediate fall on release of strain (namely the first and the third phases mentioned above) will cause an initial rise and a later similar fall in the arterial pressure due to direct transmission effect of the intrathoracic pressures to the aorta. However, since patients with heart failure already have maximal

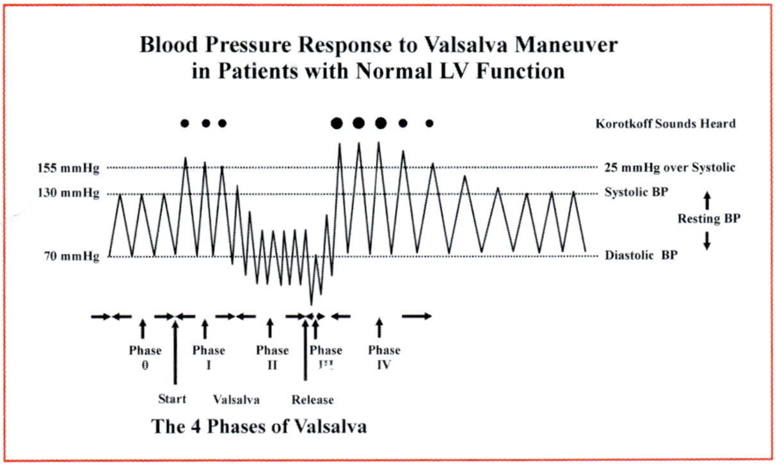

Fig. 3.1: The blood pressure response during the four phases of Valsalva maneuver in a patient with normal left ventricular function is shown diagrammatically. The phase 0 indicates the resting phase before the Valsalva maneuver. Phase I shows the increased blood pressure due to the initial increase in pulmonary venous return and the associated increased stroke volume and the increased intrathoracic pressure directly transmitted to the aorta. Phase II shows the decreased blood pressure because of decreased venous return into the thorax and therefore the heart due to the increased intrathoracic pressure preventing the venous return from the periphery. Note the increased heart rate secondary to the increased sympathetic tone. Phase III immediately after the release of the Valsalva strain shows a temporary drop in the blood pressure due to sudden decrease in the intrathoracic pressure. Phase IV shows an overshoot of the blood pressure due to the sudden return of peripherally pooled blood to the vasoconstricted arterial system (secondary to the increased sympathetic tone). The blood pressure then returns back to normal gradually. When the cuff is inflated to levels of 25 mm Hg higher than the patient's resting systolic pressure and maintained at that pressure, the Korotkoff sounds that would be heard at the various phases of Valsalva are also depicted at the top. The size of the dots reflects the expected intensities of the sounds.

sympathetic stimulation with vasoconstriction (both arterial and venous) and their ventricles are already operating on the flat portion of the Starling curve, whatever decrease that occurs in venous return due to dampening effect of strain, does not drop the stroke output very much and for the same reason following release of strain also there is no overshoot in the arterial pressure. This can be observed also in the lack of significant changes in the heart rate during strain and after release of strain. In other words, no significant tachycardia or bradycardia will be seen to develop during the Valsalva maneuver.[46,47]

The Blood Pressure response to the Valsalva maneuver in the assessment of the left ventricular function in the absence of overt Heart failure:

This consists essentially in detecting the presence or the absence of the overshoot in the BP following the release of a Valsalva strain. The presence of the overshoot would indicate a normal left ventricular function with a

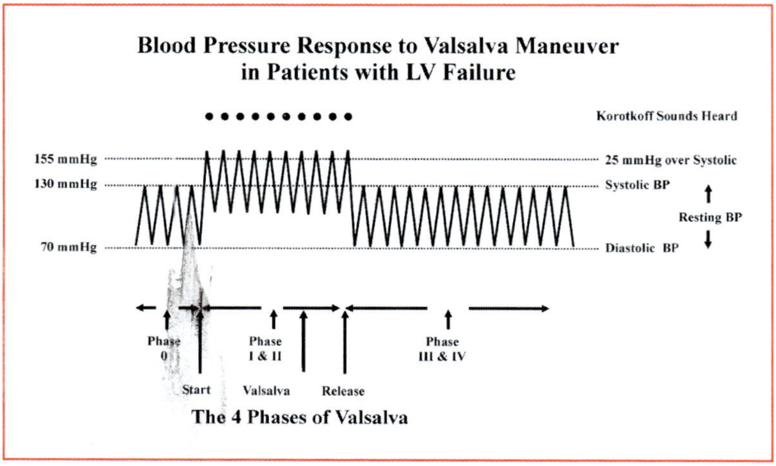

Fig. 3.2: The blood pressure response to the Valsalva maneuver in a patient with significant left ventricular dysfunction and heart failure is shown diagrammatically. Due to the chronically elevated venous pressures and the sympathetic tone, the blood pressure response to the Valsalva maneuver is different from that noted in the normal. During phases I and II, there is an elevation of blood pressure and during phase III, the overshoot does not occur. The appearance of the above tracing resembles a square wave; therefore, this type of response is called "The Square Wave Response", and indicates poor left ventricular function.

normal *ejection fraction (stroke volume over the end-diastolic left ventricular volume expressed as a percentage, normal being 60%).* Patients with left ventricular dysfunction who are not in overt failure also often have an abnormal response. They tend to have resting increase in sympathetic tone and fail to exhibit the overshoot in BP as well as the reflex bradycardia. This can be done at the bedside with the use of a BP cuff. The method involves in applying a sustained additional cuff pressure of 25 mm Hg over and above the detected systolic pressure in a patient who is supine and listening for the Korotkoff sounds while the patient is performing a Valsalva strain for 20–30 seconds. First, the systolic BP is determined. Then the cuff is inflated to 25 mm Hg above the systolic pressure and is held there while the patient is asked to perform a Valsalva strain. During strain if the patient has normal left ventricular function, there will be an initial rise due to transmission of the intrathoracic pressure to the aorta and this can be detected by the appearance of the Korotkoff sounds. The fall in BP, which occurs due to the decreased venous return during the strain phase, will lead to the disappearance of the Korotkoff sounds. During the post release phase, the Korotkoff sounds will reappear again indicating the presence of the expected overshoot in the arterial pressure. In patients with left ventricular dysfunction and high sympathetic tone but not in overt failure, however, the Korotkoff sounds may initially appear during strain, but with continued strain, the Korotkoff sounds will become inaudible and will never reappear again due to the lack of the overshoot response. Failure to achieve an overshoot of 25 mm Hg has been correlated with resting left ventricular dysfunction with decreased ejection fraction of 40 ± 10%.[48]

Blood Pressure Response to Exercise

Graded exercise stress tests using a treadmill are often carried out for assessment of functional capacity in patients with known cardiac disease as well as in the clinical assessment of patients with chest pain syndromes to rule out ischemic etiology. With dynamic exercise of the lower limbs, the venous return will increase in addition to the sympathetic stimulation that normally occurs with any physical exercise. Sympathetic stimulation will result in increase in heart rate. The cardiac output will rise secondary to the increased venous return and increase in the heart rate and in the contractility of the ventricles secondary to the increased sympathetic stimulation. This will, therefore, also result in increase in systolic BPs. In addition, there will be peripheral vasodilatation in the exercising limbs. In normal subjects, this will be accompanied by drop in diastolic BPs and the resultant increase in the pulse pressures as well. However, the extent of these responses will be related to the duration and the intensity of the exercise.

Trained individuals like the athletes differ from the untrained subjects in their response to exercise. Trained subjects raise their cardiac output with exercise by increasing the ejection fraction and use the sympathetic reserve only in the late stages of prolonged exercise. Untrained subjects, on the other hand, generally tend to increase their heart rate even with milder exercise.

It is well known that the peripheral brachial pressures often differ from the centrally recorded aortic pressures.[49] Arterial stiffness and peripheral pulse wave reflection are two important factors that contribute to this difference. Ejection of blood into the aorta by the left ventricle in systole creates a pulsatile pressure wave that travels to the periphery. At points of impedance mismatch and particularly at the high resistance arteriolar level reflection occurs.[50] The reflected wave travels backward and fuses with the incident pressure wave altering the arterial waveform. The recorded arterial pressure wave form will depend on the incident wave, the intensity of wave reflection from the peripheral sites and the timing of reflection during the cardiac cycle where the two meet and merge (*see* also Chapter 2 on Arterial Pulse). Reflection added to the incident pressure in the aorta contributes to the shape of the central aortic pressure. In general, it augments the central aortic pressure. In the more muscular peripheral arteries, the mean arterial pressure declines but both the systolic and the pulse pressures are amplified. This amplification is exaggerated during exercise[51] and reduced with increasing age.[52] While peripheral BP is usually measured, the central aortic pressure is probably more important since it determines the load that the left ventricle actually faces and also affects the coronary blood flow and the subendocardial perfusion.[53,54]

It has been known that an exaggerated BP response during dynamic exercise is predictive risk for new onset hypertension.[55] Even in nonhypertensive asymptomatic subjects, exaggerated BP response on exercise appear to have a higher risk of cardiovascular death.[56] Since the intensity of reflection is related to the arteriolar tone, vasodilatation associated with exercise will be expected to cause less amplification of pressure in the active limb, whereas in the inactive limb, the amplification may in fact be greater. It is well known that BP as measured in the arms at the brachial level tends to rise with exercise involving the lower limbs.

Exaggerated BP response to exercise probably requires some clarification. At maximal exercise like walking briskly or jogging on the treadmill at speeds in excess of 4 miles per hour (mph) with elevations ≥14° incline, can raise the BPs in some young normal subjects to levels >225 mm Hg. That could be all due to peripheral amplification without much central aortic augmentation. Exaggerated BP response becomes more meaningful when such marked rise occurs at low-to-moderate levels of exercise like corresponding to stage II of the Bruce protocol on a treadmill exercise stress test. This corresponds to walking at normal pace of about 2.5 mph at an incline of about 12°.

Hypertensive response to exercise can, however, be either due to significant peripheral amplification or due to central augmentation secondary to wave reflection and increased arterial stiffness. It is important to differentiate between the two since the latter has been known to affect the clinical outcome. Measurement of the central aortic pressure derived from the radial arterial applanation tonometry would help to differentiate peripheral amplification from central augmentation in patients with a hypertensive response to exercise. Our observations demonstrated that measurement of central aortic pressure with the radial artery applanation tonometry in the immediate postexercise phase of the treadmill exercise stress tests in fact clarifies the hypertensive response to exercise. In this study, we defined a hypertensive response to exercise as a BP achieved at Bruce stage II level of exercise to be ≥185/85 mm Hg. We also similarly arbitrarily defined significant peripheral amplification to be when the arm systolic BP exceeded the derived central aortic pressure by 25 mm Hg or more. Our study showed that patients with the maximal peripheral amplification had the least central augmentation of aortic pressures. Patients with a hypertensive response without much peripheral amplification had maximum augmentation of central aortic pressures.[57] Our study also confirmed the inverse relationship between peripheral amplification and central augmentation that has been demonstrated previously.[58] One can also express peripheral amplification as a ratio of the arm pulse pressures over the central aortic pressures. If this ratio is in excess of 1.5, it probably also means that the arterial stiffness is not increased. The prognostic significance of these findings will, however, need longitudinal observations in a larger cohort of subjects.

Determination of Pulsus Alternans

Pulsus alternans has been discussed under the arterial pulse previously. The alternation of the strong and the weaker pulse can be detected while taking BP. Corresponding to the alternating strength of the palpated pulse, one also can note alternating BP levels. During deflation of the inflated cuff to record the systolic pressure, one will be able to notice that initially the Korotkoff sounds begin to be heard only with every other stronger beat rather than with every beat as would be in the normal. With continued deflation of the cuff, there will be a doubling of the rate of the Korotkoff sounds since both the strong and the weak beats will come through. In addition, one may also note an alternating intensity of the Korotkoff sounds. In general, pulsus alternans is associated with severe left ventricular dysfunction and low cardiac output. Pulsus alternans is usually precipitated by an extrasystole. The phenomenon can be shown to develop following a premature beat in almost all patients. However, in those with normal left ventricular function it lasts only for two beats and is not noticeable clinically but may be shown by the measurement of the systolic time intervals (mentioned previously under the arterial pulse). In very severe left ventricular dysfunction, the pulsus alternans effect produced by a premature beat may persist for a long time (for several minutes). There may be instability of the calcium flux in the myocytes of the diseased heart that may account for the alternating strengths of the contraction of the myocardium in the patients with myocardial disease.[59]

Assessment of Arterial Occlusion

Assessment of Dissecting Aortic Aneurysm

The pathology usually involves some form of degeneration of the elastic fibers of the medial layers of the aorta. The condition often starts with a sudden tear of the intima of either the ascending or the descending thoracic aorta often precipitated by some form of excessive hemodynamic force such as a significant elevation in BP. The blood under pressure in the lumen finds its way through a cleavage in the medial layers of the aorta. The process may progress at a variable rate resulting eventually in a double lumen aorta made by the plane of dissection in the media, causing a false lumen in addition to the true lumen. The difference in the BPs results from the impingement of the false lumen on the true lumen, causing obstruction and the consequent lowering of the BP beyond the obstruction. Depending on the location and the degree of these obstructions to the true lumen, one may find significant differences in the pulses as well as the BPs between the two arms, between the arms and the legs as well as between the two legs. The BP differences noted may also be changing with time, since dissection may further progress resulting in either more complete occlusion of the true lumen or sometimes a distal tear of exit may reopen the previously occluded vessel. Such dynamic changes are unusual in other causes of obstruction such as due to chronic atherosclerotic vascular disease.

Atherosclerotic Vascular Disease

This condition is most commonly seen in the lower extremities, and much less frequently in the subclavian and the upper extremity vessels. Some of the subclavian stenoses may in fact be congenital rather than acquired atherosclerotic process. The BP in the arm on the side of the vascular obstruction will be lower as expected. Normally, the lower extremity BP is 10–15 mm Hg higher than both the central aortic and the arm pressures. The reasons for this increase in pressure in the lower extremities are at least two. One is their thicker and muscular walls and the second is the effect of reflection of the pressure pulses. The reasons for this increase in pressure in the lower extremities are well discussed in the Chapter 2 on Arterial Pulse.

In the lower extremity, if the BP is found to be equal to or lower than the arm then obstructive arterial disease must be considered. The obstruction may be at the level of the aorta, the iliac or the femoral. Blood pressure measurement in the lower extremity can be carried out by using a larger size cuff (8″ wide) over the thigh and auscultating over the popliteal artery. This is best done with the patient lying prone. This method probably is more accurate but may be difficult in very obese patients. To obtain a reasonably accurate systolic BP in the leg, a regular cuff can be employed above the ankle and the posterior tibial or the dorsalis pedis pulses can be palpated. When the pedal pulses are not easily felt, an ultrasound Doppler probe can be used to detect the flow and assess the peak systolic pressure. When comparisons are made, one should compare the peak pressures obtained by the same technique between the upper and the lower extremities. If one were to use the Doppler technique at the ankle, then one must obtain Doppler detected brachial or radial artery flow in the arm (preferably at the brachial artery) with the cuff over the arm for assessment of the peak pressures in the arm.

Ankle Brachial Index

The ankle brachial index (ABI) has been used extensively for the assessment of peripheral arterial disease. The method generally accepted for this purpose involves the use of ultrasound Doppler probe due to less intra- and interobserver variability. The ABI is expressed as a simple ratio of the ankle pressure over the brachial pressure. The measurement must be performed by obtaining systolic BP in both arms and the dorsalis pedis (DP) and the posterior tibial (PT) arteries at the ankle. The highest systolic BP in the arm is used most often as the denominator. The numerator for the calculation of the ABI incorporates the systolic BP of the PT and/or the DP artery separately or the average of both. The threshold value for making the diagnosis of peripheral arterial disease is a ratio $\leq$0.90.[60] A low ABI value not only implies occlusive arterial disease in the lower extremity but has also been associated with clinical coronary and carotid disease. There is an inverse relationship between ABI and risk of cardiovascular events and all-cause mortality even when adjusted for known cardiovascular risk factors.[61] Also, the risk is similar in patients with established peripheral arterial disease compared to those with established coronary artery disease.[62] In addition, a strong association has also been shown between low ABI and incident heart failure.[63]

Coarctation of the Aorta

Since coarctation of the aorta is a congenital condition, when BP discrepancies are noted, between the arm and the leg, in children or young adults where atherosclerosis is not an issue, the clinician should be alerted to the possibility of the presence of this condition. If the coarctation is in the aortic arch before the takeoff of the left subclavian artery, the pressure in the left arm will be significantly lower than the pressure in the right arm. Most coarctations usually occur after the takeoff of the left subclavian, and the upper extremity pressures will be equal. Since coarctation also causes hypertension, in younger patients with hypertension, as detected in the arm BPs, lower BPs in the legs must suggest a diagnosis of coarctation. The amount of decrease in the BPs in the lower extremities will depend on the severity of the coarctation. When the coarctation is severe, the femoral pulses may not only be delayed but also poorly felt or not palpable.

Coarctation causes hypertension as a direct result of the obstruction, limiting the size of capacitance of the aorta as well as directly raising the resistance. In addition, the decreased BP distal to the coarctation will lead to stimulation of the juxtaglomerular cells to produce more renin. The latter will increase the angiotensin II that is a potent vasoconstrictor and will result in hypertension.

Assessment of Severity of Aortic Regurgitation and Left Ventricular Function in Aortic Regurgitation

A positive Hill's sign is an exaggeration of the normal BP differential between the arm and the leg. This sign has been previously discussed in Chapter 2 on Arterial Pulse in relation to the peripheral signs of aortic regurgitation.[64] A systolic BP differential of 60 mm Hg or greater may be noted in the presence of moderate-to-severe degrees of aortic regurgitation. In those patients with aortic regurgitation when this sign is detected, serial measurements will aid in the follow-up of these patients. During follow-up, if the BP differential is found to be increasing, then it must be considered as a sign of worsening degree of aortic regurgitation. However, a gradual narrowing of the BP differential, on the other hand, would not mean an improvement in the degree of the aortic regurgitation. It might indicate in fact a progressive development of left ventricular dysfunction. When significant left ventricular dysfunction and heart failure develops consequent to long-standing aortic regurgitation, the BP differential between the arm and the leg will not be significant.

A Clinical Exercise-Manual Assessment of BP

One may attempt to guess the BP by manual palpation of the radial arterial pulse while applying pressure over the brachial artery with the thumb of the other hand so as to cause occlusion of the brachial artery. The pressure can be varied and applied as light, medium or firm. When the brachial artery gets occluded, the radial pulse will disappear. The systolic pressure must also be measured by the usual way by auscultation over the brachial artery. The amount of force that one has to exert with the thumb can be noted mentally against the recorded systolic pressures by auscultation. Generally, one can learn to correlate roughly the amount of pressure required to apply with the thumb with the level of the systolic pressures recorded. On an average, medium pressures will have to be applied when the systolic pressures are around 120–130. When the systolic pressures are <100 only light pressures will be needed. When the systolic pressures are >140, it will require much firmer compression. The important part of this exercise is to make sure that one has the pressure applied directly over the palpated brachial artery. Otherwise it will not be possible to occlude it. It also requires that one trains oneself to do this during routine measurements of BPs. The technique can be useful in situations where one has no access to a BP cuff immediately for the purposes of a quick assessment. Caution should be exercised in patients with calcified and stiff vessels that resist compression, to avoid false overestimation of the systolic BP.

Blood Pressure in the Assessment of the Relative Intensity of the First and the Second Heart Sounds

The integrity of the left ventricular function has a significant bearing on the intensity of the M1 component of the S1 (*see* Chapter 6 on Heart Sounds). When S1 and S2 are not loud enough to be palpable, the assessment of their intensity must take into account the measured BP of the patient. Extracardiac attenuating factors can lead to attenuations of the heart sounds. Since the degree of attenuation in any given patient will be expected to be similar on both S1 and S2, the intensity of S1 can be assessed only when compared to the intensity of the S2. The intensity or the loudness of the A2 component of the S2 is dependent to a large extent on the peripheral resistance, which is reflected, in the diastolic BP. A normal BP would be expected to be associated with a normal intensity of A2, a high BP would be expected to cause a loud A2 and finally a low BP would be associated with a soft A2. The A2 intensity can be graded according to the BP as probably normal, soft or loud. Then if the intensity of the M1 is compared to that of A2, one can judge its relative intensity. It can then be graded as normal, soft or loud depending on whether its intensity is equal to that of the A2, softer than A2 or louder than A2. While this exercise has some merit, its clinical value in the detection of left ventricular dysfunction is not established. Our preliminary observations suggest that the perception of the relative loudness of the M1 versus the A2 seems to be also influenced by the higher frequency content of the A2.

REFERENCES

1. Levine SR. "True" diastolic blood pressure. N Engl Med J. 1981;304:362-3.
2. Erlanger J. Studies in blood pressure estimation by indirect method Part II.The mechanisms of the compression sounds of Korotkoff. Am J Physiol. 1916;40: 82-125.
3. Rodbard S. The significance of the intermediate Korotkoff sounds. Circulation. 1953;8:600-4.
4. Cohn J. Blood pressure maesurement in shock. JAMA. 1967;199:972-6.
5. Rabbany SY, Drzewiecki GM, Noordergraaf A. Peripheral vascular effects on auscultatory blood pressure measurement. J Clin Monit. 1993 Jan;9(1):9-17.
6. Whitcher C. Blood pressure measurement. Bellville WJ, Weaver CS (Eds). New York: MacMillan; 1969.
7. Rabbany SY, Drzewiecki GM, Melbin J, et al. (Eds). Influence of vascular state on the Korotkoff sounds. Proceedings of the 13th Annual Northeast Bioengineering Conference. Philadelphia: IEEE Press; 1987. pp.166-9.
8. Tavel ME, Faris J, Nasser WK, et al. Korotkoff sounds. Observations on pressure-pulse changes underlying their formation. Circulation. 1969;39(4):465-74.
9. Drzewiecki GM, Melbin J, Noordergraaf A. The Korotkoff sound. Ann Biomed Eng. 1989;17(4):325-59.
10. The fifth report of the Joint National Committee on Detection, Evaluation, and Treatment of High Blood Pressure (JNC V). Arch Intern Med. 1993;153(2): 154-83.
11. Perloff D, Grim C, Flack J, et al. Human blood pressure determination by sphygmomanometry. Circulation. 1993;88(5 Pt 1):2460-70.
12. Frohlich ED. Blood Pressure Measurement. Can J Cardiol. 1995;11(Suppl H): 35H-7H.
13. Cavallini MC, Roman MJ, Blank SG, et al. Association of the auscultatory gap with vascular disease in hypertensive patients. Ann Intern Med. 1996;124(10): 877-83.
14. London SB, London RE. Comparison of indirect blood pressure measurements (Korotkoff) with simultaneous direct brachial artery pressure distal to cuff. Adv Intern Med. 1967;13:127-42.
15. Nielsen PE. The accuracy of auscultatory blood pressure measurements in the elderly. Acta Med Scand (Suppl). 1983;676:39-44.

16. Spence JD, Sibbald WJ, Cape RD. Pseudohypertension in the elderly. Clin Sci Mol Med Suppl. 1978;4:399s-402s.
17. Perloff JK. The physiologic mechanisms of cardiac and vascular physical signs. J Am Coll Cardiol. 1983;1:184-98.
18. Linfors EW, Feussner JR, Blessing CL, et al. Spurious hypertension in the obese patient. Effect of sphygmomanometer cuff size on prevalence of hypertension. Arch Intern Med. 1984;144(7):1482-5.
19. Manning DM, Kuchirka C, Kaminski J. Miscuffing: inappropriate blood pressure cuff application. Circulation. 1983 Oct;68(4):763-6.
20. Chockalingam A, Guest Editor. Measurement of Blood Pressure. Can J Cardiol. 1995;11(Suppl H):3H-48H.
21. Mancia G, Bertinieri G, Grassi G, et al. Effects of blood-pressure measurement by the doctor on patient's blood pressure and heart rate. Lancet. 1983;2(8352): 695-8.
22. Redman S, Dutch J. Cardiovascular responses during cuff inflation in subjects who have been sensitised to the measurement of their blood pressure. NZ Med J. 1984;97(752):180-2.
23. O'Rourke MF. Influence of ventricular ejection on the relationship between central aortic and brachial pressure pulse in man. Cardiovasc Res. 1970;4(3): 291-300.
24. Karamanoglu M, O'Rourke MF, Avolio AP, et al. An analysis of the relationship between central aortic and peripheral upper limb pressure waves in man. Eur Heart J. 1993;14(2):160-7.
25. Chen CH, Nevo E, Fetics B, et al. Estimation of central aortic pressure waveform by mathematical transformation of radial tonometry pressure. Validation of generalized transfer function. Circulation. 1997;95(7):1827-36.
26. O'Rourke MF. Arterial Function in Health and Disesae. Edinburgh: Churchill Livingstone; 1982.
27. O'Rourke MF, Kelly RP, Avolio AP. The arterial pulse. Philadelphia: Lea & Febiger; 1992.
28. Nichols WW, O'Rourke MF. McDonald's Blood Flow in Arteries, 4th edition. London: Edward Arnold; 1998.
29. Franklin SS, Gustin W 4th, Wong ND, et al. Hemodynamic patterns of age-related changes in blood pressure. The Framingham Heart study. Circulation. 1997;96:308-15.
30. Burt VL, Whelton P, Roccella EJ, et al. Prevalence of hypertension in the US adult population: results from the Third National Health and Nutrition Examination Survey 1988-1991. Hypertension. 1995;25:305-13.
31. White coat systolic hypertension: definition and prevalence by 24-hour ambulatory blood pressure monitoring; Canadian Cardiovascular Congress; 2001; Halifax, Novascotia.
32. Blood pressure control using 24-hour ambulatory blood pressure monitoring. Canadian Cardiovasc Congress; 2001; Halifax, Novascotia.
33. Karpanou EA, Vyssoulis GP, Mendrinos DS (Eds). Microalbuminuria in white coat hypertensives with isolated systolic hypertension. San Francisco, CA: American Society of Hypertension 20th Annual Scientific Session; 2005. pp. 14-18.
34. McGregor M. Pulsus Paradoxus. N Engl Med J. 1979;301:480-2.
35. Dornhorst A, Howard P, Leathart GL. Pulsus paradoxus. Lancet. 1952;1:746-8.
36. Wood P. Chronic constrictive pericarditis. Am J Cardiol. 1961;7:48-61.

37. Shabetai R, Fowler NO, Fenton JC, et al. Pulsus paradoxus. J Clin Invest. 1965; 44(11):1882-98.
38. Shabetai R, Fowler NO, Guntheroth WG. The hemodynamics of cardiac tamponade and constrictive pericarditis. Am J Cardiol. 1970;26(5):480-9.
39. D'Cruz IA, Cohen HC, Prabhu R, et al. Diagnosis of cardiac tamponade by echocardiography. Changes in mitral valve motion and ventricular dimensions with special reference to paradoxical pulse. Circulation. 1975;52:460-5.
40. Schiller NB, Botvinick EH. Right ventricular compression as a sign of cardiac tamponade: an analysis of echocardiographic ventricular dimensions and their clinical implications. Circulation. 1977;56(5):774-9.
41. Reddy PS, Curtiss EI, O'Toole JD, et al. Cardiac tamponade: hemodynamic observations in man. Circulation. 1978;58(2):265-72.
42. Shabetai R, Mangiardi L, Bhargava V, et al. The pericardium and cardiac function. Prog Cardiovasc Dis. 1979;22(2):107-34.
43. Bilchick KC, Wise RA. Paradoxical physical findings described by Kussmaul: pulsus paradoxus and Kussmaul's sign. Lancet. 2002;359:1940-2.
44. Cohn JN, Pinkerson AL, Tristani FE. Mechanism of pulsus paradoxus in clinical shock. J Clin Invest. 1967;46(11):1744-55.
45. McDonald IG, Hirsh J, Jelinek VM, et al. Acute major pulmonary embolism as a cause of exaggerated respiratory blood pressure variation and pulsus paradoxus. Br Heart J. 1972;34(11):1137-41.
46. Gorlin R, Knowles JH, Storey CF. The Valsalva maneuver as a test of cardiac function. Pathologic physiology and clinical significance. Am J Med. 1957;22:197.
47. Elisberg EI. Heart rate response to the Valsalva maneuver as a test of circulatory integrity. JAMA. 1963;186:200-5.
48. Zema MJ, Caccavano M, Kligfield P. Detection of left ventricular dysfunction in ambulatory subjects with the bedside Valsalva maneuver. Am J Med. 1983;75:241-8.
49. McEniery CM, Yasmin, McDonnell B, et al. Central pressure: variability and impact of cardiovascular risk factors: the Anglo-Cardiff Collaborative Trial II. Hypertension. [Research Support, Non-U.S. Gov't]. 2008;51(6):1476-82.
50. Nichols WW, O'Rourke MF. Wave reflections. McDonald's Blood Flow in Arteries: Theoretic, Experimental and Clinical Principles. London: Arnold; 1998.
51. Rowell LB, Brengelmann GL, Blackmon JR, et al. Disparities between aortic and peripheral pulse pressures induced by upright exercise and vasomotor changes in man. Circulation. 1968;37(6):954-64.
52. Wilkinson IB, Franklin SS, Hall IR, et al. Pressure amplification explains why pulse pressure is unrelated to risk in young subjects. Hypertension. 2001;38(6): 1461-6.
53. Bogren HG, Mohiaddin RH, Klipstein RK, et al. The function of the aorta in ischemic heart disease: a magnetic resonance and angiographic study of aortic compliance and blood flow patterns. American heart journal. [Research Support, U.S. Gov't, P.H.S.]. 1989;118(2):234-47.
54. Ohtsuka S, Kakihana M, Watanabe H, et al. Chronically decreased aortic distensibility causes deterioration of coronary perfusion during increased left ventricular contraction. J Am Coll Cardiol. 1994;24(5):1406-14.
55. Singh JP, Larson MG, Manolio TA, et al. Blood pressure response during treadmill testing as a risk factor for new-onset hypertension. The Framingham heart study. Circulation. 1999;99(14):1831-6.

56. Weiss SA, Blumenthal RS, Sharrett AR, et al. Exercise blood pressure and future cardiovascular death in asymptomatic individuals. Circulation. [Research Support, N.I.H., Extramural]. 2010;121(19):2109-16.
57. Ranganathan N, Sivaciyan V, Livanos G. Derived central aortic pressure measurement clarifies hypertensive response to exercise. Presented at High Blood Pressure Research 2011 Scientific Sessions, Orlando, FL, Sept 21, 2011.
58. O'Rourke MF, Adji A. Basis for use of central blood pressure measurement in office clinical practice. J Am Soc Hypertens. 2008;2(1):28-38.
59. Eisner DA, Diaz ME, Li Y, et al. Stability and instability of regulation of intracellular calcium. Exp Physiol. 2005;90:3-12.
60. Aboyans V, Criqui MH, Abraham P, et al. Measurement and interpretation of the ankle-brachial index: a scientific statement from the American Heart Association. Circulation. [Practice Guideline Review]. 2012;126(24):2890-909.
61. Fowkes FG, Murray GD, Butcher I, et al. Ankle brachial index combined with Framingham Risk Score to predict cardiovascular events and mortality: a meta-analysis. Jama. [Meta-Analysis]. 2008;300(2):197-208.
62. Steg PG, Bhatt DL, Wilson PW, et al. One-year cardiovascular event rates in outpatients with atherothrombosis. JAMA. 2007;297(11):1197-206.
63. Gupta DK, Skali H, Claggett B, et al. Heart failure risk across the spectrum of ankle-brachial index: The ARIC Study (atherosclerosis risk in communities). JACC Heart Fail. 2014;2(5):447-54.
64. Sapira JD. Quincke, de Musset, Duroziez, and Hill: some aortic regurgitations. South Med J. 1981;74(4):459-67.

Chapter

4 Jugular Venous Pulse

Snapshot

- Normal RA Pressure Pulse Contours
- Jugular Venous Inflow Velocity Patterns and the Relationship to the RA Pressure Pulse
- Jugular Venous Flow Events and their Relationship to Jugular Venous Pulse Contours
- Normal Jugular Venous Pulse Contour and its Recognition at the Bedside
- Individual Components of the RA Pressure Pulse, their Determinants and their Recognition in the Jugulars
- Abnormal Jugular Venous Pulse Contours as Related to Abnormal JVF Velocity Patterns
- Abnormal Jugular Contours
- Assessment of Jugular Venous Pressure
- Clinical Assessment of the Jugular Venous Pulse
- Points to Remember

The physiology of the normal jugular venous pulse contours and the pathophysiology of their alterations will be discussed in this chapter. Mechanisms of venous return and right heart filling have been of clinical interest from the days of Harvey and Purkinje.[1,2] Long before Chauveau and Marey published their recordings of the venous pulse, Lancisi had described "the systolic fluctuation of the external jugular vein" in a patient with tricuspid regurgitation.[3,4] Potain demonstrated the presystolic timing of the dominant wave of the normal venous pulse by simultaneous recording of the venous and the carotid artery pulses.[5] In the early part of the last century, the detailed studies of the venous pulse by Mackenzie helped define the waveforms, their terminology and their origins. He called the main waves "a", "c" and "v" to denote the first letters of what he thought were their anatomic sites of origins, namely the right atrium, the carotid artery and the right ventricle. He distinguished the "ventricular type venous pulse" of tricuspid regurgitation from the "auricular type" and associated it with atrial fibrillation, demonstrating also the progression of the former from the latter over time.[6,7] Since the days of Mackenzie, clinicians have studied the venous pressure and the pulse contour in different clinical conditions.[8–33] The advent of cardiac catheterization, the recording of intracardiac pressures, and the development of techniques to study blood flow velocity all contributed substantially to our understanding of the mechanisms of venous return, right heart filling and function.[10,11,13,18,20,21,24,28,30,34-46]

Since right atrial pressure pulse and the venous inflow into the right heart affect the jugular contours, a good understanding of the basics of their relationship both in the normals and in the abnormals is very meaningful and important. The discussion will be sequential under the following headings:

1. *Normal RA pressure pulse contours*
2. *Jugular venous inflow velocity patterns and the relationship to the right atrial pressure pulse*
3. *Jugular venous flow (JVF) events and their relationship to jugular venous pulse contours*
4. *Normal Jugular venous pulse contour and its recognition at the bedside*
5. *Individual components of the right atrial pressure pulse, their determinants and their recognition in the jugulars*
6. *Abnormal Jugular venous pulse contours as related to abnormal JVF velocity patterns*
7. *Mechanism of abnormal JVF velocity patterns and contours in pulmonary hypertension*
8. *Mechanism of abnormal JVF patterns and contours in postcardiac surgery patients*
9. *Mechanism of abnormal JVF patterns and contours in restriction to ventricular filling*
10. *Abnormal Jugular contours*
11. *Assessment of Jugular venous pressure*
12. *Clinical assessment of the Jugular venous pulse*

NORMAL RA PRESSURE PULSE CONTOURS

The sequential changes in the RA pressure during cardiac cycle can be considered starting with the beginning of diastole. In diastole when the tricuspid valve opens, the atrium begins to empty into the right ventricle. The diastolic filling of the ventricle consists of three consecutive phases:

Early rapid filling phase when the ventricular pressure, which has fallen quite low, compared to that in the atrium (often close to 0 mm Hg) begins to rise with the rapid tricuspid inflow.

Slow filling phase follows the early rapid filling phase when the inflow velocity begins to slow down. During this phase, the ventricular pressure actually begins to equalize with that of the atrium. The pressure where this equalization occurs is determined by the compliance of the RV and the surrounding pericardium and thorax. In the normal subjects, the pressure during this phase is usually <5 mm Hg. It can also be termed the ***pre a wave pressure*** since this phase is immediately followed by atrial contraction.

The ***pre a wave pressure*** is also the baseline filling pressure over which pressure wave build up can occur in the atrium at other periods of the cardiac cycle.

The last phase of ventricular filling occurs at the end of diastole during the atrial contraction, which raises the pressure in the atrium. The ventricular pressure follows the atrial pressure since the tricuspid valve is still open. The level to which the pressure could rise during atrial contraction (***a wave*** pressure, named after ***atrial systole***) would depend on the strength of the atrial contraction as well as the baseline ***pre a wave pressure*** and the right ventricular distensibility (compliance) (*see* below).

Atrial contraction is followed not only by atrial relaxation but also by ventricular contraction. Both events follow each other in succession during normal atrioventricular electrical conduction (during normal PR relationship). Both events lead to a fall in atrial pressure. The fall caused by atrial relaxation completes the ***a wave*** and is termed the ***x descent.***

During ventricular contraction, which follows the atrial contraction, the ventricular pressure rises and once it exceeds the pressure in the atrium, the tricuspid valve becomes closed. As ventricular systole continues, RV pressure rises and once it exceeds the pulmonary diastolic pressure, the pulmonary valve opens and ejection of blood into the pulmonary artery occurs. During this phase of ventricular systole, however, the atrial pressure continues to fall. This fall in atrial pressure is termed the ***x′ descent.*** This should be distinguished from the ***x*** descent caused by atrial relaxation.[26] *The x′ descent, on the other hand, is caused by the descent of the base of the ventricle. The contracting RV actually pulls the closed tricuspid valve and the tricuspid ring that together form the floor of the atrium.*[34,37,39,46] This movement of the base can be easily observed when one views a cine angiogram of the right coronary artery. Right coronary artery runs along the right atrioventricular groove and it can be seen to move down with each ventricular systole. Similar motion of the descent of the base can also be seen on the left side in relationship to the circumflex coronary artery, which runs along the left ventricular side of the atrioventricular groove. The descent of the base of the ventricles can be also appreciated during ventricular systole in the four-chamber views of the two-dimensional echocardiograms. The representation on the image display screen, however, is usually such that the apex of the heart is at the top. Careful observation will clearly show that the AV ring with the closed tricuspid and mitral valves moves during systole toward the ventricular side actually causing an expansion of the atrial area and dimension. The descent of the base is particularly important for the RV for its ejection, since the interventricular septum actually moves with the left ventricle during systole as will be readily observed in the two-dimensional echo image of the left ventricle in the long-axis view as well as the short-axis view.

The drop in atrial pressure during ventricular systole may be facilitated by the fall in pericardial pressures that occurs when the volume of the heart decreases during systole.[27] The preservation of the ***x′ descent*** in atrial standstill and atrial fibrillation further supports the concept that the ***x′ descent*** is unrelated to atrial relaxation.[28,40,47] The ***x′ descent,*** on the other hand, requires not only normal RV contraction but also an intact tricuspid valve.

Toward the later phase of systole when the ventricle has completed most of its ejection, the pull on the closed tricuspid valve and ring decreases. The venous inflow into RA from the venae cavae now is able to overcome the fall in atrial pressure caused by the descent of the base. This helps to build up the atrial pressure to a peak of the next wave termed the ***v wave.***

The v wave is, therefore, the venous filling wave in the atrium (named originally after ventricular systole). It occurs during later phase of ventricular systole. The level to which the ***v wave*** pressure can be built up in the presence of an intact tricuspid valve would depend not only on the right atrial distensibility or compliance but also on the baseline filling pressure which is the pre ***a wave*** pressure.

Occasionally, one can recognize a break point on the atrial pressure curve between ***the x and the x′ descent.*** This point may sometimes be termed the ***c point*** since it roughly corresponds in timing to the tricuspid valve closure. Reference to the so-called ***c waves*** are made occasionally to humps seen between ***the a and the v waves*** in the jugular venous pulse recordings made with transducers. These are mostly carotid pulse artifacts (***c*** for carotid) and they are not seen in the RA pressure pulse recordings. When seen occasionally in the RA pressure recording it may be due to a slight tricuspid valve bulge toward the right atrium during the isovolumic phase of right ventricular contraction.[6,8,25]

During later phase of systole, the ventricular pressure in fact begins to fall. Once the ventricular pressure falls below the peak of the ***v wave,*** the tricuspid valve will open and the atrial pressure again will begin to fall. This fall in atrial pressure caused by the tricuspid valve opening and the beginning of tricuspid inflow into the ventricle is termed the ***y descent.*** This completes the ***v wave.*** The ***y descent*** reaches its nadir at the end of the early rapid inflow phase of the ventricular filling in diastole. This then is the sequence, which repeats itself during each normal cardiac cycle (Fig. 4.1).

JUGULAR VENOUS INFLOW VELOCITY PATTERNS AND THE RELATIONSHIP TO THE RIGHT ATRIAL PRESSURE PULSE

From the foregoing description of the RA pressure pulse, one can easily understand that the atrial pressure falls twice during each cardiac cycle, once during ventricular systole ***(x′ descent)*** and once during ventricular diastole ***(y descent).*** The systolic descent during normal PR intervals is usually a combination of ***x*** and ***x′*** descents although the ***x′ descent*** is more prominent and the important component. The fall during ***x′ descent*** that is caused by

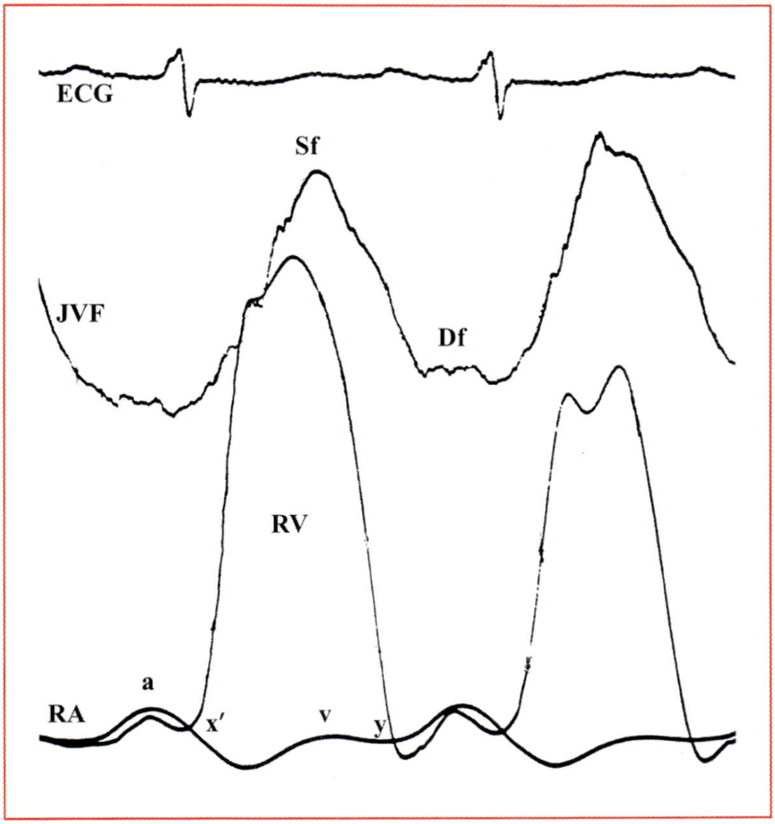

Fig. 4.1: Simultaneous recordings of ECG, Jugular Venous Flow (JVF) velocity recording, right atrial (RA) and right ventricular (RV) pressures in a subject with normal right heart hemodynamics. The RA pressure curve shows the a and the ***v waves*** with ***x′ descent > y descent***. JVF shows systolic flow velocity (Sf) > diastolic flow velocity (Df).

active ventricular systole is more dominant than the fall during the ***y descent*** that occurs during the comparatively "passive" atrial emptying in diastole when the tricuspid valve opens (across a small pressure gradient between the atrium and the ventricle). The venous return into the atrium is actually facilitated by the fall in the atrial pressure. In fact, acceleration in venous inflow velocity can be demonstrated whenever the atrial pressure falls during cardiac cycle.[40]

Although the venous inflow in the jugulars is continuous, the JVF velocity that is similar to flow velocity in the superior vena cava, in normal subjects is biphasic with one peak in systole corresponding to the ***x′ descent*** of the RA pressure pulse and a second peak in diastole corresponding to the ***y descent*** (allowing however for transmission delay) (Figs. 4.2A and B). *The systolic flow (Sf) peak is normally more dominant compared to the diastolic flow (Df) peak just as the* x′ descent *is more dominant compared to the* y descent ***in the normals.***[40] Venous inflow during atrial relaxation, under normal conditions,

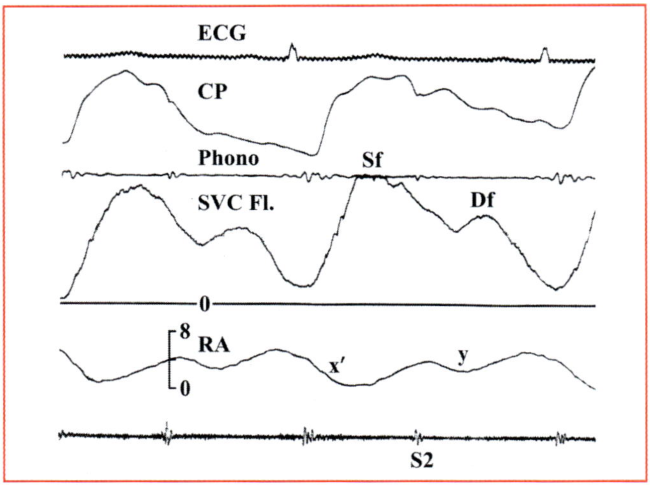

Fig. 4.2A: Simultaneous recordings of right atrial (RA) pressure, superior vena caval flow (SVC Fl) velocity in a normal subject. Also shown are ECG, carotid pulse (CP) and phonocardiogram (Phono) showing S2 for timing. All flow velocity recordings shown in this and all other figures are recorded in such a way that the velocities above the baseline zero (-0-) represent flows toward the right heart and all flow velocities below the baseline zero indicate flow direction away from the heart. The SVC flow is continuous and toward the heart and is biphasic with systolic flow velocity (Sf) greater than the diastolic flow velocity (Df). Sf corresponds to the ***x′ descent*** and the Df corresponds to the ***y descent*** in the RA pressure pulse.

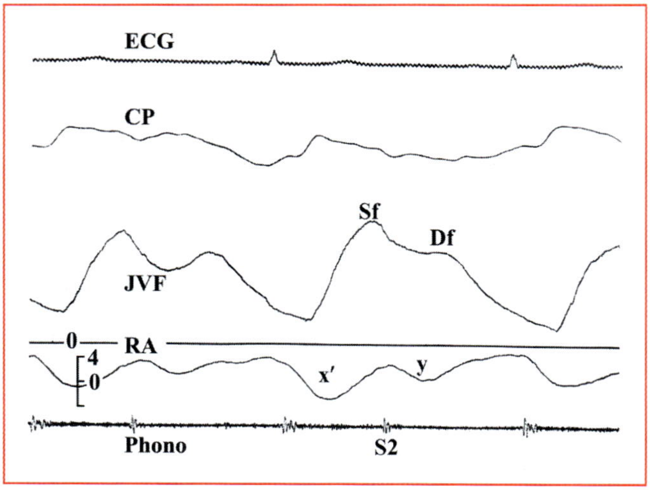

Fig. 4.2B: In the same normal patient, similar simultaneous recordings are shown except instead of the SVC flow velocity recording, transcutaneous jugular venous flow (JVF) velocity is shown. The JVF similar to the SVC flow also has a biphasic flow pattern with the ***Sf velocity*** greater than the ***Df velocity***. The peak of Sf in the JVF occurs somewhat later than that noted in the SVC Fl, almost at the time of the second heart sound (S2). The difference is due to the delay in transmission from the heart to the Jugular.

can only be seen on Doppler tracings of JVF as a notch on the upstroke of the Sf velocity, corresponding to the x descent; whereas the peak of the Sf always corresponds to the x′ descent (Fig. 4.2C). Separate atrial relaxation flow as such can be demonstrated, however, during periods of atrioventricular dissociation and when the PR interval is long.[35,36,39,40]

The Sf and the corresponding ***x′ descent*** may be somewhat diminished in atrial fibrillation. This is explainable due to the lack of atrial contraction in atrial fibrillation that may lead to a decrease in Starling effect on the ventricle, thereby diminishing the dominance of the Sf as well as the corresponding ***x′ descent***[39,40,48] (Fig. 4.3).

The forward flow velocity patterns in the jugulars could, however, be altered and become abnormal due to alterations in the right heart function. It may then lose the dominance of the Sf.[40,41,49] The relationship between the Sf and the Df velocity may be such that the ***Sf may be equal to the Df*** (Fig. 4.4). ***Sf may be less than the Df*** (Fig. 4.5) or it may become totally absent and may be replaced by ***a single Df*** (Fig. 4.6). These changes in jugular flow velocity patterns will, however, be accurately reflected by the corresponding changes in the RA pressure pulse contours of *equal x′ and y descents, x′ descent less than the y descent or a single y descent.*[40,49]

JUGULAR VENOUS FLOW EVENTS AND THEIR RELATIONSHIP TO JUGULAR VENOUS PULSE CONTOURS

Next we shall consider the JVF events as related to the jugular venous pulse contours. Although the jugular venous column is in direct continuity with the right atrium, the venous system is innervated by the sympathetic system which can influence the tone of the smooth muscles in their walls[19] and as such affect the level to which the column will rise for any given volume status of the individual and the corresponding right atrial pressure. With that background we shall consider the jugular flow events as they relate to the jugular venous pulse contour.

It is important to note that the descents or fall in pressure cause acceleration of venous inflow as stated earlier. Although more volume of blood enters the heart during diastole, the flow is slower but over a longer period of time. In systole, however, the flow is much faster over a shorter period of time (first half of systole). The column of blood in the jugulars is in direct continuity with the blood in the right atrium and right ventricle in diastole. During systole, the tricuspid valve is closed and therefore the ventricle is excluded from this system. During the slow filling phase of diastole, the flow into the jugulars at the top of the system is matched to that entering the ventricle (Fig. 4.7). This represents the baseline state at which time whatever pressure is developed is mainly determined by the ventricular distensibility (compliance) assuming that the blood volume status of the patient is normal ***(pre a wave pressure)*** (Fig. 4.7A).

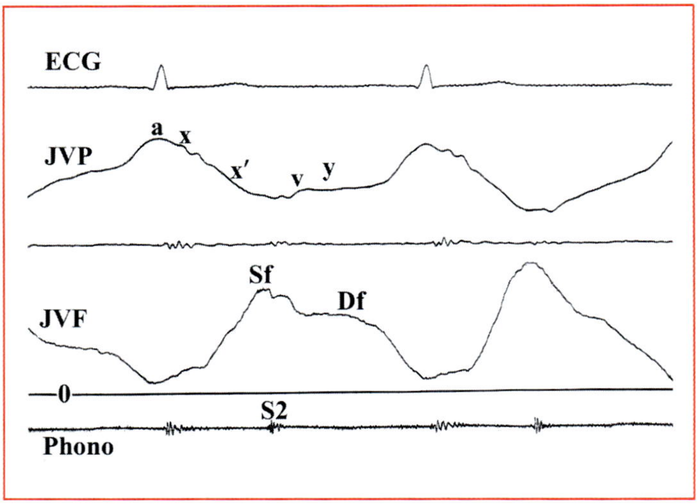

Fig. 4.2C: Simultaneous recordings of JVF, jugular venous pulse (JVP), ECG and phonocardiogram (Phono) from a normal subject. Venous inflow during ***x descent*** representing the atrial relaxation is seen as a notch at the beginning of the systolic flow (Sf). Throughout the cardiac cycle the flow is always toward the heart (above the baseline zero). JVP contour in this normal patient shows a more prominent ***x′ descent***.
Source: Modified and reproduced with kind permission of the Lippincott Williams and Wilkins from Circulation 1978;57:930-39.

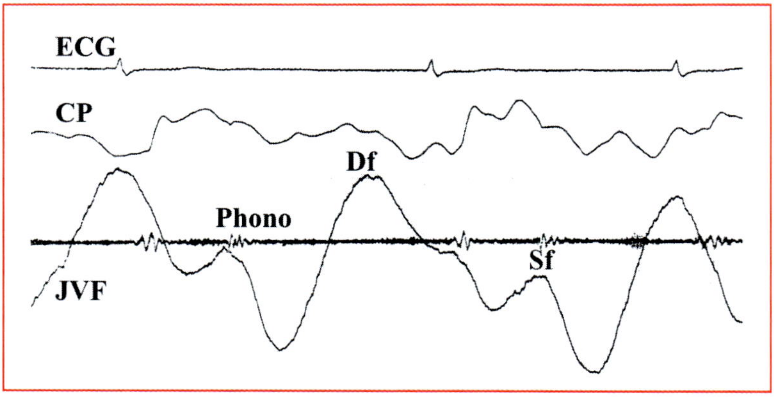

Fig. 4.3: Simultaneous recordings of ECG, carotid pulse (CP), phonocardiogram (Phono) and jugular venous flow (JVF) velocity in a patient with mitral regurgitation and atrial fibrillation. Due to lack of atrial contribution, the Starling effect is diminished leading to a decreased systolic flow. JVF shows a dominant diastolic flow (Df) compared to the less pronounced systolic flow (Sf).

With the onset of right atrial contraction, the right atrium becomes smaller and in fact is emptying. Therefore, it is unable to accept any venous return. The flow in the superior vena cava and the jugulars decelerates and almost ceases. The continuous inflow from the periphery into the system will raise the volume and the pressure thus causing the buildup of the normal

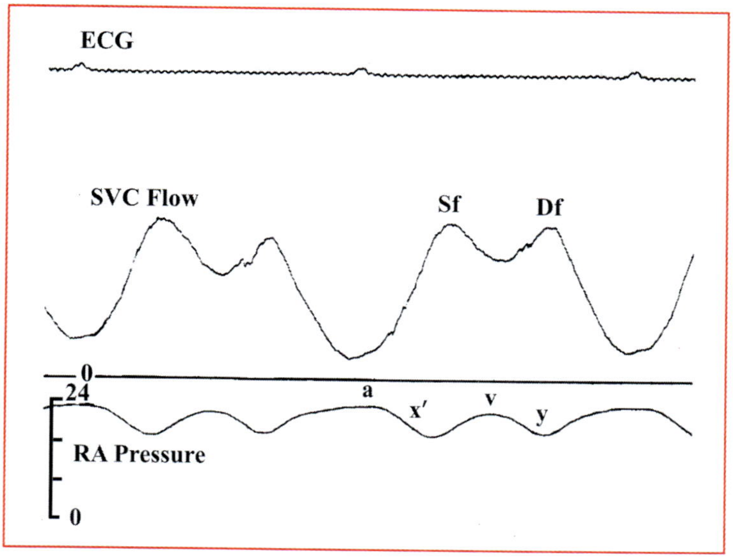

Fig. 4.4: Simultaneous recordings of ECG, right atrial (RA) pressure and superior vena caval (SVC) flow velocity from a patient with constrictive pericarditis. Note the variations from the normal. The RA pressure is high. The ***x′*** and ***y descents*** in the RA pressure tracing are equal unlike the normal and the corresponding SVC flow velocity shows a biphasic flow where the Sf and the Df are also equal.

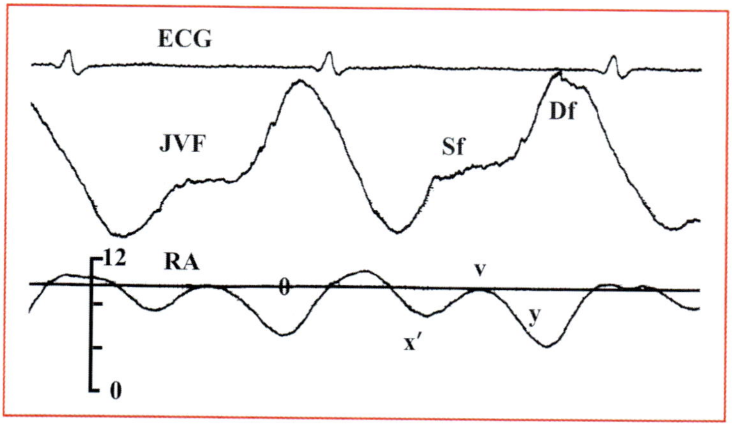

Fig. 4.5: Simultaneous recordings of ECG, right atrial (RA) pressure and jugular venous flow velocity (JVF) from another patient with constrictive pericarditis. The ***y descent*** is more prominent, compared to the ***x′ descent***, on the RA pressure tracing. The corresponding jugular venous flow (JVF) shows a more dominant Df compared to the Sf.

a wave in the jugular (Fig. 4.7B). The level, to which this may rise, will depend on the degree of deceleration of forward flow. This, in fact, will depend on the strength of the right atrial contraction and the pressure generated by it. During atrial relaxation, the atrium expands causing its pressure to fall leading to flow acceleration in the jugulars. This is a passive flow across a pressure gradient between the higher jugular pressure and lower right atrial

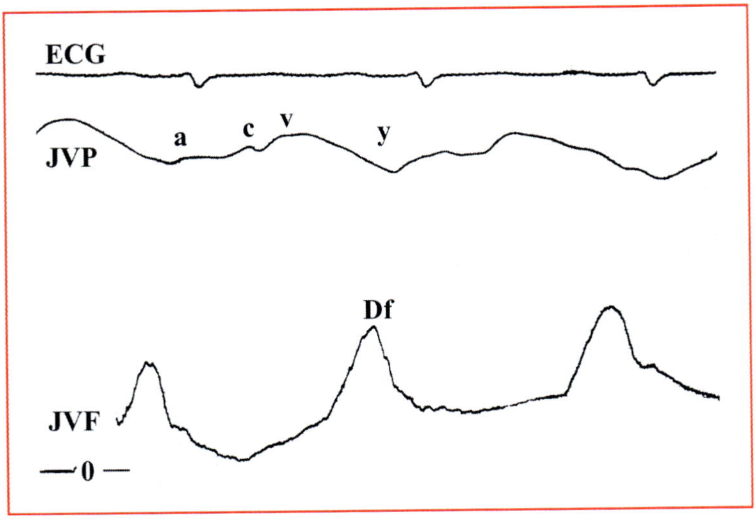

Fig. 4.6: Simultaneous recordings of ECG, jugular venous pulse (JVP) and jugular venous flow velocity (JVF) from a patient with cardiomyopathy. The flow pattern is conspicuous for the absence of a systolic flow and the JVP shows no ***x′ descent***. Instead a single peak in diastole (Df) is seen. It corresponds to a single descent in the JVP also in diastole and therefore is the ***y descent*** (see ECG for timing).
Source: Modified and reproduced with kind permission of the Lippincott Williams and Wilkins from Circulation 1978; 57:930-39.

pressure. Since the flow velocity into the atrium at this time is faster than the continuous inflow from the periphery, the jugular contour falls causing the ***x descent*** (Fig. 4.7C).

Next event to follow is ventricular systole. As explained previously this causes an active sudden drop in right atrial pressure almost like a suction effect. This accelerates the flow into the right atrium markedly. This also will lead to a further fall in the jugular contour ***(x′ descent)*** (Fig. 4.7D). Although this corresponds to the right atrial ***x′ descent,*** there is however a transmission delay.[40] The latter is accounted for by the time taken for the flow acceleration to develop in the superior vena cava and the jugulars.

During later half of systole, the descent of the base comes to a halt, thereby eliminating any further suction effect and/or drop in right atrial pressure. This will lead to reduction in flow acceleration toward the heart. The venous inflow from the periphery will now exceed the flow into the right atrium, thereby filling the system. This will lead to a rise in jugular and atrial pressures, causing the ***v wave*** to build up (Fig. 4.7E). Assuming normal blood volume, *the level to which this will rise in the jugulars will depend on three factors:*

1. *The baseline "pre a wave pressure" in the system.*
2. *The compliance or distensibility of the right atrium.*
3. *The systemic venous tone, which is predominantly influenced by the state of the sympathetic tone.*

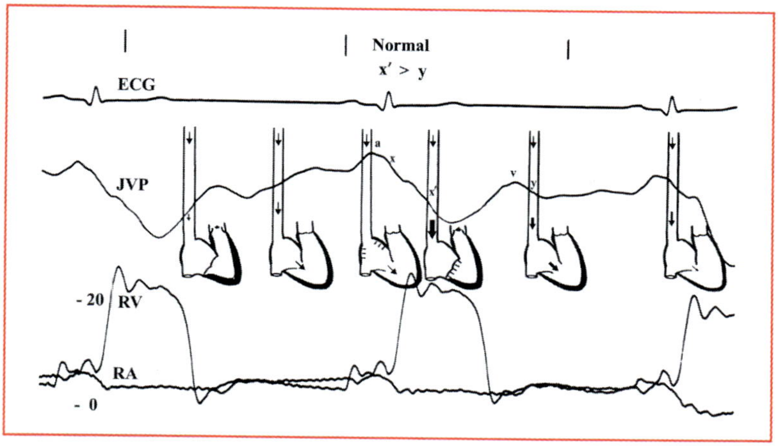

Fig. 4.7: Simultaneous recordings of ECG, jugular venous pulse (JVP) and right atrial (RA) and right ventricular (RV) pressure tracings from a patient with normal right heart hemodynamics. Superimposed are diagrammatic representations of right atrium and right ventricle during various phases of the cardiac cycle. The arrows represent blood flow velocities and help explain the changes in the JVP contour relating them to right heart physiology. The thickness of the arrows relate to the velocity of flow. The columns extending upward from the heart represents the superior vena cava (SVC) and the jugular complex. The arrows at the top of the columns represent steady flow from the periphery into the vena cava.
Source: Reprinted from Ranganathan et al. Changes in Jugular venous flow velocity after coronary artery bypass grafting. Am J Cardiol. 1989;63:725-9. Copyright (2005) with permission from Excerpta Medica Inc.

When the tricuspid valve opens with onset of diastole, the ventricular pressure having fallen to zero, allows flow through the development of a pressure gradient in the system. The acceleration of flow during this early phase of diastole is not as prominent as that which occurs during systole and therefore leads to a less prominent fall in pressure contour in the right atrium. In addition, the right atrium, being a capacitance chamber, will get smaller in the process of emptying into the ventricle and therefore the full flow velocity at the tricuspid valve is not reflected in the superior vena cava and the jugular system. This will result in the less prominent fall in the jugular contour (the ***y descent***) (Fig. 4.7F).

The normal ***a wave*** caused by the atrial contraction and the normal ***v wave*** caused by the venous filling of the atrium during later part of ventricular systole are associated with slow and small rises of pressure. They do not exceed generally 5 mmHg and are often closer to 2–3 mm Hg. Such small and slow pressure build up in the RA do not affect the jugular venous inflow velocity significantly excepting to cause deceleration. They do not ever cause reversal of forward flow.

Retrograde flow into the jugulars from the superior vena cava is always abnormal. Irrespective of the mechanisms of origin such reversal can always be shown to be associated with abnormal pressure rises in the atrium.[40] This could happen during systole in the presence of normal A-V conduction, due to tricuspid regurgitation if it is significant.[40,50] It can then eliminate the ***x' descent*** and cause an early abnormal ***v wave*** pressure rise in the atrium (Fig. 4.7G).

When the atrial and ventricular contraction are dissociated as in certain abnormal heart rhythms, however (e.g. complete A-V block with a ventricular rhythm independent and often slower than the blocked atrial complexes of sinus node origin), simultaneous atrial and ventricular contraction could occur resulting in abnormal pressure waves termed the ***"cannon" waves.*** The atrial contraction occurs against a closed tricuspid valve leading to sudden development of high atrial pressure. During the ***cannon waves,*** the high atrial pressure is associated with reversal of flow in the jugulars in systole.[40] The reversed flow into the jugulars added to the normal inflow from the periphery cause increased filling of the jugular-superior vena caval system, resulting in the abnormally prominent waves (Fig. 4.7H).

Flow reversal can also occur in diastole. Very powerful atrial contractions may occasionally result in high ***a wave*** pressure in the RA (often in the range of 15 mm Hg or more) that could also be shown to be associated with reversal of forward flow during the end-diastolic phase.[40] This could happen in tricuspid stenosis, which is a rare condition, and in patients with severe decrease in RV compliance. In the latter patients, the RV is unable to dilate completely to accept blood from the contracting right atrium and the blood has no choice but to flow back into the venae cavae (Fig. 4.10).

NORMAL JUGULAR VENOUS PULSE CONTOUR AND ITS RECOGNITION AT THE BEDSIDE

The RA pressure pulse gets transmitted through the superior vena cava to the internal jugular vein. The internal jugular vein runs underneath the sternomastoid muscle.

It extends in direction from the angle of the jaw to the hollowness between the two heads of the sternomastoid muscle attachments to the upper sternum and the medial portion of the clavicle. Often positioning the patient with a comfortable tilt of the neck with adequate light coming from the sides could make the jugular pulsations more easily visible. Sometimes having the patient lie on the left lateral decubitus position again with the head tilted somewhat could also help bring out the jugular pulsations. Directing the light source in such a way as to cause a shadow of a fixed non-moving object to fall on the skin overlying the sternomastoid will reveal the pulsations of the jugulars underneath it, since the edge of the shadow can be shown to move because of the jugular movement. The objects could be patient's chin, observers' finger or a pen held at a fixed point on the neck of the patient by the observer. Often if the light source is appropriate, one may be able to have the shadow of the laterally placed clavicular head of the sternomastoid to fall on the hollow space between the two heads of that muscle.

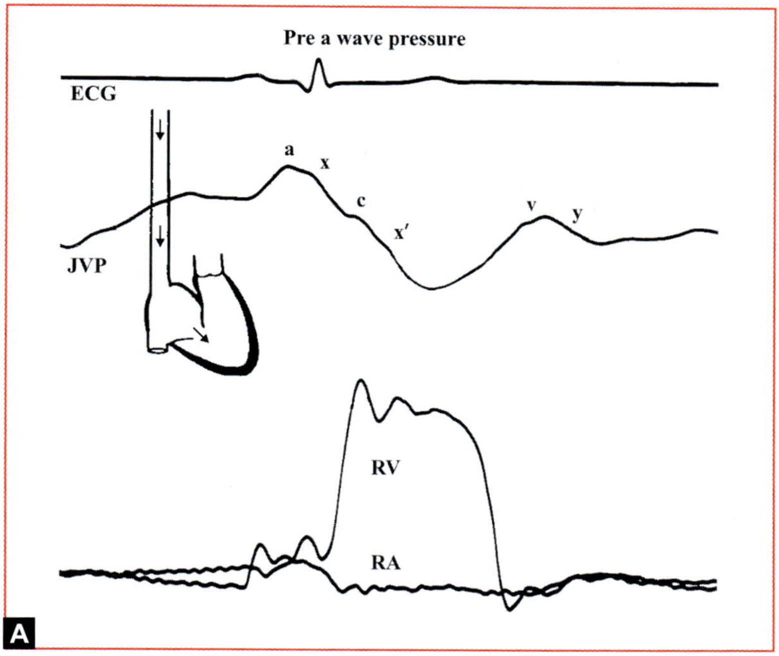

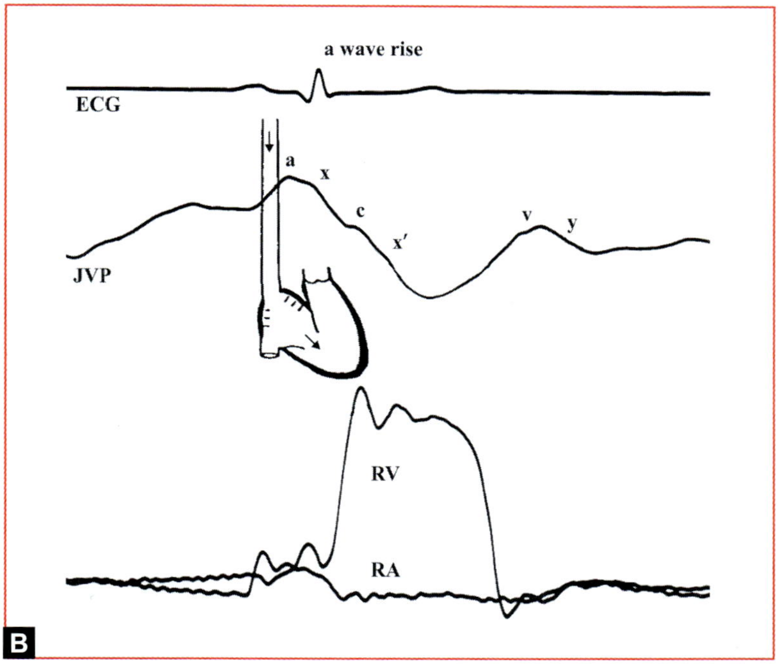

Figs. 4.7A and B: (A) In mid-diastole (slow filling phase), the tricuspid valve is open and RV and RA with SVC form a single chamber. The ventricle is almost full having gone through the rapid filling phase. The slow dilatation of RV causes slow flow rate in SVC, which is matched by inflow from the periphery. (B) When the RA contracts, it is emptying and getting smaller and cannot accept any blood at that point in time. Flow into the heart in SVC ceases. The blood coming into the system from the periphery causes a rise (a wave rise) in the jugular venous pulse.

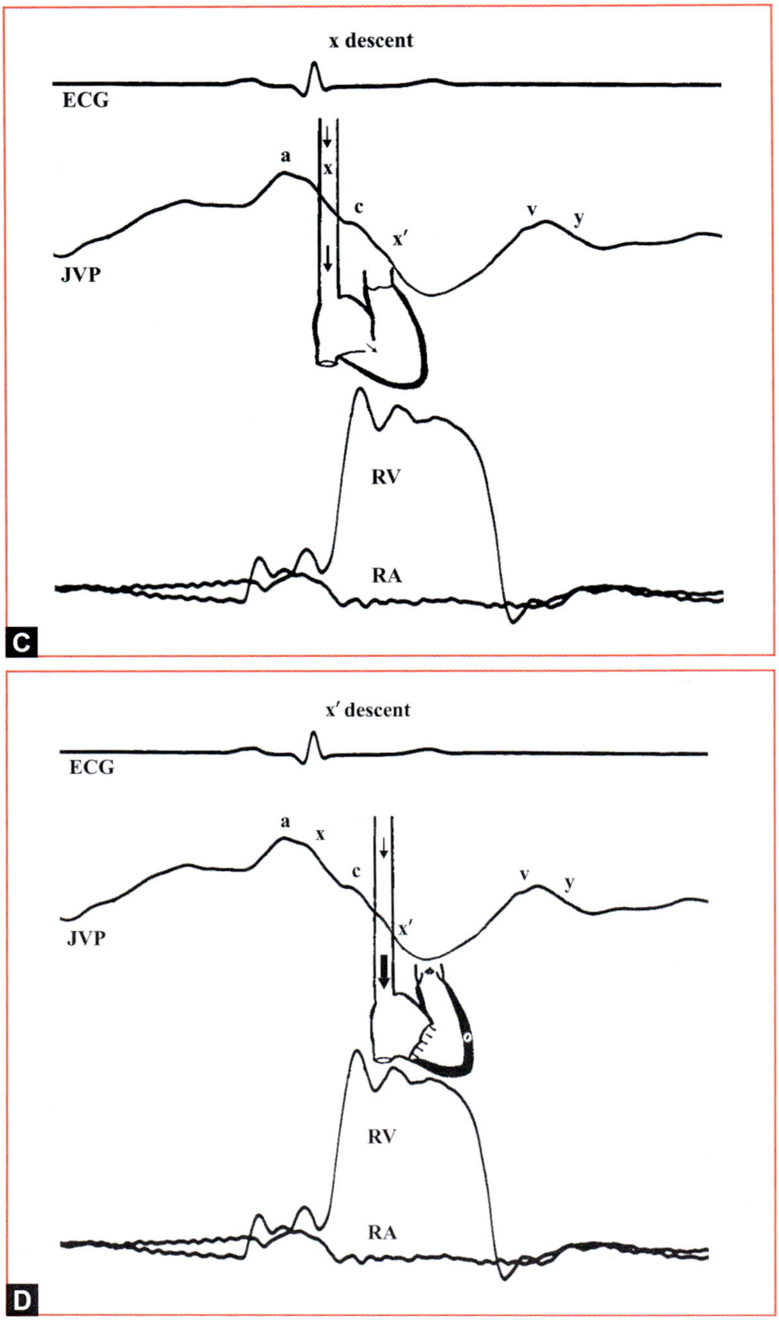

Figs. 4.7C and D: (C) After atrial systole, the RA relaxes ***(x descent)*** thus increasing its capacity and allowing blood to flow in. This flow rate in the SVC is faster than the rate at which blood is flowing into the system from the periphery, therefore the jugular pulse is seen to fall. (D) In early systole as the RV contracts, it gets smaller and pulls down the base. This causes almost a suction effect ***(x′ descent)*** and blood rushes into the RA. This rate of flow is much faster than the rate of peripheral inflow. This causes a sudden fall in the jugular pulse contour.

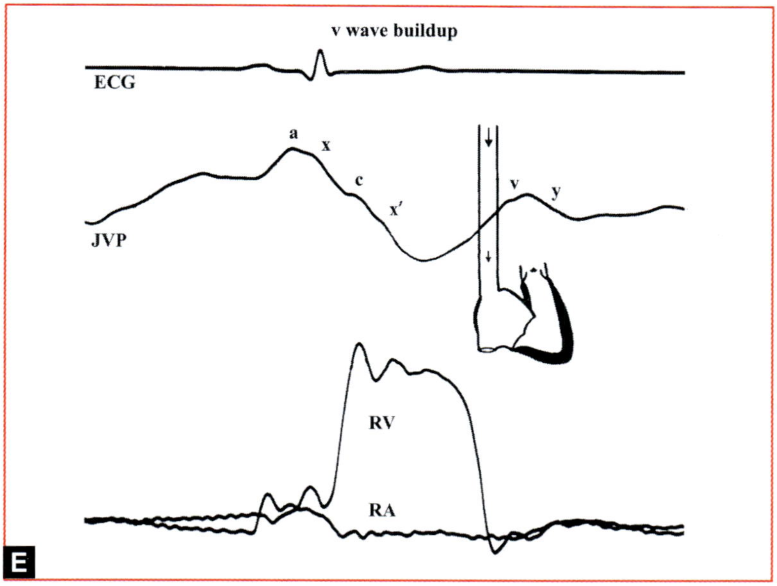

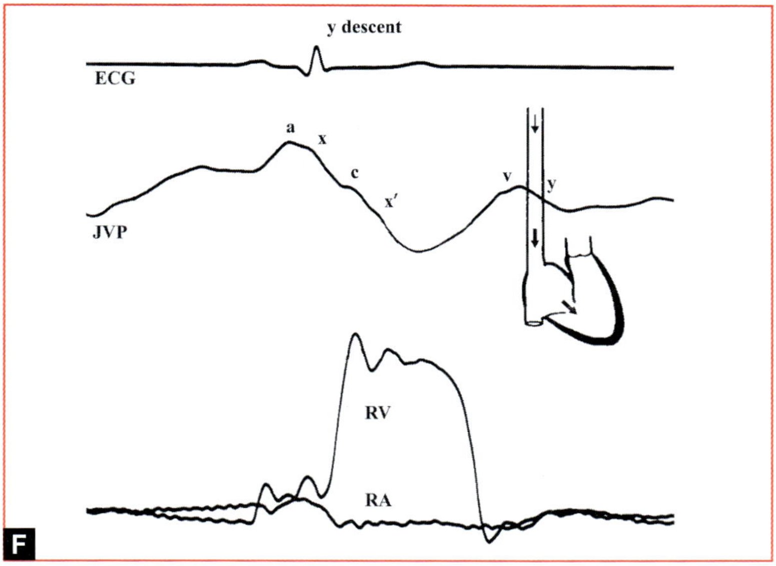

Figs. 4.7E and F: (E) Most ejection out of the ventricle occurs during the first third of systole and the maximum decrease in RV dimension occurs during this phase. During the later part of systole, the RV size does not decrease much further. The pull on the base of the RV also is not significant at this time. By this time, the RA is also full and therefore the flow in SVC is very slow and certainly slower than blood coming from the periphery. This leads to a rise the jugular column (***v wave***). (F) As the tricuspid valve opens in early diastole, blood flows passively across a pressure gradient into the RV from the right atrium. The pressure in the RA is the ***v wave*** pressure and the pressure in the RV is close to zero because of active right ventricular relaxation. The flow at the tricuspid valve is however not fully reflected in the SVC because of the capacitance of the RA, which can shrink as it were in size as it empties into the RV. The flow in the SVC is only minimally faster than the flow coming from the periphery. The difference of the two being small the y descent is not very prominent in the jugulars.

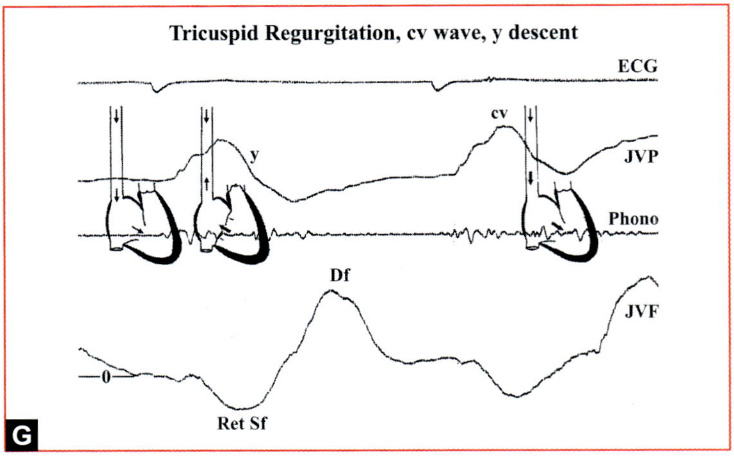

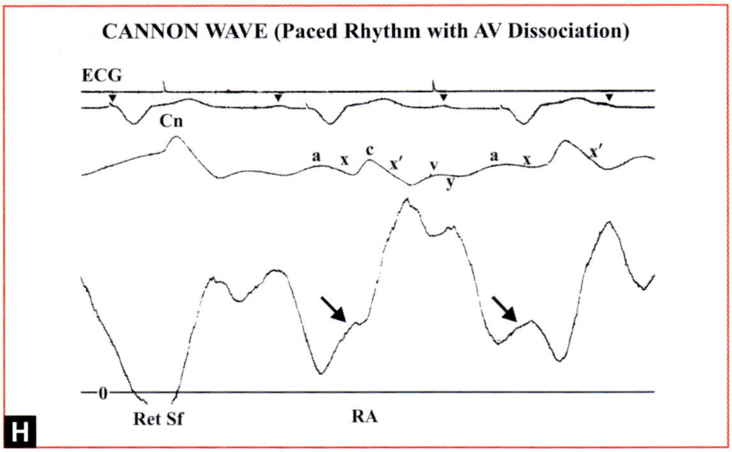

Figs. 4.7G and H: (G) Simultaneous recordings of ECG, phonocardiogram (Phono), JVP and the jugular venous flow velocity (JVF) from a patient with tricuspid regurgitation. It shows the systolic retrograde flow (Ret Sf) from the RV into the RA. This reverses the flow in SVC, giving rise to a prominent rise in jugular pulse contour ***("cv" wave).*** The Ret Sf abolishes the effect of the descent of the base during RV contraction. In addition, the retrograde flow into the RA due to RV contraction raises the v wave pressure to higher levels. During the early filling phase of diastole when the RV pressure falls to zero, there is a higher gradient of pressures between the RA and the RV, which makes the fall steep (prominent y descent). (H) Simultaneous recordings of ECG, JVP and JVFs from a patient with a permanent pacemaker. It shows a regular ventricular rhythm caused by ventricular pacing with independent P waves with atrioventricular dissociation. Arrows on ECG point to ***P waves***. The bigger arrows on JVF indicate atrial relaxation flows corresponding to ***x descents***. In the first beat, P and QRS are synchronous giving rise to retrograde flow into SVC and causing a cannon wave. Note that the duration of the cannon wave is shorter than the duration of the v wave of tricuspid regurgitation shown in (G) due to the varying P to QRS relationship, the ***x***, ***x′*** and ***y descents*** change from beat to beat. In the second beat the P and QRS relationship is basically normal with a normal PR interval and the ***x***, ***x′*** and ***y descents*** are normal. In the last beat, the PR is long and the ***x descent*** is well separated from the ***x′ descent***.

Since normal RA pressure waves (the a and the v waves) have slow rises and often of low amplitude, they are usually not appreciated in the jugulars. On the other hand, the descents in the RA pressure pulse are better transmitted and appreciated in the jugulars. They are generally *rapid movements moving away from the eye thus easily seen.* In addition, their appreciation is made easier since they reflect acceleration of flow velocity,[40,49] The descents in the internal jugular vein reflect fall in pressure in the right atrium during cardiac cycle. The reflected light intensity on the hollow area between the two heads of the sternomastoid vary when the jugular pressure rises as opposed to when the jugular pressure falls and this is easily appreciated at the bedside as well as in video recordings of jugular pulsations. When the descents occur, there is less reflected light overlying the jugulars and the area looks darker. Slight anatomic variations from patient to patient may occur. The descents may be sometimes appreciated more anteriorly at the medial edge of the sternomastoid. Sometimes it could be somewhat lateral. In some others it may be seen over a wide area in the neck.

The descents can be timed either to the radial arterial pulse or the second heart sound. The x′ descent corresponds to the systolic flow. Due to transmission delay this descent falls almost on to the second heart sound and it coincides with the radial arterial pulse. The diastolic y descent is out of phase with the arterial pulse and occurs after the second heart sound reflecting the diastolic flow velocity.[40]

In normal subjects, a single dominant descent is noted during systole (x′) due to the descent of the base corresponding to the dominant systolic flow. The y descent is often not visible in the adult although it may be noted in young subjects, pregnant women, thyrotoxic and anemic patients. In these the y descent may become visible because of its exaggeration due to rapid circulation and increased sympathetic tone. However, in these conditions due to the fact that the right ventricular systolic contraction is often normal, the ***x′ descent*** will still be the dominant descent.

As stated previously the normal ***a and the v wave*** rises are not seen but their presence can be inferred by the descents that follow. ***During normal sinus rhythm, the wave preceding x′ descent*** is the ***a wave and the one that precedes the y descent*** is the ***v wave.***

Generally, external jugular vein will not always reflect the descents. This vein usually runs superficially over the mid-portion of the sternomastoid muscle. If it should exhibit the descents that could be timed to the cardiac cycle, then one could use them for assessment of wave form and pressure much as one would normally use the internal jugular pulsations. *Jugular pulsations are easily distinguished from the arterial pulse in the neck because it moves in the opposite direction due to the usually dominant x′ descent* (Figs. 4.2C and 4.8).

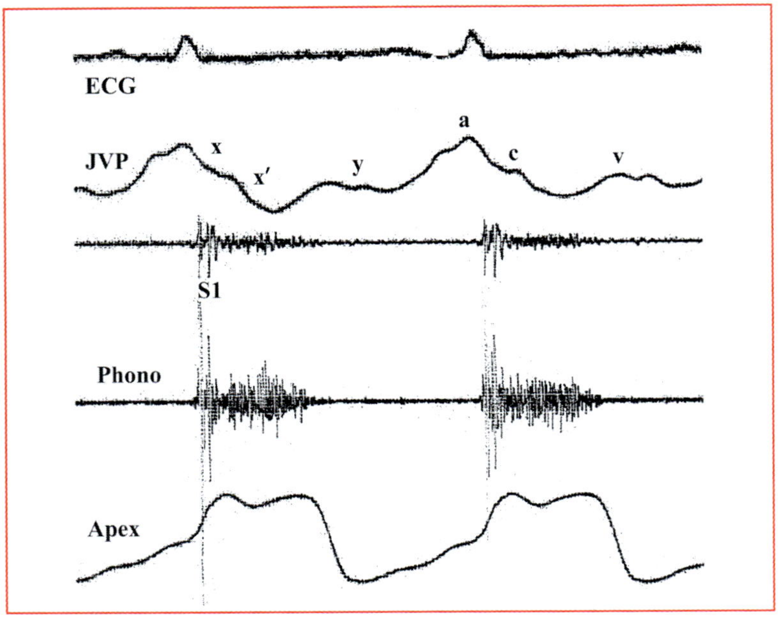

Fig. 4.8: Normal jugular venous pulse (JVP), showing a dominant fall during systole due to the ***x*** and the ***x′ descents***. The c wave in the JVP is usually a carotid pulse artifact unlike the ***c wave*** noted on the right atrial (RA) pressure tracing.

INDIVIDUAL COMPONENTS OF THE RIGHT ATRIAL PRESSURE PULSE, THEIR DETERMINANTS AND THEIR RECOGNITION IN THE JUGULARS

Pre a Wave Pressure

This is the pressure in diastole during the slow filling phase when the RV and the RA pressures become equal. During this phase, the atrium and the right ventricle are one chamber on account of the open tricuspid valve. The level at which this equalization is achieved *is determined by the compliance of the RV and the surrounding pericardium.*

The RV compliance implies the distensibility of the endocardium, myocardium as well as the epicardium. It can become abnormal and less distensible whenever pathologic processes develop in any portion of the RV wall. These processes could be in the form of hypertrophy (thickening of the myocardial fibers) such as those caused secondary to excessive pressure load (e.g. pulmonary hypertension or pulmonary stenosis). It could be in the form of inflammatory process such as myocarditis, or an infiltrative nature as in amyloidosis, or ischemia or infarction (RV infarction is usually rare but could occur when the right coronary artery gets occluded quite proximally before the RV branch origin, this is usually associated with an inferoposterior

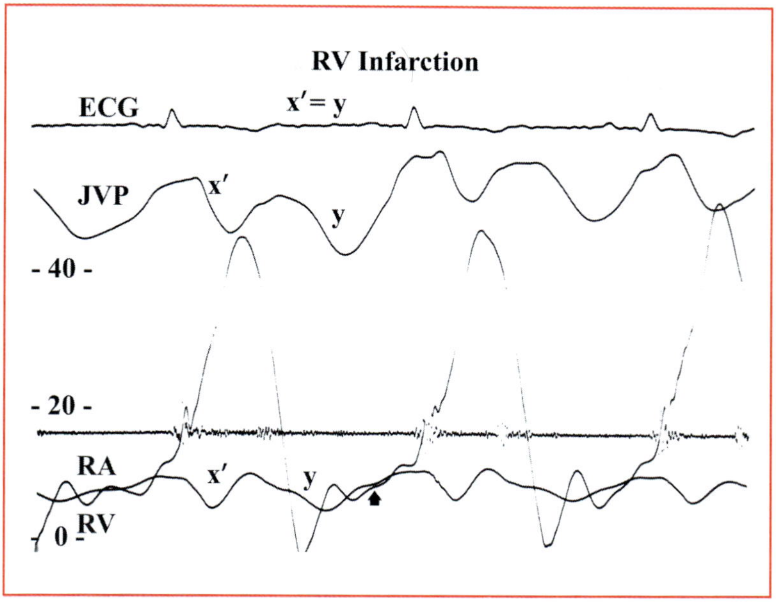

Fig. 4.9: Simultaneous recordings of RA (right atrial) and RV (right ventricular) pressures in mm Hg from a patient with RV infarction, along with jugular venous pulse (JVP). Note the double descents ***x′* = *y*** pattern in both the JVP and the RA pressure curve. Arrow points to the pre a wave pressure.

wall left ventricular infarction) or fibrosis that may supervene in the course of any of the pathologic process. This diastolic dysfunction can coexist with or without a systolic dysfunction (Figs. 4.9 and 4.11).

If the RV has developed in fact systolic dysfunction and failure, this will further aggravate the diastolic dysfunction, which often precedes systolic dysfunction. If the systolic emptying is poor, the ventricular volume will be higher at the end of systole and therefore its pressure will rise quickly to high levels with diastolic inflow.

If the RV wall is surrounded by a thick and fibrotic or calcific pericardium (e.g. chronic constrictive pericarditis) or a pericardial sac filled with fluid under some pressure (e.g. acute or subacute pericarditis with pericardial effusion), easy diastolic expansion of the ventricle will not be possible leading to a higher ***pre a wave pressure*** for any degree of filling.

The pre a wave pressure sets the baseline for the a wave and the v wave pressures.[49] If it becomes elevated as under the conditions listed above one would expect a higher ***a wave and v wave*** pressures in the atrial pressure pulse.

Elevated pre a wave pressure would be reflected in the jugulars as an elevated jugular venous pressure as judged by the assessment of the level of the top of the jugular pulsations in relation to the sternal angle.

a Wave

Irrespective of what the ***pre a wave pressure*** is, the ***a wave*** height in the atrial pressure is determined by the strength of the atrial contraction first and foremost since the ***a wave*** rise results from atrial contraction. In atrial fibrillation, both the atrial contraction and relaxation become ineffective and disorganized and feeble and thereby leading to loss of the ***a wave*** peak and the ***x descent.***[40]

The atrium tends to contract strongly when there is ***resistance to ventricular filling.*** The extreme form of resistance to ventricular filling of course would occur in tricuspid stenosis or obstruction due to a tumor (e.g. a myxoma in the atrium). These would be expected to cause very high ***a wave*** pressures.[18] In fact they do. However, these conditions are extremely rare and therefore not to be thought of first when considering causes of high ***a wave.***

The most common reason for resistance to ventricular filling is ***decreased ventricular compliance.*** The decreased compliance may be due to any pathologic process that affects the wall of the RV such as hypertrophy, ischemia, infarction, inflammation, infiltration and/or fibrosis (Fig. 4.10).

If the atrium itself becomes involved in disease process, which leads to a decrease in its systolic contraction, high ***a wave*** pressure may not be generated despite the presence of decreased ventricular compliance.

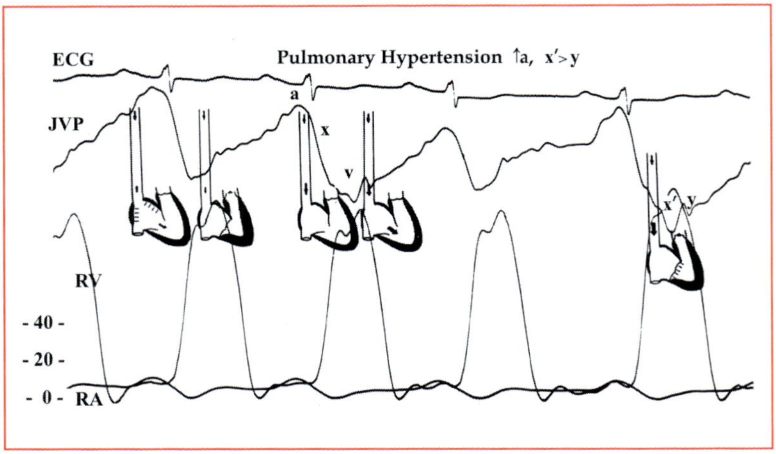

Fig. 4.10: Jugular venous pulse (JVP) from a patient with well compensated severe pulmonary hypertension with right ventricular (RV) hypertrophy and decreased compliance. The RV systolic pressure is between 90 and 100 mm Hg. Note the prominent a wave on the JVP. The a wave rise is almost as fast as the descent. The overlying diagrams depict the events at different phases of the cardiac cycle. The first diagram shows the retrograde flow into the SVC during atrial contraction. The ***x–x′ descent*** combination is still the most prominent descent.

Source: Modified and reprinted from Ranganathan et al. Abnormalities in Jugular venous flow velocity in pulmonary hypertension. Am J Cardiol. 1989;63:719-24. Copyright (2005) with permission from Excerpta Medica Inc.

Whereas the normal ***a wave*** pressure rise is slow and small and therefore not appreciated in the jugulars, ***a strong atrial contraction*** causing a quick and rapid rise in pressure ***may actually cause flow reversal*** in the jugulars and become recognizable in the jugulars as ***an abnormal sharp rising wave preceding the x′ descent*** that can be timed with the radial pulse. ***The short duration of this wave*** is another distinguishing feature.

If atrial contraction were to occur in a haphazard relationship to ventricular systole as in atrioventricular dissociation (as in complete AV block with a ventricular pacemaker driving the ventricles with atria beating on their own from sinus depolarizations), fortuitous relationship could develop that could result in simultaneous atrial and ventricular contraction. Since atrial contraction would be occurring at the time of a closed tricuspid valve due to ventricular systole, it will result in sharp and quick rise in atrial pressures termed ***"cannon waves".*** These will cause ***flow reversal*** in the jugulars[40] and be recognizable as sharp rising waves of short duration at the time of the radial pulse. They will be irregular. Rarely regular cannon waves may occur in junctional rhythms with retrograde P waves and very short PR interval (*see* Fig. 4.7H).

x Descent

The presence of ***atrial relaxation*** is the foremost prerequisite for the pressure fall termed ***x descent.*** A strong healthy atrial contraction can be expected to be followed by a good ***x descent*** (*see* Fig. 4.7C).

In terms of timing, the ***x*** descent comes just before the more dominant systolic ***x′*** descent. It usually ***precedes the x′ descent as a minor hesitation*** before the major fall during systole as observed in the jugulars during periods of normal PR relationship. ***If the PR interval is prolonged*** it could occur long before ventricular systole and in fact occur before end diastole. When it becomes ***diastolic in timing,*** it may be ***difficult to distinguish*** this at the bedside ***from*** the usual diastolic ***y descent*** in the absence of an electrocardiogram[40,49] (*see* Figs. 4.2C and 4.11).

x′ Descent

This is the major fall in atrial pressure in systole and is caused by RV contraction pulling on the closed tricuspid valve and ring.[26,40]

Its presence requires:

1. *A good RV systolic function*
2. *An intact tricuspid valve*

In fact, *a good and dominant x′ descent in the jugulars indicates good RV systolic function.* The flow velocity peak in the jugulars during the ***x′ descent*** is always dominant (*see* Figs. 4.2C and 4.7D). When there is RV systolic dysfunction, the ***x′ descent*** gets diminished and eventually may become totally absent when RV function becomes poor. *In pulmonary hypertension,*

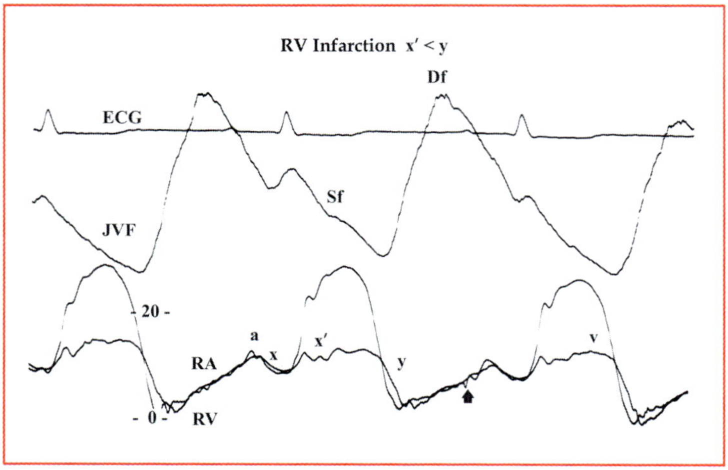

Fig. 4.11: Simultaneous recordings of jugular venous flow (JVF) velocity and right ventricular (RV) and right atrial (RA) pressures from a patient with RV infarction. Note the prolonged PR interval on ECG. Due to RV infarction, the RV contractility is poor and the ***x′ descent*** is also poor. The ***x descent*** is well separated from the ***x′ descent*** due to the long PR. Note the atrial relaxation flow on JVF corresponding to ***x descent***. The ***y descent*** is dominant and so is the corresponding Df in JVF. Small arrow indicates pre a wave pressure.

during the late stages when decompensation sets in, the x′ descent becomes diminished and eventually becomes lost (Figs. 4.12 and 4.13).[41] In acute left ventricular failure such as caused by acute myocardial infarction, the RV function may be still good as indicated by the presence of a good ***x′ descent.*** In patients with cardiomyopathy with poor ventricular function if the ***x′ descent*** is still preserved it would indicate sparing of the RV as might be the case in ischemic cardiomyopathy.[49]

While mild-to-moderate degrees of tricuspid regurgitation with normal RV systolic pressure (usually <25 mm Hg) could still be consistent with the presence of a preserved ***x′ descent,*** more than moderate degrees of tricuspid regurgitation particularly in the presence of elevated RV systolic pressure is incompatible with a well preserved ***x′ descent. Significant degrees of tricuspid regurgitation*** would clearly lead to early buildup of RA pressure and therefore counteract or ***abolish the x′ descent.*** The loss of ***x′ descent*** and early buildup of the ***large amplitude v wave*** (sometimes termed the ***"cv" wave***) followed by the diastolic ***y descent*** are characteristic of significant tricuspid regurgitation (*see* Fig. 4.7G). The ***v wave*** of tricuspid regurgitation is characteristically associated with systolic flow reversal in the jugulars. The ***v wave*** in the right atrium is clearly in such cases due to the actual regurgitant flow into the atrium. Because of its large amplitude of rise together with retrograde flow into the jugulars, *it can be recognized from a distance in the jugulars, as the large v wave ascent followed by the y descent that can be timed. The*

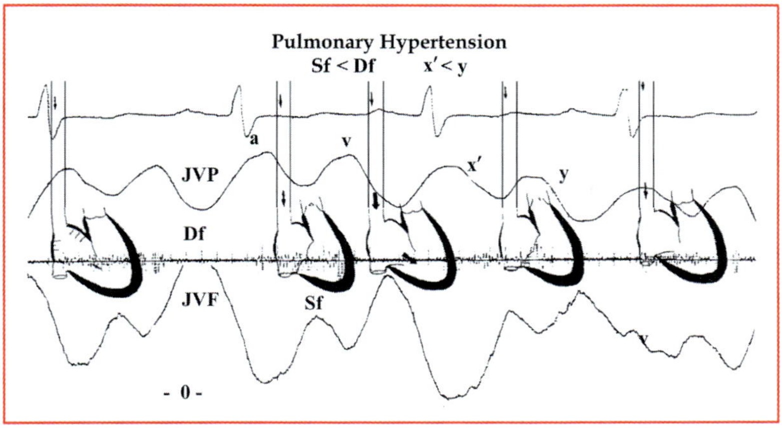

Fig. 4.12: Jugular venous pulse (JVP) and jugular venous flow (JVF) velocity recordings from a patient with pulmonary hypertension in a decompensated state. Note the more prominent ***y descent*** compared to the ***x′ descent*** in the JVP. It corresponds to the dominant diastolic flow (Df) compared to the systolic flow (Sf). The added diagrams of the heart help explain the pathophysiology of the JVP contour abnormality. Thickness of arrows refers to flow velocities.

Source: Modified and reprinted from Ranganathan et al. Abnormalities in Jugular venous flow velocity in pulmonary hypertension. Am J Cardiol. 1989;63:719-24. Copyright (2005) with permission from Excerpta Medica Inc.

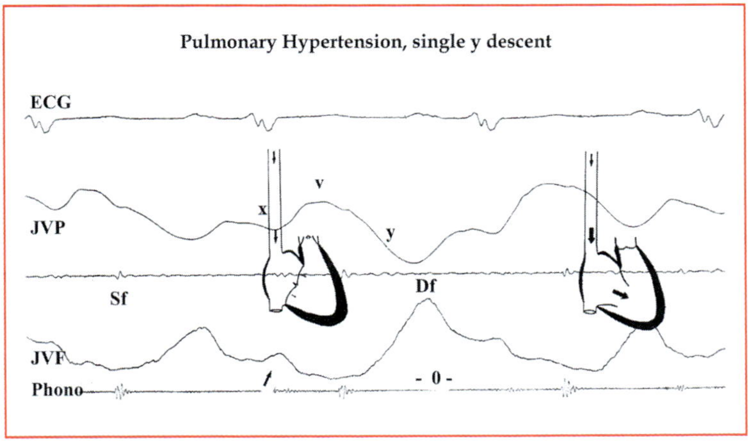

Fig. 4.13: Jugular venous pulse recording from a patient with right ventricular (RV) decompensation with pulmonary hypertension secondary to significant mitral regurgitation associated with ischemic heart disease. Note the ***x descent*** and the corresponding atrial relaxation flow (arrow). The ***x′ descent*** cannot be seen and there is a prominent ***y descent*** and a corresponding Df. There may be mild tricuspid regurgitation but not enough to overcome the buffering effect of the right atrium (RA) and no systolic retrograde flow can be seen on the jugular venous flow (JVF). The JVF tracing does not fall below the zero flow line. Diagrams have been added to explain the pathophysiology of the flow pattern.

Source: Modified and reprinted from Ranganathan et al. Abnormalities in Jugular venous flow velocity in pulmonary hypertension. Am J Cardiol. 1989;63:719-24. Copyright (2005) with permission from Excerpta Medica Inc.

rise will be systolic and can be timed with the radial pulse. Unlike the a wave, it tends to last longer, and much longer than the duration of the arterial pulse.[40]

The lack of atrial contraction in atrial fibrillation leads to a decrease in Starling effect on the ventricle. This leads to a decrease in ventricular contraction and function causing ***a diminished x′ descent*** (*see* Fig. 4.3). In recent onset atrial fibrillation with preserved RV function, the ***x′ descent*** may be still recognized in the jugulars. However in long-standing atrial fibrillation, the ***x′ descent*** tends to be absent due to coexisting RV dysfunction and some degree of tricuspid regurgitation.

Very rarely in patients with severe mitral regurgitation, the interatrial septum may be seen to bulge into the right atrium during systole. This would tend to diminish the full effect of the descent of the base on the right atrium. This decreases the ***x′ descent*** (systolic flow). This effect is termed the ***Bernheim effect*** on the atrial septum[9,40,49,51] (Figs. 4.14 and 4.15; Table 4.1).

v Wave

The ***v wave*** rise in the RA pressure in the absence of significant tricuspid regurgitation is almost always *due to venous filling of the right atrium in later part of systole* whether the actual pressure is normal or high. The normal right atrium being a capacitance chamber has good distensibility. The venous inflow from the venae cavae augmented by the ***x′ descent*** tends to build up

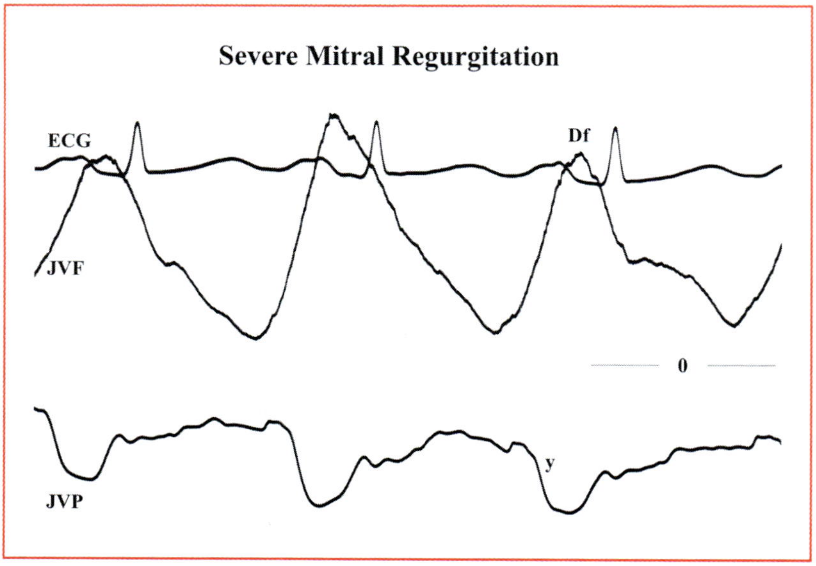

Fig. 4.14: Recordings from a patient with severe mitral regurgitation. Single diastolic flow (Df) in the jugular venous flow (JVF) velocity, corresponding to a single ***y descent*** on the jugular venous pulse (JVP). This is due to Bernheim effect.

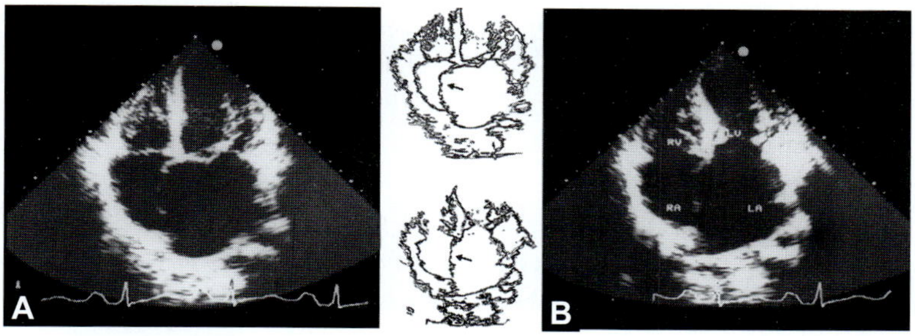

Figs. 4.15A and B: Four-chamber views of the two-dimensional echocardiograms from the same patient with severe mitral regurgitation with freeze frames in systole (A) and diastole (B) together with their line diagrams. In systole (A) indicated by the closed mitral and the tricuspid valves, the bulge of the interatrial septum into the right atrium (RA) decreasing the volume in RA is well seen. In diastole (B) as shown by the open mitral and tricuspid valves, the interatrial septum is more straight and the right atrial dimension is larger (*see* the text).

Table 4.1: Causes of decreased x′ descent.

Decreased x′ descent
Diminished right ventricular contraction
Right ventricular failure in pulmonary hypertension
Postcardiac surgery RV damage
Right ventricular infarction
Atrial fibrillation due to loss of Starling effect
Bernheim effect in severe mitral regurgitation*

*rare occurrence

a pressure that is often quite low not exceeding 5 mm Hg. In children, the circulation is rapid due to high sympathetic tone and the rapid venous inflow coming into an atrium, which is relatively small, could build up a relatively good ***v wave*** pressure. Rapid circulatory states with high sympathetic tone may also exist in conditions such as pregnancy, thyrotoxicosis and anemia[19] that also favor buildup of relatively high ***v waves.*** In pregnancy, in addition the blood volume is usually expanded. Hypervolemia, however, caused could raise the ***v wave*** pressure. Occasionally in some patients with atrial septal defect, the extra source of venous return from the left atrium across the defect together with some changes in RA distensibility could also lead to a higher than normal ***v wave*** pressure.[14,17,24]

Since the pre a wave pressure sets the baseline over which the a wave and the v wave build up naturally occur, the most common reason for pathologically high v wave pressure is an elevated high pre a wave pressure. The reason for this has been discussed previously. These include conditions such as pericardial effusion with any degree of restriction, constrictive pericarditis, pulmonary hypertension with elevated RV diastolic pressure, ischemia and/or infarcted right ventricle and cardiomyopathy. *For any given degree of elevation of pre a wave pressure and right atrial distensibility, any rise in venous tone (sympathetic tone) will allow a much further rise in the jugular v wave.*

In the jugulars, the v wave can be inferred to be present whenever a y descent is recognized. The ***v wave*** is the wave preceding the ***y descent,*** which can be timed to be diastolic. Normal ***v wave*** is not usually seen in the jugulars in the adult as recognized by the fact that the ***y descent*** is absent. *The rise of even an abnormal and elevated v wave (e.g. heart failure, constrictive pericarditis) is not usually as prominent to the observer's eyes as the fall of the y descent that follows it. The reason for this is an absence of any flow reversal in the jugulars under these conditions.* This is in contrast to the ***v wave*** of tricuspid regurgitation that always causes systolic flow reversal[40] (*see* Figs. 4.7G and 4.11).

The v waves have a larger duration and therefore when elevated are associated with higher mean right atrial pressure. Normally on inspiration, the intrathoracic pressure falls leading to an increase in the venous return. The right atrium being an intrathoracic structure is also influenced by the fall in intrathoracic pressure. In addition, the capacitance function of the right heart accommodates for the increased venous return without a rise in the RA pressure. In fact, inspiration leads to a fall in the RA pressure reflecting the fall in intrathoracic pressure. However, sometimes the RA and therefore the jugular venous pressure may actually rise with inspiration. This is termed the *Kussmaul's sign.*[20,21,52] *This sign may be identified by the fact that the v wave is more prominent during inspiration. The latter may be recognized by the inspiratory augmentation of the y descent. The Kussmaul's sign is generally indicative of decreased compliance of the right heart and/or its surrounding structures.* Thus it may be seen in a variety of conditions including heart failure, restrictive pericardial pathology with or without effusion and occasionally thoracic deformities such as kyphoscoliosis.

y Descent

The ***y descent*** being the fall in the RA pressure in diastole immediately following the opening of the tricuspid valve ***requires*** that the RV pressure in fact falls close to zero as it does normally with the early rapid filling phase of diastole. In other words, *the ventricle should not have any restriction during this early rapid filling phase of diastole,* even if it does have restriction during the later phases of diastole. This automatically excludes cardiac tamponade that implies total diastolic restriction due to high fluid pressure in the pericardial sac that allows very little or no expansion of the ventricle during diastole.

The steepness of the y descent will depend on the v wave pressure head that is present at the time of the tricuspid valve opening. The higher ***the v wave*** pressure head, the steeper and more prominent is the ***y descent,*** assuming of course that there is no tricuspid obstruction as in tricuspid stenosis (*see* Fig. 4.11). The latter condition is very rare and if it should be significant it could be expected to slow the ***y descent.***[18]

The normal ***v wave*** pressure being small, the ***y descent*** is usually not very prominent (*see* Fig. 4.8). The corresponding diastolic flow velocity in the jugulars is also slow and low. Although the small ***y descent*** may be seen in the RA pressure pulse, it is not usually seen in the jugular venous pulse. This is due to ***the capacitance function of the normal right atrium.*** The reservoir function of the atrium is such that it is able to empty into the ventricle without the top of the column actually falling much. When the right atrium gets stiff and behaves like a conduit as in postcardiac surgery patients, who have had their right atrium cannulated during surgery and therefore traumatized, this capacitance function is lost. In these patients, even the normal ***v wave*** pressure allows recognition of the ***y descent*** in the jugulars.[17,29,42,53]

Exaggerated y Descent

The ***y descent gets*** exaggerated when there is:

1. *An increased v wave pressure head*
2. *No restriction to ventricular filling during the early rapid filling phase of diastole*

This mechanism necessarily excludes cardiac tamponade, in which condition ventricular filling is restricted throughout diastole including the early rapid filling phase, despite the high ***v wave*** pressure.

Both of these conditions, namely increased ***v wave*** pressure head and absence of restriction to filling during rapid filling phase, are met under the following circumstances (Table 4.2):

1. *High sympathetic tone with rapid circulation as in children and young adults, anxiety, anemia, pregnancy, thyrotoxicosis, Paget's disease and other similar conditions*
2. *Hypervolemia as in renal failure, following rapid and large fluid infusion and pregnancy*
3. *Extra source of venous filling as in some patients with atrial septal defect as mentioned under v wave*
4. *Pericardial effusion with some restriction but without tamponade*
5. *Constrictive pericarditis that restricts expansion of RV due to thickened or sometimes calcified pericardium (Figs. 4.16 and 4.17)*
6. *Pulmonary hypertension with elevated RV diastolic pressure (see Fig. 4.12)*
7. *Ischemic or infarcted RV with elevated RV diastolic pressures (see Fig. 4.11)*
8. *Cardiomyopathy with elevated RV diastolic pressures*

Table 4.2: Causes of exaggerated y descent.
Increased ***v wave*** pressure head with NO restriction to ventricular filling during rapid filling phase
High sympathetic tone as in young children, anxiety, anemia, pregnancy, thyrotoxicosis
Hypervolemia
Extrasource of venous filling as in atrial septal defect
Pericardial effusion with some restriction
Constrictive pericarditis
Pulmonary hypertension with elevated right ventricular (RV) diastolic pressure
Ischemic and/or Infarcted RV
Cardiomyopathy
Excludes cardiac tamponade
Decreased right atrial capacitance function
Post-cardiac surgery
Bernheim effect in severe mitral regurgitation*

*Rare occurrence.

In the rare patient with severe mitral regurgitation and atrial Bernheim effect, an exaggerated ***y descent*** without elevation of the ***v wave*** pressure may occur. This is explainable by the sudden emptying of the left atrium during early diastole that causes a quick reversal of the systolic bulge of the interatrial septum.[47]

The *y descent is easily identifiable in the jugulars by its timing in diastole being out of phase with the radial arterial pulse. It can be considered exaggerated when it is equal to the x′ descent in its prominence or when it becomes more dominant compared to the x′ descent and also when it is the only descent present.*

ABNORMAL JUGULAR VENOUS PULSE CONTOURS AS RELATED TO ABNORMAL JVF VELOCITY PATTERNS

Studies from our laboratory using Doppler JVF velocity recordings and their correlation to right heart hemodynamics had established that when the forward flow velocity patterns in the jugulars lose their normal systolic dominance, they can be termed abnormal.[40,47] The flow velocity patterns of ***Sf = Df, Sf < Df and Df alone*** are abnormal forward flow velocity patterns. These correspond to the RA and the jugular venous pulse contours of ***x′ = y descent, x′ < y descent and single y descent.*** Decrease in peak ***Sf*** would imply ***decreased RV contractility (decreased x′).*** Increase in ***Df*** velocity would

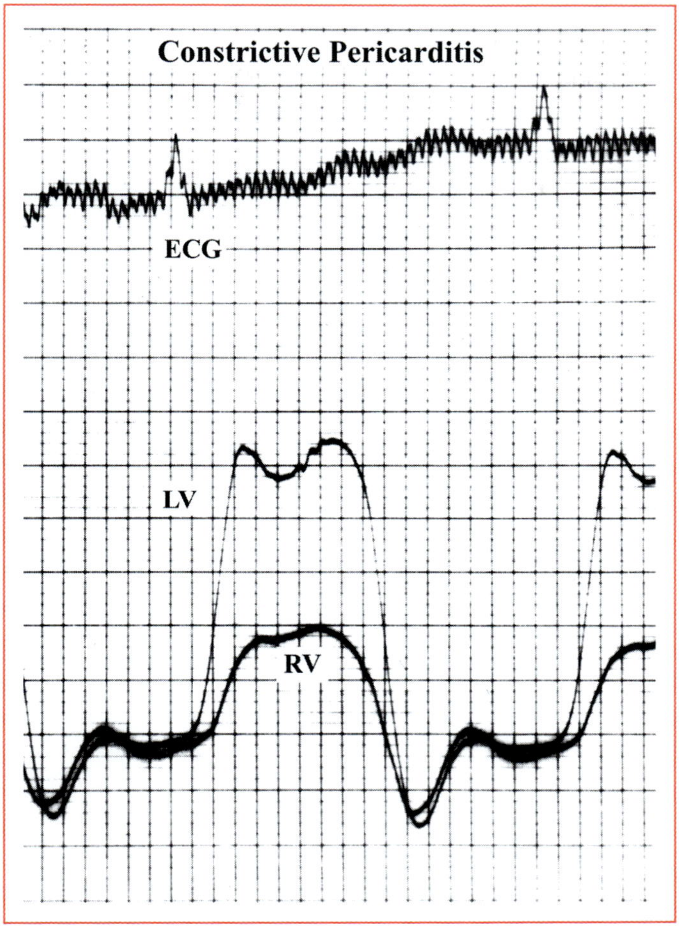

Fig. 4.16: Simultaneous recordings of the left ventricular (LV) and the right ventricular (RV) pressures from a patient with constrictive pericarditis showing the equalization of the diastolic pressures between the two sides with the typical dip followed by the plateau pattern.

imply increased ***v wave*** pressure head without restriction to forward flow in early diastole. This greater pressure gradient would cause faster emptying of the right atrial. This would be reflected in the jugulars as a greater diastolic forward flow velocity ***(increased y descent).***

Mechanism of Abnormal JVF Patterns and Contours in Pulmonary Hypertension

The majority of patients with abnormal flow patterns and pulmonary hypertension had increased RA ***v wave*** pressure implying that the Df velocity was increased (exaggerated ***y descent***). The increased ***v wave*** pressure was shown to be due to an increased RV early diastolic and ***pre a wave***

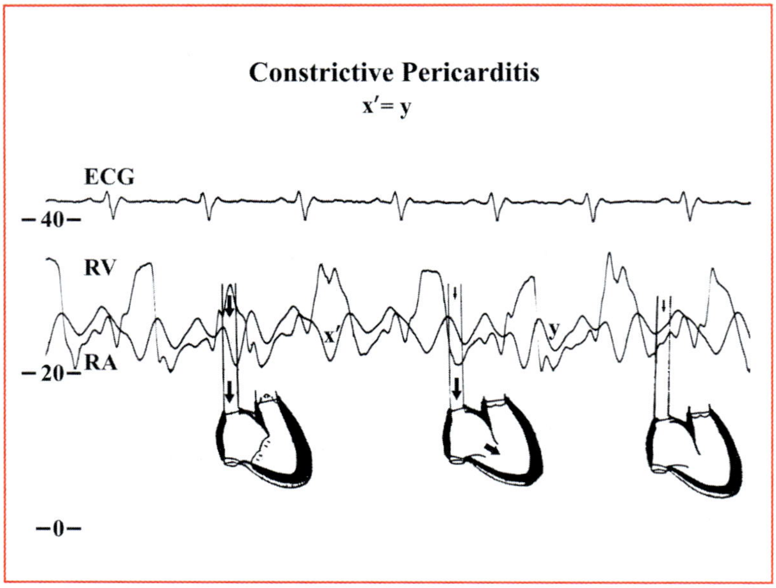

Fig. 4.17: Simultaneous right ventricular (RV) and right atrial (RA) pressures in a patient with constrictive pericarditis. Note the high RA and RV diastolic pressures. On the RA pressure tracings both the ***x′*** and the ***y descents*** are equally prominent and this would also be reflected in the Jugular pulse contour. The added diagrams explain the pathophysiology. The first shows the x′ descent, the second the ***y descent*** and the third the pre a wave period.

pressure. The incidence of congestive heart failure was higher in patients with Sf < Df and Df alone compared to the pattern where Sf = Df. This indicated that decreased RV systolic function (decreased ***x′ descent***) also played a part. This seems to be a later phenomenon in serial observations[41] (Fig. 4.18).

Mechanism of Abnormal JVF Patterns and Jugular Pulse Contours in Postcardiac Surgery Patients

In most patients who had undergone cardiopulmonary bypass, the altered flow velocity patterns are not associated with alterations in right heart pressures. Postoperatively, the right atrium seems to behave as a conduit rather than a capacitance chamber. Its capacitance function may be attenuated initially due to edema and later on probably due to stiffness caused by scarring. The loss of buffering function of the atrium as a capacitance chamber leads to full reflection of the diastolic flow velocity at the tricuspid valve to the superior vena cava and the jugulars thus exaggerating the ***y descent*** (Fig. 4.19).

When the flow velocity pattern was Sf < Df ***(x′ = y descent),*** RV dysfunction and decreased ejection fraction was demonstrated[42] (Fig. 4.20).

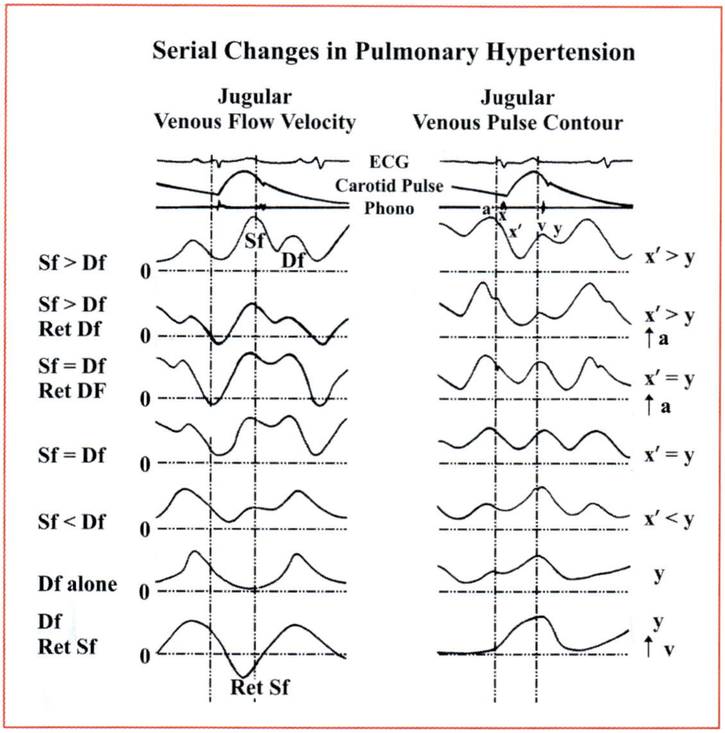

Fig. 4.18: Diagrammatic representation of the serial changes observed over time in the jugular venous pulse contour and the corresponding jugular venous flow patterns in pulmonary hypertension as the right ventricle (RV) begins to decompensate.
Source: Modified and reprinted from Ranganathan et al. Abnormalities in Jugular venous flow velocity in pulmonary hypertension. Am J Cardiol. 1989;63:719-24. Copyright (2005) with permission from Excerpta Medica Inc.

Mechanism of Abnormal JVF Patterns and Jugular Pulse Contours in Restriction to Ventricular Filling

Restriction to ventricular filling may vary in degree and may be pericardial, myocardial or endocardial in origin. Restriction in its mild form may be apparent only at the end of diastole during the atrial contraction phase. It may involve both mid- and late-diastole when more severe and when very severe, it may involve almost all phases of diastole beginning with the rapid filling phase (Fig. 4.21).

Late Diastolic Restriction

If the restriction is limited to late diastole, the only abnormality seen in right heart hemodynamics will be elevation of right atrial ***a wave*** pressure. This will be reflected in the jugular venous pulse as a prominent ***a wave*** ***(see Fig. 4.10).***

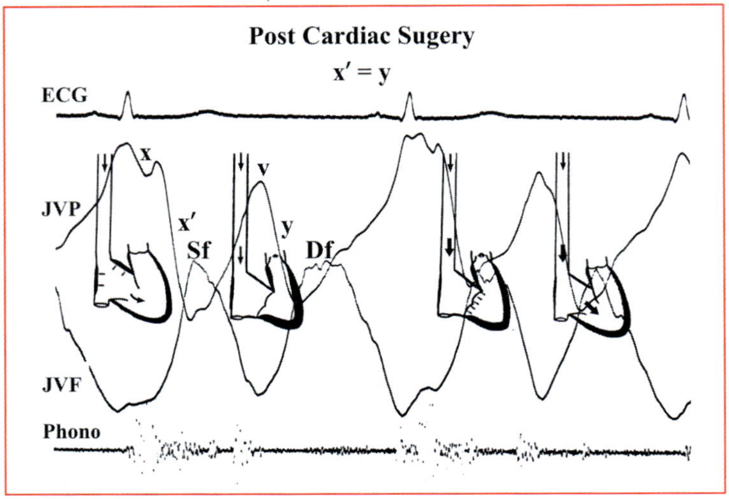

Fig. 4.19: Simultaneous jugular venous pulse (JVP), the jugular venous flow velocity (JVF), phonocardiogram and ECG in a postcardiac surgery patient showing equal ***x′*** and ***y descents***. This is an abnormal JVP contour. Superimposed diagrams help explain the pathophysiology. The right atrium (RA) rather than acting as a capacitance chamber acts only as a conduit. The size of the arrows indicating flow at the tricuspid valve and at the SVC during early diastole is equal to indicate this.
Source: Reprinted from Ranganathan et al. Changes in Jugular venous flow velocity after coronary artery bypass grafting. Am J Cardiol. 1989;63:725-9. Copyright (2005) with permission from Excerpta Medica Inc.

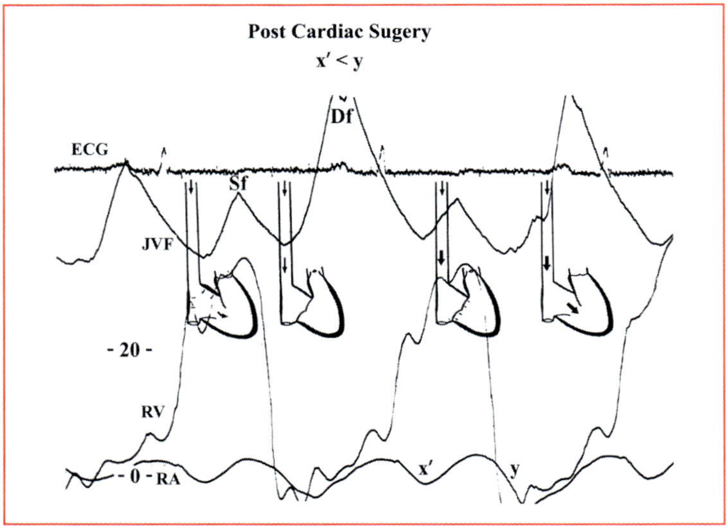

Fig. 4.20: Simultaneous recordings of ECG, jugular venous flow (JVF) velocity and the right atrial (RA) and the right ventricular (RV) pressures in a postcardiac surgery patient. The ***y descent*** on the RA pressure is more prominent than the ***x′ descent***, with the corresponding dominant diastolic flow (Df) peak in JVF.

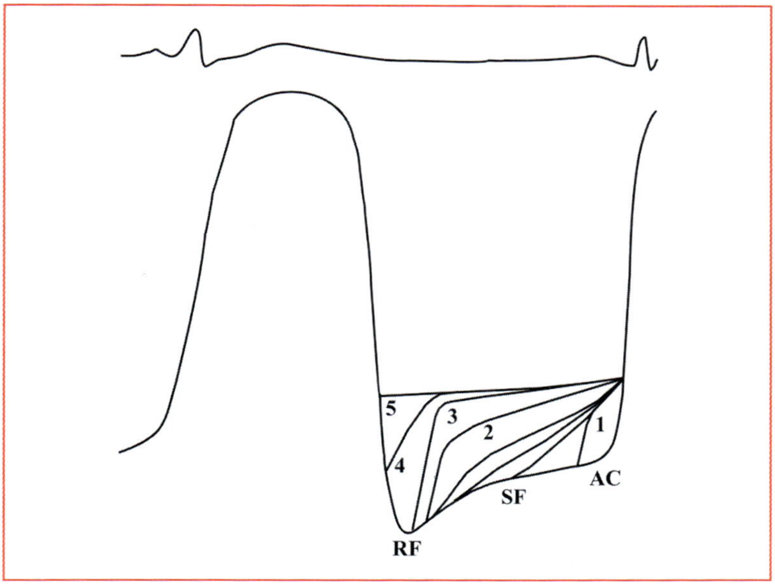

Fig. 4.21: The varying severity of restriction to diastolic ventricular filling is shown with lines to indicate the ventricular diastolic pressure elevations and their timing in diastole. In mild form, the pressure increase is during atrial contraction (AC) at end diastole (line 1). As restriction gets worse the ***pre a wave*** pressure starts to rise gradually and earlier and earlier in diastole. This progression is shown as four successive lines (lines 2). When severe, it may be total during mid- and late-diastole restricting flow into the right ventricle (RV) beginning with the slow filling phase (SF). There will be very rapid inflow only during early diastole or the rapid filling phase (RF) followed by a rapid rise in pressure with no further flow producing the classic dip and plateau or the square root pattern (line 3). This is typical for chronic constrictive pericarditis. If the restriction is severe and involves also the RF phase, the pressures rise quickly in the RV in early diastole limiting inflow altogether. This can occur in severe pericardial effusion leading to cardiac tamponade where the high intrapericardial pressure will limit ventricular expansion altogether. Line 4 depicts pre tamponade and line 5 is full tamponade with no diastolic inflow possible. Such severe elevations in diastolic pressures may rarely also occur in severe cardiomyopathy, cardiac failure and in some patients with severe right ventricular infarctions.

Mid- and Late-Diastolic Restriction

When restriction to ventricular filling encroaches more and more into mid-to-early diastole, elevation of all RV diastolic pressures would result and lead to elevations of both mean RA and ***v wave*** pressures. The increased ***v wave*** pressure-head during early diastole will lead to augmented Df (exaggerated ***y descent***). As long as ventricular function is preserved, the increased Df will equal Sf ***(x′ = y).*** In contrast, patients with myocardial dysfunction and diminished contractility will have flow patterns of Sf < Df and jugular contours of ***x′*** < ***y*** (*see* Figs. 4.4 and 4.5).

Total Diastolic Restriction

When restriction is severe and occurs throughout diastole as in tamponade, no inflow can occur into the atrium during this phase. This totally abolishes diastolic flow into the atrium. In cardiac tamponade, the four chambers of the heart are boxed within a pericardial sac under high fluid pressure. During diastole no new blood can enter the heart but blood is shifted from the atrium to the ventricle with the total volume in the boxed four chambers constant. Only time new blood can enter the heart when blood leaves this enclosed box namely during systole. Patients with tamponade, therefore, exhibit inflow only during ventricular systole, when the ventricular size is the smallest, thus allowing some expansion and filling of the atrium within the pericardial sac[47] (Fig. 4.22).

Jugular flow recordings in patients with cardiac tamponade are extremely hard to obtain due to diminished flow velocity. Thus, the only recordable forward flow would occur in systole and only during inspiration with a corresponding ***x′* descent** in the jugular pulse.[40,44] *Jugulars distend in tamponade and hardly show any descent.* If at all a descent is recognizable it will be an *x′* and may be seen only during inspiration. Usually, the venous pressure is so high that the pulsation at the top of the column would be higher than the angle of the jaw. Therefore, the pulsations cannot be seen, but flow may be recorded by Doppler to show single systolic flow. *In fact, the occurrence of a steep Y descent in patients with pericardial effusion excludes tamponade.*

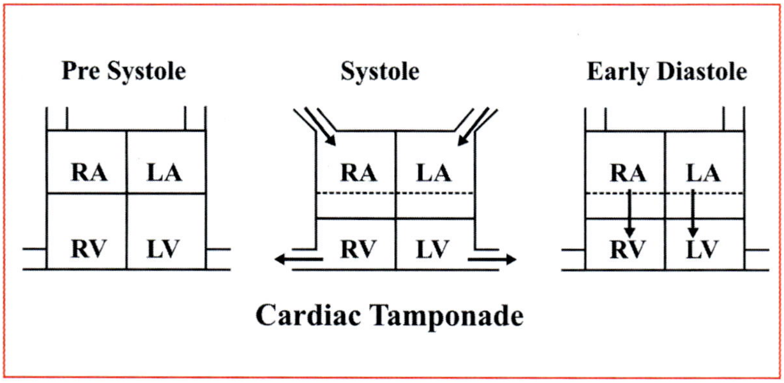

Fig. 4.22: A diagrammatic representation of the pathophysiology of the cardiac inflow and outflow in cardiac tamponade. The extracardiac pressure is so high that the heart is as if encased in a solid box at all times. The only time flow into this "box" can occur is when blood leaves the "box." This occurs during ***systole*** as blood is ejected out of the ventricles. Flow into the heart (atria) can occur only at that time (the middle diagram). In ***early diastole***, the blood is shifted from the atria into the ventricles but new blood cannot enter the heart.

If the RV filling pressures are severely elevated even in the early rapid filling phase as might happen in rare instances of constrictive pericarditis and severe cardiomyopathy, poor diastolic inflow (and correspondingly poor ***y descent***) will result despite high RA mean and ***v wave*** pressures for the simple reason that there is not enough pressure difference between the RA and RV during the early rapid filling phase. If this should happen in constrictive pericarditis, it would be accompanied by good Sf (and a corresponding ***x′ descent***),[16] whereas in cardiomyopathy, such a severe elevation of filling pressures would be associated with poor RV systolic function and therefore poor ***x′ descent.***

ABNORMAL JUGULAR CONTOURS

Double Descents in the Jugular Venous Pulse

If two descents are visible in the jugular venous pulse for each cardiac cycle, it is usually due to the x′ and the y descents unless the x descent is far separated from the x′ descent as with long PR intervals. The wave preceding the ***x′ descent*** is the ***a wave*** during sinus rhythm and the wave preceding the ***y descent*** is the ***v wave.*** In cases where double descents ***(x′ and y)*** are noted, the relative dominance of the ***x′*** versus ***y*** (systolic versus diastolic descent) will easily help in identifying the flow pattern.

The relative dominance of x′ and y descents as with relative dominance of the flow velocities are not volume dependent (Figs. 4.23A and B).[47] Therefore, even when the patients had received therapy such as diuretics with consequent fall in venous pressure, the relationship is unaltered and therefore still useful in assessment of the patient. *In the adult, it must be emphasized that it is uncommon to see both descents in the jugular venous pulse. Double descents where x′ is still dominant would generally imply that the y descent is exaggerated. Double descents where x′ = y or x′ < y generally arise either because x′ descent is decreased or the y descent is exaggerated or both, similar to the corresponding flow velocity peaks.*

Causes of decreased x′ descent as well as causes of exaggerated y descents are shown in Tables 4.1 and 4.2. Consideration of these in any given individual situation will usually help in the delineation of the problem.

Differential Diagnosis of Double Descents

A schema for the differential diagnosis and the significance of the double descents is shown in Table 4.3, both in the presence and the absence of pulmonary hypertension.

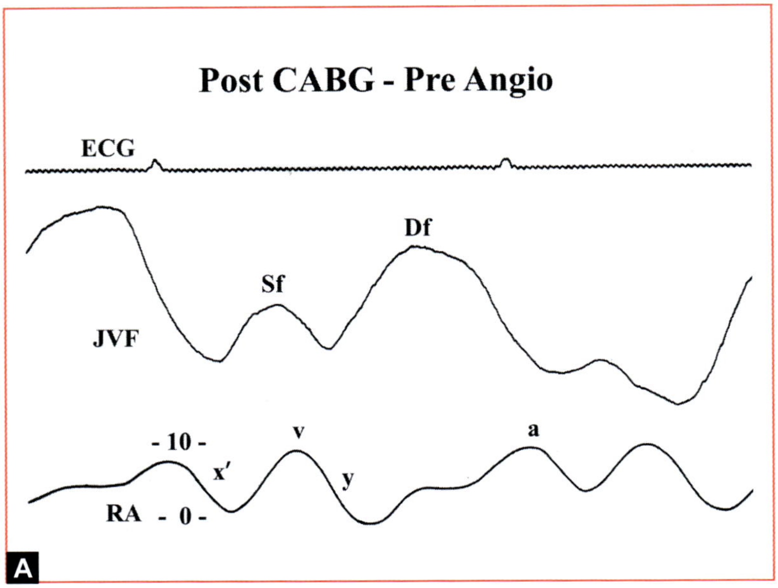

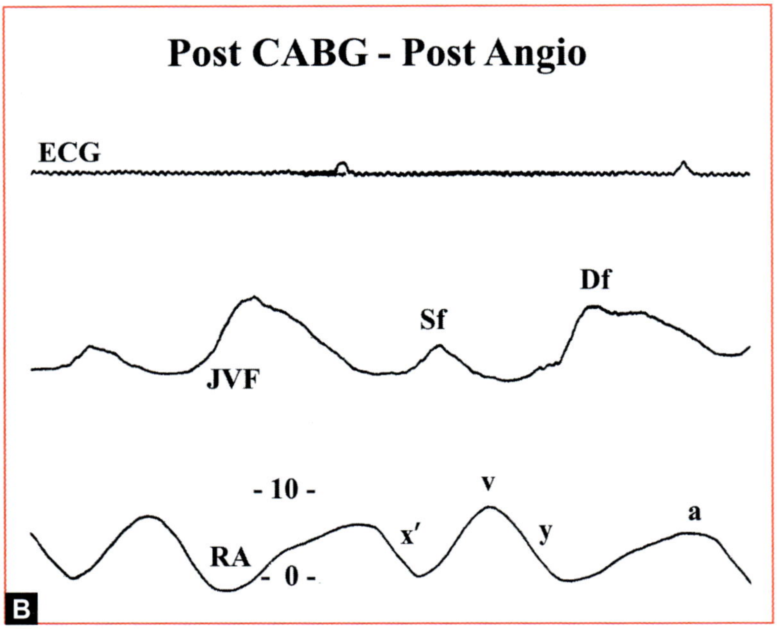

Figs. 4.23A and B: (A) Simultaneous recordings of right atrial (RA) pressure and jugular venous flow (JVF) velocity in a patient who has had coronary artery bypass grafting (CABG) taken before left ventricular angiogram. In this patient, the JVF pattern is Sf < Df and the corresponding RA pressure tracing shows ***x′* < *y***. This tends to indicate some damage to the right ventricle (RV). (B) Similar recordings in the same patient as in (A) postangiogram. The contrast material used for the angiogram presents an osmotic load and increases blood volume. This did not change the ***Sf* < *Df*** or ***x′* < *y*** relationship. This relationship is maintained despite the patient's level of hydration, thus rendering a useful means of assessing RV function.

Table 4.3: Differential diagnosis of double descents in jugular venous pulse.

In pulmonary hypertension	*In the absence of pulmonary hypertension*
x′ > y: Indicates good right ventricular (RV) function	
Compensated RV Function	Normal young adult
With increased ***a wave***	Hypervolemia
	Increased sympathetic tone
	Early pericardial effusion
	Extrasource of venous return, e.g. ASD
x′ = y: Increased v wave pressure with NO restriction to rapid filling	
Early RV decompensation	Pericardial effusion
	Constrictive pericarditis with good myocardial function
	Early/or mild RV infarction
	Early cardiomyopathy
	Postcardiac surgery due to decreased right atrial and capacitance
x′<y: Indicates decreased RV Function	
RV failure	Late stage of constriction
Mild tricuspid regurgitation	RV infarction
	Cardiomyopathy
	Post-cardiac surgery (RV damage)

With Pulmonary Hypertension

In patients with pulmonary hypertension, *the jugular pulse showing only an x′ or a dominant x′ descent would imply a compensated RV function*. In addition, if the wave preceding the ***x′ descent*** is large and rising fast, this would indicate a strong atrial contraction causing reversal of flow in end-diastole implying decreased RV compliance (Fig. 4.10 and Fig. 4.24).

If the pulmonary hypertension is severe and of long duration, the jugular pulse will change to the pattern x′ = y descent. This would imply raised RV pre a wave ***pressure*** and a secondary rise in RA and jugular v wave pressure.

With progression of pulmonary hypertension, the pattern ***x′ < y will emerge (see Fig. 4.12).*** At this stage, the RV contractility is significantly reduced and RV failure has begun.[41] Eventually RV dilatation and tricuspid regurgitation together with RV failure lead to markedly diminished or even absent ***x′ descent*** and *emergence of single dominant y descent (see Fig. 4.13 and Table 4.3).*

If the wave preceding the ***y descent*** is large and its rate of rise is prominent (the ***"cv" wave***) it would indicate systolic flow reversal of tricuspid regurgitation.

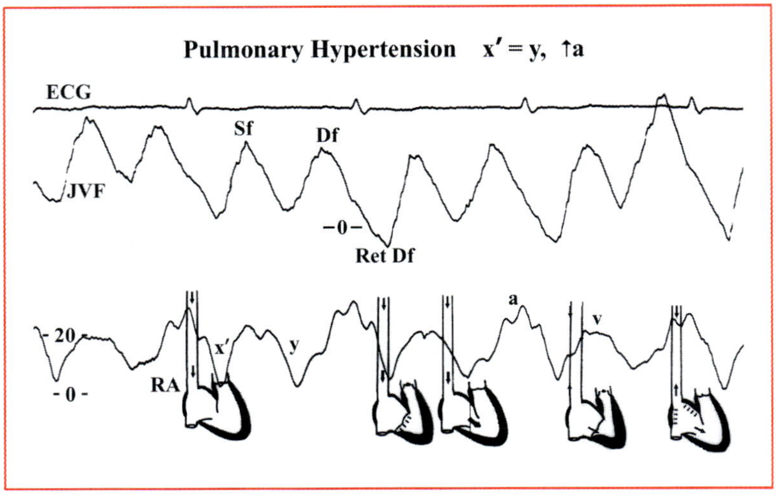

Fig. 4.24: Simultaneous recordings of ECG, jugular venous flow (JVF) velocity and right atrial (RA) pressure in a patient with pulmonary hypertension. Superimposed diagrams depict the altered pathophysiology at different phases of the cardiac cycle. The systolic and the diastolic flow peaks (Sf = Df) are equal with the corresponding RA pressure showing ***x′ = y descents***. While the right ventricular (RV) systolic function is still preserved (good x′ descent), the raised diastolic pressures in the RV secondary to RV hypertrophy and decreased diastolic compliance causes elevated RA ***v wave*** pressure, which leads to a prominent ***y descent***. The strong contraction of the RA causes also a prominent ***a wave*** (retrograde end-diastolic flow (Ret Df) in the JVF)

During this progression, before significant tricuspid regurgitation develops, the prominent ***a wave*** may in fact disappear due to deteriorating right atrial function.

Without Pulmonary Hypertension

In the absence of pulmonary hypertension also, the pattern of ***x′ > y implies normal right ventricular function.*** This can be seen in some of the conditions that lead to an exaggeration of the ***y descent*** such as the first four causes in Table 4.2.

In the absence of pulmonary hypertension ***x′ = y can be seen in:***

1. *Pericardial effusion*
2. *Constrictive pericarditis with good myocardial function*
3. *Early and mild right ventricular infarction*
4. *Early cardiomyopathy*
5. *Some patients with atrial septal defect.*

This pattern is not uncommon in the postcardiac surgery patients. It is seen less often in the current period perhaps due to improved surgical techniques. It may develop quite early after the pump run and may even persist for the life of the patient.

The dominant y descent (x' < y) pattern with or without pulmonary hypertension implies right ventricular dysfunction. In postcardiac surgery patients, this pattern is less common and would imply right ventricular damage. The pattern if noted in constrictive pericarditis implies a *late stage of constriction with myocardial dysfunction. In the presence of acute inferior infarction, this jugular pulse contour would imply right ventricular involvement.*[30] *The dominant y descent pattern is not usually seen in pure left ventricular failure of acute myocardial infarction.*

Venous Pulse Contour in Atrial Septal Defect

In adult patients with atrial septal defect, although the ***y descent*** may be visible, the ***x' descent*** remains dominant. This is due to the fact that the RV volume overload provides a strong Starling effect augmenting its contraction (Fig. 4.25). In some adult patients with atrial septal defect, the pattern of ***x' = y descent*** may be observed. This is usually due to large defects with equalization of the right atrial and the left atrial pressures with elevated RV diastolic pressures.

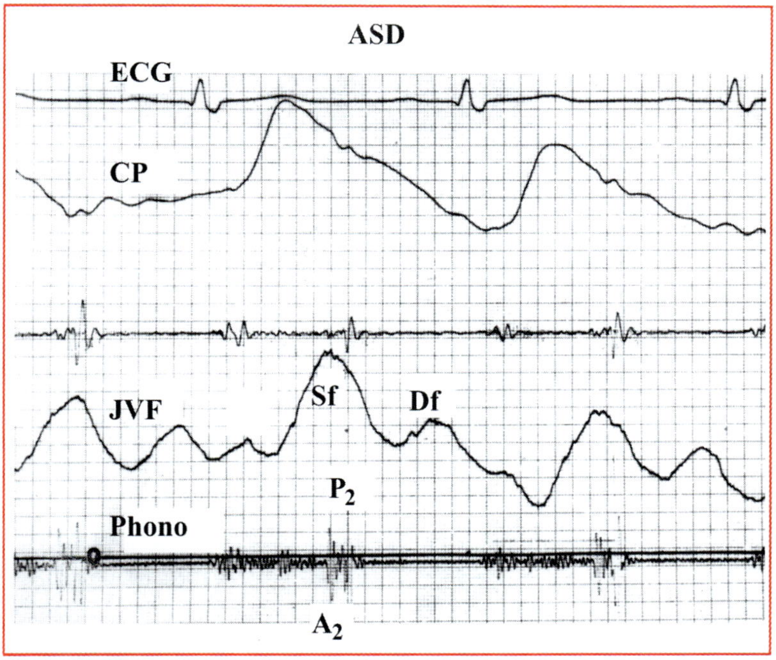

Fig. 4.25: Simultaneous recordings of ECG, carotid pulse (CP), phonocardiogram (Phono) and Jugular Venous Flow Velocity (JVF) in a patient with Atrial Septal Defect (ASD). Note the splitting of S2 (A2 and P2). The important fact is that the ***Sf > Df*** flow pattern is maintained in ASD despite increased venous return to the right heart (double source of blood—normal venous return plus shunt flow).

Venous Pulse Contour in Constrictive Pericarditis

The elevated venous pressure with ***the sharp y descent*** and deep "***y*** trough" in constrictive pericarditis has been known as ***the diastolic collapse of Friedreich*** for over a century.[20] However, ***atypical cases*** some with rapidly evolving "constrictive pericarditis" have been described that show ***only a dominant x′ descent*** despite high venous pressure.[16,54] As expected in these patients, the RV early diastolic pressure was quite high with very little pressure difference between the right atrium and the right ventricle at the time of tricuspid valve opening to account for the lack of a good ***y descent.*** This would be almost a ***hemodynamic imitation of tamponade*** to the extent that the restriction to ventricular filling also involved the early rapid filling phase.

Such a high elevation of early diastolic RV pressures in the absence of true extrinsic compression as in tamponade would imply poor systolic emptying of the right ventricle and decreased right ventricular systolic function (*see* Figs. 4.4, 4.5, 4.16 and 4.17). Rarely such a situation could occur in severe cardiomyopathy. Such patients have poor ***x′ descent.*** In fact, *in patients with severe cardiomyopathy, preservation of a good x′ descent would imply an ischemic etiology involving predominantly the left ventricle (Fig. 4.26).*

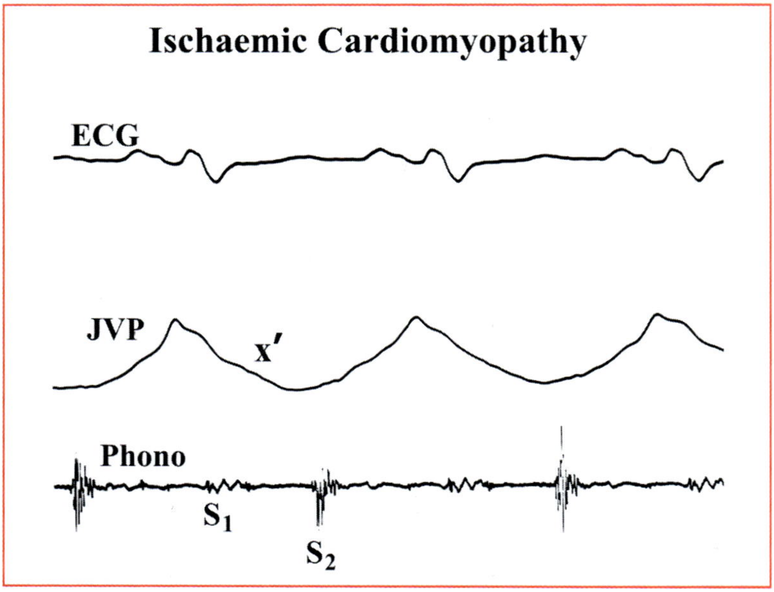

Fig. 4.26: Simultaneous recordings of ECG, jugular venous pulse (JVP), and phonocardiogram (Phono) in a patient with ischemic cardiomyopathy. The right ventricle (RV) is spared and the right heart function is normal as evidenced by the good ***x′ descent*** in the JVP.

Venous Pulse Contour in Severe Heart Failure

Patients with severe cardiac failure and poor RV systolic function will have high jugular venous pressure due to elevated ***pre a wave*** and ***v wave*** pressures. The latter will be further raised in the jugulars due to high venous tone caused by the coexistent sympathetic stimulation.[19] ***The x′ descent will be poor or lost.*** This may be aggravated by tricuspid regurgitation that may develop due to right ventricular dilatation. Atrial fibrillation may set in due to atrial overdistension. This will further diminish the ***x′ descent*** due to the loss of the Starling effect. If early diastolic pressure in the RV falls to close to zero as it should normally, then the ***y descent*** will be either dominant or the only descent noted (*see* Fig. 4.6).

If the early diastolic RV pressures were also elevated during the rapid filling phase as it may happen in severely compromised RV with very poor compliance, then the ***y descent may be also poor*** even though the ***v wave*** pressure is elevated due to very little gradient of pressure between the atrium and the ventricle. *The overall effect could be such that one would have high jugular pressure with poor descents.*

Venous Pulse Contours in RV Infarction

RV infarction may complicate acute inferoposterior infarction particularly when there is acute occlusion of a dominant right coronary artery in its proximal segment close to its origin. The RV due to its thin walls and lower systolic pressure has favorable systolic tension, which imposes less demands on oxygen compared to the left ventricle. If the hemodynamic failure is not severe with marked persistent hypotension and shock, the RV might recover most of its function. Nevertheless, during the acute phase, the ischemic dysfunction will alter both its diastolic compliance and systolic function. The extent of the functional derangement will depend on the acuteness and the extent of the ischemic insult. The latter may be modified by the severity and the chronicity of the underlying coronary atherosclerotic disease as well as the development of coronary collaterals. The hemodynamic compromise may be further complicated by disturbance in the sinoatrial (SA) node and atrioventricular (AV) nodal function caused by ischemia. The SA nodal artery is often the first branch of the right coronary artery. The AV nodal branch, however, arises further down where the right coronary artery takes the u-bend past the crux. The resulting arrhythmic disturbance may manifest as failure of sinus mechanism with development of junctional rhythms, first, second or higher degrees of SA and/or AV block. If the right atrial branches, which arise from the proximal segment of the right coronary artery, are involved in the acute occlusion, it may cause atrial infarct, compromise the right atrial function and may also result in atrial arrhythmias such as atrial fibrillation.

In addition, the ***left ventricular*** inferoposterior walls are often invariably the site of infarction and in severe cases often involve the posterior part of the interventricular septum. Acute RV dilatation might be accompanied by paradoxical septal motion. During diastole, the interventricular septum might encroach on the left side restricting its filling, and during systole bulge toward the RV and move thus paradoxically. Acute and abrupt RV as well as the LV posterior wall dilatation might also cause intrapericardial pressures to rise. The pericardial constraint might further impair both RV and LV compliance and filling. Both the posterior septal infarct and pericardial constraint would be contributing to the paradoxical septal motion noted in severe cases.

When the RV systolic dysfunction is significant, the ***x′ descent*** will be diminished or absent. If the arterial supply to the right atrium is not compromised, there could be augmented and forceful contraction of the right atrium to support RV filling. Strong atrial contraction and the accompanying good atrial relaxation would cause the ***a wave*** and the ***x descent*** to be prominent. The latter also would help to accelerate venous inflow. The altered diastolic function and decreased compliance of the RV will lead to elevation of the ***pre a wave pressure.*** This will raise the right atrial ***a wave*** and the ***v wave*** pressures and consequently the mean RA pressure. The raised RA pressures will be reflected in the jugulars as well. As long as the RV diastolic dysfunction is not severe enough to raise the early diastolic pressure in the RV, the raised ***v wave*** will be accompanied by an exaggerated ***y descent.*** Therefore, the jugulars in these patients would show a diminished or absent ***x′ descent*** with a dominant or single ***y descent.*** If the ***x descent*** is exaggerated due to forceful right atrial contraction and relaxation in the presence of normal PR interval, then it would be indistinguishable from the ***x′ descent*** at the bedside. This might actually cause the double descents with ***equal x and y.*** Sometimes, the RV annular dilatation with or without right ventricular papillary muscle dysfunction could lead to tricuspid regurgitation of variable degree raising further the right atrial ***v wave*** pressure.

When the diastolic dysfunction is severe, even the early diastolic pressure in the RV might become raised, blunting the ***y descent*** despite elevated ***v wave*** pressures. Such a profound elevation in the RV filling pressures often is indicative of severe RV infarction. This means RV diastolic filling is compromised even in the early rapid filling phase. *This of course is a hemodynamic imitator of cardiac pre tamponade-like state with total diastolic restriction.* This situation might be accompanied by RV dilatation as well as LV posterior wall dilatation. The pericardial constraint will lead to very high right atrial and jugular venous pressures. *The blood can enter the tight space only when the blood can leave the space namely during systole. In these patients, one would see very little descents in the highly elevated venous column at the bedside.* With recording of right atrial pressure, one may actually show some drop in the intra-atrial pressure during systole.

Looking for so-called ***w*** and ***m*** pattern of waveforms described by some authors in relation to the right atrial pressure recordings in the jugulars at the bedside will not be a fruitful exercise. In this context, since they also attribute the mechanism of ***the normal x′ descent*** to the fall in intrapericardial pressure due to ventricular systolic emptying, a comment again on ***the mechanism of the normal x′ descent*** needs to be made here to remove confusion. The normal ***x′ descent*** is essentially due to the descent of the base and not due to drop in intrapericardial pressure caused by ventricular systole. On the two-dimensional echocardiographic images, one can see the atrial area and consequently the volume expand with each systole as the contracting right and the left ventricles pull on the tricuspid and the mitral annulus, respectively. Furthermore, the right atrial and therefore the jugular ***x′ descent*** is selectively diminished gradually and eventually lost in chronic pulmonary hypertensive patients when RV failure sets in. In these patients, left atrial recording will confirm the presence of the normal left atrial pressure pulse contour with preserved ***x′ descent.*** This disparity between the two sides should not be there if fall in the intrapericardial pressure due to ventricular systole is the mechanism of the ***x′ descent.*** Similarly, one can observe in patients with severe left ventricular dysfunction with preserved right ventricular function, the ***x′ descent*** will be preserved until pulmonary hypertension develops and begins to alter RV function. Intrapericardial pressure will play an important part when the pericardial space is compromised *as in cardiac tamponade or situations that mimic the hemodynamics of cardiac tamponade with impediment to filling throughout diastole. This could arise in severely dilated hearts with failure and severely elevated filling pressures, rare patients with constrictive pericarditis as explained earlier and in some patients with severe RV infarction and shock.*

Venous Pulse Contours in Ebstein's Anomaly

Ebstein's anomaly is a rare congenital defect where the tricuspid valve is abnormally displaced downward toward the right ventricle. This implies that in this condition, the basal part of the right ventricle becomes atrialized. This results in ***a large right atrium, thereby increasing its capacitance.*** Sometimes the right atrium may be huge in size. The tricuspid valve may often be incompetent and lead to variable degrees of tricuspid regurgitation. In addition, the right ventricular systolic function will often be diminished. The effects of the diminished right ventricular function can be expected to decrease the ***x′ descent.*** The tricuspid regurgitation, on the other hand, depending on its severity can be expected to raise the right atrial ***v wave*** and cause the ***y descent*** to get exaggerated. Despite these changes in the RA pressure pulse contours, the jugulars may not reflect these adequately due to the ***large*** right atrial ***capacitance, which*** may have ***"a buffering effect".*** In fact, the descents in the jugulars and the jugular pulsations may be hard to see even in the relatively young patients with this defect. *It is important to consider a large-sized right atrium with high capacitance effect as part of a differential diagnosis for an inconspicuous jugular contour in the young adult.*

Rare Types of Double Descents

In the presence of a long PR interval, atrial relaxation and consequently the ***x descent*** is well separated from ventricular systole and therefore occur in diastole. This type of double descent ***(x and x′)*** may mimic the common ***x***′ and *y descents. The second of a pair of descents per cardiac cycle, however, will be systolic and correspond to the radial pulse upstroke.* With rapid heart rates, the diagnosis will require an electrocardiogram.

Two Descents in Diastole (Double Diastolic Descents)

Two descents in diastole imply the presence of an exaggerated y descent and an x descent, the latter due to long PR interval. This pattern is occasionally seen in heart failure with a dominant ***v wave*** and absent ***x***′ descent due to poor right ventricular function. The ***a wave*** is smaller and occurs early due to prolonged PR interval (*see* Fig. 4.11).

Triple Descents

Very rarely all three descents ***x, x***′ and ***y descents*** may be separately visible simulating flutter waves. This again implies prolonged PR interval.

Flutter Waves

Flutter waves may be occasionally seen in patients with atrial flutter. In this rhythm, the atria contract generally 300 times per minute with a varying ventricular rate, which in most untreated patients is usually about 150. Flutter waves are more likely to be seen only when the ventricular rate has been slowed spontaneously or secondary to therapy. ***In contrast to atrial fibrillation, the atrial contraction in patients with atrial flutter is often better organized and may generate pressure and the atrial relaxation that follow may cause visible descents.***

Single y Descent

This usually indicates poor right ventricular function. It is commonly seen in patients with chronic atrial fibrillation and congestive heart failure. When noted with a large amplitude and fast rising ***v wave*** before it, it would indicate tricuspid regurgitation. In tricuspid stenosis, the elevated ***v wave*** pressure has been described to be followed by so-called ***slow y descent.*** The slowing of the rate of fall of the ***y descent*** even if truly present is, however, not usually striking enough to be detected in the jugulars.

Exaggerated Ascents of Waves

The normal ***a*** and the ***v wave*** ascents representing low amplitude and slow rate of rise are not easily seen at the bedside. If the rise of the waves is as rapid as the descents that follow them and is associated with an increased amplitude, it *indicates retrograde flow in the jugulars, as in tricuspid regurgitation, cannon waves of atrioventricular dissociation* and in some cases with diminished right ventricular compliance and strong atrial contraction (giant ***a wave***). A large amplitude jugular ***a wave*** with rapid rise may also be expected intricuspid stenosis which is however quite rare.

ASSESSMENT OF JUGULAR VENOUS PRESSURE

The normal right atrium functions as a capacitance chamber. The mean RA pressure is often quite low and often <5 mm Hg. When assessed externally in relationship to the sternal angle with the patient's head placed at 45° upward tilt from the horizontal, the top of the moving jugular column does not exceed 4–5 cm in vertical height above the sternal angle. The recognition of the descents and their contour will make assessment of the jugular venous pressure quite easy. The top of the pulsations in the jugulars as transmitted to the skin overlying the sternomastoid muscle must be noted. Since the jugular and superior vena cava are in direct continuity with the right atrium, the estimation of the jugular venous pressure helps in the assessment of the central filling pressure in the right heart. The latter reflects the adequacy of the volume status of the patient as well as the right heart function. One must however always remember that the systemic venous or sympathetic tone influences the jugular column in addition to the right atrial pressure. *For any given volume status or filling pressure in the right atrium, the level to which the jugular column will rise will depend on the degree of the venous tone as well.*

The derivation of the right atrial mean pressure from the jugular venous pressure usually takes into account the approximate location of the mid-right atrium from the sternal angle. The sternal angle is a surface anatomic mark. The right atrium can be at a variable distance from this external reference point depending on the position of the patient. In the usual 45° upward tilt from the horizontal in which the patient is assessed this distance in vertical height from the surface sternal angle can vary between 8 and 10 cm. The higher the tilt the higher is this distance. When assessed at 90° tilt, the distance is almost 12 cm[55] (Fig. 4.27). This distance in centimeters is added to the level of jugular column in vertical height above the sternal angle in centimeters to derive the right atrial pressure in centimeters of water. The total can then be divided by 13 to get millimeters of Hg pressure.

The jugular contour unless associated with very high venous pressure will not be visible if the patient is tilted too much upward from the horizontal. In

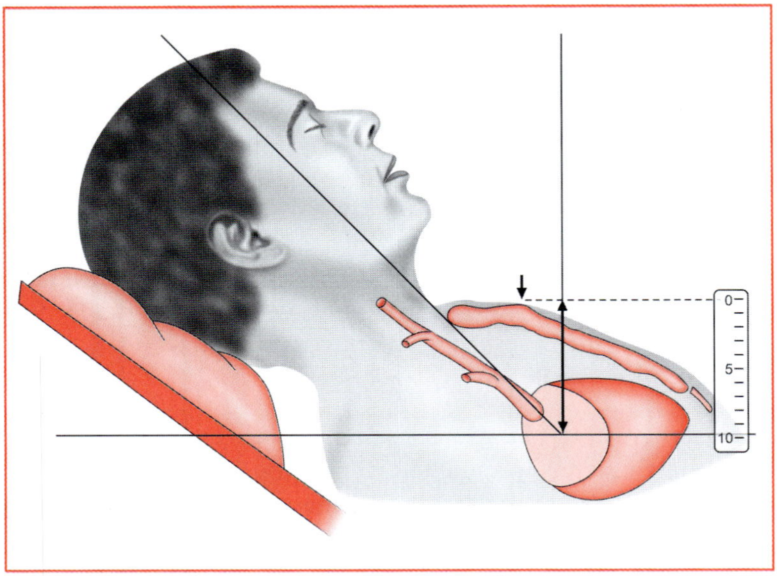

Fig. 4.27: Diagram showing a patient lying supine with the head tilted upward at 45° from the horizontal. The jugular venous pressure is measured by noting the level of the top of the moving jugular column in cm in vertical height from the external reference point of the sternal angle (SA). In this position, the mid-right atrium is about 8–10 cm in vertical height from the SA.

fact in many normal individuals, the jugular descents will be observed only when they are almost lying flat. In some of the normals, the top of the jugular column may only be visible with patient lying flat or only slightly tilted if any. While estimation of the right atrial pressure from the jugular venous pressure by adjusting for the vertical height of the right atrium from the sternal angle may be of interest, it is not absolutely necessary. One can simply have a normal range of jugular venous pressure in vertical height in centimeters from the usual external reference point of the sternal angle. Based on this normal range, one can decide whether in a given patient the jugular venous pressure is normal, low or high. A simple figure for the normal range is 4–5 cm above the sternal angle at 45° of upward tilt. In fact, this level is usually obtained only in younger subjects. In the elderly, this level is generally even lower.

Hepatojugular Reflux

When compression is applied to the abdomen, during normal respirations, the jugular venous pressure will be seen to increase transiently in normal subjects. Usually within a few cardiac cycles the pressure falls back to the pre-compression level. When the same maneuver is performed in a patient with heart failure, the venous pressure will increase and stay increased until the pressure is released. This is termed a positive ***hepatojugular reflux.***[12,32,56]

This test should be performed with care to avoid discomfort or pain to the patient. If pain is produced, then it may cause the test to become falsely positive. In addition, the patient should not hold the breath or perform a Valsalva maneuver during the compression. Finally, the compression should be applied at least for 30 seconds.

The rise in venous pressure has been attributed to rise in the intra-abdominal pressure, causing a rise in intrathoracic pressure. Subsequently, others have attributed this effect to high sympathetic tone. A positive hepatojugular reflux is known to occur in conditions with high sympathetic tone even in the absence of heart failure (e.g. thyrotoxicosis, anemia and hypoxemia).

With compression of the abdomen, the intra-abdominal pressure rises. The diaphragm is therefore forced toward the thorax. However, this in patients with normal vital capacity and normal lung reserve does not change significantly the respiratory pattern. The rise in the intra-abdominal pressure increases the venous return from the viscera in the abdomen to the thorax. In normal subjects, this increased volume is easily accommodated without any sustained rise in pressure in the venous capacitance system including the superior vena cava and the jugulars. The initial rise is usually due to a transient rise in sympathetic tone caused by some apprehension on the part of the patient when compression is applied. In states with sustained elevation in sympathetic tone, the capacitance of the thoracic great veins is reduced due to venoconstriction. This will result in sustained rise in venous pressure. In patients with heart failure, the sympathetic tone is increased therefore always resulting in a positive test.[56] If pain is caused during compression, this may raise the sympathetic tone and result in a false-positive test.

In patients with chronic obstructive lung disease, a false-positive test may be seen due to high intrathoracic pressure created by the change in the patient's breathing pattern, which opposes the upward movement of the diaphragm. This is also a sign of decreased lung reserve.

Obstruction of the Superior Vena Cava

When there is partial obstruction of the superior vena cava, the jugular venous pulsations may be still noted although the venous pressure may become elevated. When there is complete obstruction, the venous pressure will become markedly elevated, and the veins in the arms may also become distended. Superficial collateral flow will become easily visible with the flow directed toward the abdomen. At this stage, no jugular pulsations will be observed.

CLINICAL ASSESSMENT OF THE JUGULAR VENOUS PULSE

The foregoing principles of jugular physiology and pathophysiology can be simply and very easily brought to the bedside if certain points are kept in mind and applied when assessing a patient. Jugular pulse recordings obtained with electronically amplified transducers often cause artificial exaggeration of the ***a, c*** and the ***v waves.*** Recognition of the jugular pulse contours and interpretation become difficult only if the usual text book description of the ***a, c*** and the ***v waves*** based on such jugular recordings are searched for at the bedside.

POINTS TO REMEMBER

1. *Descents in the jugular venous pulse are easy to see since they are fast movements down. Objects moving away from the eyes of the observer are better seen than the ones moving toward the observer. The descents reflect flow acceleration. Normal jugular wave ascents are slow rises of pressure and therefore are hard to see. If the wave rise is prominent as well and easily seen, then they are abnormal and reflect retrograde flow in the jugulars*
2. ***Technique of recognition of the descents:*** *Internal jugular pulsations are often transmitted to the skin overlying the sternomastoid and sometimes over a wide area of the skin adjacent to it and above the clavicle. One should not get too close to the neck of the patient. In fact standing at the bedside with the patient properly positioned and feeling the radial artery pulse at the same time one should look for any fast movement down overlying the jugulars as mentioned. Rapid downward movements that synchronize with the radial arterial pulse upstroke will immediately be identified as the jugular x' descent. Simultaneous palpation of the radial arterial pulse even when one searches for the jugular pulse must be encouraged since this way, the normal* ***x' descent*** *is quickly identified. Movements of the soft tissues of the neck related to respiration can easily be distinguished as well. Sometimes the descents may be observed to move even a chain or necklace that the patient may be wearing. Throwing shadows over the skin overlying the jugulars and the sternomastoid muscle using natural light or artificial light source and watching the movement of the shadow also help in identifying the movement. Occasionally, descents may also be seen in the external jugulars due to inadequacy of the venous valves.*
3. *Arterial pulse has a fast rise, whereas the jugulars have a fast fall. That is the best way to distinguish the arterial pulsation in the neck from the jugular movement. External pressure applied below the pulsations over the sternomastoid will help to occlude the venous pulsations and not the*

carotid pulsation. When the venous pressure is high with marked tricuspid regurgitation this technique will not work. Arterial pulsation does not last long, whereas the ***v wave of tricuspid regurgitation lasts longer.***

4. *Once the descent or descents are noted, one should time them with the radial arterial pulse or the second heart sound (S2). Radial arterial pulse upstroke is the easiest and the simplest for timing. This timing with the radial pulse is not by any means like timing an Olympic photo finish or microsecond timing. In other words, one should be simply able to call each time a descent is seen as "down" "down" while feeling the pulse at the same time. This can be easily demonstrated even while teaching a group of several students at the bedside. One can be made to call the descent each time it is seen while another calls the pulse each time the upstroke is felt. The descent which is simultaneous with the pulse is the x' descent while the descent which is out of phase with the pulse is the y descent. The x' descent falls on to the S2 while the y descent comes after the S2.*
5. *In most normal adults what one will see is simply one large downward movement or descent, which will be synchronous with the pulse. This jugular contour of the normal adult can be simply described as showing* ***single x' descent.*** *It immediately implies a normal contour. In young subjects, one may see a major descent in systole with the pulse and a much smaller descent slightly after the pulse indicating the pattern of the* ***x' descent*** *followed by a small* ***y descent.*** *This contour can be described as a* ***dominant x' descent.*** *This description implies the presence of a small* ***y descent.*** *Occasionally, there may be a slight hesitation in the systolic descent due to the presence of an* ***x descent*** *(caused by atrial relaxation) quickly followed by the* ***x' descent*** *which is of course caused by the descent of the base. The combined movement will still be synchronous with the pulse indicating a normal contour.*
6. *The presence of the* ***x' descent*** *in normal regular sinus rhythm implies the presence of the* ***a wave*** *before it, although not seen to rise prominently. The presence of even a small diastolic or* ***y descent*** *(as compared to the* ***x' or systolic descent****) implies that there is a* ***v wave*** *although not rising prominently. Therefore, one needs to simply describe the descent pattern alone when the wave rises are not prominent.*
7. *Single* ***x' descent*** *or the dominant x' descent patterns in the jugulars imply good right ventricular systolic function and in addition indicates the absence of significant tricuspid regurgitation.*
8. *If two descents are seen for each cardiac cycle, these will be generally due to a combination of the x' and the y descents. Rarely, it may be due to the combination of an* ***x descent*** *well separated from the* ***x' descent*** *due to*

the presence of a long PR interval. This can only be diagnosed with the help of the electrocardiogram. This is usually not the common cause of the double descents in the jugular pulse. The more usual combination is due to the presence of both the x′ and the y descents. This is identified by the fact that the first of each pair will be systolic in timing, i.e. occurring with the radial pulse.

9. *When two descents are seen to each cardiac cycle, then one must observe the relationship of the two to decide the relative dominance of the descents. If both descents are equally prominent then the pattern is **x′ = y.** If one of them is less prominent than the other, the pattern will be **either x′ > y or x′ < y.***
10. *Double descents are clearly abnormal in the adult even when they are x′ > y. This could be normal in the young subjects and/or pregnant women. However, in these situations, the pattern has to be x′ > y.*
11. *In all cases of double descents, one should consider causes of decreased x′ descents as well as factors that may exaggerate the y descent.*
12. *The x′ descent gets decreased if there is right ventricular dysfunction in the presence of atrial fibrillation due to lack of atrial kick and in the presence of significant tricuspid regurgitation.*
13. *Exaggerated y descent requires an increased v wave pressure head with no restriction to ventricular filling in early diastole. This mechanism excludes cardiac tamponade in which filling restriction occurs throughout diastole.*
14. *Since double descents can occur with and without the context of pulmonary hypertension, they may be approached accordingly. These are discussed in detail in the text. Since jugular contour abnormalities are not specific for pulmonary hypertension, diagnosis of pulmonary hypertension must be made on the basis of other clinical findings such as a loud or palpable pulmonic component of the second heart sound, sustained subxiphoid right ventricular impulse and/or electrocardiographic evidence of right ventricular hypertrophy. Absence of these signs does not necessarily exclude the presence of pulmonary hypertension and therefore further tests may have to be taken to exclude or confirm the presence of pulmonary hypertension. Two-dimensional echocardiogram particularly with the Doppler assessment for tricuspid regurgitation jet if identified will often help in this respect. Peak tricuspid regurgitation velocity if identified can be related to the pressure difference between the right ventricle and the right atrium. The pressure difference is approximately four times the velocity squared (pressure gradient = $4V^2$).*
15. *In the presence of pulmonary hypertension, the relative dominance of the x′ versus the y descent reveals the adequacy or otherwise of the right*

ventricular systolic function. The x' > y pattern is indicative of compensated right ventricular function. When it is x' = y, it probably means beginning right ventricular dysfunction. The pattern x' < y definitely is a late pattern, indicating RV decompensation.

16. *In the absence of pulmonary hypertension x' = y is usually normal for a postcardiac surgery patient. In the patient who has not had previous cardiac surgery, other conditions such as pericardial effusion with some restriction, constrictive pericarditis, cardiomyopathy or mild or early RV infarction in the context of acute inferior myocardial infarction need to be considered. Similar pattern can also be seen in some patients with atrial septal defect. If the pattern were x' < y, it would in addition indicate significant RV systolic dysfunction.*
17. *If the descent is single and is out of phase with the radial pulse, the pattern can be described as single y descent. It indicates significant right ventricular dysfunction. This is the common pattern seen in patients with chronic atrial fibrillation and heart failure with right ventricular dysfunction.*
18. *Prominent rises of either the a wave or the v wave in the jugulars imply flow reversal in the jugulars. If it is seen to precede the x' descent, it must be the a wave and if it precedes a y descent, then it must be the v wave of tricuspid regurgitation.*
19. *The a wave as opposed to the v wave has a shorter duration like a flicker. They occur regularly in the context of resistance to ventricular filling with a strong atrial contraction, causing end-diastolic flow reversal. They can occur irregularly due to simultaneous right atrial and right ventricular contraction in situations of atrioventricular dissociation. In this instance, they are termed "cannon waves".*
20. *The v wave, on the other hand, precedes the y descent. When a single y descent is noted then one must try to assess the prominence of the wave rise preceding it. If it were of large amplitude and rising actively as well, it would indicate the presence of tricuspid regurgitation. It will be seen to rise with the arterial pulse but will last longer than the arterial pulse in duration. The v wave of tricuspid regurgitation is often visible from a distance and may be seen well with the patient sitting up. It indicates quite clearly systolic flow reversal in the jugulars.*

REFERENCES

1. Harvey W. Exercitatio Anatomica de Motu Cordis et Sanguinis in Animalibus, Frankfurt, Gugliemi Fitzeri, 1628 (English translation by Leake C.D. Springfield: Thomas, 1949).
2. Purkinje JL. Uber die Saugkraft des Herzens Ubersicht der Arbeiten und Veranderungen der schlesischen Gesellschaft fur vaterlandische Kultur in Jahre. 1843:147.

3. Chauveau A, Marey E. Appareilles et experiences cardiographiques par l'emploi des instruments enregistreures a indications continues. Mem Acad Med. 1863; 26:268.
4. Lancisi JM. Motus Cordis et Aneurysmatibus. Rome; 1728.
5. Potain PCE. Des mouvements et des bruits qui se faissent dans les veines. Mem Soc Med Hop Paris. 1867;4:3.
6. Mackenzie J. The study of the Pulse. London: Pentland; 1902.
7. Mackenzie J. The interpretation of the pulsations in the jugular veins. Am J Med Sci. 1907;134:12.
8. Wiggers. CJ. Modern Aspects of the Circulation in Health and Disease. Philadelphia: Lea & Febiger; 1923.
9. Russek HI, Zohman BL. The syndrome of Bernheim. Am Heart J. 1945;30:427.
10. Bloomfield RA, Lauson HD, Cournand A, et al. Recording of right heart pressures in normal subjects and in patients with chronic pulmonary disease and various types of cardio-circulatory disease. J Clin Invest. 1946;25:639.
11. Hansen AT, Eskildsen P, Gorzsche H. Pressure curves from the right auricle and the right ventricle in chronic constrictive pericarditis. Circulation. 1951;3:881.
12. Burch GE, Ray CT. Mechanism of the hepatojugular reflux test in congestive heart failure. Am Heart J. 1954;48:373.
13. Wilson RH, Hoseth W, Sadoff C, et al. Pathologic physiology and diagnostic significance of the pressure pulse tracing in heart in patients with constrictive pericarditis and pericardial effusion. Am Heart J. 1954;48:671-83.
14. Reinhold J. Venous pulse in atrial septal defect: a clinical sign. Brit Med J. 1955;1:695.
15. Cossio P, Buzzi A. Clinical Value of the venous pulse. Am Heart J. 1957;54:127.
16. Gibson R. Atypical constrictive pericarditis. Brit Heart J. 1959;21:583.
17. Hartman. H. The jugular venous tracing. Am Heart J. 1960;59:698-717.
18. Perloff JK, Harvey PW. Clinical recognition of tricuspid stenosis. Circulation. 1960;22:346-64.
19. Sharpey-Schafer EP. Venous tone. Brit Med J. 1961;2:1589.
20. Wood P. Chronic constrictive pericarditis. Am J Cardiol. 1961;7:48.
21. Lange RL, Botticelli JT, Tsagaris TJ, et al. Diagnostic signs in compressive cardiac disorders. Constrictive pericarditis, pericardial effusion, and tamponade. Circulation. 1966;33:763-77.
22. Colman AL. Clinical examination of the jugular venous pulse. Springfield: Thomas; 1966.
23. Wood P. Diseases of the heart and circulation. Philadelphia: JB Lippincott Company; 1968.
24. Tavel ME, Bard RA, Franks LC, et al. The jugular venous pulse in atrial septal defect. Arch Intern Med. 1968;121:524-9.
25. Rich LL, Tavel ME. The origin of the jugular C wave. N Engl J Med. 1971;284: 1309-11.
26. Constant J. The X prime descent in jugular contour nomenclature and recognition. Am Heart J. 1974;88:372.
27. Holt JP, Rhode EA, Kines H. Pericardial and Ventricular pressure. Circ Res. 1960;8:1171.
28. Harley A. Persistent right atrial standstill. Brit Heart J. 1976;38:646.
29. Matsuhisa M, Shimomura K, Beppu S, et al. Post-operative changes of jugular pulse tracing. J Cardiogr. 1976;6:403.

30. Jensen DP, Goolsby JP, Jr, Oliva PB. Hemodynamic pattern resembling pericardial constriction after acute inferior myocardial infarction with right ventricular infarction. Am J Cardiol. 1978;42:858-61.
31. Coma-Canella I, Lopez-Sendon J. Ventricular compliance in ischemic right ventricular dysfunction. Am J Cardiol. 1980;45:555-51.
32. Constant J. Bedside Cardiology, 3rd edition. Boston: Little Brown; 1985.
33. Matsuhisa M, Shimomura K, Beppu S, et al. Jugular phlebogram in congenital absence of the pericardium. Am Heart J. 1986;112:1004-10.
34. Brecher GA. Cardiac variations in venous return studied with a new bristle flowmeter. Am J Physiol. 1954;176:423.
35. Brawley RK, Oldham HN, Vasko JS, et al. Influence of right atrial pressure pulse on instantaneous vena caval blood flow. Am J Physiol. 1966;211:347-53.
36. Pinkerson AL, Luria MH, Freis ED. Effect of cardiac rhythm on vena caval blood flows. Am J Physiol. 1966;210:505-8.
37. Wexler L, Bergel DH, Gabe IT, et al. Velocity of blood flow in normal human venae cavae. Circ Res. 1968;23:349-59.
38. Froysaker T. Abnormal flow pattern in the superior vena cava induced by arrhythmias. A peroperative flowmetric study in man. Scand J Thorac Cardiovasc Surg. 1972;6:140-8.
39. Kalmanson D, Veyrat C, Chiche P. Atrial versus ventricular contribution in determining systolic venous return. A new approach to an old riddle. Cardiovasc Res. 1971;5:293-302.
40. Sivaciyan V, Ranganathan N. Transcutaneous Doppler jugular venous flow velocity recording. Circulation. 1978;57:930-9.
41. Ranganathan N, Sivaciyan V. Abnormalities in jugular venous flow velocity in pulmonary hypertension. Am J Cardiol. 1989;63:719-24.
42. Ranganathan N, Sivaciyan V, Pryszlak M, et al. Changes in jugular venous flow velocity after coronary artery bypass grafting. Am J Cardiol. 1989;63:725-9.
43. Shabetai R, Fowler NO, Guntheroth WG. The hemodynamics of cardiac tamponade and constrictive pericarditis. Am J Cardiol. 1970;26:480-9.
44. Rittenhouse EA, Barnes RW. Hemodynamics of cardiac tamponade: early recognition from jugular venous flow velocity. J Surg Res. 1975;19:35-41.
45. Nelson RM, Jenson CB, Smoot WM. Pericardial tamponade following open heart surgery. J Thorac Crdiovasc Surg. 1969;58:510.
46. Gabe IT, Gault JH, Ross J, Jr, et al. Measurement of instantaneous blood flow velocity and pressure in conscious man with a catheter-tip velocity probe. Circulation. 1969;40:603-14.
47. Ranganathan N, Sivaciyan V. Jugular venous flow velocity pattern, application to bedside recognition of jugular venous pulse contour and right heart hemodynamics. Am J Noninvas Cardiol. 1993;7:75-88.
48. Kalmanson D, Veyrat C, Chicke P. Venous return disturbances induced by arrhythmias. A transcutaneous, instantaneous, flowmetric study at the site of the jugular vein. Cardiovasc Res. 1970;4:279-90.
49. Ranganathan N, Sivaciyan V. Jugular Venous Flow velocity pattern application to bedside recognition of Jugular venous pulse contour and right heart hemodynamics. Am J Noninvas Cardiol. 1993;7:75-88.
50. Froysaker T. Anomalies of the superior vena caval flow pattern in patients with tricuspid insufficiency. Scand J Thorac Cardiovasc Surg. 1972;6:234-45.
51. Bernheim P. De la stenose ventriculaire droite. Rev Gen Clin Therap J Pract. 1915;29:721.

52. Bilchick KC, Wise RA. Paradoxical physical findings described by Kussmaul: pulsus paradoxus and Kussmaul's sign. Lancet. 2002;359:1940-2.
53. Wann LS, Morris SN, Tavel ME. Effects of cardiopulmonary bypass on the jugular venous pulse. Am Heart J. 1977;94:262-4.
54. Kesteloot H, Denef B. Value of reference tracings in diagnosis and assessment of constrictive epi- and pericarditis. Br Heart J. 1970;32:675-82.
55. Saunders DE Jr, Adcock DF, Head DS. Relationship of sternal angle right atrium in clinical measurement of jugular venous pressure. J Am Coll Cardiol. 1988;11(2):89A.
56. Constant J, Lippschutz EJ. The one minute abdominal compression test or "the hepatojugular reflux," a useful bedside test. Am Heart J. 1964;67:701.

Chapter

5 Precordial Pulsations

Snapshot

- The Mechanics and Physiology of the Normal Apical Impulse
- Physical Principles Governing the Formation of the Apical Impulse
- Normal Apical Impulse and its Determinants
- Assessment of the Apical Impulse
- Left Parasternal and Sternal Movements
- Right Parasternal Movement
- Pulsations over the Clavicular Heads
- Pulsations over the Second and/or Third Left Intercostal Spaces
- Subxiphoid Impulse
- Practical Points in the Clinical Assessment of the Precordial Pulsations

In this chapter, the pulsations of the precordium will be discussed in relation to their identification, the mechanisms of their origin and their pathophysiologic and clinical significance.

Precordial pulsations include the "apical impulse", left parasternal movement, right parasternal movement, pulsations of the clavicular heads, pulsations over the second left intercostal space and subxiphoid impulses.

THE MECHANICS AND PHYSIOLOGY OF THE NORMAL APICAL IMPULSE

Since during systole the heart contracts, becoming smaller and therefore moving away from the chest wall, why should one feel a systolic outward movement (the apical impulse) at all? Logically speaking there should not be an apical impulse.

Several different methods of recording the precordial motion had been used to study the apical impulse in the past going back to the late 19th century.[1,2] Among the more modern methods, the notable ones are the recordings of the apexcardiogram,[3-17] the impulse cardiogram[18] and the kinetocardiogram.[19-21] While the apex cardiography records the relative displacement of the chest wall under the transducer pickup device that is often held by the examiner's hands, the proponents of the impulse cardiography and the kinetocardiography point out that these methods allow the recording of the absolute movement of the chest wall since the pickup device is anchored to a fixed point held in space away from the chest. The kinetocardiograhy uses a flexible metal bellows probe coupled by air transmission to the manometer. The impulse cardiogram, on the other hand, utilizes a light metal rod with a flag at one end, held by light metal springs attached to a Perspex cone. The light metal rod with the flag is coupled directly to a photoelectric cell, the instrument being held rigidly in a metal clamp fixed to a stand. Despite its limitations, the apex cardiography has been extensively studied with simultaneous left ventricular pressures obtained through high fidelity recordings with the use of catheter tipped micromanometers.[8,14,15] These studies have demonstrated clearly that the upslope of the apexcardiogram corresponds closely to the rise of the pressure in the left ventricle during the isovolumic phase of systole. The summit of the systolic upstroke of the apexcardiogram (the E point) in the normal subjects occurs about 37 ms after the opening of the aortic valve and roughly 40 ms after the development of the peak dP/dt of the left ventricular pressure in the normal subjects.[15] These observations are also consistent with the findings obtained using the kinetocardiography.[20] When the apical impulse is recorded by kinetocardiography, it is seen to begin about 80 ms after the onset of the QRS in the electrocardiogram and about 10 or 20 ms before the carotid pulse upstroke. These observations indicate, therefore, that the apical impulse begins to rise during the pre-ejection phase of the left ventricular contraction and must therefore involve part of the isovolumic phase of systole and the peak movement must involve the early rapid ejection phase of systole.

Timed angiographic studies of Deliyannis and coworkers[22] show that the portion of the heart underlying the apex beat is usually the anterior wall of the left ventricle which moves forward during early systole and moves away and backward from the chest wall during mid-late systole. They suggest that the forward movement of the left ventricle in early systole is caused by the contraction of the middle circular fibers, which are confined to the upper three-fifth of the normal heart. The falling away of the apex of the left ventricle in late systole is attributed to the contraction of the spirally oriented fibers overlying the apex of the left ventricle, since in the normal heart, the middle circular fibers do not extend to the apex. They further suggest that in left ventricular hypertrophy, the middle circular fibers extend to the apex completely, thereby preventing the movement away of the apex from the chest wall in mid-late systole (according to these authors accounting for a sustained duration of the apical movement when there is underlying left ventricular hypertrophy).

A variety of explanations have been given for the presence of the normal apical impulse. The common explanation is that the heart rotates counter clockwise along its long axis during contraction, making the left ventricle to swing forward to hit the chest wall.[23-25] This twisting motion has been observed in the beating heart when exposed at surgery. This rotation is along the axis of the left ventricle. Torsional deformation of the left ventricular mid-wall in human hearts with intramyocardial markers has in fact been demonstrated. This appears to have some regional non-uniformity. Torsional deformation appears to be maximal in the apical lateral wall, intermediate in the apical inferior wall and minimal in the anteroapical wall. Torsional changes were less at the mid-ventricular level compared to the apical segments with similar regional variation. The exact cause of the regional variations is not defined. The possible causes suggested by these authors include variations in the left ventricular fiber architecture as well as the asymmetric attachment of the left ventricle to the mitral annulus posteriorly and the aortic root anteriorly.[26] The papillary muscles together with the underlying left ventricular myocardium contract during systole to keep the mitral leaflets together in the closed position, preventing their eversion into the left atrium with the rising intraventricular pressure. In the process, the closed mitral apparatus must exert an opposite pull on the individual papillary muscle groups. It is possible that the asymmetric attachment of the mitral apparatus to the left ventricle may result in an asymmetric pull on the papillary muscles with a stronger pull on the anterolateral papillary muscle group and the underlying left ventricular myocardium compared to the pull exerted on the post-eromedial papillary muscle group. This might also be a contributory factor in the accentuated torsional changes seen in the apical lateral walls. In addition, during the phase of isovolumic contraction, it has been shown that there is an increase in the external circumference of the left ventricle together with a decrease in the base to apex length.[27] However, these changes during systole alone are still insufficient to explain the apical impulse, which must result from hitting of the inside of the chest by the left ventricle.

Since during systole all fibers contract and while the ventricular walls thicken all around, the overall size becomes smaller the moment ejection begins and therefore the heart would not be expected to come closer to the chest wall. Thus, the genesis of the apical impulse is poorly explained by these mechanisms alone.

The formation of the apical impulse is perhaps better understood when simple principles of physics are also considered, since they are applicable in relation to the heart and the great vessels. Stapleton refers to these indirectly when he states that the apical impulse "probably represents recoil movement that develops as left ventricular output meets aortic resistance".[20]

PHYSICAL PRINCIPLES GOVERNING THE FORMATION OF THE APICAL IMPULSE

The heart is essentially a pump connected to the aorta and the pulmonary artery both of which are conduits of fluid (blood). Therefore, pure physical principles of hydrodynamics should be sufficient to explain the mechanism of the apical impulse formation with one important anatomic consideration which is the fact that the aorta is essentially a coiled pipe (aortic arch) and fixed posteriorly at the descending segment:

Newton's third law of motion indicates that for every action there is equal and opposite reaction. This effect is easily demonstrated in the simple physics experiment illustrated (Figs. 5.1 and 5.2). Similarly, as the left ventricle contracts and the intracavitary pressure rises during the isovolumic contraction phase (after the mitral valve closure and before the aortic valve

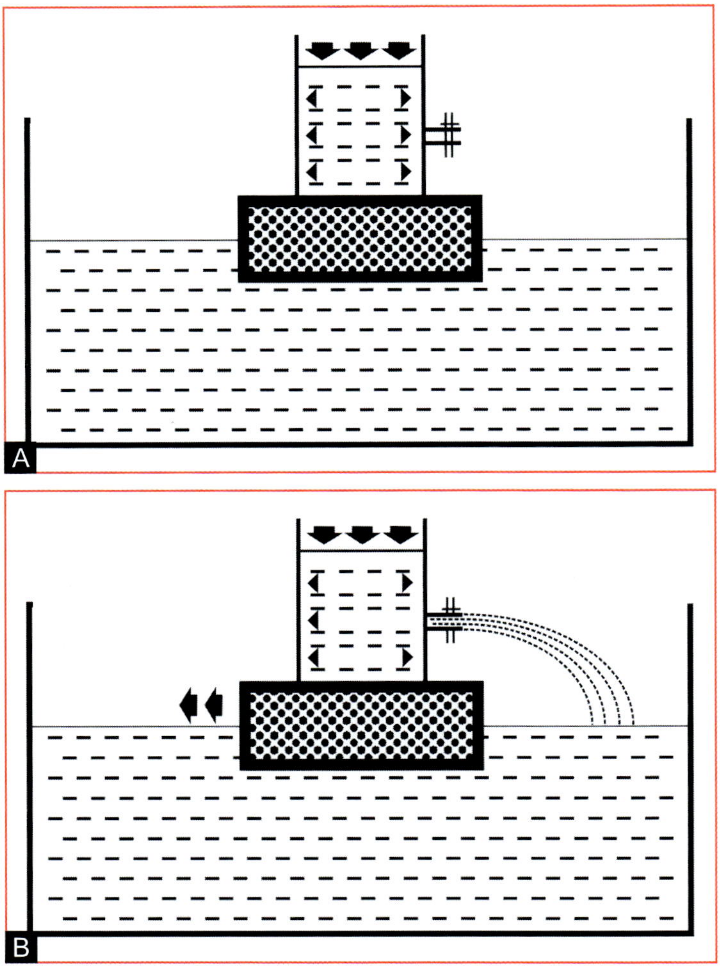

Figs. 5.1A and B: (A) Atmospheric pressure (bold arrows) exerted on water in the beaker is evenly distributed on all sides of the beaker (short arrows in beaker) and the system is in equilibrium. (B) When the tap on the beaker is opened and the water runs out, the forces pushing on the left side of the beaker are no longer balanced by equal and opposite forces, therefore the beaker and the cork it is sitting on will move to the left.

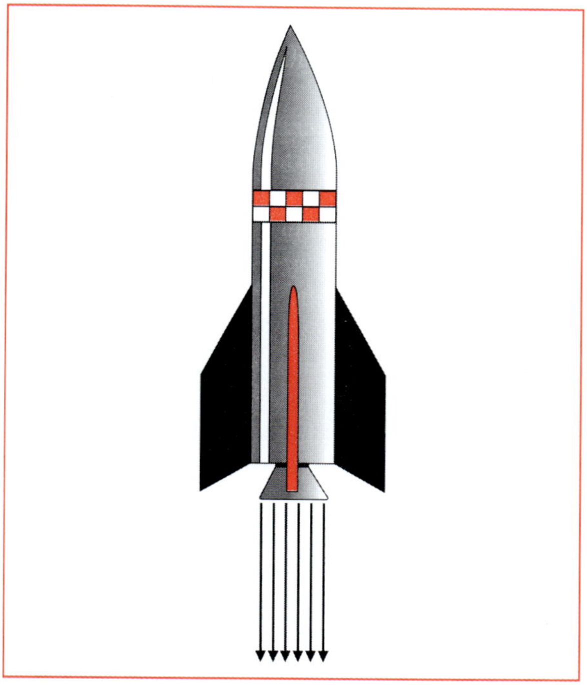

Fig. 5.2: Rocket propulsion is also based on the same principle of Newton's third law of motion. As the pressure escapes from the bottom of the combustion chamber of the rocket the forces pushing up are no longer balanced by equal opposing forces and push the rocket upward.

opening), this pressure is equally distributed on all the walls of the left ventricle including the apex and the closed aortic valve. There could be some change in shape and possibly torsional deformation during the time of the peak acceleration of the left ventricular pressure development. No appreciable motion of the heart, however, occurs because forces on the opposing walls balance out. This equilibrium is disturbed once the aortic valve opens and the ejection begins. As in the physics experiment, similar to the beaker's movement in the direction opposite to the flow of water, the unopposed force on the apex of the left ventricle will move the left ventricle downward (Figs. 5.3A and B).

Ejection of fluid under pressure into a coiled pipe will have a tendency to straighten out the pipe as is commonly observed with the coiled garden hose as the water is turned on. Aorta representing a coiled pipe, ejection of the left ventricular stroke volume into the aorta under pressure will have a tendency to straighten the aortic arch. The aortic arch being anatomically fixed posteriorly (descending segment of the arch) only its anterior portion (the ascending segment of the arch) can recoil. This recoiling force will move the left ventricle upward and forward toward the chest wall[20] (Fig. 5.3C).

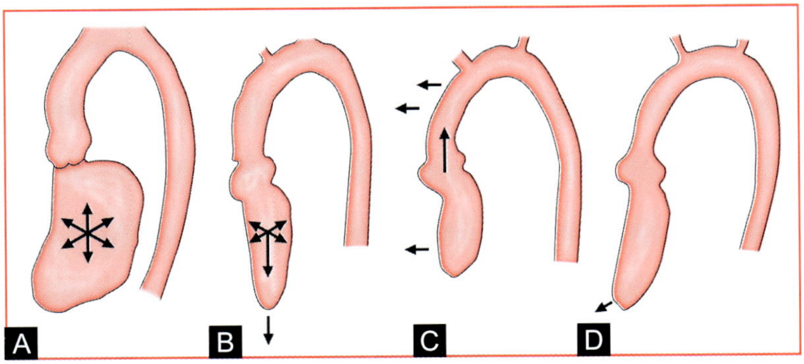

Figs. 5.3A to D: (A) During isovolumic contraction, pressure in the left ventricle rises and is equally distributed on all walls of the left ventricle and no appreciable movement occurs. (B) As the aortic valve opens and blood is ejected out into the aorta, the force against the apex is no longer balanced by equal and opposite force and pushes the heart downward. (C) As the aortic valve opens and a large volume is ejected under pressure into the aorta during systole, the aortic arch being a coil will have a tendency to uncoil (recoil) thus pulling the left ventricle, which is attached to it, outward and forward with it. (D) The combined effect of the two forces on the left ventricle causes it to move downward and forward, giving rise to the apical impulse.

The resultant effect of the two forces described above will move the apex of the left ventricle toward the chest wall during systole despite the fact that the left ventricle is contracting and becoming smaller (Fig. 5.3D). *The force and the extent of the resultant impulse that is felt on the chest wall by the examining hand as the apical impulse will be determined by both the cardiac function as well as the extra cardiac attenuating factors.*

The force with which the heart will move and hit the inside of the chest wall will depend on the two physical principles discussed above. The velocity of ejection, which is a reflection of the force of myocardial contractility under any given preload and afterload or impedance to ejection, is an important determinant of the momentum attained by the heart as it moves toward the chest wall according to Newton's third law of motion. The amount of blood ejected into the aorta for each beat (the stroke volume) as well as the peak systolic pressure reached will determine the amount of recoil of the aorta, thus adding to the momentum of the heart. The force of the moving heart will compress the soft tissues between the ribs, allowing the impulse to be transmitted to the outside where it is felt.

The transmission of the apical impulse can be affected by the characteristics of the chest wall. It is well known that the apical impulse may not be felt in patients with certain chest wall deformities, obese patients with thick chest walls, and those with stiff and fixed rib cage (e.g. ankylosing spondylitis and some elderly patients).[23,24] Intervening lung tissue may also interfere with proper transmission of the impulse by absorbing the force as a cushion as it commonly happens in patients with chronic lung disease.[24] Similarly, large pericardial and/or pleural effusion on the left side can cushion the force and prevent its transmission.

NORMAL APICAL IMPULSE AND ITS DETERMINANTS

If an iron ball caused the impact on the inside of the chest wall it would maximally compress the soft tissues of the chest wall transmitting all the momentum to the outside of the chest wall. On the other hand, if the impact on the inside of the chest wall were caused by a cotton ball, which itself would become compressed by the impact, thus resulting in no appreciable impulse on the outside.

The same difference of transmission would be noted if the inside of the chest wall was to be impacted by the side of a balloon as opposed to the nipple at the tip of a balloon, which is not fully inflated. The nipple being soft cannot compress the tissues and instead will get compressed easily. Both the nipple and the inflated portion of the balloon form one single chamber having the same pressure. Applying Laplace's law where,

Tension = *P* (pressure) x *r* (radius) for a thin walled cylindrical shell, and

If the wall has a thickness, the circumferential wall stress is given by **Lame's equation**, as follows:

$$\text{Tension} \propto \frac{\text{P (pressure)} \times \text{r (radius)}}{\text{2h (wall thickness)}}$$

It becomes obvious that the difference in the radii of the nipple and the body of the balloon account for the difference in their wall tensions and therefore their respective compressibility (Fig. 5.4). *The apical impulse that is felt during systole is similarly a reflection of the relative non-compressibility of the wall of the left ventricle due to the developed wall tension.*

In a normal left ventricle during a normal cardiac cycle, the left ventricle has maximum volume or radius at the end of diastole. However, the end-diastolic pressure being relatively low (around 12 mmHg), the wall tension is relatively low, and also there is no appreciable motion of the heart. As the pressure rises during the isovolumic contraction phase, the left ventricular wall tension will also rise reaching a peak just before the opening of the aortic valve (E point in Figure 5.5).

Once ejection begins, the heart moves as explained previously bringing the tense left ventricular wall against the chest wall. The left ventricular wall tension, however, will begin to fall with onset of ejection and decrease as the ventricle becomes smaller in systole. The systolic thickening of the wall during this phase also will tend to reduce the wall tension further. Since the left ventricle ejects most of its volume during the early part of systole (first third), the tension would have reached a low level by the end of this phase.

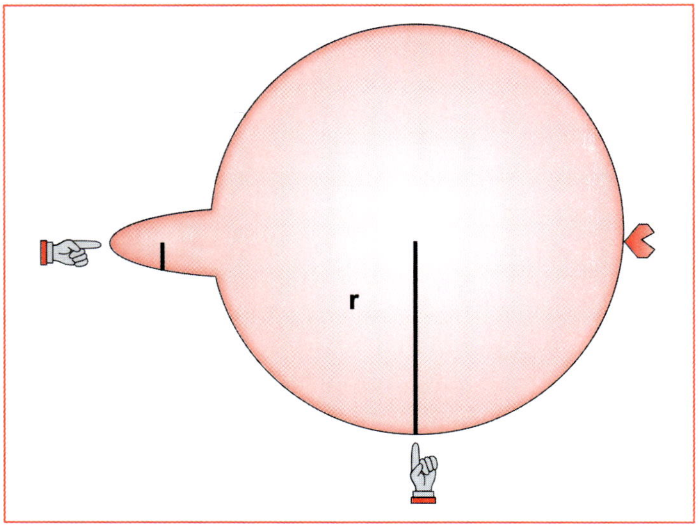

Fig. 5.4: A partially inflated balloon has the same pressure in the body of the balloon as well as in the nipple. However, the resistance felt by the poking finger is different in the body compared to the nipple. This is due to differences in the wall tension caused by differences in the radii (r) by Laplace's law.

The wall tension will continue to fall in late systole primarily due to fall in the ventricular pressure, as the myocardium begins to relax.

The apical impulse in the normal heart reflects faithfully the tension curve just described.[17] *Therefore, the impulse is felt during the first third of systole only, reaching a peak at the approximate timing of the first heart sound and moving away from the palpating hand long before the second heart sound is heard.*[18]

ASSESSMENT OF THE APICAL IMPULSE

The apical impulse by definition is the lateral most point of systolic outward motion that can be felt on the chest wall.[23] The term "point of maximal impulse" should not be confused with this and in fact should not be used to describe the apical impulse.[20]

The following features should be ascertained when assessing the apical impulse:

1. *Location*
2. *Area*
3. *Which ventricle is causing the impulse?*
4. *Character:*
   a. *Dynamicity*
   b. *Duration*
   c. *Extra humps and timing*
5. *Palpable sounds and murmurs in the area of the apical impulse.*

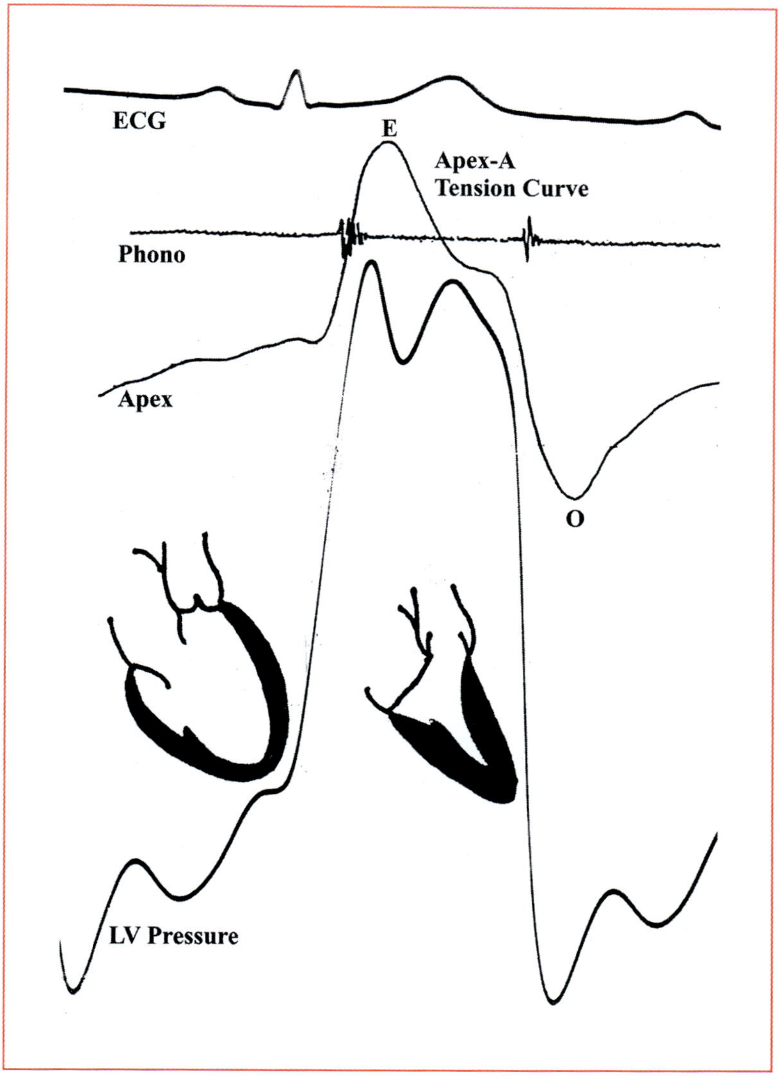

Fig. 5.5: Simultaneous recording of electrocardiogram (ECG), phonocardiogram (Phono), apexcardiogram (Apex) and left ventricular (LV) pressure curve. Also shown is the left ventricular outline in diastole and systole. The apexcardiogram that is a recording of the apex beat normally felt, basically depicts a tension curve taking into account both the pressure and the radius of the LV.

Location

The normal apical impulse being formed by the left ventricle is generally felt at the fifth intercostal space in the mid-clavicular line. The location should be assessed in the supine position or better still with the patient sitting erect. In the erect position, the normal apex is usually located about 10 cm to the left from the mid-sternal line.[22–24] Since the mid-sternal line is easily definable

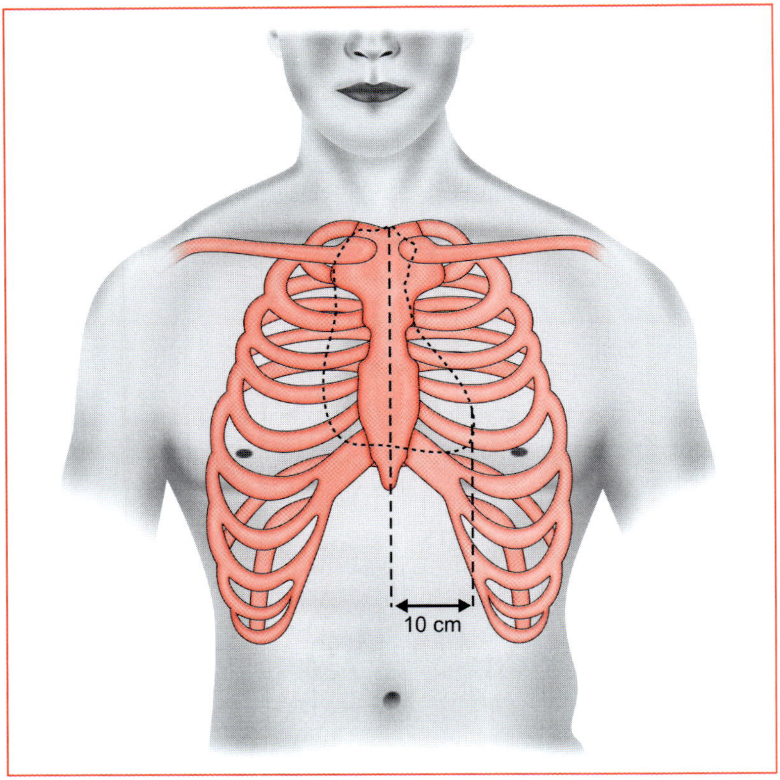

Fig. 5.6: The position of the normal apex beat is about 10 cm from the mid-sternum.

and the erect position corresponds to the way in which a chest X-ray is taken to assess the cardiac silhouette, this is probably more accurate when one tries to ascertain whether or not there is cardiomegaly (Fig. 5.6). In the left lateral decubitus position, the heart may be slightly displaced laterally due to gravity and may give the false impression of a laterally displaced apical impulse. Therefore, this position is not useful in determining the actual location. The implication of a truly laterally displaced apical impulse is that the heart is enlarged.[23] In very large and dilated hearts, the apical impulse may be displaced to the posterior axillary line and this area may be better approached from behind the patient. Medially placed apical impulse may be observed in some thin patients with vertical hearts, which is a normal variant.

Area

The normal apical impulse occupies a small area approximately the size of a quarter (2.5–3.0 cm in diameter). Its width usually fits two fingerbreadths horizontally and felt over one intercostal space vertically. This small area stems from the fact that the normal left ventricle is conical in shape and probably the apex of the cone with its small area comes into contact with the chest wall. When the left ventricle is enlarged its shape becomes more spherical and allows greater area of contact with the chest wall resulting in an enlarged area of the apical impulse. As opposed to the location of the apical impulse, the area or the size can be assessed in the left lateral decubitus position. This maneuver bringing the heart closer to the chest wall accentuates the impulse allowing more precise determination of its characteristics. In fact, it is recommended that all features to be assessed regarding the apical impulse be carried out in the left lateral decubitus except, of course, its location. A wide area apical impulse (>3.0 cm in diameter) is more valuable indicator of cardiomegaly than its actual location[28] (e.g. left ventricular aneurysm involving the anterior wall, abnormal and enlarged right ventricle forming the apex, a thin patient with a vertical heart developing cardiomegaly may have a wide area apical impulse still placed in the "normal" location).

Which Ventricle is Causing the Apical Impulse?

The heart during systole becoming smaller generally withdraws from the chest wall except for "the apex" for the reasons explained above. The effect of this withdrawal on the chest wall can be observed as an inward movement of the chest wall during systole called **"Retraction"**. Although the heart basically is comprised of two separate pumps (right and left ventricles), these two pumps operate normally at two vastly different pressures. Left ventricular systolic pressures being approximately five times higher than that of the right ventricle, its wall tension is much higher, resulting in the increased wall thickness of the left ventricular chamber. The effect of the increased muscle mass on the left side leads to dominance of the left-sided hydrodynamic forces described above. This results in the left ventricular apex as the only area of normal contact during systole. The rest of the heart essentially retracts from the chest wall. In a normal heart, this retraction of the chest wall can be observed to be located medial to the apical impulse and involving part of the left anterior chest wall.[20] Even the right ventricle that is anatomically an anterior structure gets normally pulled away from the chest wall due to its own contraction (becoming smaller) and more importantly the septal contraction also pulling the right ventricle posteriorly. *This retraction observed in normal patients is located medial to the apical impulse.*[23,24] It can be best appreciated with patients in the left lateral decubitus position with a palpating finger only on the apical impulse with clear view of the rest of the precordium for proper observation of the inward movement of the retraction (opposite in direction to the outward movement of the apical impulse). *This "medial retraction" identifies and indicates that the left ventricle forms the apical impulse.* The extent of the area of medial retraction may be variable depending on both cardiac and extra cardiac factors such as the compliance of the chest wall. It may sometimes be noted only over a small area very close to the apex beat. Nevertheless if it is medial to the apical impulse, it still identifies the apex beat to be that caused by the left ventricle (Figs. 5.7A to C).

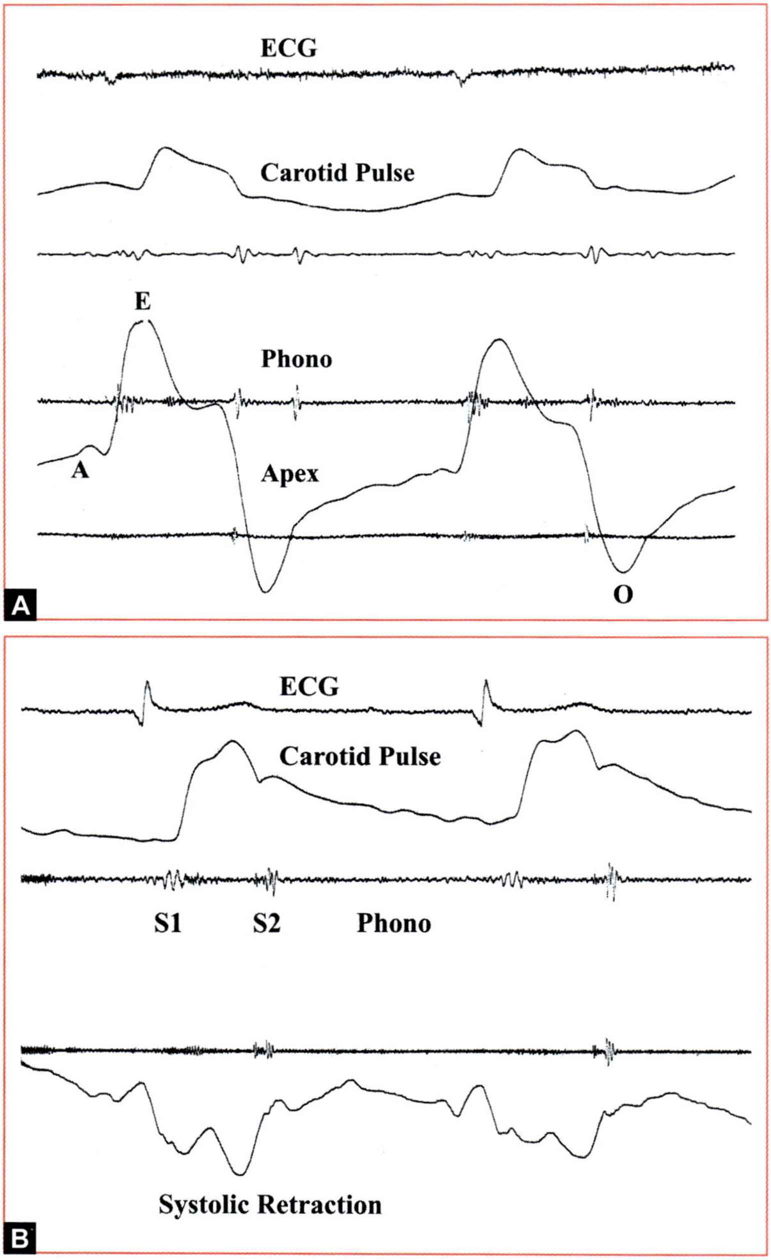

Figs. 5.7A and B: (A) Normal apexcardiogram (Apex) showing a small "A" wave caused by atrial contraction (not palpable). This is followed by a rapid rise peaking at point E (onset of ejection), corresponding to the onset of the carotid pulse upstroke. The apex beat moves away rapidly from the recording transducer as well as the palpating hand during the last two-thirds of systole ending at "O" point corresponding to mitral valve opening. (B) Simultaneous recordings of ECG, carotid pulse tracing, phonocardiogram (Phono) and recording from an area medial to the Apex beat showing systolic retraction, indicating that, in this patient, the apex beat is formed by the left ventricle.

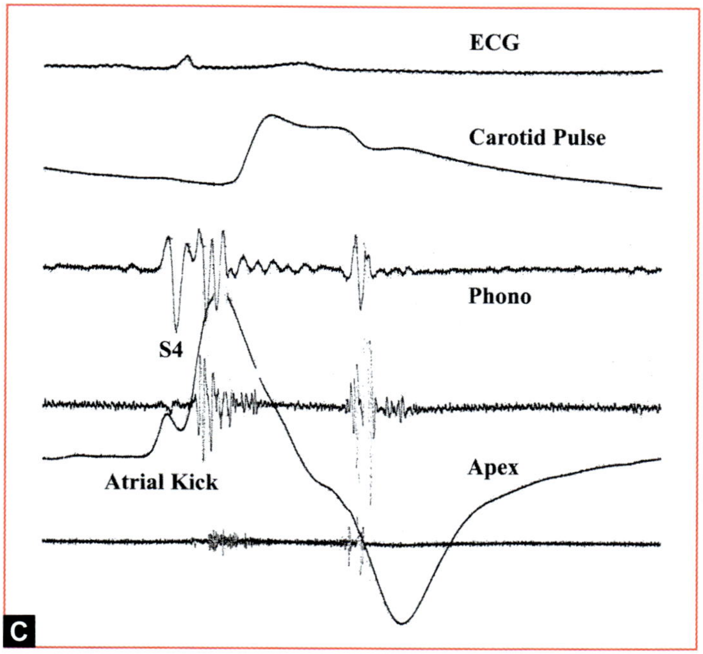

Fig. 5.7C: (C) Apexcardiogram of a patient with coronary artery disease with normal left ventricular systolic function. The amplitude and the duration of the systolic wave of the apex beat are normal. The downstroke of the Apex starts at the upstroke of the carotid pulse (very early systole). The "A" wave is exaggerated (atrial kick) due to a strong atrial contraction evoked by the increased stiffness of the left ventricle (decreased diastolic compliance) producing the S4 recorded on the phonocardiogram.

When right ventricular forces are exaggerated and become dominant due to high pressures as in pulmonary hypertension and/or excess volume in the right ventricle causing enlarged right ventricle (as may be seen in conditions of left-to-right shunt through an atrial septal defect where the right ventricle receives extra volume of blood due to the shunt flow in addition to the normal systemic venous return), the right ventricle may form the apical impulse. Usually in these states, the left ventricular forces are also diminished due to underfilling of the left ventricle (e.g. atrial septal defect, pulmonary hypertension). In this situation, the hydrodynamic forces, which lead to the formation of the apex beat being right ventricular, result in elimination of normal area of medial retraction. It may in fact be replaced by an outward movement of the precordium from the sternum to the apex area. In such patients the area of the chest wall lateral to the apical impulse will have the inward movement during systole.[20,23,29] This ***"lateral retraction"*** is again best observed when care is taken to have a clear view of the lateral chest wall with the palpating finger on the apex beat. *The presence of "lateral retraction" identifies the apical impulse to be formed by a right ventricle, which is an abnormal state.*

The usefulness of identifying the retraction and thereby determining the ventricle forming the apical impulse lies in the fact that all informations derived from the assessment of that apex beat pertain to that ventricle (e.g. a wide area apex beat with medial retraction implies left ventricular enlargement).

When both the right and the left ventricles are enlarged, then both of them may produce palpable impulses each with its own characteristics (the left ventricular impulse with an area of retraction that is medial to it and the right ventricular impulse overlying the lower sternal area with an area of retraction lateral to it).[23] The apical impulse being the lateral most impulse will be left ventricular. The retraction will therefore be in between the two impulses, therefore termed the ***median retraction.***

Character

The character of the apex beat is assessed in terms of its *dynamicity; duration and whether the impulse is single, double or triple.*

If the apical impulse cannot be felt or seen, it stands to reason that one cannot assess its character. This may be due to both cardiac and extra cardiac factors. In fact in patients with thick chest walls, obese patients and patients with chronic obstructive pulmonary disease where one does not expect to be able to feel the apical impulse, mere palpability alone, may indicate cardiomegaly.

Dynamicity

The normal apical impulse is generally felt as a short and quick outward movement, which is usually barely visible but often better felt than seen. Once the impulse is felt then it becomes easier to see the movement of the palpating finger along with the underlying chest wall in contrast to the surrounding area of the chest wall. Unless this method is followed, mistakes are often made confusing a palpable loud heart sound in the apical area as the apical impulse. Sometimes beginners describe such palpable sounds as "diffuse apex beat". This term should never be used to describe the apical impulse in any circumstance since it does not convey any useful information.

When the movement of the apical impulse is exaggerated with large amplitude as well as being rapid then the impulse is described as "hyperdynamic". Placing a stethoscope head on the area of the impulse and observing its movement can easily confirm this feature. In contrast to the normal, hyperdynamic apical impulse can be easily seen without having to palpate. In very thin chested young adults, exaggerated amplitude may be present but this should not be confused with hyperdynamicity.

A hyperdynamic apical impulse implies "volume overload" state of the ventricle involved. This usually results from a large stroke volume being ejected with increased force and velocity due to Starling mechanism. A hyperdynamic left ventricular impulse therefore suggests conditions that are ***associated***

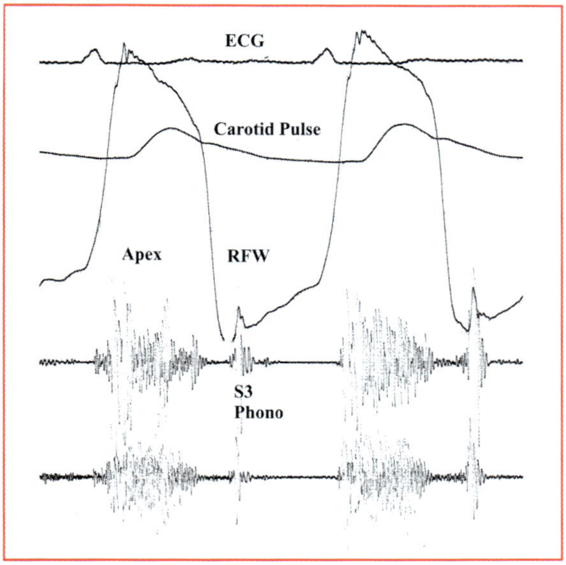

Fig. 5.8: Apexcardiogram (Apex) of a patient with severe mitral regurgitation with a hyperdynamic left ventricular apical impulse. Prominent rapid filling wave (RFW) in early diastole and a corresponding S3 recorded on the phonocardiogram together with the systolic murmur of mitral regurgitation.

with increased diastolic volumes.[24,25] The conditions that cause this may be systemic or cardiac. The systemic causes are usually associated with increased cardiac output such as seen in anemia, thyrotoxicosis, Paget's disease, pregnancy, Beriberi and arteriovenous fistulae. The cardiac causes are usually not accompanied by high cardiac outputs. These include mitral regurgitation, aortic regurgitation, ventricular septal defect, and aortopulmonary communications (e.g. persistent ductus arteriosus). In these conditions, the left ventricle receives extra volume of blood during diastole in addition to the normal pulmonary venous return (Fig. 5.8).

If the apical impulse is right ventricular and is hyperdynamic, then "volume overload" of the right ventricle must be considered as in tricuspid regurgitation, atrial septal defect and pulmonary regurgitation.

Duration

The duration of the apical impulse (how long the outward movement lasts during systole?) can only be assessed properly by simultaneous auscultation during palpation of the apex beat. By relating the time at which the apical impulse moves away from the palpating hand to the timing of the second heart sound is heard, one can assess whether the duration of the apical impulse is normal or prolonged.[17,18,23,24] *The apical impulse with a prolonged duration is termed "sustained".* The term "heave" to describe the apical impulse should never be used since it conveys no clear-cut meaning and is interpreted differently by different observers.

Normal apical impulse rises rather quickly and reaches a peak at the time of the first heart sound and moves away rapidly from the palpating hand so that the second heart sound is heard long after the apex beat has disappeared. If an apical impulse is not palpable in the supine position it is crucial to repeat the examination in the left lateral decubitus position. In our experience, this does not affect the duration of the impulse.[24] *In fact, we recommend that the duration of the apical impulse be determined in this position in all patients.*

When the impulse is felt to recede from the palpating hand as the second heart sound is being heard then the duration is prolonged and the apical impulse is sustained. Sustained left ventricular thrust during the second half of systole has been noted to be associated with an increase in left ventricular mass and volume.[7,30,31] *In addition, sustained apical impulse has been known to be associated also with significant left ventricular dysfunction*[6,7,17,31]

The sustained duration of the apical impulse implies that the wall tension in the ventricle forming the apex (usually the left ventricle) is maintained at a high level for greater part of systole.[17] This can occur as a result of increased pressure or increased volume being maintained throughout systole. *This is contrary to the general belief and teaching that sustained impulse results from a hypertrophied ventricle.*[18,22,23,25] If one relates wall tension according to Lame's modification of Laplace's formula, hypertrophy if anything should help normalize increased wall tension caused by either pressure or volume increase during systole. While the increased wall tension is a powerful stimulus for hypertrophy to occur, sometimes such hypertrophy may not fully normalize the wall tension.

The wall tension may be kept at a high level during systole by increased intraventricular systolic pressure. This is encountered in patients with significant outflow obstruction (e.g. aortic stenosis) or severe systemic hypertension. This can occur even when the ejection fraction (EF) is normal (EF is the percentage of the diastolic ventricular volume that the ventricle ejects with each systole). The normal left ventricle ejects at least 60% of its contents with each systole. In other words, the normal EF is about 60% ***in these patients*** (Figs. 5.9A and B). Since there is increased impedance to ejection in such cases, the ventricle takes longer to eject its volume as opposed to normal when most of the volume is ejected by the first third of systole.

In the absence of significant outflow obstruction and/or severe hypertension (systolic pressures over 180 mm Hg), a sustained apical impulse would imply the second important cause of prolonged duration of elevated wall tension, which would result from poor systolic emptying. This is seen for instance in patients with left ventricular dysfunction (grade III with EF between 30% and 49% and grade IV with EF < 30%) (Figs. 5.9C and D).[17] *The most important corollary of this is that a non-sustained apical impulse implies normal left ventricular EF.*[17]

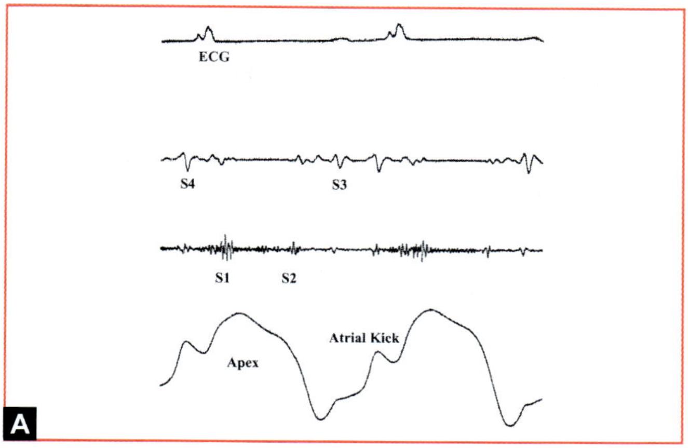

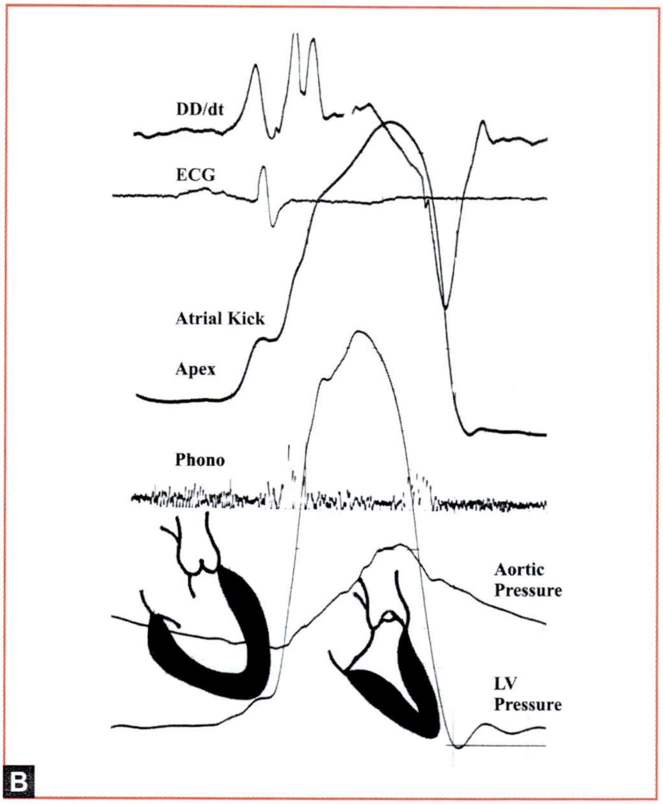

Figs. 5.9A and B: (A) Apexcardiogram (Apex) of a patient with aortic stenosis with a sustained apical impulse. The fall occurs beginning with the second heart sound (S2). A prominent atrial kick and a corresponding S4 are noted. Also S3 was heard in this patient with some early signs of heart failure. (B) Simultaneous recordings of electrocardiogram (ECG), phonocardiogram (Phono) and Apex, with its first derivative (DD/dt) in a patient with aortic stenosis. The recording of the left ventricular (LV) and aortic pressures shows the significant systolic gradient due to the obstruction. Also shown are the LV outlines in diastole and systole depicting the hypertrophied LV with normal systolic decrease in LV size. Note the atrial kick and the sustained apical impulse with the downstroke starting at the timing of S2.

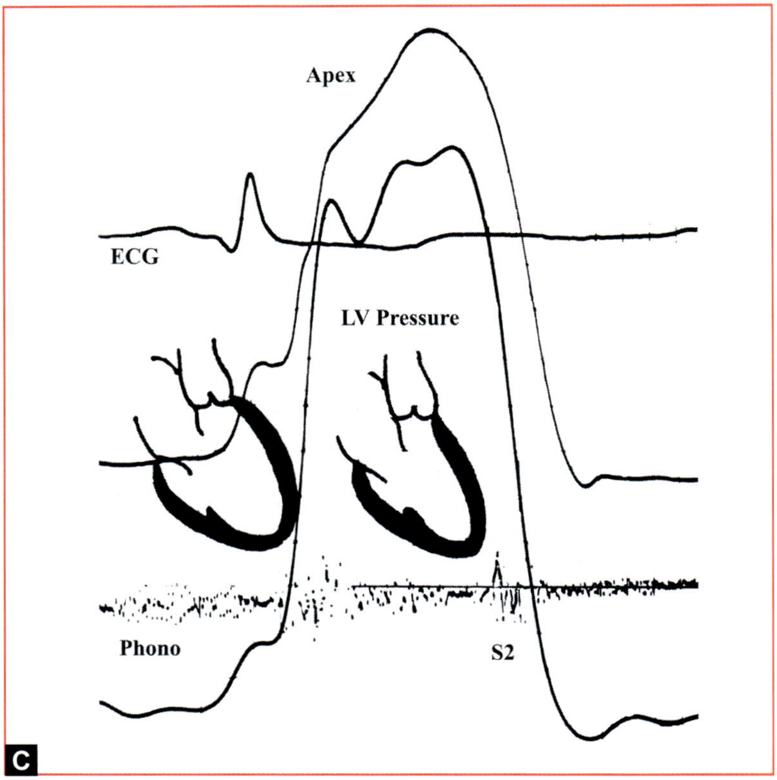

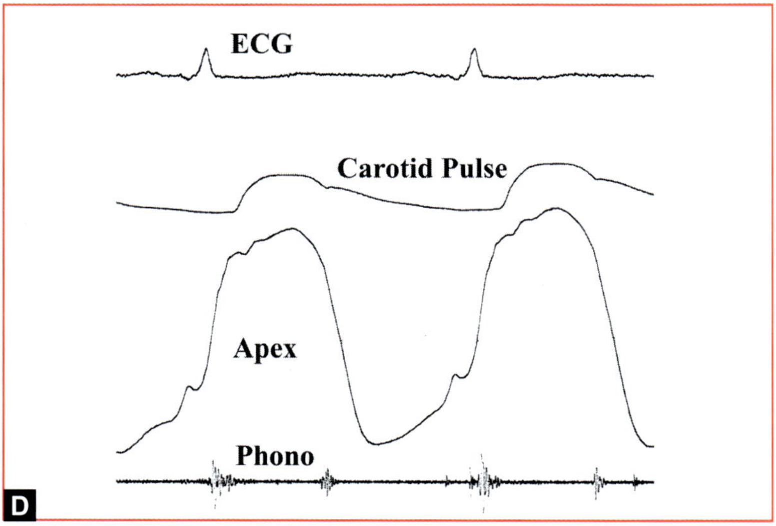

Figs. 5.9C and D: (C) Simultaneous recordings of ECG, Phono and Apex and LV pressure in a patient with coronary artery disease and LV dysfunction. Left ventricle outlines in diastole and systole depicts the lack of decrease in LV dimensions, reflecting significant LV dysfunction and decreased ejection fraction. Apex recording shows sustained duration with the downstroke beginning close to S2. (D) Sustained Apex in a patient with ischemic heart disease and significant left ventricular dysfunction.

Extra Humps and Their Timing

Atrial kick: The normal apical impulse has a single outward movement, which is palpable. The rise in left ventricular wall tension during end of diastole caused by atrial contraction may be recorded even in the normal subjects by sensitive instruments ("A" wave in the apexcardiogram), which is not palpable (*see* Fig. 5.7A). However, in patients with decreased ventricular compliance (stiff ventricles that offer resistance to expansion in diastole), the atrium compensates for this by generating a stronger or forceful contraction resulting in higher pressure. This produces an exaggerated "A" wave that may become palpable as an extra hump giving a double apical impulse also called an ***"atrial kick or hump."***[9,23] While this corresponds to an audible fourth heart sound (S4), it is not a palpable S4. This type of double apical impulse is easily recognized at the bedside as a step or hesitation in the upswing of the apical impulse. It can also be brought out by holding a tongue depressor over the apical impulse. Extra length of the tongue depressor helps to amplify the movement making it visible. The presence of an atrial kick, therefore, implies decreased ventricular compliance. The latter can occur as a result of hypertrophy, scarring, infiltrative process, ischemia or infarction. The forceful atrial contraction acts as an effective booster pump enhancing the contractility and output of the ventricle.[25,32] *It also implies a healthy atrium, sinus rhythm and no obstruction to ventricular inflow (no mitral stenosis in case of a left ventricular apex* and no tricuspid stenosis in case of right ventricular apex). The presence of an atrial kick in patients with aortic valvular stenosis and/or hypertension would imply significant stenosis or hypertension[33] (Figs. 5.10A and B). Atrial kick may sometimes give the impression of a sustained apical impulse if assessed casually.[17,20] Therefore, care should be taken to assess the duration of the impulse in the presence of an atrial kick since it has a significant implication with regard to the assessment of systolic ventricular function. In ischemic heart disease, atrial kick may be the only palpable abnormality. This indicates decreased ventricular compliance and preserved systolic left ventricular function and EF (grade I with EF 60% and over or grade II left ventricular function with EF between 50% and 59%). If the atrial kick is associated with a sustained apical impulse, then it indicates moderate left ventricular dysfunction (grade III with EF between 30% and 49%). In patients with sustained apical impulse without atrial kick who are still in sinus rhythm, the degree of left ventricular dysfunction is generally severe (grade IV with EF < 30%)[17] This occurs as a result of poor atrial function secondary to over distension or fibrosis of the left atrium.

Rapid filling wave: The second cause of a double apical impulse is the presence of an exaggerated rapid filling wave, which becomes palpable. The ventricular filling during diastole occurs in three phases. When the atrioventricular valves open in diastole, the initial inflow from the atria into the

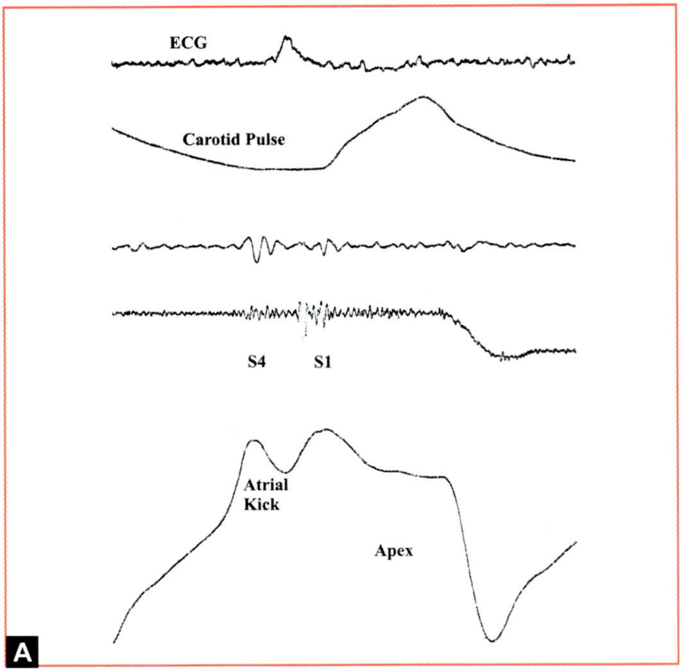

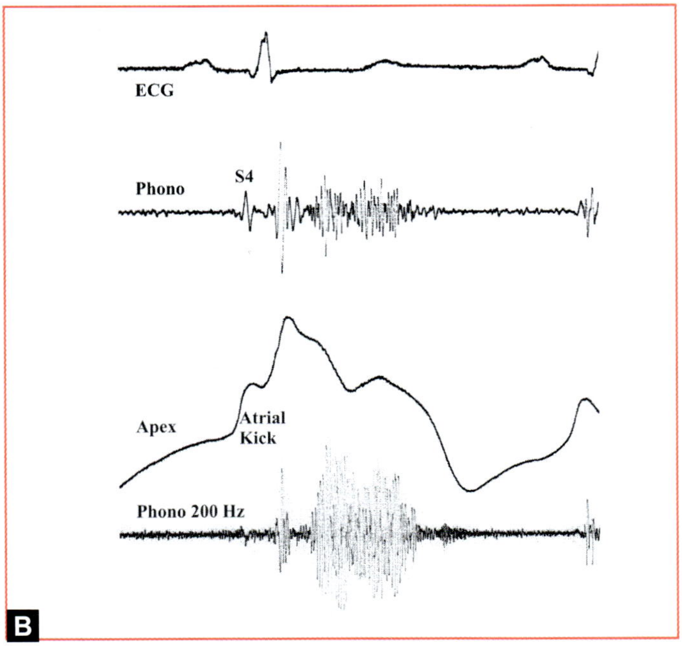

Figs. 5.10A and B: (A) Apexcardiogram (Apex) in a patient with aortic stenosis (AS) and palpable atrial kick. Note the corresponding S4. The duration of the Apex is sustained and the upstroke of the carotid pulse is delayed due to AS. (B) Apex recording in a patient with hypertrophic obstructive cardiomyopathy (HOCM) with palpable atrial kick. Phonocardiogram (Phono) shows the corresponding S4 as well as the murmur caused by the left ventricular outflow obstruction.

ventricles is quite rapid and so this phase is termed the rapid filling phase. The second phase of filling is the slow filling phase when the inflow volume and velocity slow down and the pressure in the ventricle becomes equalized to the atrial pressure. This slow filling phase lasts until the atrial contraction occurs toward the end of diastole. When a large volume of blood enters the ventricle during the early rapid filling phase, it can cause an exaggerated rapid filling wave, thereby producing an extra hump in early diastole. This is seen in ventricular volume overload states (e.g. severe mitral or aortic regurgitation).[25] This is felt as a gentle rebound after the initial rapid down stroke of the apical impulse from the palpating hand (as "a step" in the downswing of the apex beat) (Figs. 5.8 and 5.11). It may be associated with a third heart sound (S3) or short diastolic inflow rumble (not mitral stenosis). But it is not a palpable S3.

Mid-systolic retraction: The third cause of a double apical impulse is "mid-systolic retraction", giving rise to two systolic humps instead of the usual single systolic impulse. This type of double impulse is noted only in some patients with ***hypertrophic obstructive cardiomyopathy (HOCM)*** with significant subaortic dynamic obstruction and rarely in some patients with severe prolapse of the mitral valve leaflets with ***insignificant*** mitral regurgitation.[20] This is detected by appreciating the fact that both the humps occur

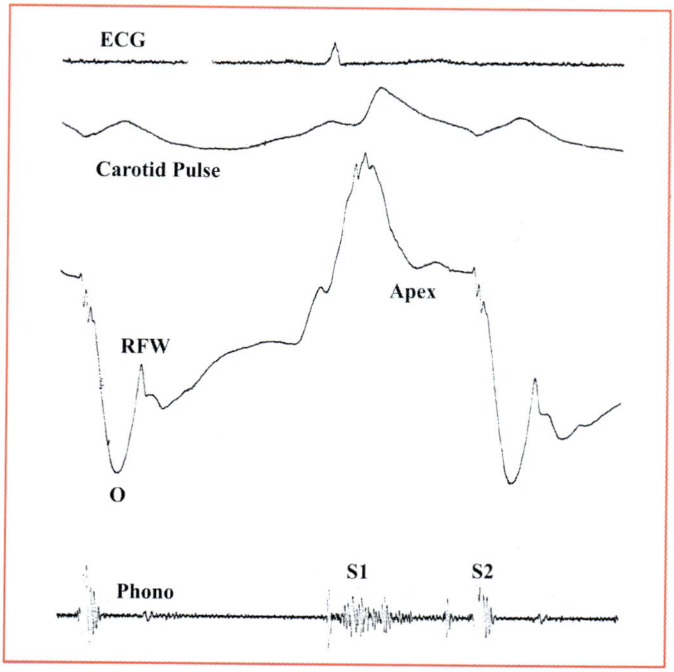

Fig. 5.11: Apexcardiogram in a pregnant woman showing an exaggerated rapid filling wave (RFW) indicating an increased volume returning to left ventricle in early diastole.

during systole. In HOCM, the initial hump is due to the rapid early ejection. In mid-systole, as obstruction develops due to the sudden anterior motion of the anterior mitral leaflet coming into contact with the interventricular septum, ejection momentarily stops. This causes the left ventricle to fall away from the chest wall, thus causing the mid-systolic retraction. In late systole as the ventricle starts relaxing, the obstruction disappears, leading to resumption of ejection of blood into aorta. This causes the second hump in systole.

Similar type of momentary and sudden decrease in ejection into the aorta may occur in mitral valve prolapse. This results from large redundant leaflets, which suddenly prolapse into the left atrium when the ventricular size becomes smaller during ejection. The blood in the ventricle preferentially goes in the direction of the left atrium due to the lower pressure in the atrium in comparison to the pressure in the aorta. If the prolapse is not associated with significant mitral regurgitation, then ejection into aorta resumes once the prolapse reaches its anatomic limits, causing the second systolic hump (Fig. 5.12).

In very rare instances one may actually feel a ***"triple apical impulse."***[20] This is usually due to a combination of an atrial kick together with the presence

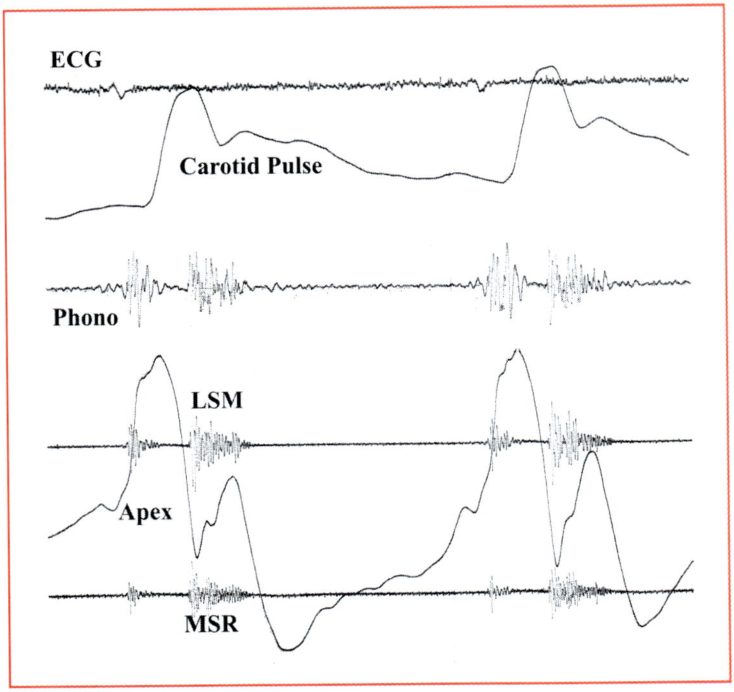

Fig. 5.12: Apexcardiogram (Apex) of a patient with mitral valve prolapse showing mid-systolic retraction (MSR). Note the late systolic murmur (LSM). The two peaks may be felt as a double impulse.

of a mid-systolic retraction. Such combination is only possible in HOCM and therefore is diagnostic of this condition (Fig. 5.13). This indicates the decreased compliance due to the idiopathic hypertrophy and the significant subaortic dynamic obstruction. The triple impulse is not seen in mitral valve prolapse since the ventricular compliance is not decreased in this disorder. Although one may think that a triple impulse may be possible in mitral prolapse as a result of mid-systolic retraction and a palpable rapid filling wave, this combination is not likely since palpable rapid filling wave requires significant mitral regurgitation. This, in turn, will preclude the presence of a mid-systolic retraction.

Palpable Sounds and Murmurs in the Area of the Apical Impulse

Occasionally, a loud first heart sound may be palpable in the region of the apex beat and may be actually mistaken for the apex beat itself. This may occur in patients with mitral stenosis which has led to the description of

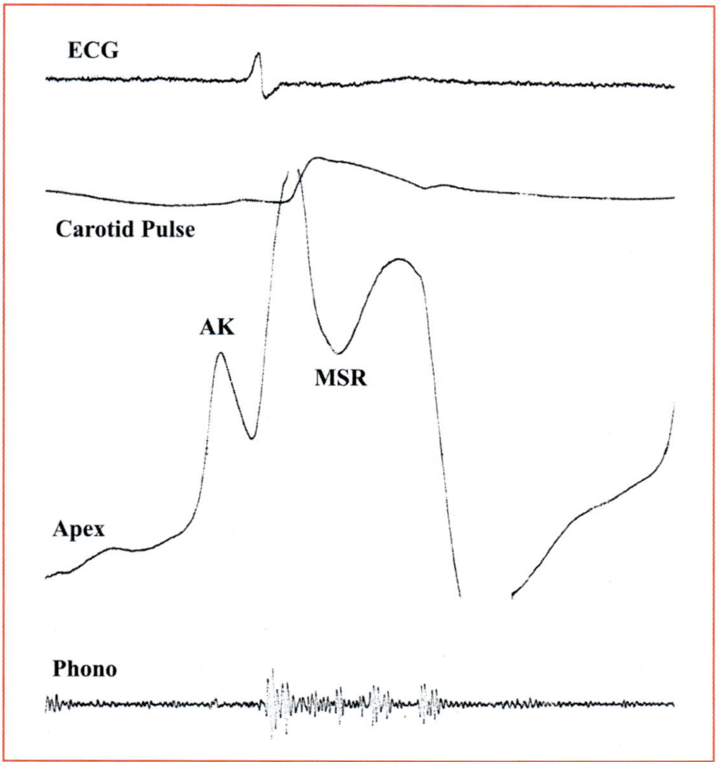

Fig. 5.13: Apexcardiogram (Apex) of a patient with HOCM showing triple apical impulse. The first impulse is the atrial kick (AK) followed by early and late systolic humps separated by a mid-systolic retraction (MSR).

so-called tapping apical impulse of mitral stenosis.[18] In general, the apical impulse when properly identified in uncomplicated mitral stenosis will be expected to be a normal left ventricular impulse.

Palpation in the apex area may also help in detecting loud murmurs, which cause palpable thrills. The significance of this is in the grading of the loudness of the murmurs.

LEFT PARASTERNAL AND STERNAL MOVEMENTS

Both the sternal and the left parasternal regions should be carefully assessed for either visible or palpable movements. The movements can either be outward systolic impulse or an inward systolic retraction.[20] The recognition of whether it is outward or inward during systole is best assessed with timing of systole by the simultaneous palpation of the arterial pulse.

Causes of the Outward Systolic Left Parasternal/Sternal Movement

1. A right ventricle that has either high pressures (e.g. pulmonary hypertension) and/or high volume load (e.g. atrial septal defect)
2. A right ventricle held forward by a large left atrium (e.g. mitral stenosis)
3. A right ventricle pushed forward by systolic expansion of the left atrium in severe mitral regurgitation[20,34]
4. Abnormal left ventricular anterior wall expansion in systole due to an aneurysm or akinetic/dyskinetic segments during ischemia.[20,24]

Causes of the Left Parasternal/Sternal Systolic Retraction

1. Normal systolic retraction in some patients.
2. *When the area of retraction is wide and exaggerated, then left ventricular volume overload as with mitral regurgitation or aortic regurgitation must be suspected.* In these conditions, the left ventricle receives extra volume of blood (regurgitant volume) in diastole in addition to the normal pulmonary venous return. The retraction tends to be more exaggerated in patients with isolated aortic regurgitation as opposed to mitral regurgitation for similar degrees of volume overload. This is due to the systolic expansion of the left atrium in mitral regurgitation, which opposes the retraction caused by left ventricular systole. *In fact, excessive sternal retraction rules out severe mitral regurgitation. On the other hand, it may be commonly observed in significant aortic regurgitation (Fig. 5.14).*[20]
3. When the sternum is made flail due to trauma or surgery (post-median sternotomy), it may exaggerate the normal systolic retraction.
4. *Sometimes the only visible or palpable precordial movement will be just a systolic retraction without a definable apical impulse. This occurs in*

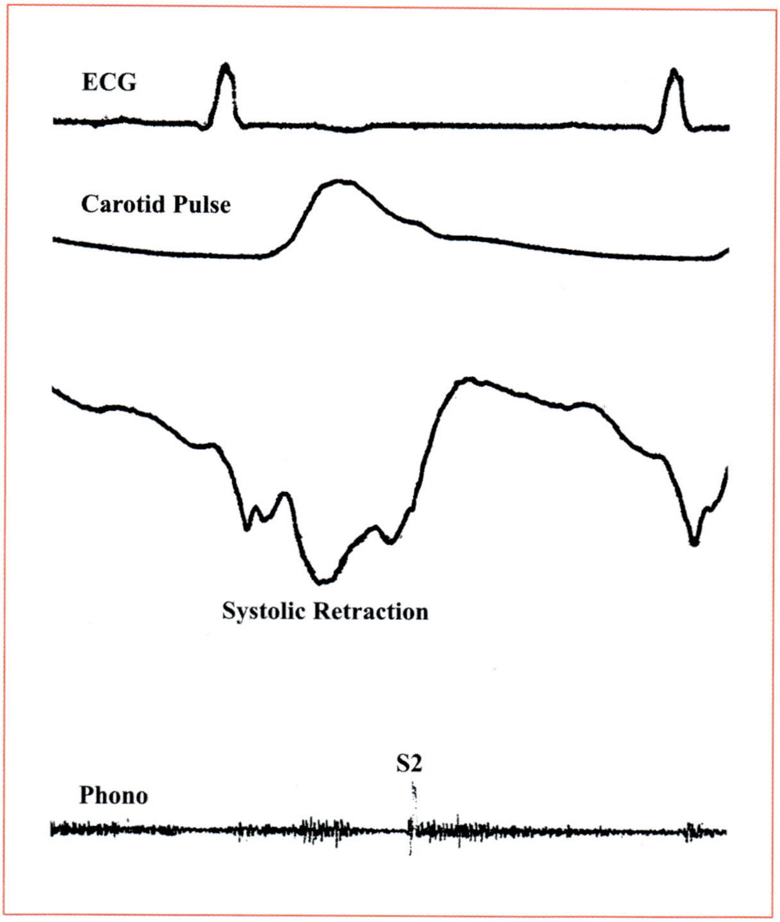

Fig. 5.14: Marked systolic retraction in a patient with significant aortic regurgitation. The recording was made with the transducer medial to the apical impulse over the lower left parasternal area.

two conditions: constrictive pericarditis and Ebstein's anomaly. In both of these conditions, the left ventricle is relatively underfilled. In constrictive pericarditis, the systolic retraction of the chest overlying the ribs in the left axilla has been known as the Broadbent sign.[32] In Ebstein's anomaly, the right atrium is usually huge due to partial atrialization of the right ventricle due to a congenital downward displacement of the tricuspid valve attachment and the tricuspid regurgitation that accompanies it.

RIGHT PARASTERNAL MOVEMENT

Any outward systolic impulse in this region should imply aortic root dilatation as in aortic aneurysm and/or dissection.

PULSATIONS OVER THE CLAVICULAR HEADS

Pulsations of the clavicular heads indicate the presence of abnormal dilatation of the aortic arch (e.g. aneurysm).

PULSATIONS OVER THE SECOND AND/OR THIRD LEFT INTERCOSTAL SPACES

This region anatomically overlies the pulmonary outflow tract. Pulsations in this area may be felt in patients with pulmonary artery dilatation with or without pulmonary hypertension. Pulmonary artery dilatation may occur either on an idiopathic basis or due to excess pressure (pulmonary hypertension irrespective of the cause) or excess volume flow through the pulmonary outflow (e.g. atrial septal defect with large volume flow due to left-to-right shunt at the atrial level).

SUBXIPHOID IMPULSE

Subxiphoid region should be palpated by placing the palm of the hand over the epigastrium with the fingertips pointing up toward the patient's head. Gentle pressure is applied downward and upward. Often as a good rule, the patient should be asked to take a deep inspiration in order to move the diaphragm down. This facilitates the palpation of the right ventricle.[2,25] If the impulse were palpable pushing the fingertips downward (toward the feet) as opposed to lifting the palmar aspect of the hand, it would indicate a palpable right ventricular impulse. Transmitted abdominal aortic pulsations will cause the impulse to strike the palmar aspect of the hand. *Unlike the sternal and parasternal movement discussed previously, subxiphoid palpation is very specific for a right ventricular impulse.*

In the normal adult, there is never a detectable right ventricular impulse by subxiphoid palpation. Therefore, if a right ventricular impulse is detected subxiphoid in an adult it should indicate either a pressure and/or volume overload of the right ventricle. Its character should be determined as discussed previously in relation to the apex beat, namely the dynamicity, duration and whether the impulse is single or double (Fig. 5.15).

PRACTICAL POINTS IN THE CLINICAL ASSESSMENT OF THE PRECORDIAL PULSATIONS

1. *The traditional methods of inspection and palpation together with auscultation are necessary for the proper assessment of the precordial pulsations and in particular the apical impulse. In the supine position, with the patient's precordium well exposed under proper lighting conditions (preferably natural light source from the sides), one should inspect*

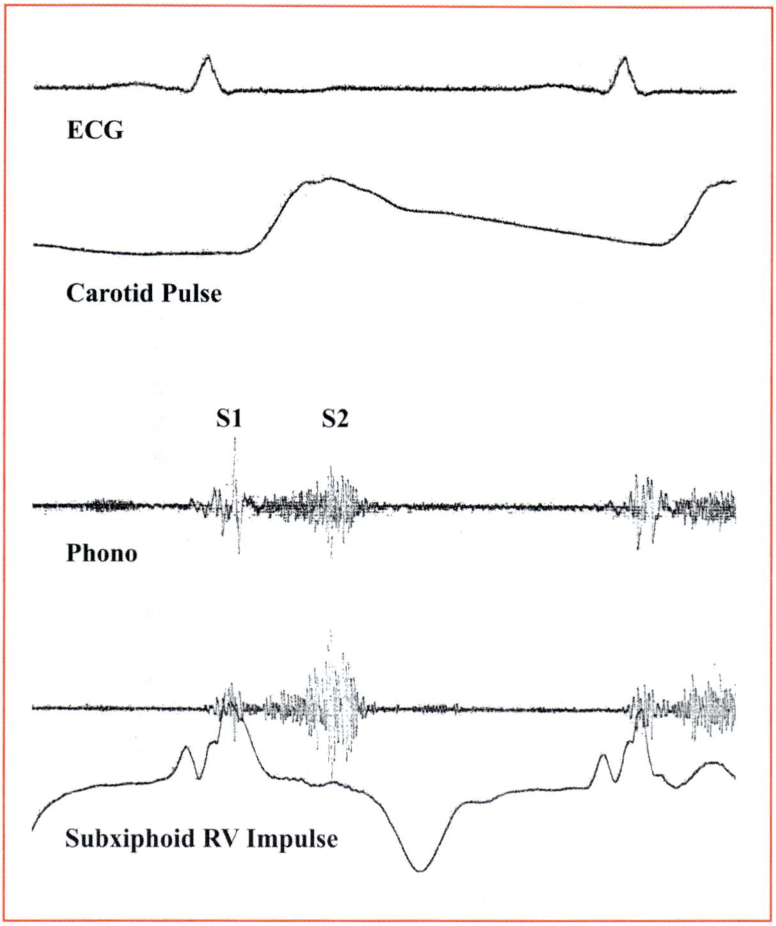

Fig. 5.15: Recording of a subxiphoid right ventricular impulse in a patient with combined aortic stenosis and hypertrophic obstructive cardiomyopathy and severe secondary pulmonary hypertension. It is similar to the apical impulse in its characteristics.

carefully for movements of the chest wall over all areas of the precordium including the sternal area, the left parasternal area, the right parasternal area, the apical area, the basal portions overlying the second and third interspaces, and the sternoclavicular junction. Any observed movement should then be timed with simultaneous palpation of the radial pulse upstroke to determine whether the observed movement is outward during systole or inward during systole. It is needless to say that if the movement is outward during systole then it will be synchronous with pulse upstroke.

2. *In normal patients, it is uncommon to see exaggerated movements over the precordium inward or outward during systole. Rarely in very young and thin chested subjects, one may see active movements over the apical*

area. The parasternal and the sternal regions in most normals are very quite. The normal inward retraction of this region is usually difficult to feel. It may only be seen over a small area adjacent and medial to the apex area or the apical impulse.

3. *When the area of retraction overlies a larger area of the parasternum or the sternum, then conditions that may predispose to such situations must be considered. These include left ventricular volume overload states such as aortic and mitral regurgitations. The retraction of the parasternal and the sternal region may in fact be excessive and easily visible in significant and isolated aortic regurgitation, since in these patients the excess diastolic volumes of the left ventricle (due to both the normal pulmonary venous return coming through the mitral inflow as well as the additional regurgitant flow coming from the insufficient aortic valve) provide strong Starling effect increasing the force of left ventricular contraction. In addition, in isolated aortic regurgitation, the left atrium will not be enlarged and therefore will not offset the degree of the retraction as it often does in mitral regurgitation, which will cause left atrial expansion during systole. The left atrium being the posterior chamber, its expansion will tend to push the rest of the heart forward during systole. This will limit the degree of the retraction seen in mitral regurgitation. The excessive sternal retraction seen in patients with significant aortic regurgitation may be mistaken for right ventricular movement with sternal lift if one does not take care to time the movement with simultaneous palpation of the carotid or the radial arterial pulse. The timing with the arterial pulse will show the sternal movement to be inward during systole.*
4. *In severe mitral regurgitation, the left atrial expansion may cause a sternal lift but this will tend to be slightly delayed in onset when compared to the onset of the left ventricular apical impulse in the same patient if both impulses are simultaneously palpated. This will be in contrast to a true right ventricular movement over the sternum, which will rise at the same time as the left ventricular apical impulse.*
5. *The following points are important to remember while assessing the apical impulse:*
   a. *The apical impulse is the lateral most point of systolic outward movement that is felt over the precordium. The apical impulse that is palpable must be an area of the chest wall that can be both felt and seen to move forward during systole as assessed by a palpating finger. The apical impulse may be palpable only intermittently due to respiratory variations. It may be felt well most often at end expiration when the lungs are deflated. However in some patients, the descent of the diaphragm with respirations may have an effect on the mediastinum. This may variably affect the palpability of the apex beat. However, it*

may be best felt only when it is against an intercostal space as opposed to being behind a rib. This may happen at any phase of respiration.

b. *While defining the apical impulse one must be able to conclude as follows:*
   i. *It is palpable (meaning that the area can be both seen and felt to move under the palpating finger).*
   ii. *It is barely palpable meaning that one feels a sensation of outward movement but not enough to see it clearly.*
   iii. *It is not palpable.*

   Mistaking a palpable sound over the apical area, mostly caused by a loud first heart sound for the apical impulse can be avoided if one looks for the actual area of movement of the chest wall underneath the palpating finger. Often the loud sound may be picked up by the palm of the whole hand over the apical area and the lower left sternal region.

c. *The location of the apical impulse is best assessed with the patient sitting upright, when palpable it will give some clue regarding the presence or absence of cardiomegaly. However in a substantial number of patients, the apical impulse will be palpable only in the left lateral decubitus position.*

d. *All other important points to be determined regarding the apical impulse (such as its area or dimension, the location of the retraction whether medial or lateral to the apex, the character whether it is sustained in duration, its dynamicity, the determination of extra humps and even the detection of any palpable sounds or murmurs over the apical area) are best felt and determined in the left lateral decubitus position of the patient.*

e. *The presence of medial retraction identifies a left ventricular impulse while lateral retraction indicates a right ventricular impulse. One can sometimes stick one end of a tongue blade with a tape over the area of the apical impulse or hold it against it while observing for area of retraction adjacent to it. The tongue blade is a valuable simple tool and can also be used to observe for the contour of the apical motion for the detection of the presence of any extra humps such as an atrial kick.*

f. *Retraction may sometimes be median with two areas of outward systolic impulse. One of these will be laterally placed and is obviously the apical impulse formed by the left ventricle and the other will be the right ventricular impulse, which will be medial to the area of retraction. In such a situation, both impulses will rise simultaneously. Each of the two respective impulses must be assessed further in the same manner in which the apical impulse is characterized.*

g. *The duration of the apical impulse is best determined with the whole palm of the hand palpating and timing at the same time by auscultation over the nearby area or the third or the fourth left interspace near the left sternal border. The normal apical impulse comes out with the first heart sound and recedes away from the palpating hand very rapidly, and it is therefore hard to latch onto it for any length of time. One cannot even know when it recedes since it does so swiftly. If one can tell when it begins to fall away from the palpating hand, then its duration is already prolonged. If it is felt to recede as one hears the second heart sound then it is definitely sustained. A sustained left ventricular impulse in the absence of significant hypertension (BP systolic above 180) or aortic stenosis often picked up by delayed upstroke of the carotid pulse (see Chapter 2 on Arterial Pulse) would be indicative of decreased left ventricular systolic function (grade III with EF between 30% and 49% or grade IV with EF < 30%). (Left ventricular function can be graded by measurements of EF that is obtained by dividing the stroke volume by the end-diastolic volume of the left ventricle).*

   A non-sustained impulse would favor normal systolic function with normal EF (60% or more) or only mild dysfunction with EF between 50% and 59%.

h. *The dynamicity of the apex beat can be best appreciated by placing the head of a stethoscope over it to see how large and rapid the movement of the chest wall is underneath it. If the movement is large and rapid then it will be reflected by the movement of the stethoscope head.*

i. *While palpating for the contour and the detection of the presence of any extra humps such as the atrial kick, it is important to feel gently since excessive pressure could fail to detect them by filtering out lower frequency vibrations. The atrial kick is detected by the presence of a hesitation or a step in the outward movement of the apical impulse. The exaggerated rapid filling wave during diastole is felt, on the other hand, as a gentle rebound after the initial rapid down stroke of the apical impulse from the palpating hand (as "a step" in the downswing of the apex beat).*

6. *Left parasternal and sternal areas must be inspected carefully for movement with simultaneous palpation of the radial pulse. This will help in the appreciation of any exaggerated retraction over these areas if present. Parasternal and in particular sternal movement must be assessed further with palpation using the palm of the hand and having the patient breathe out and holding their breath at end expiration. This helps to deflate the lungs and reduce the attenuation caused by the expanded lungs.*

7. *Subxiphoid palpation, on the other hand, for right ventricular movement is done with the palm of the hand placed with the tips of the*

fingers pointing toward the head of the patient. The patient should be asked to take a deep breath so that the diaphragms can descend and with it the right ventricle. If right ventricle is palpable, then it will produce an active motion, which will hit the fingertips. If the impulse hits the palmar aspect of the fingers then it must be transmitted aortic pulsation and not the right ventricular impulse. In the adult, the normal right ventricle never produces a palpable subxiphoid impulse while one may feel this in children and adolescents.

REFERENCES

1. Potain C. Du rhythme cardiaque appele' bruit de galop. Bull Soc Med Hop Paris. 1875;s2:12:137-66.
2. Mackenzie J. The Study of the Pulse, Arterial, Venous and Hepatic and of the Movements of the Heart. Edinburgh, London: Young J Pentland; 1902.
3. Benchimol A, Diamond E. The normal and abnormal apexcardiogram. It's physiological variation and its relation to intracardiac events. Am J Cardiol. 1963;12:368.
4. Tafur E, Cohen LS, Levine HD. The normal apexcardiogram, its temporal relationship to electrical, acoustic and mechanical cardiac events. Circulation. 1964;30:381.
5. Tavel ME. Campbell RW, Feigenbaum H, et al. The apexcardiogram and its relationship to hemodynamic events within the left heart. Br Heart J. 1965;27:829.
6. Lane FJ, Carrroll JM, Levine HD, Gorlin R. The apexcardiogram in myocardial asynergy. Circulation. 1968;37:890.
7. Sutton GC, Prewitt TA, Craige E. Relationship between quantitated precordial movement and left ventricular function. Circulation. 1970;41:179-90.
8. Craige E. Clinical value of apex cardiography. Am J Cardiol. 1971;28:118-21.
9. Gibson TC, Madry R, Grossman W, et al. The A wave of the apexcardiogram and left ventricular diastolic stiffness. Circulation. 1974;49:441-6.
10. Mc Ginn FX, Gould L, Lyonn AF. The phonocardiogram and apexcardiogram in patients with ventricular aneurysm. Am J Cardiol. 1968;21:467.
11. Prewitt T, Gibson D, Brown D, et al. The "rapid filling wave" of the apex cardiogram. Its relation to echocardiographic and cineangiographic measurements of ventricular filling. Br Heart J. 1975;37:1256-62.
12. Wayne HH. The apexcardiogram in ischemic heart disease. Calif Med. 1972; 116:12.
13. Venco A, Gibson DG, Brown DJ. Relation between apex cardiogram and changes in left ventricular pressure and dimension. Br Heart J. 1977;39:117-25.
14. Willems JL, De Geest H, Kesteloot H. On the value of apex cardiography for timing intracardiac events. Am J Cardiol. 1971;28:59-66.
15. Manolas J, Rutishauser W, Wirz P, et al. Time relation between apex cardiogram and left ventricular events using simultaneous high-fidelity tracings in man. Br Heart J. 1975;37:1263-7.
16. Manolas J, Rutishauser W. Diastolic amplitude time index: a new apexcardiographic index of left ventricular diastolic function in human beings. Am J Cardiol. 1981;48:736-45.
17. Ranganathan N, Juma Z, Sivaciyan V. The apical impulse in coronary heart disease. Clin Cardiol. 1985;8:20-33.

18. Mounsey JP. Inspection ad palpation of the cardiac impulse. Prog Cardiovasc Dis. 1967;10:187-206.
19. Eddlemann EE. Kinetocardiographic changes in ischemic heart disease. Circulation. 1965;31:650-5.
20. Stapleton JF, Groves BM. Precordial palpation. Am Heart J. 1971;81:409-27.
21. Schweizer W, Bertrab RV, Reist P. Kinetocardiography in coronary artery disease. Br Heart J. 1965;27:263-8.
22. Deliyannis AA, Gillam PMS, Mounsey JPD, et al. The cardiac impulse and the motion of the heart. Br Heart J. 1964;26:396.
23. Constant J. Inspection and palpation of the chest. In: Bedside Cardiology, 2nd edition. Boston: Little Brown and Co; 1976. pp. 100-33.
24. Abrams J. Precordial palpation. In: Horwitz LD, Groves BM (Eds). Signs and Symptoms in Cardiology. Philadelphia: JB Lippincott; 1985. pp. 156-77.
25. Perloff JK. The physiologic mechanisms of cardiac and vascular physical signs. J Am Coll Cardiol. 1983;1:184-98.
26. Hansen DE, Daughters GT 2nd, Alderman EL, et al. Torsional deformation of the left ventricular midwall in human hearts with intramyocardial markers: regional heterogeneity and sensitivity to the inotropic effects of abrupt rate change. Circ Res. 1988;62(5):941-52.
27. Hawthorne EW. Dynamic geometry of the left ventricle. Am J Cardiol. 1966; 18:566-73.
28. Eilen SD, Crawford MH, O'Rourke RA. Accuracy of precordial palpation for detecting increased left ventricular volume. Ann Intern Med. 1983;99:628-30.
29. Boicourt OW, Nagle RE, Mounsey JP. The clinical significance of systolic retraction of the apical impulse. Br Heart J. 1965;27:379-91.
30. Conn RD, Cole JS. The cardiac apex impulse. Clinical and angiographic correlations. Ann Intern Med. 1971;75:185-91.
31. Mills RM Jr, Kastor JA. Quantitative grading of cardiac palpation. Comparison in supine and left lateral decubitus positions. Arch Intern Med. 1973;132:831-4.
32. Wood PW. Diseases of the Heart and Circulation. Philadelphia: JB Lippincott; 1956. p. 411.
33. Epstein EJ, Coulshed N, Brown AK, et al. The "A" wave of the apex cardiogram in aortic valve disease and cardiomyopathy. Br Heart J. 1968;30:591-605.
34. Basta LL, Wolfson P, Eckberg DL, et al. The value of left parasternal impulse recordings in the assessment of mitral regurgitation. Circulation. 1973;48: 1055-65.

Chapter 6 Heart Sounds

Snapshot

- Principles of Sound Formation in the Heart
- First Heart Sound (S1)
- Clinical Assessment of S1 and its Components
- Second Heart Sound
- Normal S2
- Abnormal S2
- Clinical Assessment of S2
- Opening Snap
- Clinical Assessment of the OS
- Third Heart Sound (S3)
- Clinical Features of S3
- Clinical Assessment of S3
- Fourth Heart Sound (S4)
- Clinical Assessment of S4

PRINCIPLES OF SOUND FORMATION IN THE HEART

In the past, many theories have been advanced to explain the origins of sounds during cardiac cycle. These included simple concepts explaining sound originating from the actual contact of valve cusps upon closure. When it was realized that the strength of contraction of the left ventricle had a significant effect on the intensity of the first heart sound, the myocardial theory of the origin of the sound was postulated. Some of the theories even had suggested extracardiac origin of sounds such as the third heart sound (S3). It is now however well established by several investigators and accepted that the formation of all sounds in the heart can be explained by a "unified concept."[1-10]

It is a common experience that a pipe half-filled with water, held between our two palms of the hands, produces sound when it is moved back and forth splashing the water. We all have heard banging sounds sometime produced in the water pipes of the plumbing systems of our homes. The latter is seen when air gets introduced into the plumbing system. In both the examples given above, the mechanism of sound production is the same. When the moving column of water in either case comes to sudden stop or marked deceleration, the energy of the column dissipates and in the process generates vibration of the pipes as well as the column of water. These vibrations, when in the audible range, are heard as sounds. The intensity of the sound will very much depend on the initial energy of the moving column of water. Of the two examples, the sounds in the second case are usually very loud and may be heard within the entire house. This is mainly because the water pressure in the system is approximately 40 pounds per square inch.

Similarly, all the sounds of the heart are formed when a moving column of blood comes to a sudden stop or decelerates significantly. The intensity of a heart sound will depend on the level of energy that the moving column of blood has attained. The sudden deceleration causes dissipation of energy which results in the production of vibrations affecting the contiguous cardiohemic mass.[3] The factors affecting the acceleration and deceleration of columns of blood involved in the formation of the various heart sounds are different and may be many. These will have to be considered for each sound separately taking into account the physiology and the pathophysiology of the phase of the cardiac cycle involved.

FIRST HEART SOUND (S1)

The first heart sound occurs at the onset of ventricular contraction. To better understand the physiology of the first heart sound, one needs to know the cardiac events that occur around the time of the first heart sound (S1). At the end of diastole, the atrium contracts and gives an extrastretch and filling to the ventricle. This is immediately followed by the ventricular contraction. When the ventricular pressure rises and exceeds the atrial pressure, the mitral and the tricuspid valve leaflets become apposed and close. As the ventricular pressures continue to rise and exceed that of the aorta and the pulmonary artery, the semilunar valves open and the ejection phase begins. All these events occur at rapid succession over a short period of time and contribute to the production of the first heart sound. As a result of this, S1 is relatively wide and is made of many components, which overlap each other. These components are "atrial", "mitral", "tricuspid" and "aortic".[2,5,7,10-14]

Atrial Component

The energy of the column of blood pushed by the atrial contraction gets dissipated as the column decelerates against the ventricular walls. This deceleration is gradual in most normal subjects due to good compliance and distensibility of the ventricles. Therefore the sound generated by this has very low frequency and is not audible. This will be discussed further in relation to the fourth heart sound (S4). However when the PR interval on the electrocardiogram is short, this component can occur very close to the onset of the ventricular contraction and actually be part of the first heart sound and contribute to its duration. Aside from this, it has no clinical significance.[11,14]

Mitral Component

This is the most important component of S1. It corresponds in timing to the closure of the mitral valve leaflets.[10,12] However, the mere apposition of the valve leaflets does not produce the sound. As the ventricle starts contracting, the pressure rises and imparts energy into the mass of blood within its cavity. When the pressure in the ventricle just exceeds that of the atrium, the column of blood is put into motion. Since the aortic pressure is much higher than the atrial pressure and the aortic valve remains closed at this time, the blood contained in the ventricle can only rush toward the atrium. Because of the anatomic construction of the mitral valve similar to that of a parachute, the leaflets are lifted by the moving blood into a closed position. The papillary muscles contracting and pulling on the chordae tendineae prevent leaflet eversion into the atrium. The closed leaflets held back by the papillary muscles reaching the limits of their stretch, stop the column of blood from moving into the atrium. This sudden deceleration of the column of blood causes the mitral component or the M1 (Figs. 6.1 and 6.2A and B). The energy

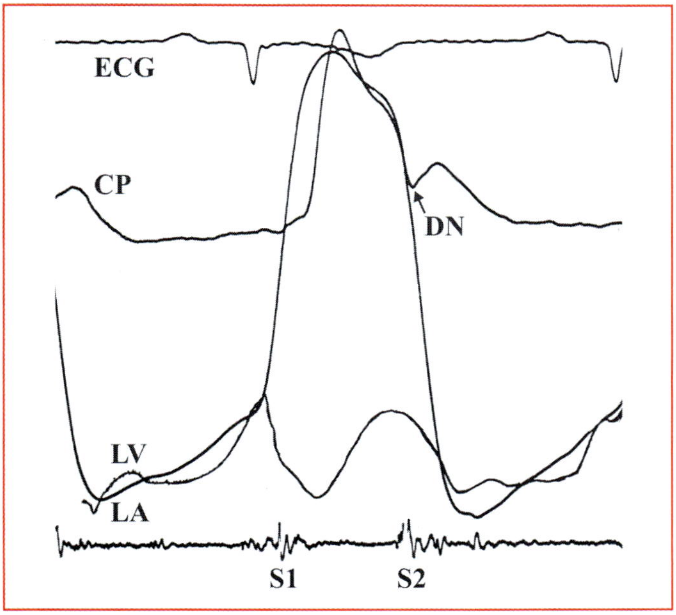

Fig. 6.1: Simultaneous recordings of electrocardiogram, carotid pulse (CP), left ventricular (LV) and left atrial (LA) pressures. When the rising LV pressure exceeds the LA pressure, the column of blood contained in the ventricle is put into motion since the aortic valve is still closed at this time. Since the LA pressure is relatively low, the column of blood will tend to rush toward the LA. The anatomic construction of the mitral valve is such that the leaflets are closed and prevented from eversion by the contraction of the papillary muscles. The valve closure leads to sudden deceleration of the moving column of blood. The resulting dissipation of energy leads to the production of the mitral component of the first heart sound. The rise of CP indirectly reflects aortic pressure rise. However, there is a transmission delay. DN denotes dicrotic notch.

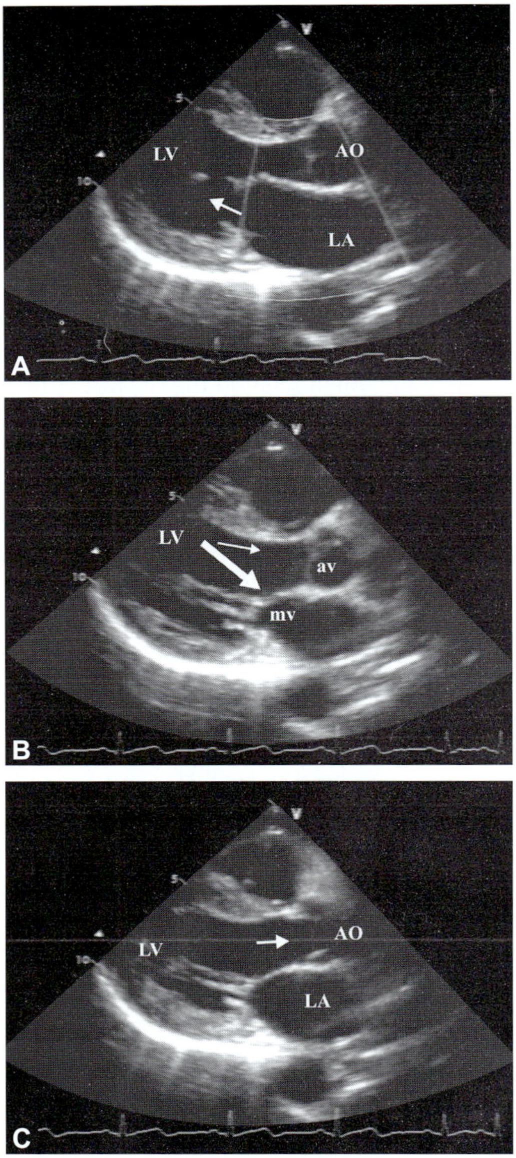

Figs. 6.2A to C: Stop frames from the two-dimensional echocardiographic recordings taken in the parasternal long axis from a normal subject showing the left ventricle (LV), mitral valve (mv), left atrium (LA), aorta (AO) and the aortic valve (av) at end-diastole (A), onset systole (B) and onset ejection (C). The heads of the arrows indicate the direction of movement of the column of blood in the left heart. At end-diastole, the diastolic filling of LV is nearly completed. With the onset of systole, the rising LV pressure puts the column of blood into motion, with the main direction ***(thicker arrow)*** toward the low pressure LA, where it gets decelerated by the closure of the mv. This leads to production of the mitral component. When the rising LV pressure exceeds the aortic pressure with further contraction of the ventricle, the av opens and ejection phase begins. When the ejected column of blood hits the walls of the AO, deceleration occurs again leading to the production of the aortic component.

dissipation causes vibrations of the column of blood as well as the entire surrounding structures, i.e. the mitral valve structures and the ventricular wall.[15] The mechanism of sound formation of M1 is very similar to that of the sound produced by the parachute filling with wind as it stretches and causes the deceleration of the moving mass of air, or by the sail of a sailboat that snaps when filled with a gust of wind.

Tricuspid Component

Tricuspid component (T1) is obviously similar in its origin to the M1 due to the occurrence of similar cardiac events involving the right sided structures namely the tricuspid valve leaflets and the right ventricular wall. However, these events occur at much lower pressures and are slightly delayed. The effects of the mechanical events of the right ventricle begin slightly later than that of the left ventricle. Therefore, the T1 follows the M1.[13] It must be noted that this component, because of the lower pressures, is usually low in frequency. The T1 in the normal adult subjects although may be recordable, may contribute to the duration of S1 but may not be audible as a distinct component.[16,17]

Aortic Component

The aortic component (A1) is usually the second component of audibly split S1 in the adults.[7,17] After the closure of mitral and tricuspid valves, the ventricular pressure continues to rise during the phase of isovolumic contraction. When the pressure exceeds the aortic and pulmonary diastolic pressures, ejection phase begins as the semilunar valves open. The column of blood ejected into the aorta as it hits the aortic walls decelerates and when the deceleration is significant, it results in an audible sound (Fig. 6.2C).[18]

Normal S1

Since the major and the most important component of S1 is M1, the S1 is usually heard loudest at the apex and the lower left sternal border around the fourth left intercostal space. The sound is usually low pitched and longer in duration compared to the sharper, shorter and higher frequency second heart sound (S2). It can be timed to occur at the onset of a carotid pulse or the apical impulse and it is a useful way of distinguishing it from S2. It can be mimicked by the syllable "Lubbb" as opposed to the sharper S2, which sounds like "dub." It may be audibly split into two components in some patients when the separation exceeds at least 20 ms. When such a split is heard, it could be due to M1-T1 in children and young adolescents and is usually due to M1-A1 in the adults (Fig. 6.3). The T1 component tends to be maximally heard over the sternum and the left sternal border and not usually over the apex, which is formed by the left ventricle in the normal subjects. Tricuspid component

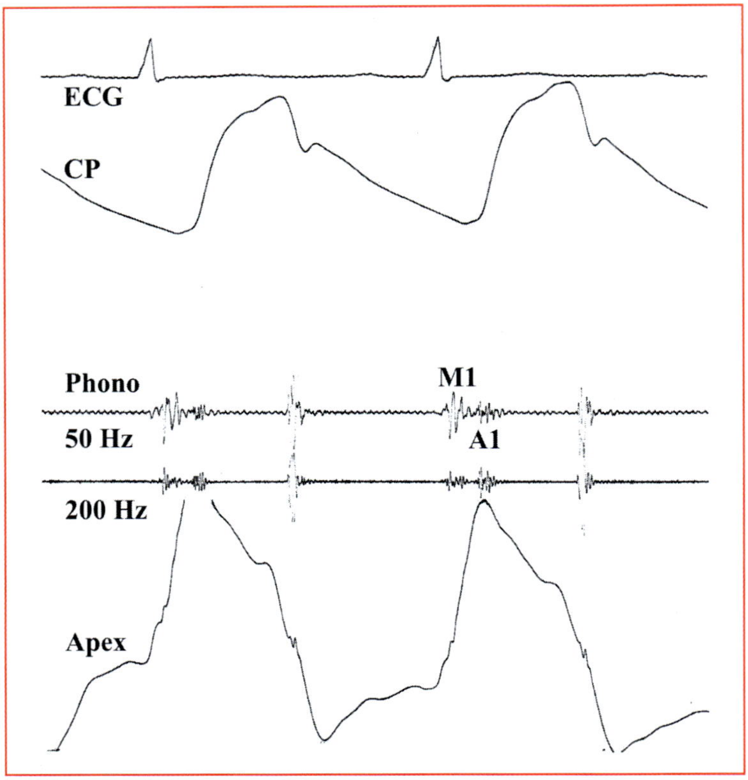

Fig. 6.3: Phonocardiogram recorded at the lower left parasternal area close to the apex showing two distinct components of the normal first heart sound namely the mitral component M1 and the aortic component (A1). The M1 precedes the onset of the carotid pulse whereas the A1 occurs with it. Note that the externally recorded carotid pulse tracing has a pulse transmission delay. Simultaneously recorded ECG, the carotid pulse and the apexcardiogram are shown to indicate the timing. The abbreviations used in this and other such illustrations are as follows: (ECG: Electrocardiogram; CP: Carotid pulse tracing; Apex: Apexcardiogram; Phono: Phonocardiogram; Hz: Cycles per second).

also tends to get louder on inspiration due to greater volume and Starling effect during inspiratory phase of respiration on the right side. The A1 on the other hand does not vary with respiration and is just as loud over the apex.

It must be pointed out that not all patients have a split S1 that is audible. This may be due to various factors involved in the production of the T1 and the A1. The normal T1 may not be loud enough to be audible. The A1 which occurs after the isovolumic contraction phase, may be too narrowly split to be heard as separate distinct sound especially when the isovolumic phase is short. The other reason may be that the orientation of the left ventricular axis in relation to the aortic axis may be such that the ejected blood easily flows out into the aorta without much deceleration at the walls. When the axial orientations form less of an obtuse angle, the chances are more for greater deceleration and formation of audible A1 component. Such variations in the axial orientations can be observed in angiographic or two-dimensional (2D) echocardiographic studies in most patients.

Intensity of S1 (Loudness)

The intensity of S1 is obviously related to the intensity or loudness of the individual components namely the M1, T1 and A1. Since the major determinant of S1 intensity is M1, we shall consider this first.

Mitral Component Intensity (M1)

Since the M1 component corresponds to the mitral valve closure and is produced by sudden deceleration and dissipation of energy of the moving column of blood in the left ventricle, its intensity will depend on the energy imparted to that column of blood by the contracting ventricle. The level of energy imparted will depend on the degree of acceleration achieved by the contracting myofibrils at the time of mitral valve closure. As the ventricle begins to contract, more and more myofibrils are recruited which help in achieving faster rate of pressure rise (dP/dt) in the ventricle.

The mitral valve will close only when the pressure in the contracting left ventricle reaches and just surpasses the pressure in the left atrium. If the atrial pressure were high at the time of mitral valve closure, the ventricle would have achieved a high dP/dt. If the atrial pressure were low on the other hand at the time of mitral valve closure, the dP/dt achieved by the left ventricle would be similarly low. *The energy in the moving column of blood in the left ventricle, which is dissipated upon closure of the valve, is dependent on the dP/dt achieved by the left ventricle at the time of closure. The higher the dP/dt achieved by the contracting left ventricle at the time of mitral valve closure (the pressure crossover point), the louder will be the intensity of the M1.*[6,12,19,20] *The corollary of this implies the lower the dP/dt is at the time of mitral closure the softer will be the intensity of M1.*

The dP/dt achieved at the time of mitral closure will depend on the contractility of the left ventricle and the left atrial pressure. The left atrial pressure at the time of mitral valve closure may be high for one of the following reasons:

1. *Mitral stenosis or mitral obstruction*
2. *Incomplete atrial relaxation at the time of valve closure (short PR interval)*
3. *Short diastoles in atrial fibrillation*
4. *Heart failure*
5. *Mitral regurgitation*

However not all of the above are associated with a loud M1.

M1 in Mitral Stenosis or Obstruction Secondary to Atrial Myxoma

It used to be thought that the loud S1 (M1) that is characteristic of severe mitral stenosis was caused by closure of the valve that was kept wide open by high left atrial pressure. Some even may have thought that calcification of the leaflets contributed to the intensity upon closure.

In mitral stenosis, S1 (M1) is loud because the valve closure occurs at a time when the d*P*/d*t* in the ventricle is high as a result of a higher pressure crossover point (Figs. 6.4 and 6.5). In some patients with very severe mitral stenosis usually associated with heavily calcified valves, the M1 may not be loud. This probably stems from the fact that the left ventricles in such patients are grossly underfilled from the mitral obstruction and therefore are unable to achieve good contractility and d*P*/d*t*.

In left atrial myxoma, which causes mitral obstruction, the M1 will be loud for the same reason as in mitral stenosis.

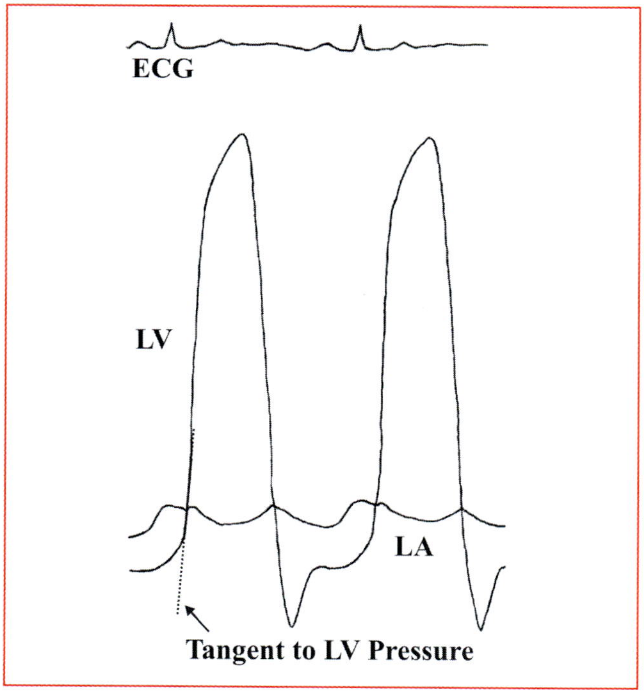

Fig. 6.4: Diagrammatic illustration of the left ventricular (LV) and the left atrial (LA) pressure curves in a patient with mitral stenosis showing the diastolic pressure gradient between LA and the LV reflecting the mitral stenosis. When the rising LV pressure with the onset of systole exceeds that of the LA, the mitral valve will close. Note that the tangent to LV pressure drawn at the point of the crossover of the two pressure curves during this phase of LV systolic pressure rise is steep showing that the ventricle has achieved by this time a faster rate of contraction and higher dP/dt.

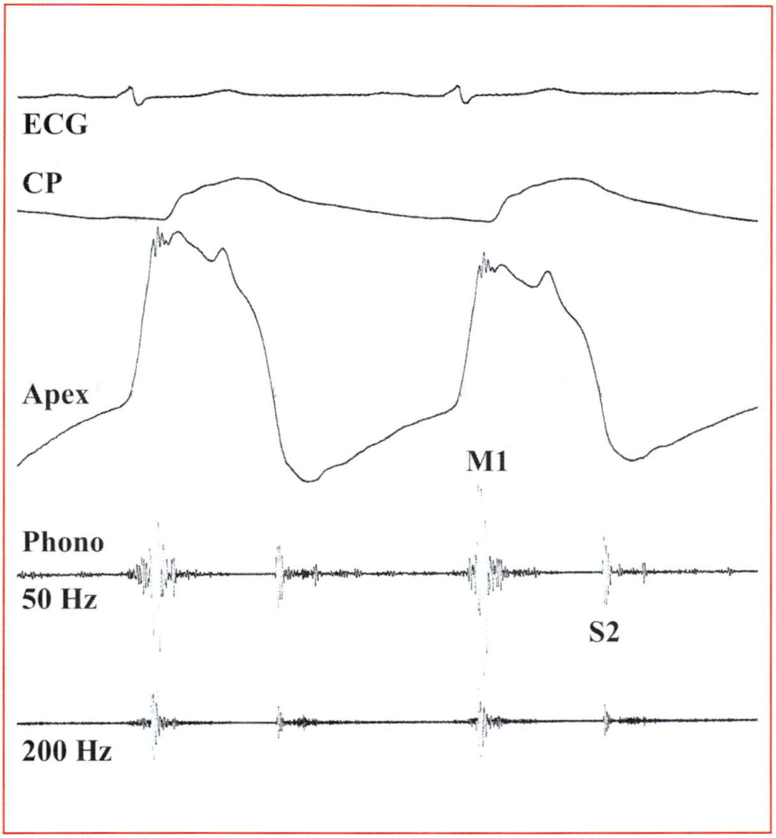

Fig. 6.5: Phonocardiographic recording from a patient with mitral stenosis showing the loud intensity first heart sound caused by the loud ***mitral component.***

Mitral Component (M1) and PR Intervals

After left atrial contraction, if the left ventricle begins to contract before the left atrium had a chance to fully relax, the left atrial pressure will be high at the time of pressure crossover and mitral closure. This is likely to occur when the PR interval is short. This will result also in a louder M1 component (Fig. 6.6A). The corollary to this means that a long PR interval will result in a soft M1 (Fig. 6.6B). This is due to complete relaxation of the left atrium before the left ventricular contraction and maximal fall in the left atrial pressure resulting in a very low pressure crossover point where the dP/dt achieved by the left ventricle will be low.

When the PR interval changes as in atrioventricular (AV) dissociation (e.g. complete AV block), or type I second degree AV block (Wenckebach), the intensity of M1 will also vary according to the PR interval. It will be louder with shorter interval and softer with longer intervals (Fig. 6.7).

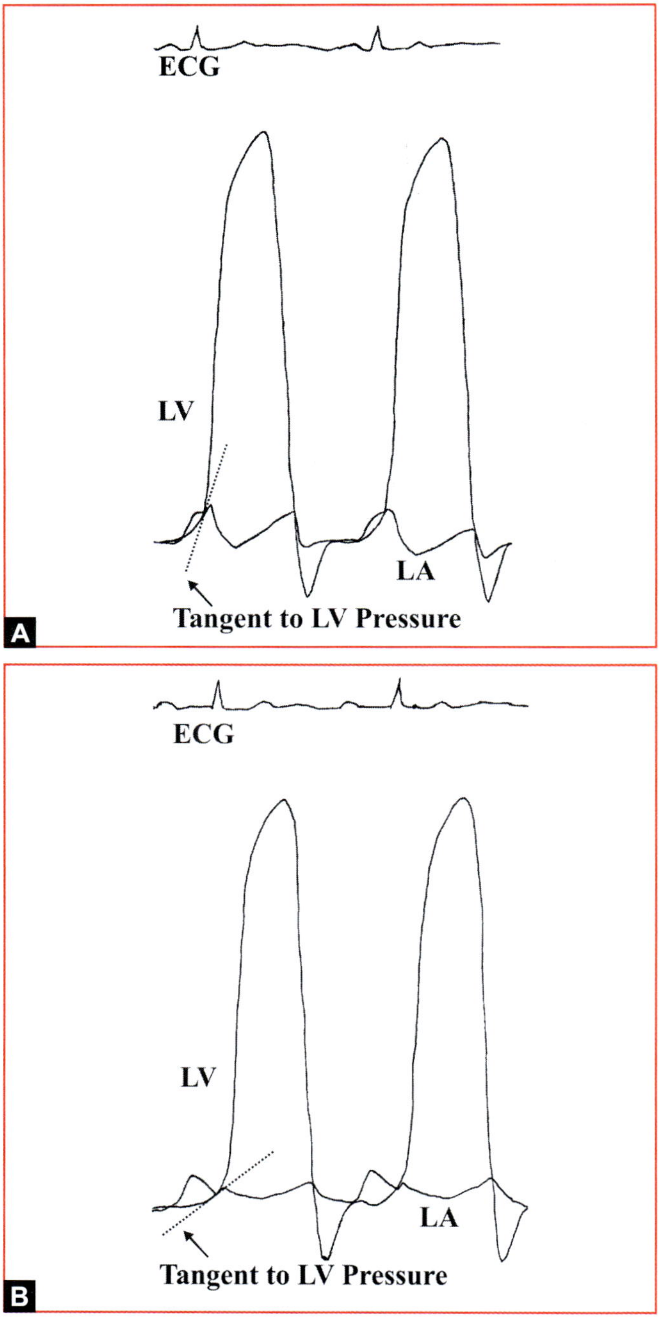

Figs. 6.6A and B: Diagrammatic illustrations of the superimposed left ventricular (LV) and the ***left atrial*** pressure curves to show the differences in the slope of the LV pressure rise at the point of the crossover of the two pressures with the onset of systole caused by short PR interval shown in (A) and long PR interval shown in (B). The slope is steeper when the PR is short whereas it is flatter when the PR is long. This will result in mitral component to be loud when the PR is short whereas it will be soft when PR is long.

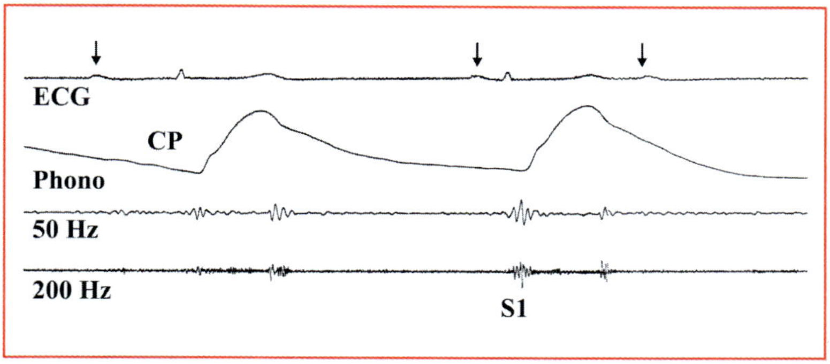

Fig. 6.7: Phono tracing from a patient with complete atrioventricular (AV) block recorded from the apex area. Arrows show the non-conducted P waves in the ***electrocardiogram.*** The effect of the variations in the PR interval caused by the A-V block on the first heart sound (S1) intensity can be seen. The first beat with long PR has a poor S1 intensity whereas the second beat with a shorter PR has much better S1 intensity.

Mitral Component (M1) and Short Diastoles in Atrial Fibrillation

Variable M1 intensity is also characteristic of atrial fibrillation. The mechanism however relates to the varying diastolic filling and its effect on contractility as well as varying levels of atrial pressure at the time of mitral closure. Following shorter diastoles while the filling of the left ventricle may be poor leading to decreased Starling effect and contractility, the left atrial pressure does not have a chance to fall to lower levels. This results in a higher left atrial pressure. Since these two will have opposing effects on M1 intensity, usually the higher left atrial pressure effect dominates causing louder M1 with shorter diastoles.

Mitral Component (M1) in Heart Failure

Although the left atrial pressure in heart failure is invariably elevated, this does not always result in a loud S1. The marked decrease in contractility of the left ventricle results in a poor d*P*/d*t* development at the time of mitral closure. In these patients often there is a high sympathetic tone and high levels of catecholamines. These tend to compensate and attempt to improve the contractility of the myocardium. At times this may in fact succeed in improving the initial rise in left ventricular pressure although the effect may not be sustained throughout systole. This may be sufficient to produce reasonable intensity of S1. In very severely damaged hearts, such compensation often does not result in any significant improvement in the d*P*/d*t* and therefore the S1 (M1) is very soft and sometimes inaudible.

Mitral Component (M1) in Mitral Regurgitation

Since the intensity of M1 is dependent also on sudden deceleration of the moving column of blood in the left ventricle, the presence of significant mitral regurgitation would preclude such sudden deceleration. This in effect may lead to a softer M1. On the other hand, the mitral regurgitation may raise the mean left atrial pressure and therefore the pressure crossover point. It also presents a volume overload effect for the left ventricle thereby increasing its contractility through the Starling mechanism. These two effects will tend to increase the intensity of the M1. Therefore, the M1 intensity in mitral regurgitation in any given patient will depend on the severity of the mitral regurgitation, the acuteness of its onset and the underlying left ventricular function. The opposing effects of these on the M1 may result in a normal M1 intensity.

In acute mitral regurgitation, the left atrial pressure usually rises much higher due to a relatively non-compliant left atrium. This in a patient with ruptured chordae with relatively normal left ventricular function may tend to favor production of a good intensity of M1 as long as the mitral regurgitation is not too severe. In severe mitral regurgitation however, there will be hardly any deceleration possible due to the valvular insufficiency. Similarly, in a patient with ruptured papillary muscle and acute myocardial infarction the M1 will be inaudible. This is not only due to decreased myocardial contractility but also mainly due to the wide-open nature of the mitral regurgitation and ***poor or no deceleration of the column of blood.***

Lesions that Interfere with the Integrity of the Isovolumic Phase of Systole

The importance of the integrity of the isovolumic systole for the preservation of the intensity of the M1 has been pointed out by Shah previously.[12] This essentially pertains to the fact that for a good intensity M1 to occur the column of blood needs to accelerate toward the mitral valve for it to be decelerated by the closure. The cited examples of lesions that interfere with the integrity of the isovolumic phase of contraction include significant mitral regurgitation, significant aortic regurgitation, large ventricular septal defect and large ventricular aneurysm. In these entities, the moment the left ventricular pressure rises, the ejection phase begins with transfer of blood out of the contracting left ventricle. The M1 in wide-open mitral regurgitation will be soft as pointed out earlier. Mitral component in aortic regurgitation is of particular interest.

Mitral Component (M1) in Aortic Regurgitation

Aortic regurgitation being also a volume overload situation for the left ventricle, will lead to increased contractility and therefore would be expected to have a good amplitude of S1 (M1). In severe and acute type of aortic valve regurgitation however, the left ventricular diastolic pressures often rise to very high levels to the point that the pressure in the left ventricle may equal the aortic diastolic pressure and exceed that in the left atrium before ventricular systole begins. This will essentially result in ***pre-mature mitral valve closure.*** In some instances, the mitral leaflets could be incompletely closed with perhaps some diastolic bulging into the left atrium under the high left ventricular diastolic pressure allowing some diastolic mitral regurgitation. However, with the onset of ventricular systole, the leaflets may be fully closed with papillary muscle contraction even before significant pressure rise, at a time when the developed d*P*/d*t* in the left ventricle will be still low. Since the left ventricular and aortic diastolic pressures are often equal, there will be very little or no isovolumic phase of contraction. The moment the ventricular pressure begins to rise faster, the ejection will occur with column of blood essentially moving toward the aorta. Since the mitral valve had already closed before this, there will be no acceleration of column of blood toward the left atrium and therefore no deceleration to cause a sound. This will lead to a very soft and inaudible M1 (S1)[20-23] (Figs. 6.8A and B).

Tricuspid Component Intensity (T1)

The T1 intensity is usually soft in the normal adults and therefore not easily audible. However, its intensity may be increased under the following circumstances:

Increased RV Contractility

Tricuspid component intensity may be increased when there is increased right ventricular contractility as may be seen with right ventricular volume overload causing increased Starling effect (Fig. 6.9). These states include most commonly left to right shunt through an atrial septal defect. In tricuspid regurgitation although the volume overload is present, the regurgitation does not allow adequate deceleration of the column of blood, therefore the T1 intensity is not generally increased. In congenital pulmonary regurgitation with normal pulmonary pressures and normal RV function, the T1 intensity will be increased. Iatrogenic pulmonary regurgitation as may often occur following operative repair of Tetralogy of Fallot, the T1 intensity may not be increased particularly if there is associated right ventricular damage. Similar consideration will apply also in patients with pulmonary regurgitation secondary to pulmonary hypertension.

Higher Right Atrial Pressure at the Time of Tricuspid Valve Closure

1. In ***tricuspid obstruction*** caused by either tricuspid stenosis (which is rare) or by tumors such as atrial myxoma, the right atrial pressure will be elevated and this will lead to a higher pressure crossover point on the right side. This will result in higher d*P*/d*t* achieved by the right ventricle at the time of tricuspid valve closure resulting in loud T1.

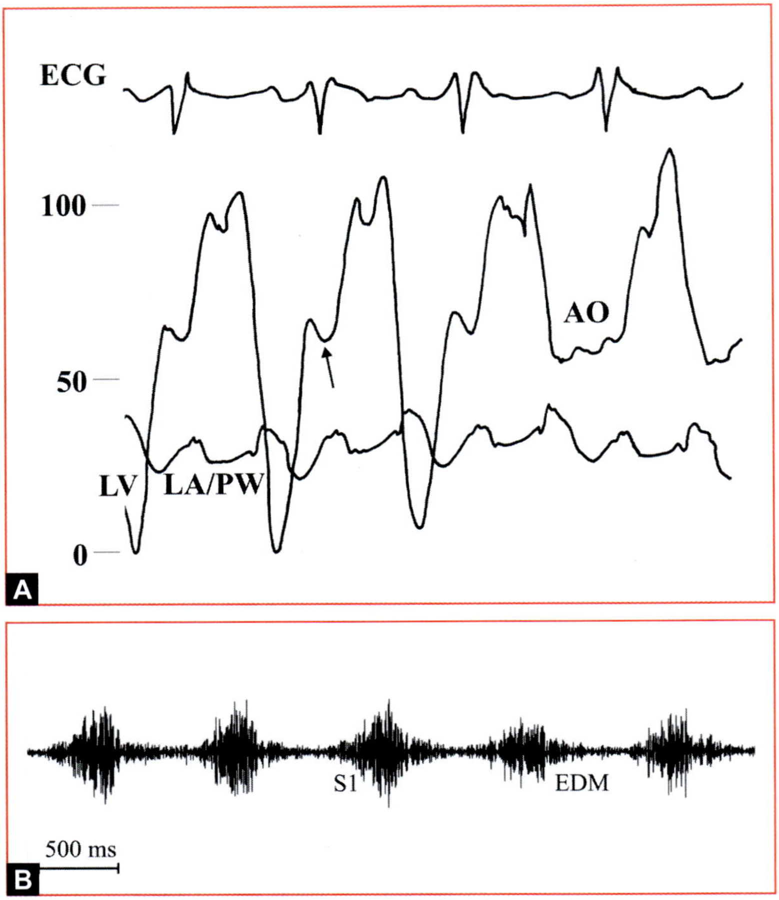

Figs. 6.8A and B: (A) Simultaneous recordings of indirect left atrial (LA) pressure (the pulmonary ***capillary wedge*** pressure) and the left ventricular (LV) pressure from a patient with acute severe aortic regurgitation (shown in the first two beats). The recording catheter is withdrawn to aorta to show the aortic (AO) pressure (fourth beat). The diastolic pressure in the LV rises quite abruptly and in the middle of diastole exceeds the level of the LA pressure thereby closing the mitral valve pre-maturely before the onset of systole. This will result in a poor intensity S1 [shown in (B)]. The arrow points to the end-diastolic pressure in the LV, which is almost equal to the diastolic pressure in the AO. (B) Digital display of the magnetic audio recording from a patient with severe aortic regurgitation recorded close to the apex area. Note the crescendo-decrescendo systolic ejection murmur followed by the ***early diastolic murmur*** of the aortic regurgitation. The former is due to large stroke volume ejected from the left ventricle as a result of the volume overload. The first heart sound is soft and is poorly recorded.

2. ***When the tricuspid valve is abnormally large and redundant*** as seen in some patients with ***Ebstein's anomaly,*** the actual deceleration of the column of blood may occur slightly later because of the redundancy. By this time the right ventricular d*P*/d*t* may have reached a steeper slope

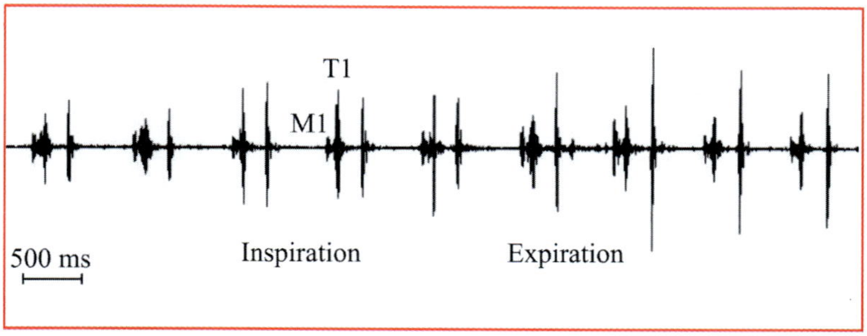

Fig. 6.9: Digital display of the magnetic audio recording from a 16-year-old young man with a large and slightly redundant tricuspid valve taken at the lower left sternal border area. Two components (mitral component M1 and tricuspid component T1) of the first heart sound are seen of which the second component gets intensified on inspiration showing that it is the T1.

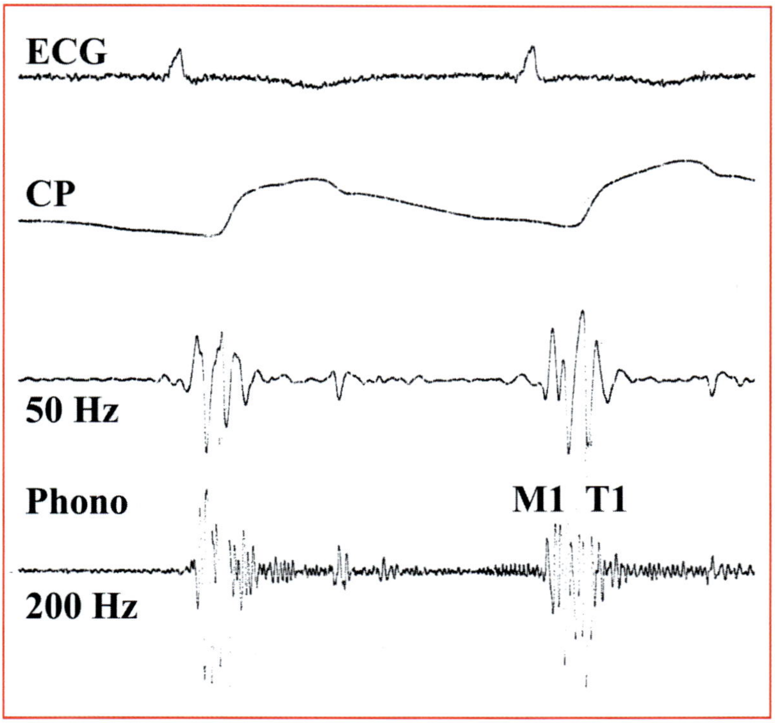

Fig. 6.10: Phono recording from a patient with Ebstein's anomaly of the tricuspid valve recorded from the lower left sternal area showing a delayed louder intensity tricuspid component T1.

contributing to an increased intensity of T1 (Fig. 6.10). ***The sail sound*** described in some patients with Ebstein's anomaly represents the louder delayed T1.[24]

Aortic Component Intensity (A1)

The A1 may or may not be present depending on whether or not the ejected jet during the onset of ejection decelerates sufficiently against the wall of the aortic root to cause a sound. This is perhaps purely determined by the anatomy. When present it usually is coincident with the onset of pressure rise in the central aorta. The only controlling factor determining its intensity will be the left ventricular contractility.

Aortic component may be increased in the presence of hyperdynamic states such as anemia, thyrotoxicosis and Paget's disease.

Aortic Ejection Sound and Click

Certain conditions may lead to effective deceleration of the ejected jet at the onset of systole resulting in a loud, sharp and clicky sound. These may either arise from the aortic root, as is the normal A1 or arise from the aortic valve. Sometimes however, the sound may not be as clicky. This may occur at the usual timing of normal A1 or slightly later. When it arises as a result of exaggeration of the normal A1, it will occur at the onset of aortic pressure rise. Strong inotropic agents (e.g. isoproterenol and norepinephrine) can be shown to increase the amplitude of the aortic root ejection sound. On the other hand, methoxamine which lacks the inotropic effect will decrease the amplitude.[18]

The most common causes of these aortic ejection sounds and/or clicks are as follows:

1. ***Bicuspid aortic valve*** where the cusps are often unequal in size and the opening may be eccentric resulting in **an eccentric *jet*.** The latter would therefore be expected to decelerate against the wall of the aorta. The direction of the jet may be almost perpendicular to the aortic wall resulting in a sharper and louder sound. The timing of this is usually similar to the normal A1 or delayed only to a slight degree (Figs. 6.11A to C).
2. **Congenital aortic valvular stenosis:** In congenital aortic valvular stenosis, the aortic valve is often domed. When the aortic valve is domed and stenosed and does not freely open, the deceleration may occur against the doming valve itself.[25] The sound often in these instances will be clicky. The aortic ejection clicks have been shown to correspond to the timing of the maximal doming. The click precedes the onset of the aortic stenosis murmur and in timing occurs at 20–30 ms after the onset of the aortic pressure rise. It occurs at the anacrotic shoulder of the aortic pressure pulse (Fig. 6.12). When the stenosis is severe and the valve is immobile and calcified, aortic ejection clicks are not heard. The presence of the ejection click in obstruction of the left ventricular outflow tract will suggest a valvular origin of the stenosis.[18,26]

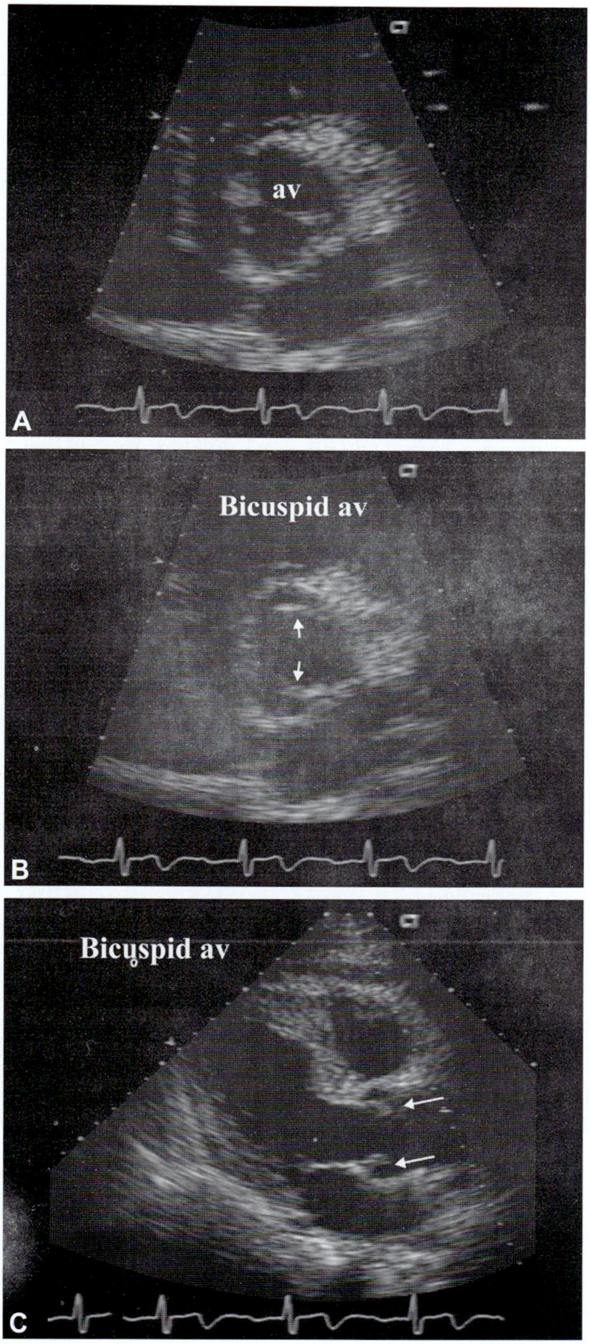

Figs. 6.11A to C: Figures (A to C) are stop frames from two-dimensional echocardiogram taken from a patient with a bicuspid aortic valve and aortic ejection click. The short axis shows the two cusps in the closed position in (A) and in the open position in (B). The aortic valve cusps are seen to be slightly domed in systole (arrows) as observed in the parasternal long axis shown in (C).

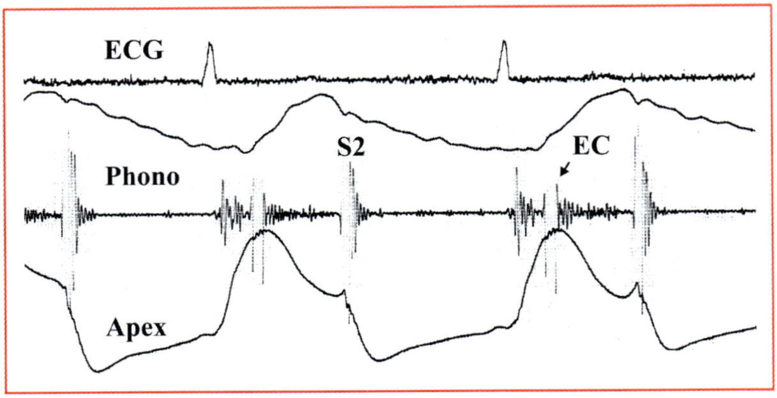

Fig. 6.12: Phono recording from a patient with congenital aortic valve stenosis with domed bicuspid aortic valve. Note that the aortic ***ejection click*** is slightly delayed and seen to correspond to the anacrotic hump on the ***carotid pulse.***

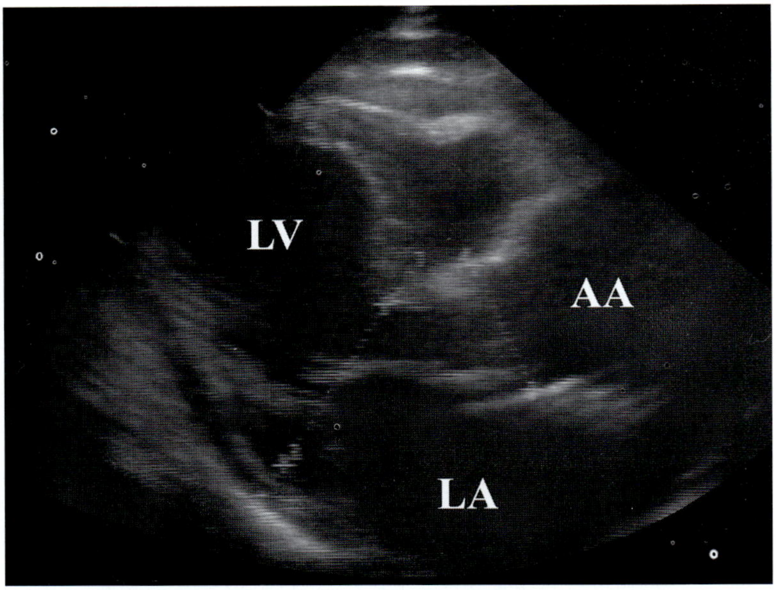

Fig. 6.13: Stop frame from the two-dimensional echocardiogram from a patient taken in the parasternal long axis showing dilated aneurysmal ascending aorta (AA) just above the aortic valve. Note that the orientation of the AA is such that it is at a 90° angle to the longitudinal axis of the ***left ventricle.***

3. In aortic root aneurysm, the column of ejected blood will make close to a 90° angle with the wall of the aorta due to distortion caused by the aneurysmal dilatation (Fig. 6.13). Aorta also may be non-compliant. This will result in more of a clicky sound usually later in time than the normal A1 (Fig. 6.14)

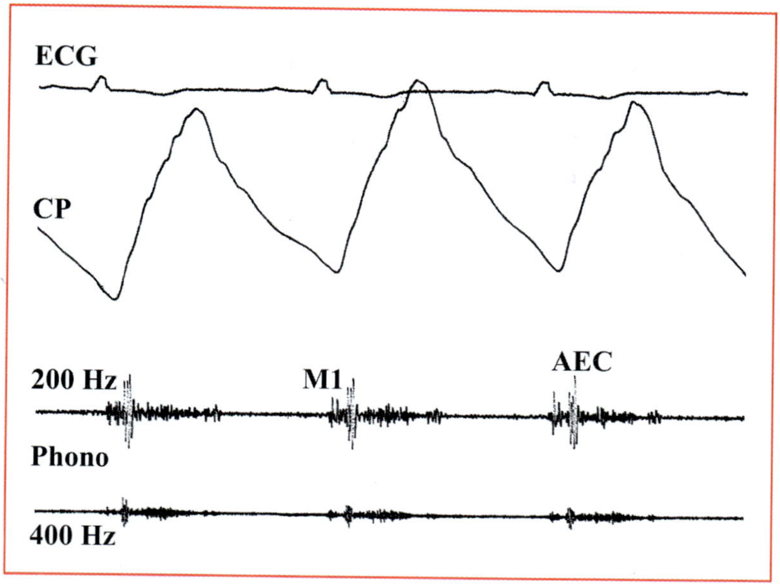

Fig. 6.14: Phono recording from a patient with hypertension and dilated aortic root taken at the lower left sternal border area showing an ***aortic ejection click.***

Aortic ejection sounds and clicks when present are usually heard over the left sternal border and the apex. However when caused by aortic root aneurysm they may be louder at the second and third right intercostal space at the sternal border.

Pulmonary Ejection Sound and Click

Since the normal pulmonary pressures are low there is no audible or recordable normal pulmonary ejection sound. Therefore when a pulmonary ejection sound or click is heard it is always pathological.

There are usually two causes of pulmonary ejection clicks which are as follows:[27]

1. Dilated Pulmonary Artery: Pulmonary artery may become dilated as a result of severe long-standing pulmonary hypertension or be of idiopathic origin with normal pulmonary pressures. The ejected column of blood because of distortion caused by dilatation of the root will be decelerating against the wall of the pulmonary artery causing a clicky sound. This click as with all other right-sided events will increase in intensity with inspiration.
2. Congenital Pulmonary Valvular Stenosis: *In congenital pulmonary valvular stenosis, the click occurs with the maximal doming of the valve.* The deceleration of the column of blood is against the domed valve. The mechanism is similar to that observed in aortic valvular stenosis except

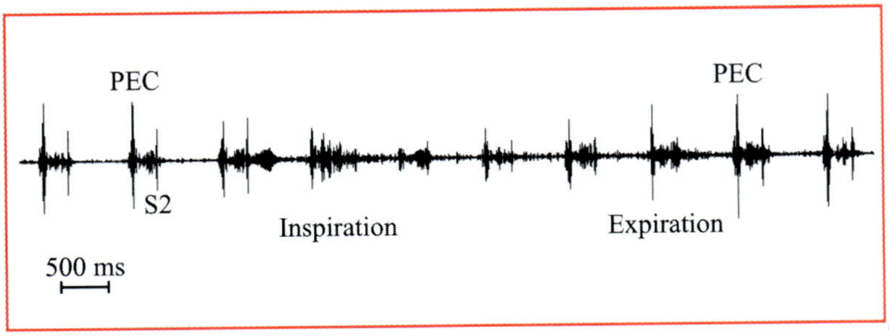

Fig. 6.15: Digital display of the magnetic audio recording from a patient with congenital pulmonary valve stenosis taken from the lower left sternal area showing the pulmonary ejection click ***(PEC)***. Note that the sharp sound which begins the systolic murmur ***(PEC)*** is seen to become very soft and almost disappear on inspiration becoming clicky and sharp on expiration.

it is present invariably in all patients. The pulmonary valve is usually very pliable and never calcified. *This click however has a unique variation with respiration, which in fact helps identify its origin. The click becomes softer or even inaudible on inspiration[28] (Fig. 6.15). This is the only exception to the rule that the right-sided events get exaggerated with inspiration.* In these patients the pulmonary artery pressure is usually very low. During inspiration the increased venous return into a hypertrophied and somewhat non-compliant right ventricle, raises the right ventricular end-diastolic pressure during right atrial contraction. This may exceed the pulmonary artery diastolic pressure. This, in effect, would cause the doming of the pulmonary valve even before the ventricular contraction starts. Thus with ventricular systole as the column of blood is set into motion, the valve being maximally domed, there is no sudden deceleration against the valve itself, therefore no sound.

Pulmonary ejection clicks are maximally loud over the second and third left intercostal space at the left sternal border. However, when they are loud they can be heard over a wide area of the pre-cordium including the xiphoid region.

CLINICAL ASSESSMENT OF S1 AND ITS COMPONENTS

When assessing the S1 at the bedside, one should assess the following:

1. *Intensity or loudness*
2. *Variability of intensity (loudness)*
3. *Presence of more than one component (split S1)*
4. *Quality*
5. *Location of maximal loudness*
6. *Effect of respiration.*

Intensity or Loudness

Since loudness can vary due to non-cardiac factors such as body shape or chest wall deformities or the presence of pulmonary disease, these should be taken into account in assessing the true loudness, which may be attenuated.

The loudness of the sound however can be graded using the system of grading murmurs, which allows six categories of loudness: the grades I-III are not loud enough to be palpable whereas grades IV-VI are loud and palpable. The grade I sound requires tuning in, to mentally filter out room noise from the actual sound. The grade II sound is audible the moment the auscultation is begun even without having to concentrate and eliminate the room noise. This is the usual intensity heard by beginners. The grade III sound is the loudest sound audible, which however is not palpable. The grade IV sound is although palpable, but requires full contact of the stethoscope against the chest wall for audibility. The grade V sound requires only the edge of the stethoscope to touch the chest wall to hear the sound. The grade VI sound however can be heard with the stethoscope slightly but completely off the chest wall.

When S1 intensity is graded using the system mentioned above, all grades IV-VI are abnormal. Even grade III sound may be significant in some patients. However it is difficult to diagnose a true decrease in S1 intensity due to extracardiac factors, which attenuate the sound. Other methods to overcome part of this problem have been discussed in Chapter 3 in relation to the blood pressure and the assessment of ventricular function.

When S1 is loud, it is important to locate the area of maximal loudness, which may be possible by palpation. If the apical impulse is left ventricular as defined by the presence of medial retraction, and the maximal loudness of S1 is at the apex then one can safely assume that the M1 is the loud component. But it is important to remember that the other components of S1 can at times be the loudest and may become palpable. Occasionally, ejection clicks (both aortic and pulmonary) when very loud may also become palpable. These will have to be identified by other features on auscultation.

Variability of Intensity

Variations in S1 intensity from cycle to cycle are usually due to variations in M1. There are four basic causes for variations in M1 intensity.

a. *Atrioventricular* ***dissociation:*** *Where the PR relationship may vary haphazardly from beat to beat. The shorter PR intervals will have louder M1 whereas the longer PR will have softer M1. This phenomenon can occur in complete AV block, patients with electronic pacemaker, and also in ventricular rhythms.*

b. *In* ***Mobitz type I second degree AV block*** *the S1 intensity may become progressively softer as the PR lengthens before the dropped beat and pause.*
c. ***Atrial fibrillation:*** *Where the diastolic filling periods keep changing constantly causing various degrees of Starling effect and variations in left atrial pressure at the time of mitral valve closure.*
d. ***Pulsus alternans:*** *Where due to instability of intracellular calcium shifts, the contractility alternates between weak and strong beats. This usually occurs only in severe cardiomyopathies.*

Components of S1 and Its Quality

One should on auscultation determine whether or not there is more than one component of S1 that is audible (split S1). Then one should try to ascertain the origin of each component and compare their relative loudness. At the same time, any clicky quality of the components should also be noted. Such clicky quality to S1 or one of its components should alert one to the presence of aortic or pulmonary ejection click. Normal M1 is not clicky although a mechanical mitral prosthetic ball valve usually would cause a clicky M1 at the time of its closure.

When one of the components of S1 is very loud, it can have a masking effect on the other component thereby appearing on auscultation to have only a single component. When the S1 is loud, one should not always assume this to be due to loud M1. It is important to identify its features thereby identifying its origin. The M1 and the A1 will be maximally loud at the apex and will not change with respiration. Same rule applies also to the aortic ejection click although it may be equally loud at the second right intercostal space. The T1 on the other hand is loudest at the lower left sternal border and over the xiphoid area and can be noted to increase in loudness on inspiration. Occasionally when the right ventricle is very large and forms the apex of the heart (lateral retraction present) then the T1 may be loudest over the apex.

It is also important to note that a loud pulmonary ejection click being very close in timing to the normal S1 may be mistaken for one of its components. However this can be easily solved by the fact that ***it will get softer on inspiration*** and may sometimes be audible only on expiration. The maximal loudness of a pulmonary ejection click is usually over the second and third left intercostal spaces.

When A1 is clicky and/or loud enough to cause a good split S1, one can further confirm it to be M1 and A1 by observing the effect of standing. Standing by reducing the venous return, will tend to lower the left atrial pressure and the left ventricular end-diastolic pressure. While there may be a slight rise in heart rate secondary to the sympathetic stimulation, the decreased filling pressure will lead to a slower rate of pressure rise in the left ventricle. This will imply some lengthening of the isovolumic contraction phase. The A1, which comes at the onset of ejection therefore coming after the end of isovolumic contraction phase, will be somewhat delayed from the M1 thereby making the split somewhat wider on standing.

SECOND HEART SOUND

The S2 occurs at the end of the ejection phase of systole. It is related to the closure of the semilunar valves. Since there are two semilunar valves, aortic and pulmonary, there are also two components for the S2 namely the aortic component (A2) and the pulmonary component (P2).

Mechanism of Formation of S2

As the blood is ejected into the aorta and the pulmonary artery during systole (stroke volume), the aortic and the pulmonary pressures rise and these two vessels get distended. At the end of systole, as the ventricular pressures begin to fall, the elastic components of the great vessels maintaining a higher pressure result in a pressure gradient which drives the columns of blood back into the ventricles. The columns of blood in the great vessels preferably flow toward the ventricles at this time because of the lower resistance with the dropping ventricular pressures compared to the periphery. The reverse flow of the columns of blood in the aorta and the pulmonary artery parachutes the cusps of the aortic and the pulmonary valves closing them. The sudden deceleration of the columns of blood against the closed semilunar valves results in dissipation of energy, causing the A2 and the P2 components of the S2 (Figs. 6.16A to D).

NORMAL S2

The S2 is usually sharper, crisper and shorter in duration compared to S1. This is due to the fact that the semilunar valve closures occur at much higher pressures than the AV valves and the dissipated energy in the columns of blood is much greater. In normal young subjects one can often hear both components of S2 (A2 and P2). The S2 will therefore be heard as a split sound. The first of the two components is the A2. The higher impedance (i.e. resistance to forward flow) in the systemic circulation results in earlier acceleration of reverse flow in the aortic root causing the aortic valve to close earlier.[29,30]

The pulmonary arterial bed is larger and offers markedly less resistance to forward flow. This will make the tendency to reverse flow to occur later and slower compared to the left side. In addition, it is also possible that the lower pressures achieved by the right ventricle during systole may actually result in a slower rate of relaxation of the right ventricle compared to the left

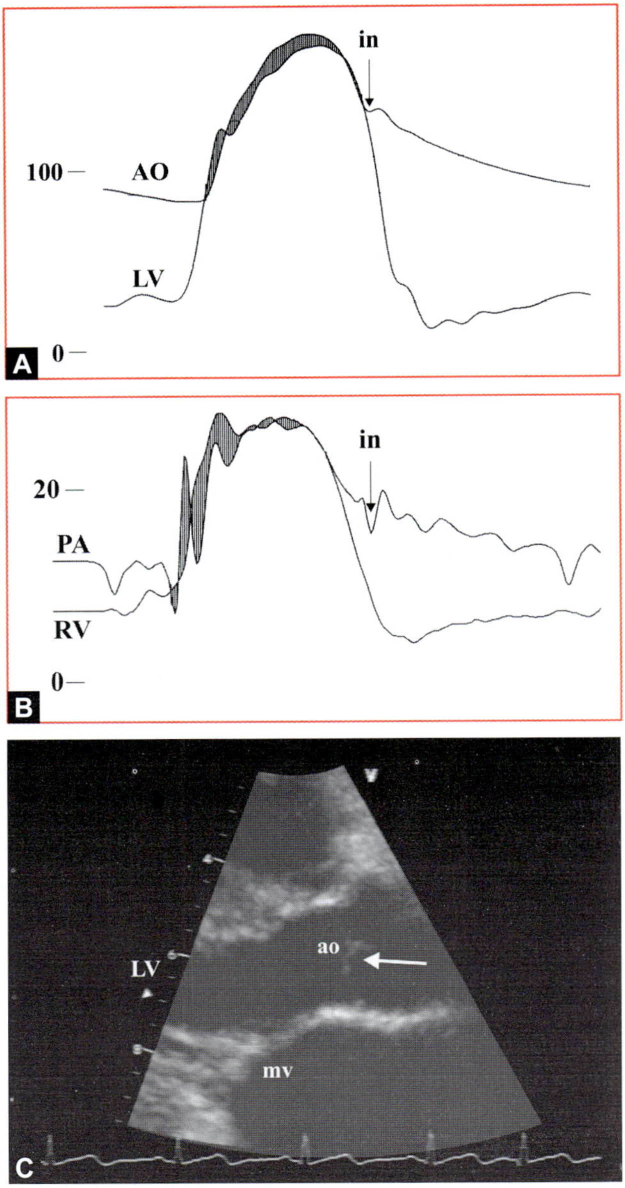

Figs. 6.16A to C: (A and B) Simultaneous left ventricular (LV) and aortic (AO) pressure and simultaneous right ventricular (RV) and pulmonary artery (PA) pressure are shown in (A) and (B), respectively. The falling ventricular pressure at the end of systole leads to the development of a pressure gradient between the AO and the LV on the left side and between the PA and the RV on the right side. The aortic and the pulmonary components of the second heart sound occur at the time of the respective incisura (in) in the AO and PA pressures. (C) Stop frame from a two-dimensional echocardiogram from a normal subject taken at the parasternal long axis showing the aortic valve in the closed position causing the deceleration of the column of blood which is trying to enter the left ventricle from the aorta as a result of the pressure gradient at the end of systole between the AO and the LV.

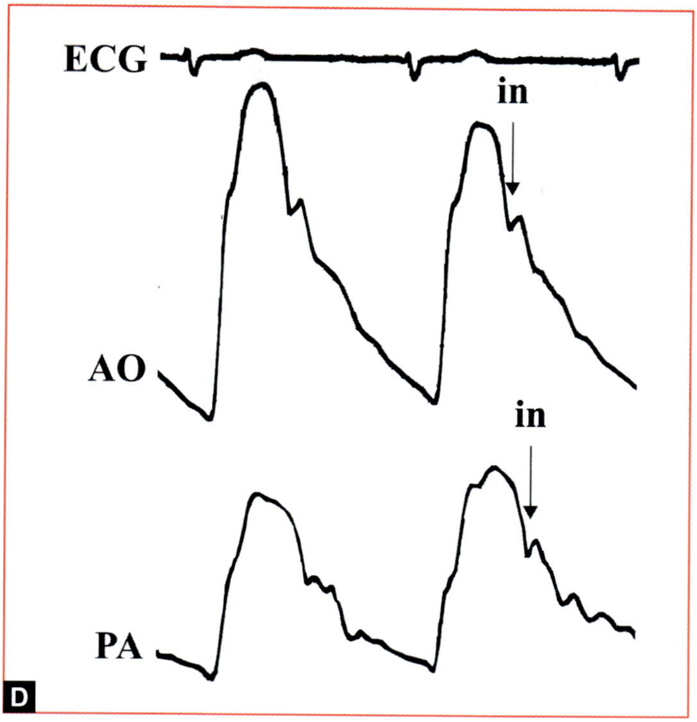

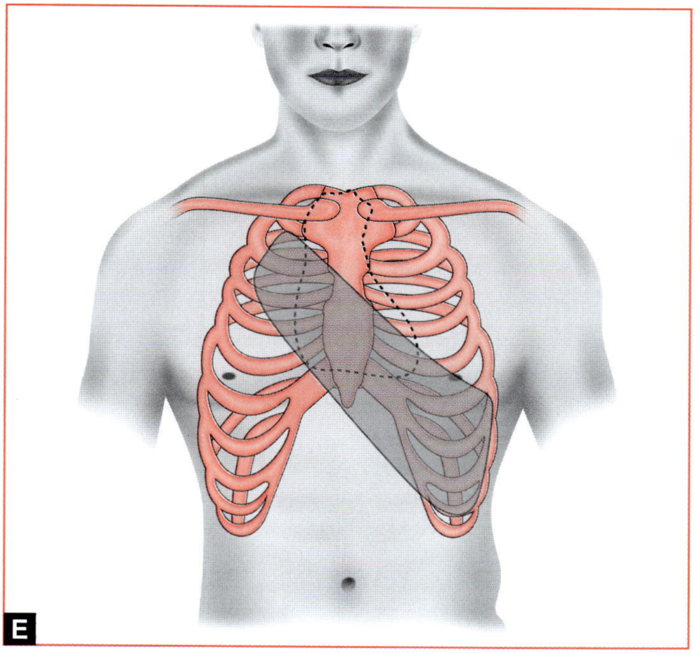

Figs. 6.16D and E: (D) Recording of the simultaneous AO and PA pressures show that the incisura (in) in the AO occurs earlier than in the PA. (E) The diagram of the chest showing the true aortic area, which is the Sash area (shaded area) extending from the second right interspace to the apex.

ventricle. For these reasons, the P2 component occurs later. The A2 component is normally heard over the true aortic area, which is *the Sash area (the area extending from the second right intercostal space at the sternal border to the apex)* (Fig. 6.16E). The P2 on the other hand is heard over the second and the third left intercostal spaces near the sternal border. Therefore the splitting of the normal S2 is best appreciated at the second and third left intercostal spaces. The relative loudness of the two components is such that *in the normal, the A2 is always louder than the P2 mainly because the systemic arterial resistance is normally 10 times higher than the pulmonary arterial resistance.*[4,16,30]

Normal Respiratory Variations of A2-P2 Split

In normal subjects the splitting is often best recognized on inspiration since the two components tend to move away from each other causing them to separate better. On expiration they tend to move closer to each other. This often results in them becoming single or if they are still separated the splitting is very narrow (Figs. 6.17A and B). During inspiration, there is increased venous return to the right heart due to the fall in the intrathoracic pressures. There is also expansion of the lungs resulting in decreased resistance in the pulmonary circulation. The expansion of the lungs also increases the pulmonary vascular capacity therefore leading to a slightly decreased left sided filling. These changes affect both components of the S2 in terms of their timing making the A2 to come earlier and the P2 to be delayed. However, the A2 is affected to a very small degree since the systemic resistance is not affected by respiration. The P2 on the other hand is delayed on inspiration for two reasons, one is the increased volume on the right side and the second is the fall in the pulmonary resistance on inspiration. The former will result in increase in the right ventricular ejection time. The latter will allow easier forward flow resulting in slower tendency for reversal. On expiration, with rise in the intrathoracic pressure, the venous return to the right heart decreases and the right ventricular ejection time will shorten. The lungs collapse, the pulmonary capacity will diminish and the resistance will rise. These changes will result in P2 to come early on expiration.[4,16,31,32]

The normal respiratory variation is not as prevalent in the elderly as it is in the younger patients.[32] This may be due to decreased compliance of the chest wall, great vessels and the relatively increased impedances in both systemic and pulmonary circulations.

ABNORMAL S2

The abnormalities of S2 may occur as a result of changes in the intensity of the individual components or changes in their timing. The latter often may lead to abnormal respiratory variations.

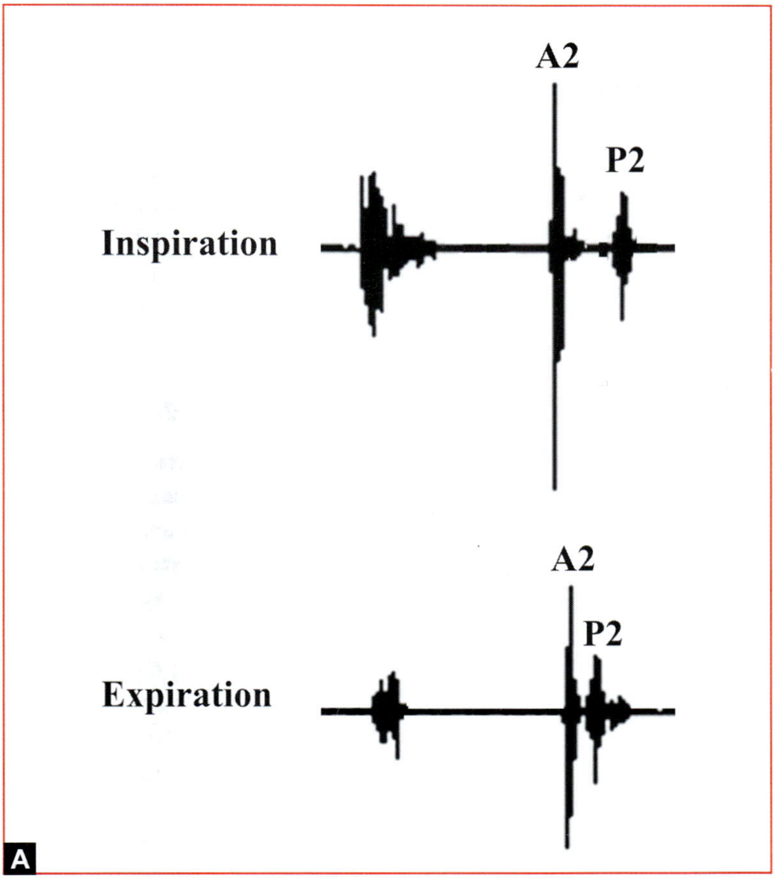

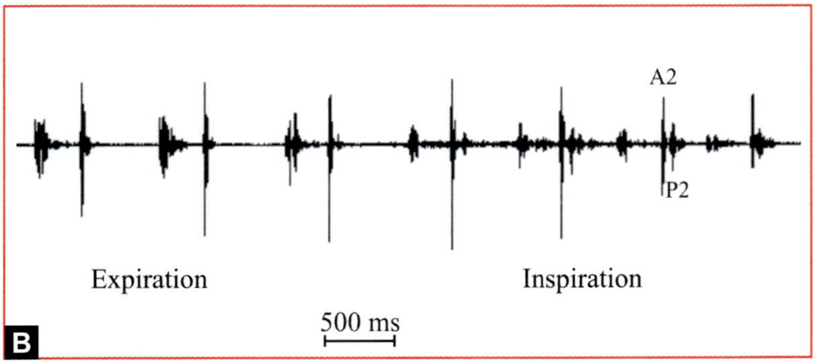

Figs. 6.17A and B: (A) Diagram showing the two components of the second heart sound (S2) and their variation with respiration in the normals. The normal sequence is that the aortic component (A2) occurs before the pulmonary component (P2). On inspiration, the A2 comes slightly earlier but the P2 is significantly more delayed widening the split. The reverse occurs on expiration with the split becoming quite narrow. (B) Digital display of the magnetic audio recording from a normal young subject taken from the third left intercostal space at the left sternal border showing the normal S2 split on inspiration into A2 and P2 and essentially a single S2 on expiration.

Intensity of S2

The loudness or intensity of the S2 can be determined by the grading system previously alluded to in relation to S1. The sounds with loudness grades IV-VI would be abnormal and increased. When S2 is either inaudible or is of grade I in loudness, it could be considered decreased when S1 or other sounds are normal.

Intensity of A2

The A2 intensity is dependent on the amount of energy that the column of blood in the aortic root attains in its attempt to flow toward the ventricle (assuming the integrity of the aortic valve). This in turn is dependent on the stroke volume, aortic elasticity and most importantly the peripheral resistance. When the stroke volume is either normal or increased, the peripheral resistance becomes the major determinant of the intensity. When there is increased peripheral resistance, the diastolic pressure in the aorta remains higher than normal. When the left ventricular pressure falls due to the onset of ventricular relaxation in late systole, the maintained higher pressure in the aorta provides a greater pressure head to act on the column of blood in the aortic root. The higher pressure head trying to move the column of blood in the aortic root toward the left ventricle imparts greater energy. Thus when it decelerates it causes a louder A2. *Thus in systemic hypertension, A2 becomes louder, may be palpable and may become musical in quality due to maintained vibrations under high tension. The sound mimics the beating on a tambour.*

In patients with ***severe heart failure*** and poor stroke volume, A2 can become soft and rarely inaudible despite high peripheral resistance. The poor stroke volume causes poor distension of the elastic components of the aortic root and therefore the energy in the column of blood closing the valve is very low. These patients often have low pulse pressure and low amplitude arterial pulse.

In ***severe aortic stenosis,*** the stroke volume is ejected slowly and over a longer period and also leads to poor distension of the aortic root, leading to often a lower intensity A2 and this may be inaudible.

Aortic Component (A2) Intensity in Aortic Regurgitation

Aortic regurgitation can occur as a result of valvular disease or aortic root pathology. Aortic regurgitation leads to increased stroke volume. The peripheral resistance is usually low due to compensatory mechanisms. *The large stroke volume causes greater distension of the aortic root and therefore would cause a greater amount of energy in the column of blood in the aortic root trying to close the valve. The degree of deceleration achieved by the reversing column of blood will depend on the anatomic cause and the severity of the regurgitation. Despite significant aortic regurgitation, because of increased energy in the column of blood, the A2 intensity is often well preserved. The lower peripheral resistance will have a tendency to reduce the intensity of A2. The two effects often may balance each other. However, in very severe (wide open) regurgitation, A2 intensity may decrease significantly due to poor deceleration.* When patients with aortic regurgitation develop left ventricular failure, their stroke volume will be reduced to normal levels and their A2 may become soft or inaudible.

Sometimes ***A2 may be louder than normal for anatomic reasons*** namely conditions that make the aorta anterior and closer to the chest wall. These include a thin chest, straight back syndrome with decreased anteroposterior diameter, transposition of the great vessels (congenitally corrected or uncorrected) and Tetralogy of Fallot where in addition the P2 may be attenuated due to a deformed pulmonary valve.

Intensity of P2

The P2 intensity similar to the A2 intensity is dependent on the stroke volume, pulmonary artery elasticity and the pulmonary arterial resistance. When the right ventricular stroke volume is significantly increased as *in left to right shunts through an atrial septal defect, the P2 may become louder although not reach the level of palpability unless significant pulmonary hypertension is also present. Along with the increased size of the right ventricle,* this may also contribute to ***the audibility of the P2 over a wider area of the precordium.*** Pulmonary artery remains always elastic except in severe pulmonary hypertension. The major determinant of increased P2 intensity is in fact the pulmonary arterial resistance. ***In pulmonary hypertension,*** whether acute or chronic, the pulmonary arterial resistance is increased due to vasospasm (increased vascular tone). As well when the pulmonary hypertension is chronic, structural changes occur in the arterial wall with medial hypertrophy and increased intimal thickening which make the pulmonary arterial system stiff and less elastic. The increased resistance raises the pulmonary arterial systolic and diastolic pressures. The RV relaxation may be impaired taking a longer time for the right ventricular systolic pressure to fall. In addition, the increased pulmonary pressures provide a greater pressure head. *The higher pressure head together with increased resistance to forward flow acts to impart greater energy and velocity to the column of blood in the pulmonary root in its attempt to flow toward the right ventricle.* Therefore when it decelerates, it produces a *louder intensity P2. When the P2 becomes palpable (grades IV-VI), it invariably indicates severe pulmonary hypertension.*

Because of low pressures on the right side, the P2 is often soft and occasionally not audible. In significant pulmonary stenosis, the stroke volume may be quite low and this together with very low pulmonary arterial pressures may lead to a very low intensity P2 that may be inaudible.

Abnormal Timing of A2 and P2 Components

The time of occurrence of the individual components A2 and P2 may be delayed if the duration of systole is lengthened either due to electrical or mechanical delays or if the onset of flow reversal in the aortic root or the pulmonary artery is delayed due to changes in impedance to forward flow.[4,32–36]

Electrical Delay

When there is an electrical conduction defect such as a bundle branch block, the affected side will lengthen the electrical portion of the duration of the electromechanical systole. This in turn will result in the delayed occurrence of the individual A2 and P2 components. Left bundle branch block (LBBB) will cause A2 delay and right bundle branch block (RBBB) will cause P2 delay (Figs. 6.18A and B). Similar conduction defect can also be produced artificially by pacing either ventricle, which will produce late activation of the non-paced ventricle. In other words, right ventricular pacing will cause LBBB effect and left ventricular pacing will cause RBBB effect. Transient bundle branch block effect can also occur during ventricular ectopic beats. The site of origin of the ectopics will determine which of the two ventricles will be delayed in excitation. Right ventricular ectopics will have LBBB and left ventricular ectopics will have RBBB morphology and effects respectively.

Mechanical Delay

The mechanical portion of systole may be delayed when there is ***significant outflow obstruction.*** This would result in ***high intraventricular pressure,*** which is required to overcome the obstruction. *The time taken for the pressures to fall below the level of the pressure in the great vessel* (aorta or the pulmonary artery) then would be ***lengthened.*** The reversal of flow at the aortic or the pulmonary root would start later because of the delay and this in turn would delay the occurrence of the individual component of S2 on the affected side (Fig. 6.19).

Similar delay may also be caused in ischemic ventricular dysfunction where the ischemic muscle fibers may lag in the onset of contraction and therefore maintain the developed intraventricular pressures for a longer period preventing its fall. Since ischemia often involves primarily the left ventricle, this type of delay is more likely to affect the A2.

The A2 and the P2 components usually coincide in timing with the incisural notch on the aortic and the pulmonary artery pressure curve respectively (see Figs. 6.16A and B). In general, the duration of the electro-mechanical systole on the left side and the right side is about equal under normal circumstances if the duration of the electro-mechanical systole is defined as the interval from the beginning of the electrical activation (QRS onset) to the respective time when the ventricular pressures fall below the level in the great vessels (aorta and the pulmonary artery).

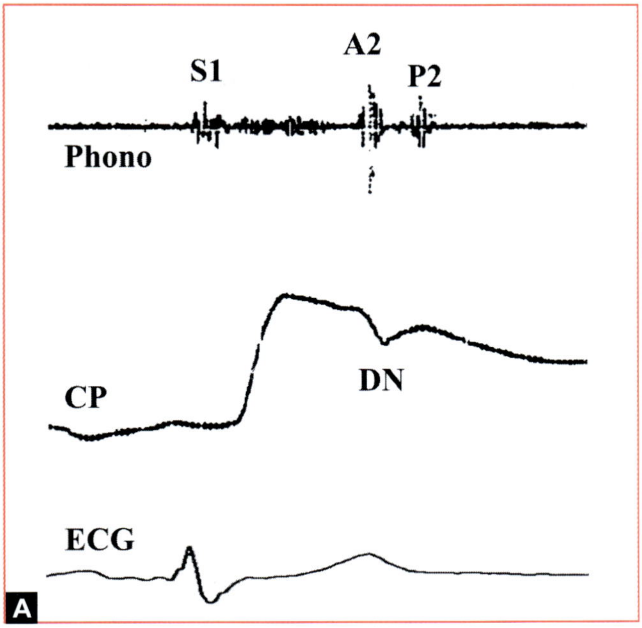

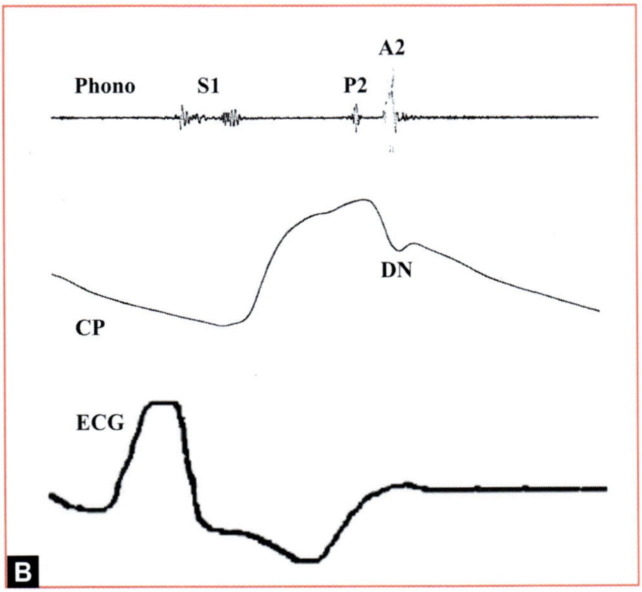

Figs. 6.18A and B: (A) Diagram to show the delayed pulmonary component (P2) producing a wide spilt of the second heart sound (S2) in right bundle branch block, which causes electrical delay of conduction to the right side. Note that the sequence is normal with aortic component (A2) occurring first followed by P2. The component that is closest to the dicrotic notch (DN) on the carotid pulse (CP) is A2. The DN lags slightly behind due to the pulse transmission delay. (B) Diagram to show the abnormal sequence of the S2 components caused by the electrical delay due to left bundle branch block. ***Pulmonary component*** occurs before A2. The A2 is the component closest to the DN on the CP.

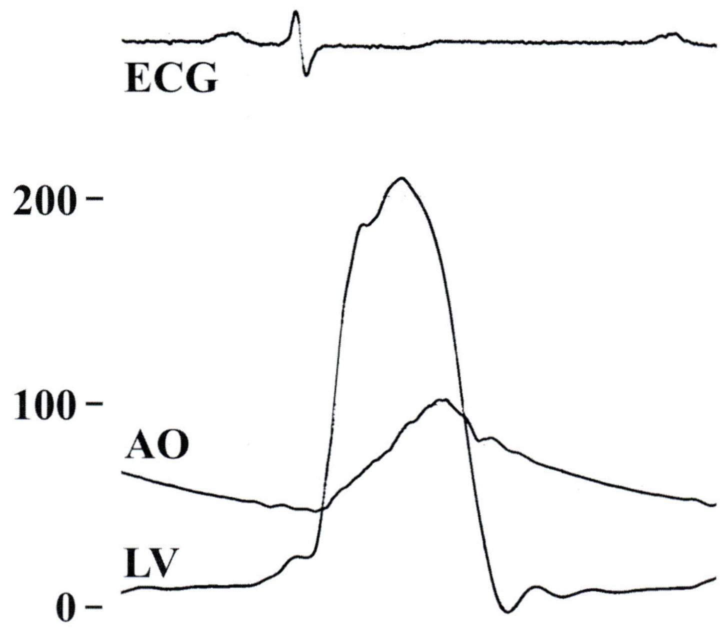

Fig. 6.19: Simultaneous left ventricular and aortic (AO) pressures from a patient with severe aortic valve stenosis. Note that the severe mechanical obstruction leads to high intraventricular pressure, which will take longer to fall to the level of the AO pressure thereby delaying the aortic component.

Right ventricular myocardial dysfunction may develop with time in pulmonary hypertension when it is severe. The rate of rise of the right ventricular systolic pressure as well as its decline during relaxation may become slower. This may selectively increase the duration of systole on the right side relative to the left side contributing to a delayed P2.[30] Similar situation tends to develop more readily in acute pulmonary hypertension.

Delay Secondary to Effects of Impedance

Impedance refers to the resistance to forward flow of blood in the great vessels. If the impedance to forward flow is low, as the ventricular pressures begin to fall below that of the great vessels, the tendency for reversal of flow at the aortic or pulmonary root will be delayed. Therefore the occurrence of the A2 or the P2 will be delayed depending on which circuit is affected. If the impedance is high then the reversal tendency will be earlier causing earlier occurrence of the affected component. This can be understood easily by *the analogy of an automobile in motion and how far it is likely to travel after the application of the brakes.* This will not only depend on the momentum of the vehicle but also on the character of the road surface whether wet, slippery or rough, whether there is a slope and if so whether the gradient is down or up as well as the resistance offered by the wind velocity and direction. The combined effects of these factors constitute the impedance to the moving automobile and will determine how far the vehicle will travel and how long before it will eventually halt. The impedance to forward flow in the great vessels is provided by *the combined effects of various factors. These include the vascular capacity, and how filled the system is, the vasomotor tone of the vessels (the systemic or the pulmonary vascular resistance), the viscosity of the blood.* In the normal adults, the aortic or the systemic impedance is approximately 10 times higher than the pulmonary impedance. This is a major factor which contributes to the earlier occurrence of A2 compared to P2. This is because the pulmonary vascular capacity is large; the pulmonary vascular resistance is low compared to that of the systemic side.[30]

When the ventricular pressure in late systole begins to fall below that in the aorta or the pulmonary artery, it leads to the development of a pressure gradient between the great vessel and the ventricle. The lower ventricular pressure favors the column of blood in the aorta and the pulmonary artery to flow towards the respective ventricle. However, the flow may still continue forward if the impedance is low. This will be reflected by the delay in the incisural notch of the aortic or the pulmonary pressure curve as measured from the point in time when the falling intraventricular pressure reaches the level of the incisural pressure (which is the pressure at which the aortic and the pulmonary valves close respectively). This delay in the incisural notch has been termed as the ***"Hang out" interval*** by some investigators[29] (Figs. 6.16A and B and Fig. 6.20). This interval is quite small on the aortic side averaging 15 ms whereas it is usually considerably longer (between 30 and 80 ms) on the pulmonary side almost completely accounting for the normal A2-P2 separation.

Since the systemic impedance is high at basal state, change in impedance enough to cause an appreciable effect on the A2 timing must be significant. On the other hand, small changes of the pulmonary impedance, which are usually low, may have an effect on the P2 timing since the percentage change will tend to be higher. *Thus with normal inspiration the expansion of lungs will increase the pulmonary vascular capacity thereby lowering the pulmonary impedance considerably in terms of percentage change.* This is one of the important contributing factors for the normal inspiratory delay of P2.

In pulmonary hypertension, the ***increased pulmonary impedance*** has the effect of shortening the delay of the incisural notch ***making the P2 occur earlier*** due of course to the earlier occurrence of the flow reversal at the pulmonary root. This will be expected to cause ***a narrower split of S2*** (Fig. 6.21).

In patients with left to right shunts through a ventricular septal defect, who eventually develop severe pulmonary hypertension secondary to the occurrence of pulmonary vascular disease, the shunt becomes reversed leading to cyanosis. In these patients who are termed to have the ***Eisenmenger's syndrome,*** the systemic and the pulmonary impedance are about equal and would result in a single S2.[37]

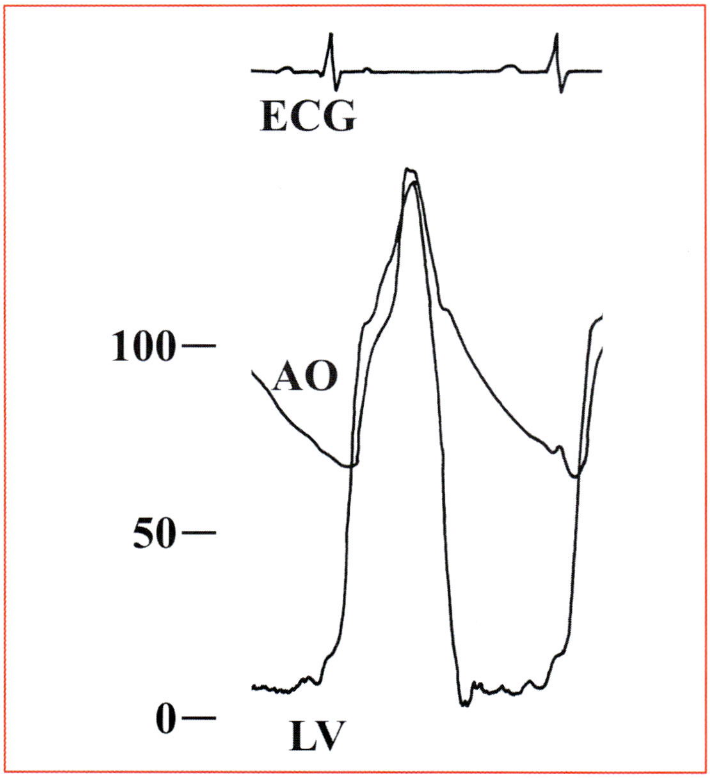

Fig. 6.20: Simultaneous ***left ventricular*** and aortic (AO) pressures from a patient with chronic aortic regurgitation. The aortic component (A2) will occur simultaneously with the incisural notch (in) in the aortic pressure. Note the slight delay between the ventricular pressure at the level of the incisura (in) on the AO recording and the actual occurrence of the incisura (A2 timing). This delay has been termed by some as the hang out interval, which reflects the impedance of the circuit. The hang out interval on the pulmonary side will be more since the pulmonary impedance is normally very low.

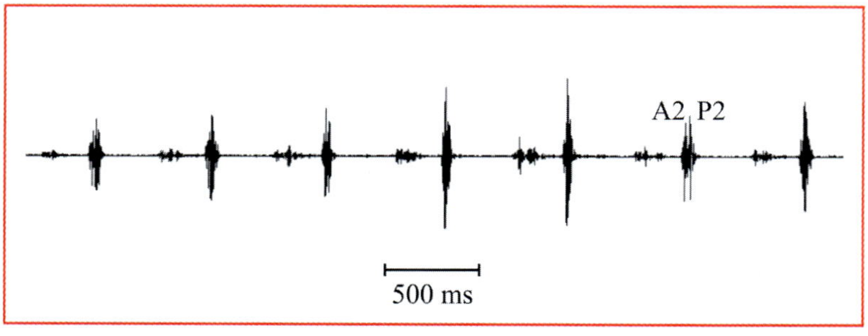

Fig. 6.21: Digital display of a magnetic audio recording from a patient with significant pulmonary hypertension with compensated right ventricular function, taken from the third left intercostal space at the left sternal edge. Pulmonary component occurs much earlier due to high pulmonary impedance causing a very narrow split of second heart sound.

Effect of Delayed Occurrence of the S2 Components on the Respiratory Variation of S2 Splitting

When the A2 is delayed, however the delay is caused, if the delay is long enough then the sequence becomes altered namely a P2-A2 sequence is produced instead of the normal A2-P2 sequence. On inspiration when there is more volume on the right side as well as a significant drop in pulmonary impedance the P2 will be delayed. This delayed P2 will come closer to the already delayed A2 and may actually fuse and may become single S2. On expiration, the reverse will occur with the P2 now coming earlier due to decreased volume being ejected by the right ventricle and a rise in the pulmonary impedance due to decreasing pulmonary vascular capacity secondary to collapsing lungs. This will then result in a split S2 on expiration ***(persistent or audible expiratory splitting).***[33] Since the two components tend to come together on inspiration and separate from each other causing a split S2 on expiration, it is termed the ***paradoxical or reversed splitting of S2***[36] (Figs. 6.22A and B).

If the P2 is delayed on the other hand, the sequence will still be normal, A2 followed by P2.[35] However, the P2 will tend to be separated from A2 all the time. The separation will be greater on inspiration when the P2 gets normally delayed and the separation may be narrower but maintained even on expiration. In other words, there will be a persistent expiratory split of S2 with normal physiologic widening of S2 split expected due to inspiration. This can also be termed as a ***wide physiologic splitting of S2.***

Delayed A2

The causes of a delayed A2 component can be considered also under the three general categories.

Left Bundle Branch Block

When there is left bundle branch block, the mechanical onset of contraction will be delayed due to the delay in electrical activation. The depolarization wave will have to reach the left ventricle through the "working class" myocardial cells, which is a slow process as opposed to conduction through the normal His-Purkinje fibers. If the disease process in the left bundle system is focal and very proximal at its origin then the electrical wave front may latch on to the normal Purkinje fibers of the distal divisions of the left bundle and this may speed up the process of activation. The resulting electromechanical delay may not be severely prolonged. However when the disease process in the left bundle branch is more extensive and involves the distal divisions, then the delay can be significant. Thus varying degrees of electromechanical coupling may occur in different regions of the left ventricular myocardium. This will

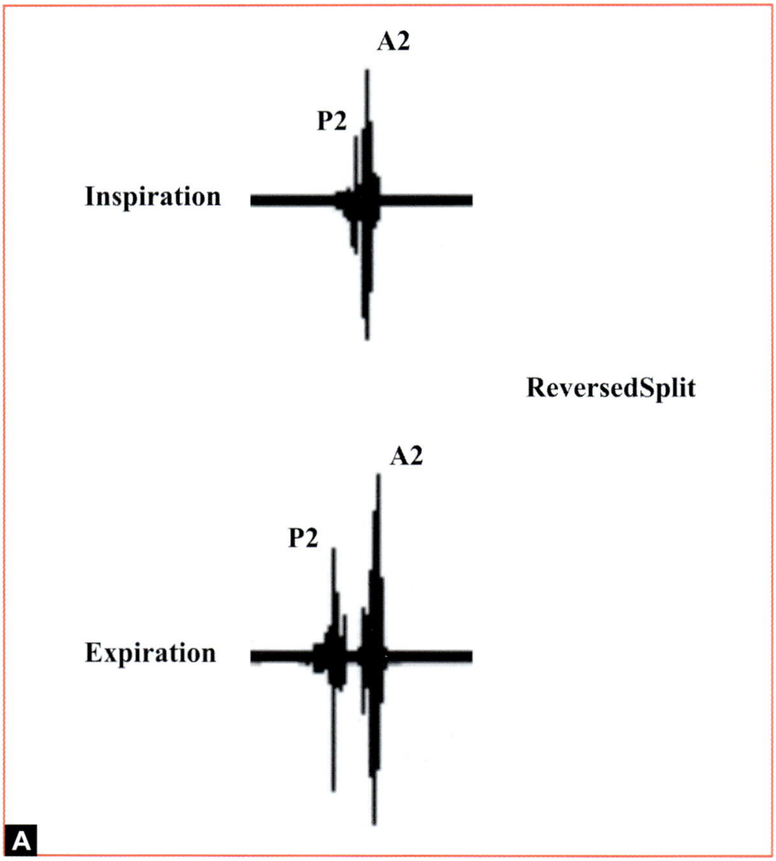

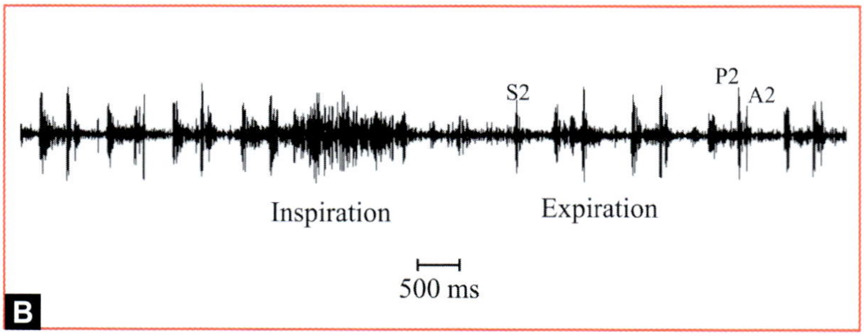

Figs. 6.22A and B: (A) Diagram shows a reversed sequence of the second heart sound (S2) components caused by delayed aortic component (A2) producing a paradoxical split with respiration. The normal inspiratory delay of the pulmonary component (P2) makes the two components come together on inspiration with very little or no obvious split. On expiration, the opposite occurs with P2 coming earlier so as to make an audible split. (B) Digital display of a magnetic audio recording from a young patient with significant left to right shunt through a persistent ductus arteriosus taken from the third left interspace showing a paradoxical split of S2 caused by very low systemic impedance making a delayed A2 component. The noise in the baseline gets exaggerated due to inspiration. The S2 becomes single for at least two beats after the end of inspiration. On expiration, there is on the other hand a clear split of S2.

lead to the delayed onset of contraction in the affected segments of left ventricular myocardium. The QRS duration may therefore show varying degrees of prolongation, 0.12 second or more. If electromechanical coupling is variably delayed then the rise in ventricular pressure during isovolumic phase will not be smooth and orderly. This will lead to lengthening of isovolumic contraction and a slower rate of rise of pressure. This may occur independent of the underlying myocardial function. In fact, in the majority of such patients with more extensive disease, the measurement of the individual components of the duration of the electromechanical systole will show not only lengthening of Q-S1 interval (electrical delay), but also lengthening of isovolumic contraction phase (the interval between S1 and the onset of ejection as assessed by aortic pressure recording).[33,34]

Mechanical Delay

Aortic valvular stenosis: When the obstruction is significant and fixed as in severe aortic valvular stenosis, the left ventricular pressure often rises to very high levels in systole. This is a necessity to overcome the obstruction for the ejection to occur. The high intraventricular systolic pressure takes a longer time to fall below that of the aorta and the ejection continues slowly and is maintained for a longer period. This prolongation in ejection contributes to the delayed occurrence of the A2. The sequence will be reversed. The P2 may be actually buried in the end portion of the systolic ejection murmur, which is often long in significant aortic stenosis. The A2 may be soft and may be the only audible component of S2. The reversed splitting and the reversed sequence, which can be theoretically expected, may not be noticeable clinically.

Hypertrophic obstructive cardiomyopathy: In this disorder, the interventricular septum is markedly hypertrophied. The ejection is often rapid at the onset. The rapid ejection of blood has a Venturi effect on the anterior mitral leaflet, which together with the interventricular septum forms the left ventricular outflow tract. This in effect pulls the anterior mitral leaflet from its initial closed position to an open anterior position moving toward the septum ***(systolic anterior motion).*** This systolic anterior motion actually leads the anterior leaflet to come in contact with the interventricular septum in mid-systole. This results in the outflow obstruction. This leads to almost cessation of ejection and development of mitral regurgitation because of the open mitral orifice and lower left atrial pressure. The obstruction thus developed in mid-systole is maintained until later part of systole when the Venturi effect wears off and the anterior leaflet moves back to its closed posterior position. The ejection resumes during this late phase. Thus the ejection gets prolonged causing delayed A2. The reverse sequence and the reversed splitting of S2 may in fact be clinically appreciated in this disorder when the obstruction is severe.[36]

Severe hypertension: In severe hypertension, the left ventricle often has to eject blood overcoming significant rise in the peripheral resistance. Very high levels of intraventricular systolic pressure may take a longer time to fall to the level of pressure in the aorta. In addition, often there may be impairment in both the onset of relaxation as well as in the rate of relaxation resulting in slower rate of fall in the intraventricular pressure. Also there may be coexisting ischemia aggravated by high pressures increasing the myocardial oxygen demand. Ischemia will further aggravate the poor relaxation in addition to prolonging the mechanical systole (see under "Ischemia"). For all these reasons, the occurrence of A2 may be delayed significantly. The sequence may be reversed resulting in reversed splitting of S2. *This usually requires a relatively well preserved overall left ventricular systolic function since significant decrease in systolic function would mean decreased ejection fraction and diminished stroke volume. This will tend to shorten the duration of the mechanical systole and not lengthen it.*

Ischemia: Ischemic myocardial dysfunction often involves pre-dominantly the left ventricle. The ischemic portion of the myocardium may have *delayed electrical activation and/or delayed onset of mechanical contraction contributing to prolongation of mechanical systole delaying the A2.* In the presence of ischemic left ventricular dysfunction, segmental or regional variations may also come into play since coronary lesions are often non-uniform. The non-ischemic areas will begin the contractile process raising the ventricular pressure. The delayed contraction of the ischemic areas occurring after the contraction of normal segments will help to maintain the ventricular pressure preventing its fall, although the peak pressure attained may in fact be lower. This in turn will prolong the duration of mechanical systole causing delayed A2. *The same is however not expected in the case of completed infarction. In this instance, the infarcted area will not contract at all causing no prolongation of the duration of mechanical systole. Therefore in patients with acute myocardial infarction, the presence of a reversed splitting of S2 should indicate significant coexisting ischemia.* Transient paradoxical splitting may occur during angina pectoris in some patients reflecting the ischemic left ventricular dysfunction.[33]

Decreased Systemic Impedance

The systemic impedance is normally high and therefore in order for the A2 to be delayed on account of impedance change, the aortic impedance must become very low. Such situations are not very common. Reversed splitting of S2 is occasionally encountered in patients with large left to right shunts at the aortic level through a persistent ductus arteriosus[36,38] (Fig. 6.22B). This is explainable by the fact that the aortic outflow impedance is considerably reduced in such patients due to the communication to the pulmonary artery and its branches. Decreased impedance has been considered to play a part for the delayed A2 seen in some patients with aortic stenosis and significant post-stenotic dilatation as well as in some patients with chronic severe aortic regurgitation.[36]

Delayed P2

The causes of a delayed P2 component can also be approached under the same three categories as mentioned above.

Right Bundle Branch Block

The right bundle branch is a long thin fascicle running under the endocardium on the right ventricular side of the inter-ventricular septum. It crosses the right ventricular cavity through the muscle bundle called the moderator band and arborizes as Purkinje network at the base of the anterior right ventricular papillary muscle. The conduction through the right bundle can be interrupted very easily even by some mechanical pressure as applied through a catheter placed in the right heart. The lesions causing RBBB need not be therefore extensive. The delayed electrical activation of the right ventricle in complete RBBB with QRS width of 0.12 second by itself can cause the delay in the P2. Rarely delayed mechanical contraction with prolongation of the isovolumic contraction on the right side may also play a part.

Left ventricular pacing and left ventricular ectopics also by producing late activation of the right ventricle can be associated with delayed P2.

Mechanical Delay

Right ventricular outflow obstruction: In pulmonary stenosis (infundibular or valvular), the elevated right ventricular systolic pressure will take a longer time to fall to the level of the pulmonary artery prolonging the duration of the mechanical systole on the right side. This would result in a delayed P2. The mechanism is very similar to that described with reference to aortic stenosis. The delay however may vary with severity.

Effects of Impedance

Pulmonary hypertension: ***The effects of increased pulmonary impedance*** in significant pulmonary hypertension will be expected to cause an ***early occurrence of P2*** that should result in a ***narrowly split S2*** (*see* Fig. 6.21). This is what happens in general in the early stages of chronic pulmonary hypertension. At this stage, the right ventricular myocardial performance is still normal despite the high pulmonary pressures.

The mechanical ***effects*** of chronic pulmonary hypertension on the left ventricular myocardial performance ***may vary not only with the severity***

but also with the duration of the pulmonary hypertension and the development and adequacy of compensation. Right ventricular hypertrophy developing over a long period when the process is chronic may be adequate to maintain normal systolic function. However, *before actual systolic dysfunction develops leading to right ventricular failure, the diastolic function will become impaired* very similar to what one finds in left ventricular dysfunction and failure. The right ventricle will manifest the diastolic dysfunction by the slower rate of relaxation in later part of systole and during the isovolumic relaxation phase. The systolic dysfunction may also be reflected in slower rate of rise of the systolic pressure during the isovolumic phase of contraction. *The slower rate of rise and decline of right ventricular systolic pressure would lead to the prolongation of right ventricular mechanical systole relative to the left side.* This often can be observed to be associated with the development of abnormal contours in the jugular venous pulsations where jugular descents show less prominence of the ***x′ descent*** and more dominance of the ***y descent*** compared to the usually dominant systolic ***x′ descent.*** In other words, the jugular contour will show ***x′ = y, x′ < y or single y descent*** as opposed to ***single x′ or x′ > y descent*** contour which is normally seen with the preserved right ventricular function. These changes indicate the development of right ventricular dysfunction.[39] In such instances, the relative lengthening of duration of right ventricular systole compared to that of the left side would result in a delayed P2. This is not uncommon when decompensation develops in chronic pulmonary hypertension.[30,40,41] The net effect will of course lead to a wide split S2. Rarely the splitting may be relatively fixed as well. The latter has been attributed to the inability of the right ventricle to increase the stroke volume on inspiration.[42]

Right ventricle is also not an efficient chamber in handling sudden rise in pulmonary artery pressures and resistance as seen in ***acute pulmonary embolism.*** Similar myocardial dysfunction may develop in some patients with acute pulmonary embolism causing a ***delayed P2,[43] and the effects of the delayed P2 may persist for several days*** and may be observed to improve and become more normal when full clinical recovery occurs.

Decreased pulmonary impedance: The pulmonary impedance is generally low even in the normal as discussed earlier. However, in some instances the impedance becomes considerably lower due to increased pulmonary vascular capacity. This is the case with atrial septal defect with large pulmonary arteries and branches due to the long-standing high pulmonary flow due to the left to right shunt.

Persistent wide splitting of S2 in patients who have had their atrial septal defect corrected is also probably a reflection of their increased pulmonary vascular capacity with decreased pulmonary impedance. An increased pulmonary vascular capacitance can occasionally be the cause of a wider split S2 which fails to close on expiration in some normal adults.[35]

Idiopathic and post-stenotic dilatation of the pulmonary artery: In idiopathic dilatation of the pulmonary artery as well as in post-stenotic dilatation of pulmonary artery accompanying mild to moderate pulmonary valvular stenosis, there is probably some deficiency of the elastic tissue in the pulmonary artery, which may be even responsible for the excessive dilatation. This may result in slower elastic recoil of the pulmonary artery partly accounting for the delayed P2. In addition, the increased capacitance may have a lowering effect on the impedance.[30,33,44]

Early A2

In severe mitral regurgitation, the A2 may occur early. Mitral regurgitation offers an extra outlet for the left ventricle to empty during systole reducing considerably the resistance to ejection. Mitral regurgitation presents a volume overload on the left ventricle since the left ventricle has to accept the regurgitant volume as well as the normal pulmonary venous return during diastole. The increased volume would increase the left ventricular contractility by its Starling effect. This together with an extra outlet for the left ventricle would cause more rapid and faster ejection. This will have the effect of making the A2 occur early.

The effect of an early A2 is to make a relatively wide separation of A2 and P2. The splitting of S2 may be recognizable as a persistent expiratory split of S2. This often tends to occur only when the mitral regurgitation is severe and either acute or subacute as seen for instance with ruptured chordae tendineae.[33] The clinical conditions, which may result in such mitral regurgitation, are usually non-rheumatic in origin.

Early P2: The effect of high pulmonary impedance in significant pulmonary hypertension has been mentioned earlier, which makes the P2 occur earlier than normal. However, this effect cannot make P2 come earlier than A2. The result of an earlier-than-normal timing of P2 will be to make a narrower split of S2 on inspiration, which will close on expiration and become single S2.

Abnormal Respiratory Variations of A2-P2 Split

The normal respiratory variation of S2 split with A2 coming earlier and P2 occurring later on inspiration, and the reverse on expiration, depend on the inspiratory increase in venous return increasing the right ventricular volume, as well as an expanding lung increasing the pulmonary vascular capacity. The former would increase the right ventricular ejection time and the latter would decrease the pulmonary impedance. Such a normal separation of the A2 from the P2 during inspiration is usually not noticeable in the normal adult particularly in the elderly. *Even in the young adult, A2-P2 split will usually disappear and be replaced by a single S2 on expiration when the patient is examined in the standing position. If the A2-P2 split persists on expiration in the standing position but narrower than what is observed on inspiration, then one has a relatively wide physiologic splitting of S2.* While this could be a normal variant in some, in most individuals one needs to consider the causes of a delayed P2 to account for the wide physiologic splitting. Both the normal split and the relatively wide split of S2 require a normal A2-P2 sequence.

When the A2-P2 separation occurs on expiration and the S2 becomes single on inspiration then a delayed A2 mechanism is in place causing abnormal sequence of P2-A2. This of course is termed *the reversed or paradoxical splitting of S2.*

When the A2-P2 separation remains relatively fixed and not appreciably change with respiration, then one has a *fixed splitting of S2,* which usually occurs in *atrial septal defect* (Figs. 6.23A to C). The communication between the two atria and the flow through the defect compensates for changing venous return on both inspiration and expiration. *The inspiratory increase in right ventricular volume is associated with a decrease in the amount of shunt into the right atrium from the left side. On expiration, the venous return diminishes and this is associated with an increase in the shunt flow through the atrial septum. In other words, the right ventricular volume is more or less the same on both inspiration and expiration.* Thus the right ventricular ejection time remains the same on both inspiration and expiration accounting for the relatively fixed S2 split. The A2-P2 sequence remains normal in atrial septal defect.[45,46]

CLINICAL ASSESSMENT OF S2

Second heart sound is a sharper crisper sound and can be mimicked by the syllable "dub". It marks the end of systole and beginning of diastole. With normal heart rates, diastole of course is longer than systole. If the jugular contour is normal and visible in the patient then the S2 can be noted to coincide with the systolic descent or ***the x′ descent*** of the jugular pulse. The ***x′ descent*** is noted to fall onto the S2. Since the ***x′ descent*** can be timed also independently with the radial arterial pulse with which it coincides, it can be used to focus one's attention on the S2 at the time of auscultation. This may help the beginner providing a visual marker for the S2 timing and appreciation of its components.

When assessing the S2, one needs to pay attention to the intensity as well as define the nature of the individual components and their variation with respiration. Trying to pose a series of questions (*see* questions given below) and trying to answer them in a systematic manner is a useful bedside method to adapt.

1. *Is the S2 single or split?*
2. *If split sometimes and single at other times, is the patient breathing in or out during split?*

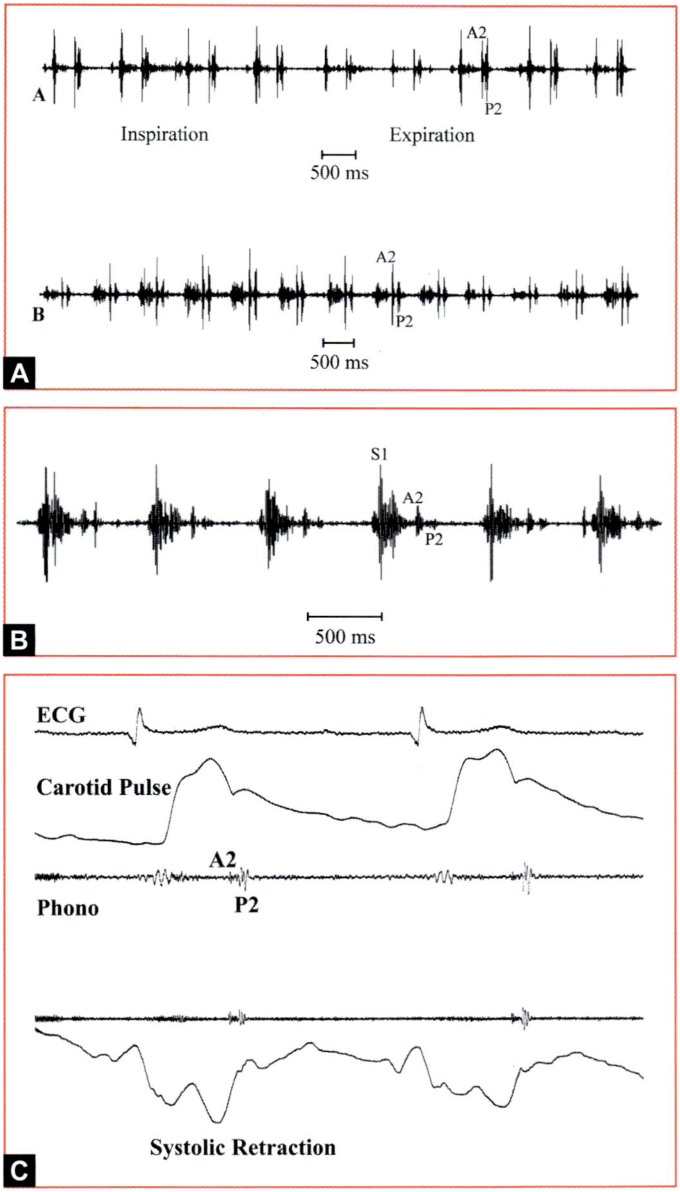

Figs. 6.23A to C: (A) Digital display of the magnetic audio recordings from two different patients with secundum atrial septal defect taken from the lower left sternal border region. Both show a relatively fixed split of second heart sound (S2). In Figure 6.23A, the split is somewhat narrower while in Figure 6.23B, it is wider. (B) Digital display of a magnetic audio recording from a patient with a secundum atrial septal defect showing a split S2 at the apex. The first heart sound has high amplitude due to a loud tricuspid component. It is followed by an ejection systolic murmur. This patient had a large right ventricle, which formed the apex beat. (C) Phono recording from a patient with atrial septal defect taken at the apex area showing a split S2. Systolic retraction is seen on the simultaneous ***Apex*** recording. This area of retraction was lateral to the apical impulse caused by the enlarged right ventricle.

3. *If split all the time, is it wider sometimes and narrower at other times or remain about the same all the time?*
4. *If wider sometimes and narrower at other times, is the patient breathing in or out when the wider split is heard?*
5. *If more or less equally separated components all the time and no variation is appreciated, is it the same or does it close with patient in standing position to maximize the respiratory variation in volume on the right side?*
6. *When the S2 is split, how wide an area over the precordium the split S2 is heard?*
7. *Is the split heard over the lower left sternal border region? Does it extend over the xiphoid area?*
8. *Is the split heard over the apex area?*
9. *If heard over the apex area, is the apical impulse palpable and if so whether the apical impulse is left ventricular or right ventricular in origin?*
10. *What is the grade of loudness of the S2?*
11. *Which is the area of the maximum loudness?*
12. *Is it palpable?*
13. *Where is it best palpated?*
14. *If split which component is louder—A2 or P2?*
15. *If split and cannot assign the respiratory variation clearly, is it possible to detect the sequence whether A2-P2 or P2-A2?*

Split S2

The normal A2 is heard over a sash area extending from the second right intercostal space to the apex area. The normal P2 is heard over the second and third left intercostal spaces. *Thus a normal split of the S2 is best heard over the second or the third left intercostal space where both components are audible.* Often asking the patient to take a breath-in may actually bring in too much noise caused by the breath sounds. It may actually interfere with the assessment of the split whether present or not and if present to further assess the variation and their relationship to the phase of the respiration. Thus *it may be easier to listen to the S2 and identify its components whether split or not and then merely observe the relationship to normal breathing.* Occasionally one may be able to direct the patient to breathe to a medium effort without making too much respiratory noise. But this may be more difficult than watching the effect of the normal respirations.

The A2 is equally loud at the left ventricular apex as it is in the second right intercostal space and in fact it may be loudest at the apex occasionally. Aortic component is never palpably loud unless significant systemic hypertension is present. The intensity of the A2 does not vary with respiration.

Pulmonary component on the other hand is never heard normally beyond the second and third left interspace, and when heard over the lower sternal border region and or to the xiphoid region, would indicate either a louder intensity P2 as in pulmonary hypertension or the right ventricle is enlarged due to a volume overload state such as in atrial septal defect or tricuspid or pulmonary regurgitation. For the same reason, the P2 is not usually audible at the normal apex area, which is usually formed by the left ventricle and identified as such by the presence of a medial area of retraction. On the other hand, if the apex is formed by an enlarged right ventricle as identified by the presence of a lateral area of retraction, then the normal P2 could be audible over the apex area.

Pulmonary component often can be noted to increase in intensity with inspiration. The increased volume in the right side provides presumably a greater right ventricular stroke volume distending the pulmonary root to a greater degree.

A palpable P2 in the second left intercostal space usually indicates pulmonary hypertension. This often correlates to a pulmonary systolic pressure of at least 75 mmHg. Grade III A2 and a Grade III P2 fusing on expiration may occasionally become palpable. If this happens, the S2 palpability will be restricted to expiration. But *if S2 were palpable throughout inspiration and expiration in the second left intercostal space then it would definitely indicate pulmonary hypertension even if there were coexistent systemic hypertension.* This stems from the fact that a palpable A2 is not felt maximally at the second left intercostal space. On the other hand, the location of maximal loudness of P2 is second left intercostal space. *The exception when an A2 may be actually palpable at the second left interspace is transposition of the great vessels (whether congenitally corrected or not) where the aortic root is anterior, superior and leftward.*

In young thin adults or adolescents and in children due to the thinner chest wall, the P2 may be normally audible over a larger area than in the normal adult. As well they will tend to have an easily audible split of the S2 and sometimes it could be wide. When examined in the erect position, the respiratory variations become maximal and can often be identified to become closer on expiration if not actually becoming single. In the elderly above the age of 60 years, however it is unusual to hear a good split of S2 due to poor chest wall compliance as well as age-related increases in the pulmonary impedance. Therefore split S2 in the elderly is often abnormal and deserves clarification.

Sequence Identification

In the normal, the A2 precedes P2. While A2 is heard over the apex, the P2 is usually not heard at the normal apex, which is formed by the left ventricle. If one auscultates over the second or third left intercostal space and hears a split S2 and then quickly changes over to apex with the rhythm of the split S2 in mind, one may be able to detect which of the two components is dropped or not heard at the apex. If the first of the two components is dropped at the apex then the sequence will have to be P2-A2. If the second component of the split is dropped, then the sequence will be A2-P2. These conclusions stem from the fact that the normal P2 is the one that is not heard at the apex. This technique can occasionally work much easier particularly with practice. Sometimes it may be easier than trying to assess the relationship to respiratory phases. It is particularly useful when the split is very wide and does not close on expiration and the patient is being examined in situations where it is not possible to adapt an erect or standing position such as in critically ill patients.

Rule of the S2 Split at the Apex

In view of the above observations, one can easily state that a split S2 at the apex is abnormal (Figs. 6.23B and C) and should make one consider the following possibilities:

a. That the P2 is loud and may indicate the presence of pulmonary hypertension.

b. If the P2 is not loud and there is no evidence of pulmonary hypertension, then the right ventricle may be enlarged as in volume overload and consider lesions such as an atrial septal defect.

c. Pulmonary component is normal and probably audible at apex due to a thin chest as in children.

d. The split S2 effect is mimicked by a normal single A2 followed by another sound such as an opening snap (OS) or S3.

Persistent or Audible Expiratory Split of S2

A split S2 that is audible on expiration is often a clue to some abnormality of the timing of the individual A2 and P2 components (Fig. 6.23A). It may indicate one of the following three possibilities:

1. *Relatively wide physiologic split of S2 with normal sequence and one must consider the causes of a delayed P2.*
2. *Reverse or paradoxical split of S2 and abnormal P2-A2 sequence and one must consider the causes of a delayed A2.*
3. *Relatively fixed split of S2 as in atrial septal defect.*

In the normal adult, the S2 split can be made to close on expiration particularly if assessed in the erect position with either patient sitting or standing. This allows for maximum variation of right ventricular volume changes with inspiration and expiration. Thus in most normal adults it would be abnormal to get a persistent S2 split on expiration when examined in this position. *Therefore one should never diagnose abnormal persistent expiratory split of S2 unless the patient has been examined in the erect and preferably standing position.*

Often applying the technique of sequence detection particularly if the split is not heard at the apex area, one may be able to narrow down the possibilities. *Even if the split is heard at the apex and the apex is formed by the left ventricle, then the concept that the P2 must be softer at the apex than at the second or third left intercostal space can be applied to detect the component that gets softer as one approaches the apex, listening and inching the stethoscope from the base to the lower left sternal border region and then to the apex.* A reverse sequence is detected if the first of the two components gets softer at the apex. Then causes of the A2 delay must be considered. A normal sequence is detected if the second of the two components gets softer at the apex. Then causes of delayed P2 must be considered. These deductions are made on the basis that the apex in the given patient is left ventricular in origin.

In atrial septal defect, the persistent expiratory split may or may not be associated with a wide splitting of S2. *Splitting can be fixed and yet narrow in atrial septal defect particularly if the pulmonary flow is markedly increased and the pulmonary bed is relatively overfilled and behaves like a system with high impedance.* This will tend to bring the P2 forward causing a narrower split. The development of some degree of *pulmonary hypertension also may contribute* to increased impedance and a narrower split. Nevertheless, it will be relatively fixed and not appreciably change with respiration. One must carefully assess the patient with the patient in the erect or standing position before concluding about a fixed split. *Occasionally the pulmonary systolic murmur due to flow may not be impressive and often the diagnosis of atrial septal defect hinges on diagnosing a fixed split S2.*

Partial anomalous pulmonary venous drainage into the right atrium may also cause a wide and sometimes relatively fixed split of S2. This lesion often coexists with an atrial septal defect and rarely may be an isolated anomaly. The clinical features often resemble atrial septal defect.[42] When it occurs with an intact atrial septum, fixed splitting does not occur.[47,48]

Patients with primary pulmonary hypertension developing some degree of decompensation, may have a wide persistent split of the S2 and the variation with respiration may be minimal and therefore may mimic a relatively fixed splitting of atrial septal defect. *Sometimes the effect of a post-Valsalva strain may help to distinguish the two.* During the strain phase of the Valsalva maneuver, the patient attempts to breathe against a closed glottis. This leads to increased abdominal and intrathoracic pressures, which prevents normal venous return, which would lead to considerable decrease in the right heart volume. Following the release of the Valsalva strain, there is a sudden drop in the intrathoracic and the abdominal pressure, which leads to sudden increase in the venous return. This would markedly increase the right heart volume for a few beats, diminishing again afterward. In the normal, the splitting may increase over 20 ms immediately following the release of strain. A few seconds later, the S2 splitting may become narrower or single.[46]

In atrial septal defect, the flow through the septal defect from the left atrium to the right side will compensate for the changes in the venous return more or less keeping the right ventricular volume the same. Therefore, the S2 split will remain relatively the same.[46] On the other hand, in primary pulmonary hypertension, the S2 split will be much wider immediately after release due to increase in the duration of right ventricular systole due to the abnormal behavior of the right ventricle in handling the volume load and the split will become narrower after a few beats when the venous return decreases. Exercise also may help distinguish pulmonary hypertension from atrial septal defect. Exercise will widen the split in right ventricular failure from pulmonary hypertension and will not do so in atrial septal defect.[16]

OPENING SNAP

After the closure of the semilunar valves, which is associated with the occurrence of the S2, the ventricles continue to relax and the ventricular pressures continue to fall. When the ventricular pressure falls below that of the atrium, the isovolumic phase of relaxation comes to an end and the atrio ventricular valves open to begin the phase of diastolic filling. If an artificial mechanical prosthetic valve had been used to replace the native valve, let us say the mitral valve, then one can often hear an opening click at this time of the cardiac cycle, which will follow the S2. Since such an artificial prosthetic mitral valve will also make a sharp closing click corresponding to the timing of S1 (Fig. 6.24), then one will actually hear a cadence or rhythm made by the clicky S1 followed by S2 and an opening click. ***The rhythm is Click.....Two...Click.***

Unlike the artificial mechanical prosthetic valve, when the normal mitral and tricuspid valves open, there is usually no formation of sounds with it. This is mainly because the valve opening results in the individual leaflets to move away from each other more or less symmetrically resulting in no real deceleration of the moving column of blood from the atria against the leaflets themselves in their attempt to enter the ventricles. However, when the valves are stiffened and fused at the commissures resulting in some degree of stenosis as seen in rheumatic mitral stenosis, then one may hear a sound associated with the opening of the mitral valve. The sound is often snapping and sharp in quality and hence termed the OS.[49-51] It has been discussed previously in relation to S1, that the M1 in mitral stenosis is loud and snapping. *The OS can be considered the reverse of the closing snap, which is the loud M1 in Mitral stenosis* (Figs. 6.25A and B). The presence of a loud M1 followed by a normal S2 and a sharp OS gives rise to a recognizable cadence: ***One.....Two...O......... Lubb.....Pa...Ta.........***

Similar sound can also occur in rheumatic tricuspid stenosis but the latter is very rare and therefore need not be discussed further.

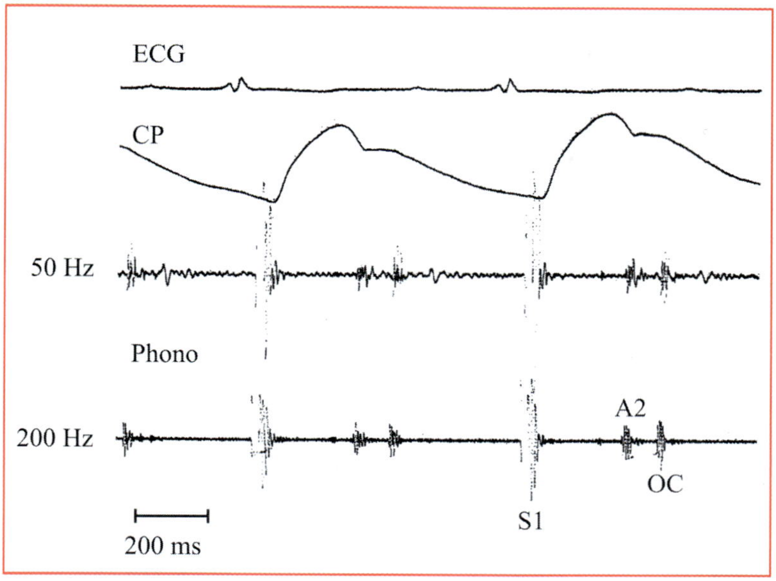

Fig. 6.24: Phono recording from a patient with a mechanical mitral valve prosthesis taken from the lower left parasternal area showing clicky sharp sounds associated with opening and closure of the mechanical valve. The closing of the valve causes a clicky sharp ***first heart sound*** and when it opens it produces a sharp ***opening click*** after the ***second heart sound***.

The Mechanism of Formation of the OS

In mitral stenosis, the commissural fusion results in anatomic distortion of the mitral valve, and the valve behaves like a stiffened funnel. The tethering of the leaflets at the commissures does not allow free opening of the leaflets. Both the anterior and the posterior leaflets tend to move together in the same direction anteriorly. If there is no excessive calcification of the main body of the anterior leaflet, it will be seen to actually bow anteriorly toward the ventricular septum with the opening motion of the valve at the onset of diastole (Fig. 6.26). During systole when it closes it will have the shape almost like a hockey stick particularly when seen on a 2D echocardiogram. The column of blood from the left atrium begins to enter the left ventricle when the pressure in the ventricle falls below that of the *v wave* peak in the left atrial pressure, which will lead to opening of the valve. Because of the distorted orifice and incomplete separation of the leaflets, part of the column of blood will actually be oriented against the body of the anterior leaflet instead of being oriented toward the orifice. When the leaflet excursion comes to its anatomic limits because of its commissural tethering, this part of the column of blood will be decelerated suddenly along with the leaflet. The dissipated energy at this time can be expected to produce the sound. Since in mitral stenosis, the left atrial pressure is often elevated, the column of blood moving from the left atrium

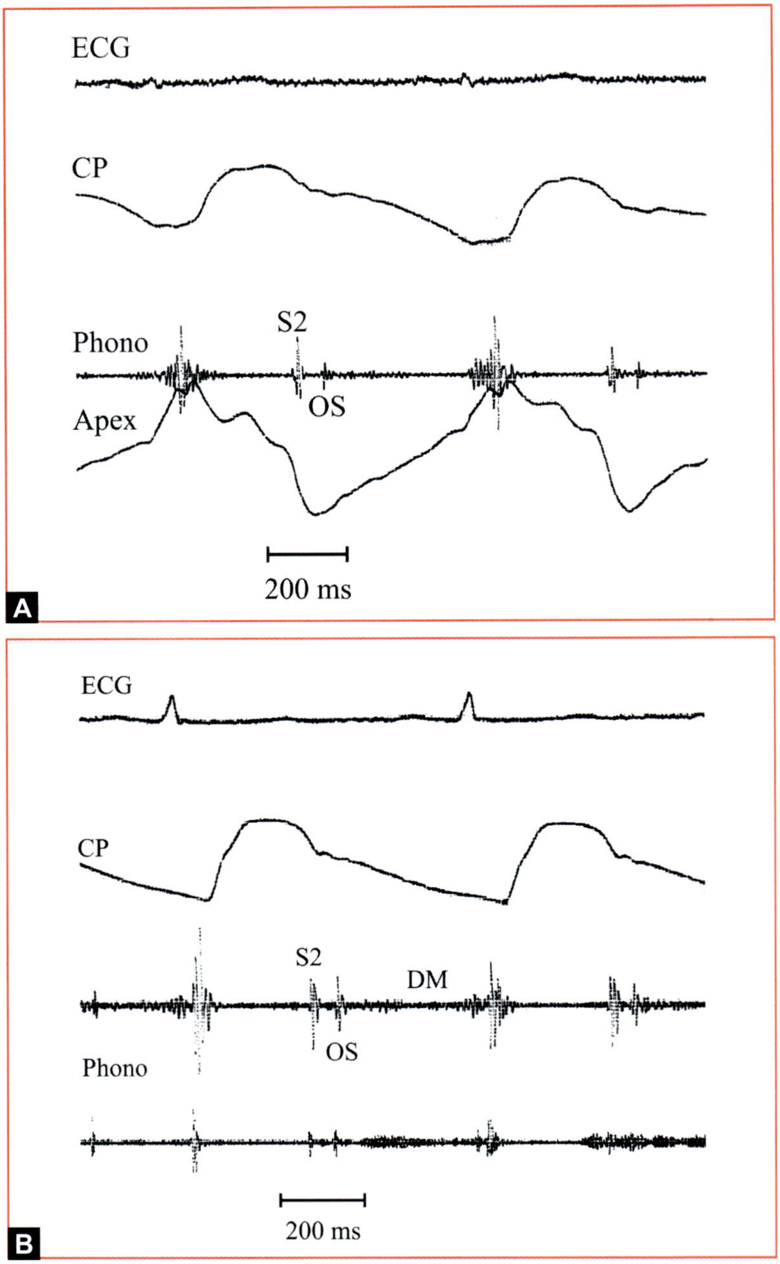

Figs. 6.25A and B: (A) Phono recording taken at the apex area from a patient with rheumatic mitral stenosis who has had a previous mitral valve commissurotomy for relief of the obstruction. The first heart sound (S1) is relatively loud. Note a sharp sound following the second heart sound (S2), which is the opening snap (OS). The OS occurs almost simultaneously with the most nadir point of the Apex tracing which is termed the O point. (B) Phono recording from another patient with mitral stenosis taken close to the apex area showing the loud S1 followed by the S2 and the OS. Also seen is the ***diastolic murmur*** of the mitral stenosis.

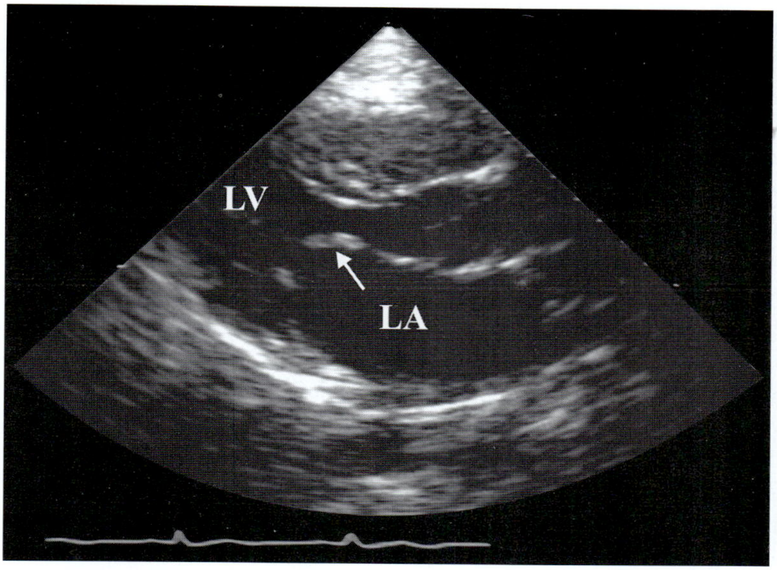

Fig. 6.26: Stop frame of a two-dimensional echocardiogram from a patient with mitral stenosis in the parasternal long axis at the onset of diastole showing the typical bowing of the anterior mitral leaflet (arrow). Note that the leaflet tip is pointing posteriorly due to tethering caused by the stenosis making a funnel-like opening. Part of the column of blood trying to enter ***the left ventricle*** from the ***left atrium*** during diastole is oriented toward the belly of the leaflet. When the leaflet excursion reaches its anatomic limits caused by the tethering, this column of blood gets suddenly decelerated. This leads to the production of the opening snap.

is under a higher pressure gradient than normal. Therefore there is relatively greater energy in the moving column contributing to a louder sound. Characteristically when the valve is relatively mobile, it leads to the production of the sharp snapping OS.[51-53]

Opening Snap in the Absence of Mitral Stenosis

Rarely excessive flow across the mitral valve in certain clinical conditions can be associated with the presence of an OS associated with the opening of the mitral valve in the absence of mitral stenosis. These include pure mitral regurgitation, ventricular septal defect, persistent ductus arteriosus, tricuspid atresia with large atrial septal defect and thyrotoxicosis.[54-56] In atrial septal defect, the torrential flow across the tricuspid valve may be associated with a tricuspid opening snap.[56]

Congenital mitral stenosis is not usually associated with OS since these valves are abnormal and not pliable.

Timing of the OS and the S2-OS Interval

The OS will be expected to occur at the end of the isovolumic phase of relaxation. The latter has an average duration of 60 ms at least. The ***S2-OS interval*** then must be usually expected to be at least 50 ms or longer. In general the OS may occur anywhere between 50 and 110 ms after S2. The OS has been reported to follow A2 by a delay ranging 30–150 ms.[56] The interval *will depend on the level of the aortic pressure, the rate of isovolumic relaxation and the left atrial v wave pressure peak.* Of these three, the most important determinant is the level of the peak left atrial pressure. Thus if the left atrial ***v wave*** is higher, then the OS will occur earlier than when the left atrial *v wave* is lower (Fig. 6.27A). Since the height of the left atrial pressure is indirectly related to the severity of the mitral stenosis, *the more severe the stenosis, the higher will be the left atrial pressure and earlier the OS will occur after the S2* (Fig. 6.27A). The S2-OS interval can be either short, i.e. close to 60–70 ms, medium, i.e. close to 80–100 ms or long, i.e. between 100 and 120 ms.

A ***short S2-OS*** interval can be simulated by the syllables, ***Lubbb ...pa.. da.*** when said as fast as possible. It can be medium and may simulate the syllables, ***Lubbb...pa....ta*** when said as fast as possible. When it is ***late***, it will be mimicked by ***Lubbb...pa......pa*** again said as rapidly as possible.

It can also be easily visualized that the extent of the excursion of the leaflet before its sudden tensing due to the tethering will vary according to the severity of the mitral stenosis as well. The more severe the stenosis, the less will be the extent of the excursion and therefore the earlier will be the OS (Fig. 6.27B).

Since besides the left atrial pressure, the aortic pressure as well as the rate of isovolumic relaxation controls the S2-OS interval, this interval may not predict always accurately the severity of mitral stenosis especially in the elderly patients and in the presence of hypertension. This interval will vary in atrial fibrillation due to the varying diastolic lengths. The longer cycles will be followed by lower left atrial pressure due to longer time for left atrial emptying and the next systole will also be more likely to have a lower left atrial pressure. Thus following long diastoles, the S2-OS interval will be longer. In the presence of low cardiac output and a very large left atrium, one may have a long S2-OS interval even with significant mitral stenosis. In view of these confounding factors, a short S2-OS interval may be more helpful than a wide S2-OS interval in predicting the degree of mitral stenosis.

Maneuvers that make the left atrial pressures to fall such as making the patient stand up from a supine position will make the OS come later (Fig. 6.28). The reason for this is the decreased venous return that occurs with assuming the erect posture, which will lower the left atrial pressure.

Following supine exercise, the S2-OS interval shortens due to rising left atrial pressure. Postexercise S2-OS interval of less than 60 ms will be suggestive of significant mitral stenosis.[56]

The Intensity of OS

In general, the presence of a good intensity OS requires a fairly mobile valve. When the stenosis is relieved by surgical mitral valve commissurotomy, the

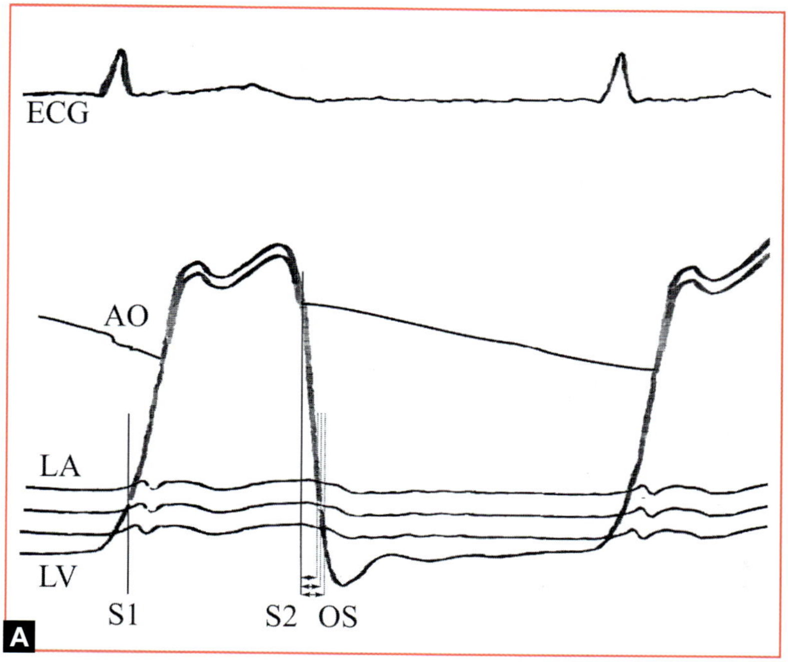

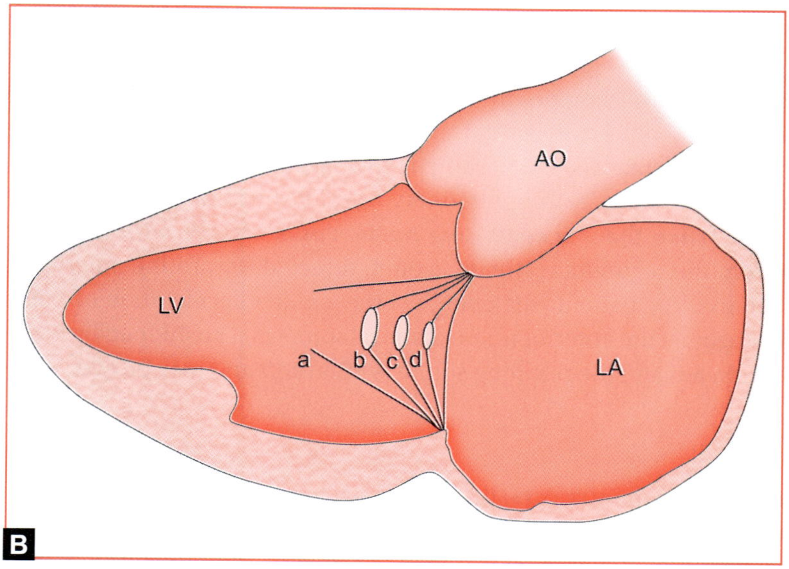

Figs. 6.27A and B: (A) Diagram showing simultaneous left ventricular (LV) and left atrial (LA) pressures in mild, moderate and severe degrees of mitral stenosis. The more severe is the stenosis the higher will be the left atrial pressure. The opening snap (OS) occurs at the end of the isovolumic relaxation phase of the left ventricle when the LV pressure falls just below the LA pressure. The OS will therefore tend to occur earlier with higher LA pressure and later with lower LA pressure. Thus the second heart sound-OS interval is short with severe mitral stenosis and long with mild mitral stenosis. (B) Visual representation of the excursion of the mitral leaflets in mitral stenosis of different degrees of severity: (a. Normal, b. Mild, c. Moderate, d. Severe).

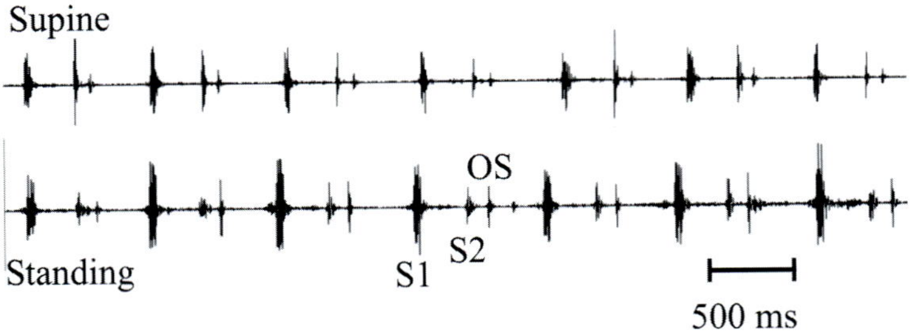

Fig. 6.28: Digital display of a magnetic audio recording from a patient with mitral stenosis taken at the lower left parasternal region showing the variation in the second heart sound-opening snap (S2-OS) interval between supine and standing position. The S2-OS interval is slightly longer on standing than when supine. The fall in the left atrial pressure caused by the upright posture makes the OS come later after S2. The aortic component-pulmonary component split however will either narrow considerably or become single S2 on assuming an upright position.

OS will not be always abolished since there may be still enough tethering of the leaflets at the commissures with all the anatomic pre-requisites for the OS production. When it is excessively restricted due to heavy calcification, the OS is unlikely to occur.

When there is severe mitral stenosis with very low cardiac output and decreased stroke volume, the OS intensity may be diminished due to the low flow. When there is significant pulmonary hypertension associated with severe mitral stenosis, the accompanying large right ventricle and low flow due to obstruction at the pulmonary arterioles will also tend to make the OS soft. ***When there is coexisting aortic valve disease with aortic regurgitation,*** the regurgitant stream is often directed toward the anterior mitral leaflet. In these patients the energy of the sudden deceleration of the mitral inflow against the anterior mitral leaflet is somewhat cushioned by the regurgitant stream and the resulting sound is often ***soft*** and may be even absent.

CLINICAL ASSESSMENT OF THE OS

The OS is generally maximally loud somewhere between the lower left sternal border and the apex. When it is very loud, it could be heard over a wide area including the base. At the apex, it coincides with the onset of the diastolic murmur of the mitral stenosis. The presence of OS following the S2 almost always simulates a wide split S2. In addition, a good intensity OS tends to be often associated with a loud S1. Thus when one hears a loud S1 and what sounds like a wide split S2, one should always suspect an OS and attempts then should be made to confirm or rule out its presence. This essentially consists in looking for ***the specific features of the OS,*** which are as follows:

1. *It is maximally loud between the left sternal border and the apex.*
2. *It is sharp and generally high in frequency.*
3. *Its intensity may slightly vary with respiration becoming slightly softer on inspiration due to less blood flowing through the left side and slightly louder on expiration due to increase in flow through the left heart. It behaves similar to A2 in this regard. It is different from P2, which will become louder on inspiration.*
4. *Second heart sound-opening snap interval tends to remain relatively the same with inspiration and expiration. Sometimes the P2 coming earlier on expiration may give one the impression that the S2-OS interval is widening.*

   A wide paradoxical split of LBBB may sometimes be confused with S2-OS. In the absence of LBBB however, if the second component of a wide split should increase in loudness at the apex or the split should become wider on expiration, it is unlikely to be a delayed P2 and an OS should then be suspected as the cause of the split.
5. *When the patient's posture is changed from supine to sitting with feet dangling or better still to a standing position, the OS will be found to come later. In other words, the fall in the left atrial pressure that accompanies the erect position due to the decreased venous return will make the OS occur later and this will make the split wider than when supine. The A2-P2 split will do the opposite since any decrease in venous return will make the P2 come earlier. This simple observation will often help in distinguishing between the two. Occasionally however the OS may become too soft all together on standing due to significant drop in output and flow across the mitral valve particularly in severe mitral stenosis.*
6. *The most definite way of recognizing the presence of OS is the ability to appreciate all three components on inspiration namely A2, P2 and the OS. This tends to happen in most patients when it is specifically looked for. The effect of such a triple sound on auscultation is very unique and once heard anyone can appreciate it.* ***The tripling or trilling on inspiration*** *with a simple split on expiration can be picked up over the second to fourth left sternal border area depending on how wide the area is where the P2 is audible in the given patient (Fig. 6.29).* ***The trill usually sounds like an effect of beating on a snare drum. It also can be mimicked by a triple clicking on the commonly used mouse attachment on any modern day computer.***

A late OS when soft may mimic an early S3. The distinctions will be discussed under section S3.

THIRD HEART SOUND (S3)

After the opening of the mitral and the tricuspid valves, blood flows into the ventricles from the atria during diastole. *Diastolic filling of the ventricle is*

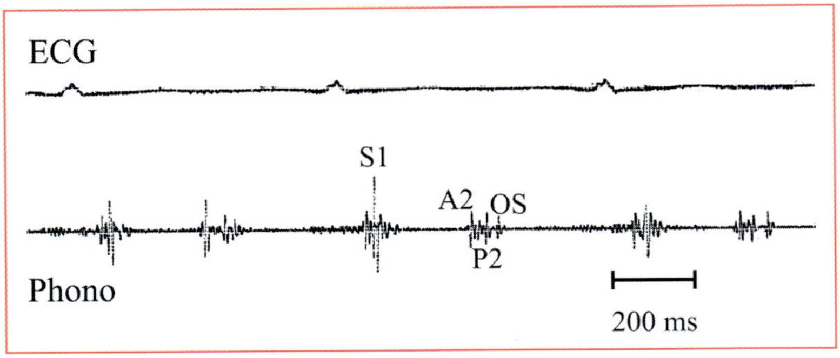

Fig. 6.29: Phono recording from a patient with mitral stenosis taken from the third left interspace showing the split S2 with ***aortic component*** and ***pulmonary component*** as well as the ***opening snap*** making a triple sound (trill) which is easily recognized.

divisible into three phases, an early rapid filling phase (RFP) followed by a slow filling phase or diastasis and at the end by the atrial contraction phase. The early phase of the ventricular filling is characterized by sudden vigorous expansion associated with rapid inflow of blood. The peak of this filling period may be accompanied by a sound, which is termed the third heart sound or S3.

Diastolic Function

The RFP of diastole is a very dynamic process, which begins with the active ventricular relaxation. Henderson wrote in 1923, "In the heart, diastolic relaxation is a vital factor and not merely a mechanical stretching like that of a rubber bag".[57] It begins at the latter half of systole and involves the isovolumic relaxation phase and the early ***RFP.*** It involves actin-myosin cross bridge dissociation by the re-uptake of Ca^{++}. Relaxation is an active process since it is ***energy dependent*** and requires ATP and phosphorylation of phospholamban (one of the proteins involved in the modification of sarcoplasmic calcium ATPase function) for uptake of calcium into the sarcoplasmic reticulum. Metabolic control of this complex process is through coronary perfusion, neurohumoral and cardiac endothelial activation. For instance, cyclical release of nitric oxide has been noted to occur most marked sub-endocardially peaking at the time of relaxation and diastolic filling. In addition, the intrinsic viscoelastic properties of the myocardium are also important. Fibrosis that accompanies hypertrophy probably plays a role in the impairment of relaxation.[58-60]

Just as force of contraction is alterable due to variation in filling or preload and afterload (the systolic load that the left ventricle has to face after it starts to contract), similarly *mechanical factors can also alter the rate of relaxation.*[61] *Five types of loading affecting relaxation are recognized. One slows the rate of relaxation and four tend to increase the rate of relaxation*[62-64] *(Fig. 6.30).*

1. Increase in volume or pressure in early phase of systole tends to slow relaxation.

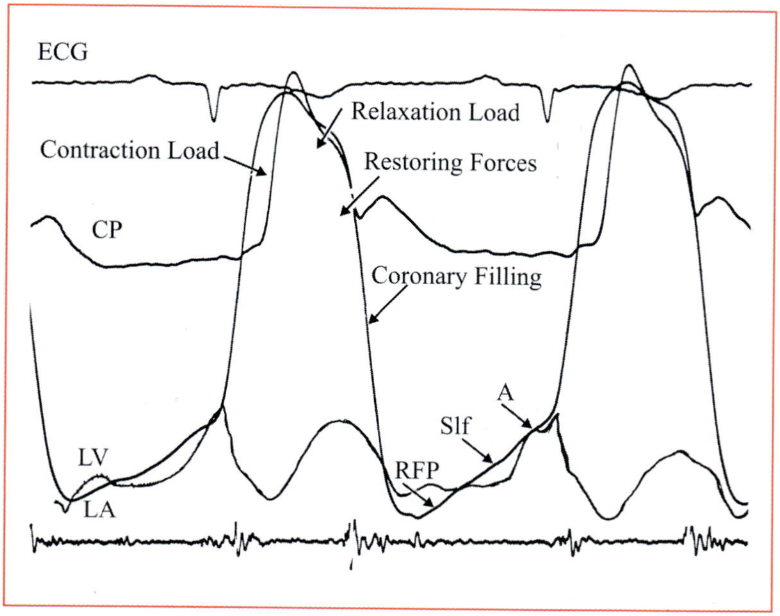

Fig. 6.30: Diagram of simultaneous left ventricular (LV), left atrial (LA) pressures and the ***carotid pulse*** indicating the various mechanical forces affecting the relaxation of the left ventricle operating at different phases of the cardiac cycle. While increase in volume or pressure in early systole ***(contraction load)*** slows relaxation, the same in later systole ***(relaxation load)*** hastens it. Restoring force resulting from the deformation of contraction and the ***coronary filling*** during isovolumic relaxation improve relaxation. When the LV pressure falls below that of the LA, diastolic filling begins. Diastole consists of three phases, the early rapid filling phase (RFP), followed by the ***slow filling phase*** and finally the atrial contraction (A) phase. Active expansion during RFP is favored by increasing wall stress (*see* the text).

2. On the other hand, increases in volume or pressure in late systole hasten relaxation.
3. The deformation caused by contraction itself provides a stored potential energy, which contributes to the restoring forces.
4. During the period of isovolumic phase of relaxation, coronary filling begins and acts to improve relaxation.
5. Finally, the prevailing wall stress affects the rate of relaxation during the early RFP of diastole.

The load effects on the rate of relaxation have been studied in isolated muscle clamp experiments as well as in canine hearts studied with microcomputer-assisted pumps. In these studies, effect of volume increments in specific portion of systole has demonstrated the same phenomenon.[63,65] The potential energy gained by contraction is thought to act through cytoskeletal proteins such as titin, which get compressed. During diastole, they expand like springs, expending this stored energy and provide a recoiling force for the myocardial filament to regain its length.[59] Three clinical examples will be considered.

Hypertrophic Cardiomyopathy with Obstruction

The nature of this condition is such that it is accompanied by impairment of relaxation. The fibrosis that accompanies the hypertrophy may be expected to contribute to this.[60] In addition, one can expect some load-dependent alteration in relaxation as well. In hypertrophic cardiomyopathy with obstruction, the mid-systolic obstruction will lead to increased pressure in the left ventricle which will act as an increased "contraction phase" load. In addition, these patients have a very high ejection fraction and low end systolic volume. This leads to poor late systolic relaxation load. Both these factors could also contribute to poor relaxation.

Post-extrasystolic Beat

It is common knowledge that the beat following an extrasystole is stronger and forceful but it is usually not recognized that ***this post-ectopic beat has slower relaxation.*** If one records the rate of ventricular pressure rise and fall (dP/dt), it will be seen that the peak negative dP/dt reflecting the rate of relaxation is smaller in the post-ectopic beat compared to the normal beat (Fig. 6.31). The reasons for this are probably two-fold, one there is an excess of calcium made available to the myocardial cells from the extrasystole and the cells are somewhat calcium overloaded. This will be expected to slow relaxation. The second reason is perhaps also the poor relaxation phase load in the post-ectopic beat due to near complete ejection.

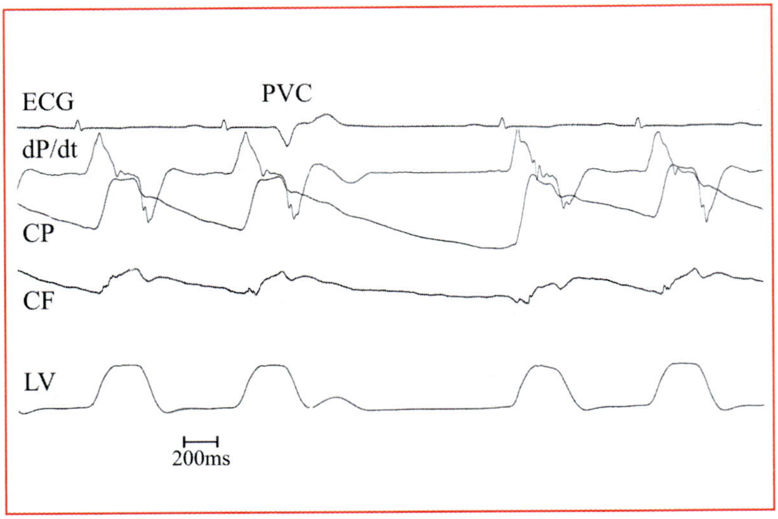

Fig. 6.31: Simultaneous left ventricular pressure and its first derivative ***(dP/dt)*** shown along with the ***carotid pulse*** and ***electrocardiogram.*** Note that the first beat following the premature ventricular beat has a significant decrease in the rate of relaxation as shown by the depth of the negative dP/dt.

Mild LV Dysfunction

In a study of LV function using characteristics of the apical impulse as measured by apexcardiography,[66] we observed that *the rate of isovolumic relaxation slope was slower in patients with mild LV systolic dysfunction* whereas this slope was *not abnormally slow when the ventricular systolic function was moderately or severely depressed.* In the presence of significant systolic dysfunction, the ejection fraction is reduced. This leads to an increased end-systolic volume. It is conceivable that this may act as a "relaxation phase" load, which could indirectly help in improving relaxation. It is known that the rate of LV relaxation as measured by peak negative dP/dt is impaired in patients with ischemic heart disease and known systolic dysfunction and decreased ejection fraction.[67] The diastolic time intervals like the isovolumic relaxation time and other non-invasive measurements however are affected by many factors and they do not consistently gauge LV relaxation.[68] Perhaps this is the reason that this non-invasive measurement by apexcardiography failed to pick up the abnormality in the presence of significant LV dysfunction.

Finally, both the process of calcium inactivation and the load effects on the rate of relaxation could be variable and not uniform through the entire myocardium depending on the pathologic process.[62] This is best exemplified by ischemic heart disease, which is often segmental.

Early Rapid Filling Phase

The RFP of diastole is part of this active phase of relaxation. The S3, when present, occurs at the end of this period. The rate of expansion of the ventricle during this phase is conditioned by the prevailing load or wall stress increasing with the increasing wall stress. The latter can be defined by the ***LaPlace relationship*** where the wall stress or the wall tension is directly proportional to the pressure and the dimension or the radius and inversely related to the wall thickness. This phase begins at the onset of mitral and tricuspid valve opening. The peak pressure head driving the filling of the ventricle is the peak **v wave** pressure in the atrium since the ventricular pressure is close to zero at the beginning of this phase. *During this phase of filling, the ventricle receives volume and expands and its walls continue to thin.* This means that there is an increasing wall stress from the beginning of this phase (which is at the mitral opening) to the end of this period. *Thus this period of filling accelerates under increasing rate of active expansion favored by the increasing wall stress, which characterizes this period. If the v wave height is increased for any reason then this will add to the wall stress achieved further hastening relaxation and expansion[62] (Fig. 6.30).*

Slow Filling Phase and Atrial Contraction Phase

As opposed to the early RFP of diastole, *the period of slow filling or diastasis and the atrial contraction phase are influenced by compliance, which is mainly secondary to the passive elastic properties of the myocardium (Fig. 6.30).* Compliance can be expressed for the whole ventricle in terms of volume–pressure relationship (dV/dP) or the converse which is expressing it as unit pressure change for unit increase in volume (dP/dV). The latter is termed chamber stiffness. When the same is expressed for individual muscle fiber, it is called muscle stiffness (measured by stress-strain relationship, force per unit area/fractional change in dimension).[69–73]

Factors that affect the compliance of the ventricle are as follows:

1. *Completeness of relaxation*
2. *Chamber size*
3. *Thickness of the wall*
4. *Composition of the wall (inflammation, infiltrate, ischemia or infarction, scars, etc.)*
5. *Pericardium*
6. *Right ventricular volume/pressure and their effects on the LV compliance*

The ventricle can become stiff and offer ***more resistance*** to expansion when the overall *size is small* as in children. It also is ***stiffer when the process of relaxation is impaired*** for any reasons mentioned above, e.g. hypertrophic cardiomyopathy with obstruction, ischemic heart disease due to ischemia. The degree of ***decrease in compliance*** when there is ***hypertrophy of the myocardium depends on the cause of hypertrophy.*** When there is physiologic hypertrophy as seen in the athletes, the decrease in compliance is slight. The decrease in compliance when the hypertrophy is due to pressure load as in significant hypertension or outflow obstruction (e.g. aortic stenosis), the decrease in compliance is more marked. Profound decrease in compliance tends to occur in hypertrophic cardiomyopathy. In addition, *any pathologic process (ischemia, scars, inflammation, infiltrative process and others)* that affects the myocardium can alter the compliance of the ventricle by making ***the affected segments stiff.*** Ischemia is particularly of interest. It makes the ischemic segments relax poorly. The segments become stiff due to incomplete relaxation.[74] This affects the overall distensibility of the ventricle when the ischemia is significant. ***The decreased compliance leads to increased diastolic filling pressure when the ventricle fills during diastole.*** The increased diastolic pressure is transmitted to the atrium since the mitral valve is open during diastole and the increased left atrial pressure is in turn transmitted to the pulmonary capillary bed. This increased pulmonary alveolar capillary pressure leads to the production of symptoms of dyspnea during an episode of angina. The increased diastolic pressure in the ventricle however gives a greater stretch on the non-ischemic segments and increases their contractility thereby preserving the forward cardiac output.

If for any reasons the ventricle becomes stiff or less compliant, then the expansion during the slow filling period becomes difficult and slower. The compensation for this inadequate ventricular filling is provided by a stronger than normal contraction of the atrium during the atrial contraction phase assuming that the atrium is healthy.

Mechanism of Formation of the S3

Third heart sound occurs at the end of the RFP of diastole.[75,76] The column of blood entering the ventricle during this phase is under the pressure head provided by the ***v wave*** pressure in the atrium. This phase of diastolic expansion is generally rapid and vigorous for reasons discussed above. But *in almost all hearts, this rapid expansion suddenly changes to a period of slower expansion.* Thus there is a tendency almost in all hearts for the moving column of blood entering the ventricle during the RFP to decelerate somewhat toward the end of this period (Fig. 6.32). *When the transition becomes more abrupt then this will be expected to affect the moving column of blood causing it to decelerate more abruptly. The factors that are likely to make the transition more abrupt in general are those that decrease the compliance of the ventricle.*[77-80]

The energy achieved by the moving column of blood during the active RFP of diastole is related to the rate of relaxation, the velocity and the volume of blood entering the ventricle and the pressure head provided by the v wave

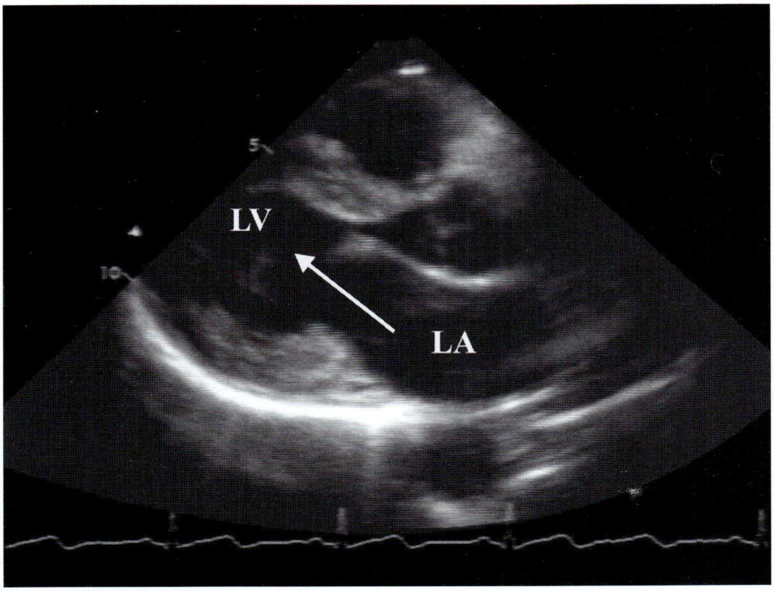

Fig. 6.32: Stop frame of a two-dimensional echocardiogram taken from a normal subject in the parasternal long axis at the end of the rapid filling phase of diastole when the moving column of blood (arrow) entering the ***left ventricle*** from the ***left atrium*** gets suddenly decelerated due to the fact that the rapid expansion suddenly changes to a period of slower expansion. Factors that make the transition more abrupt tend to produce a third heart sound (*see* the text).

peak in the atrium. When the momentum achieved by the moving column of blood is significant and the transition from the early RFP to the slow filling phase more abrupt, due to decreased ventricular compliance however brought about, then the deceleration will occur more suddenly and the dissipation of energy will result in the production of an audible sound within the ventricle. The sound will obviously occur at the peak of the rapid filling wave and this of course is the S3. Intraventricular pressure and transmitral flow studies in dogs have demonstrated a small but consistent reverse transmitral gradient to always accompany this deceleration.[81] *In addition, the sounds accompanying the flow deceleration could be recorded inside the ventricles, as well as over the epicardial surface of the exposed ventricles ruling out the external origin theory of S3.*[82] The whole hemic mass including the blood, the mitral structures as well as the ventricular wall and the papillary muscles probably participate in the vibration.

Physiologic S3

This occurs in children and in pregnant women and in other conditions that are associated with rapid circulation such as anemia and thyrotoxicosis. ***In children, the rapid inflow and the small size of their hearts together*** contribute to the development of S3 (Fig. 6.33). The small size offers an increased

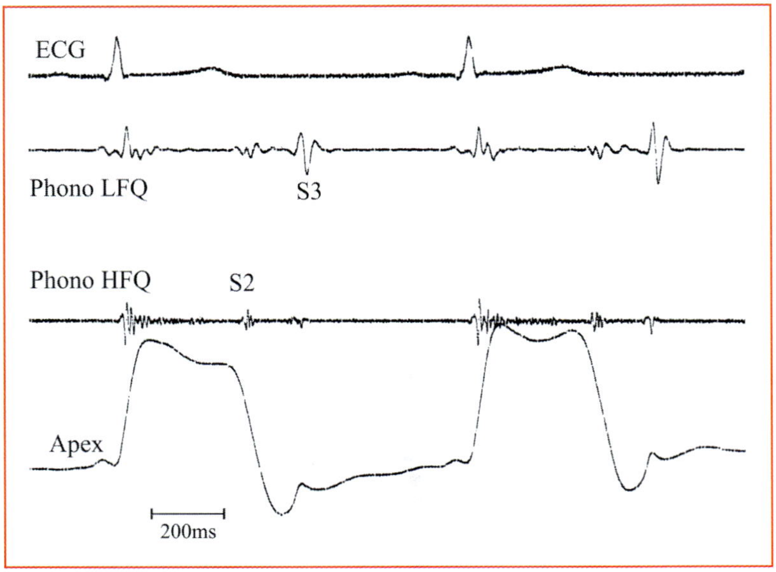

Fig. 6.33: Phono recording from a young subject taken at the apex area along with an ***apexcardiogram (Apex)*** showing a physiologic third heart sound (S3). The S3 is well seen in the low frequency range of 25-50 Hz. It is not as prominent in the ***high frequency*** range of 200 Hz. The S3 is seen to coincide with the peak of the rapid filling wave (arrow) in diastole.

resistance to expansion initially like a balloon when one tries to blow it up. Once expanded, then there is not much resistance to further filling. Physiologic S3 however is rare after the age of 35 years. In pregnant women, the blood volume is increased and in addition there is a relatively rapid circulation and increased sympathetic tone. The compliance need not be decreased. *In the presence of rapidly moving large volume of inflow, the transition from the rapid expansion to slow expansion may be sufficient to cause enough deceleration to produce the S3.*

Third Heart Sound (S3) in Ventricular Volume Overload

In volume overload states such as mitral and tricuspid regurgitations, the inflow volume during diastole into the ventricle is larger since the regurgitant blood into the atrium as well as the usual venous (systemic or pulmonary) return will enter the ventricle during diastole. The ventricle is also hyperdynamic in its contraction in these states due to the Starling effect caused by the large volume of diastolic filling. The relaxation following such stronger contraction will also be expected to be very rapid due to better restoring forces. In addition, the *v wave* peak pressure in the atrium will be higher due to the regurgitation (through the mitral and the tricuspid valves). For these reasons, *the inflow into the ventricle will be not only large in volume but also will be moving with greater velocity achieving greater energy.* In fact, an apexcardiogram obtained in patients with volume overloaded left ventricle will often show an exaggerated large rapid filling wave with an overshoot (Figs. 6.34A and B). The response of the ventricles to chronic volume overload is to dilate and enlarge. This is accompanied by increased compliance. Therefore, the *deceleration is mainly brought about from the rapid expansion to slow expansion alone.* The S3 in these states may in fact have enough duration and sounds ***like a short murmur.*** In late stages when the ventricles have developed secondary hypertrophy and focal fibrosis particularly in the sub-endocardial regions, then the resulting decrease in compliance will also play a part in the production of the S3. Similar situations are also likely to occur and result in left sided S3 in large left to right shunts through persistent ductus arteriosus and ventricular septal defects. In these conditions, the increased pulmonary flow received through the communication has to exit through the pulmonary veins into the left atrium.

In atrial septal defect with large shunts, the increased flow from the left atrium into the right atrium causes a RV volume overload. Similar considerations apply. However, since the right ventricle is more compliant than the left ventricle, increased flow through the tricuspid valve alone will not be sufficient to produce a right-sided S3. However, one can expect to hear a tricuspid inflow murmur in diastole instead.[83]

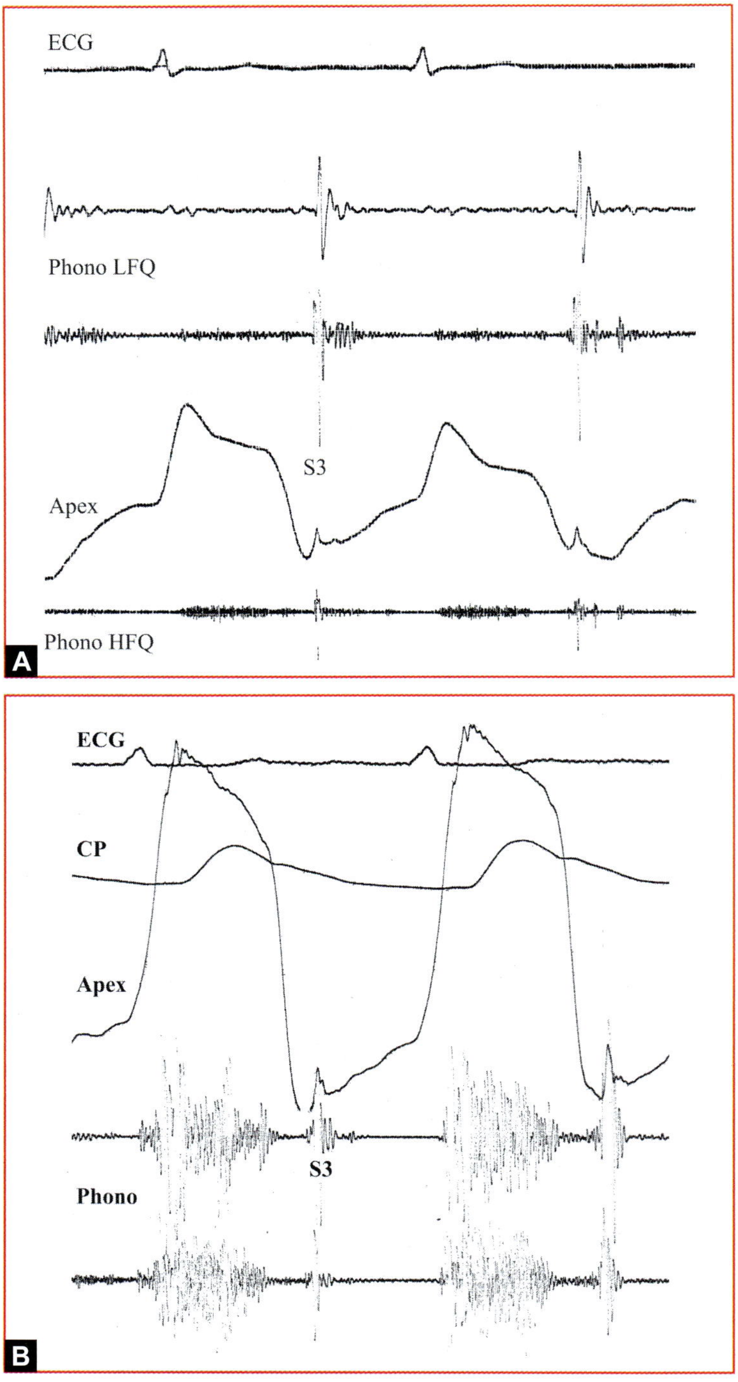

Figs. 6.34A and B: Phono recordings taken from the apex area along with recording of the apical impulse ***(Apex)*** from two patients both with significant mitral regurgitation causing left ventricular volume overloads. In both, overshoot of the rapid filling phase can be seen on the ***Apex*** coinciding with the ***third heart sound*** on the ***phono.***

Third Heart Sound (S3) in Ventricular Dysfunction

In patients with significant LV dysfunction of whatever etiology, *the LV diastolic pressure will rise due to decreased ventricular compliance.* Since during diastole the mitral valve is open, the ***rise in*** the LV ***pre a wave*** pressure will raise the baseline left atrial pressure. This will indirectly raise the level of both ***a and v waves*** in the left atrium. The ***increased*** left atrial ***v wave*** pressure (in heart failure, cardiomyopathy or in the post-myocardial infarction state) will aid in the development of greater energy acquired by the moving column of blood during the RFP. The ventricular ***compliance is generally decreased*** in these conditions due to the pathologic processes involving the myocardium. Thus the set-up is there for the production of S3 in these states (Fig. 6.35). When the symptoms and signs of heart failure improve with therapy there will be an associated fall in the LV diastolic and the left atrial pressures. Often at this time, the S3 will become soft or inaudible. *If S3 remains relatively loud*

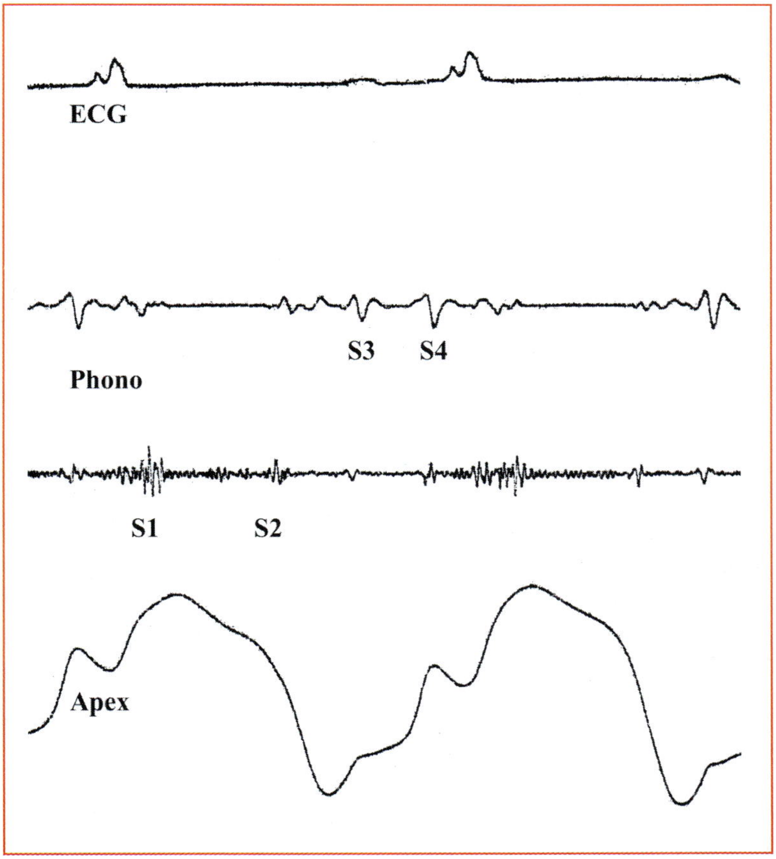

Fig. 6.35: Phono recording from a patient with severe aortic stenosis and left ventricular failure taken from the apex area along with the recording of the apexcardiogram. The ***Phono*** shows both the ***fourth heart sound and the third heart sound.***

after the symptoms of dyspnea and edema have improved with associated radiologic clearance of signs of failure, then it indicates *marked decrease in LV compliance. This is usually not a good prognostic sign.*

Third heart sound in acute myocardial infarction usually occurs when there is a large infarct associated with LV failure. If improvement in symptoms and signs of failure is accompanied by the disappearance of S3, then it usually is a good prognostic sign. A loud persistent S3 in the post-infarction state may be due either to significant mitral regurgitation or a marked decrease in compliance due to extensive myocardial damage. Occasionally both of these may be playing a role.

In patients with ventricular aneurysm, S3 is not usually seen in the absence of heart failure. Also, S3 is uncommon in acute ischemia unless it is severe enough to produce hemodynamic deterioration with or without mitral regurgitation secondary to papillary muscle dysfunction.[76]

In significant pulmonary hypertension when the right ventricle begins to fail, a right-sided S3 is likely to develop. The mechanism involves essentially similar principles as discussed under LV dysfunction above. The rise in RV ***pre a wave*** pressure leads to raised baseline pressure in the right atrium. This will add to the ***v wave*** pressure in the right atrium. With RV dilatation, the tricuspid ring will get eventually stretched leading to the development of tricuspid regurgitation. This adds further to the ***v wave*** pressure height in the right atrium. This is slightly different from the left side where the mitral valve does not get fully stretched by LV dilatation since only the posterior annulus, which is attached to the ventricle, gets stretched. Anteriorly the mitral valve is attached to the aortic root. The latter does not stretch with LV dilatation. Thus, mitral regurgitation does not usually arise from LV dilatation alone. The increased right atrial ***v wave*** pressure head together with significant decrease in compliance of the right ventricle brought about by the hypertrophy caused by the pulmonary hypertension provide the set-up for the right-sided S3. Right-sided S3 in general requires not only increased flow across the tricuspid valve but also significant elevation of right atrial pressure usually seen in the context of pulmonary hypertension during the stage of decompensation.

Right ventricle does not tolerate acute rises in pulmonary artery pressure however. Thus, in acute pulmonary thromboembolism, right ventricle will dilate acutely and this may produce not only tricuspid regurgitation but also cause steep rises in the systolic and the diastolic pressures in the right ventricle. The latter by raising the right atrial pressure will provide the necessary conditions for the right-sided S3.

Third Heart Sound (S3) in Constrictive Pericarditis (Pericardial Knock)

In chronic constrictive pericarditis, the thickened and fibrosed, sometimes even calcified pericardium, surrounds the ventricles like steel armor not allowing their full expansion. *The ventricles generally are able to expand only during the phase of the rapid inflow.* Once the peak of this expansion is reached then further expansion is often impossible due to the thickened and unyielding pericardium. *The diastolic pressure in the ventricles will abruptly rise to high levels and plateau thereafter until the end of diastole giving the classic square root sign to the ventricular pressure curves. In classic constrictive pericarditis, both the LV and RV diastolic pressures* will in fact be ***equal*** under resting conditions (Fig. 6.36). The raised diastolic ventricular pressures will be transmitted to the respective atria. This of course is the reason for the raised ***v wave*** pressure head for the rapid filling period. The rapid inflows will be abruptly decelerated by the decreased compliance of the ventricles caused by the abnormal pericardium producing the S3.[84]

The degree of cardiac compression may slightly vary in different patients. The RFP may also be slightly shortened. The S3 therefore may occur ***slightly earlier*** than usual. The sound also may be somewhat sharper[84] (Fig. 6.37). It is sometimes called a ***pericardial knock.*** However, in the majority the S3 is

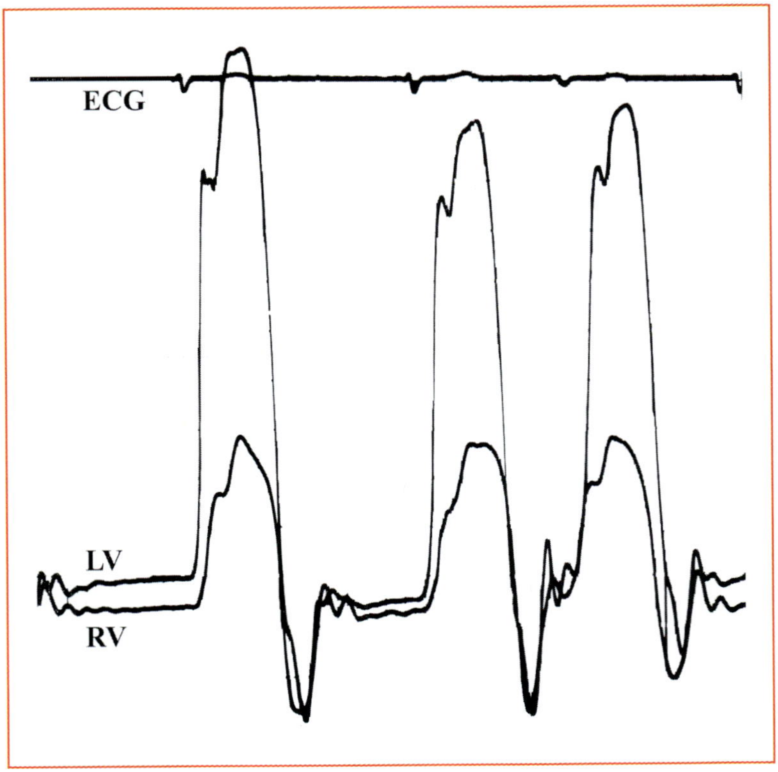

Fig. 6.36: Simultaneous recording of ***left ventricular*** and ***right ventricular*** pressures from a patient with severe chronic constrictive pericarditis showing the raised diastolic pressures with equalization between the two sides along with the typical dip and plateau pattern ***(the square root sign).***

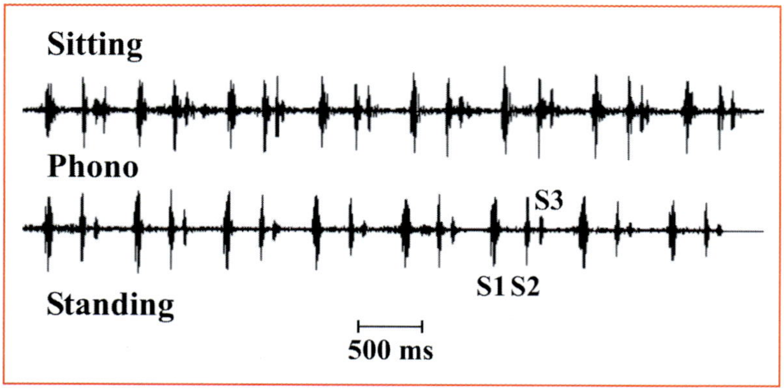

Fig. 6.37: Digital display of a magnetic audio recording from a patient with chronic constrictive pericarditis taken from the left lower parasternal area showing an early third heart sound which persists even in the erect position ***(standing)*** due to high atrial pressures.

quite similar in character to the usual S3 most likely because the constriction does not shorten the RFP and begins to impede filling only at the end of the RFP.

Third Heart Sound (S3) in Atrial Myxoma (Tumor Plop Sound)

In atrial myxoma, one may hear an S3-like sound termed the **tumor plop**. The sound is actually produced when the tumor plops into the ventricle in diastole. The tumor is usually attached by a stalk to the interatrial septum. For instance, in the case of a left atrial myxoma, the tumor may in fact protrude and come in the way of the mitral inflow causing mitral orifice obstruction. This of course also leads to elevation of the left atrial pressure as in mitral stenosis. The elevated left atrial ***v wave*** pressure initiates a vigorous expansion during the RFP. When the opening of the mitral valve occurs, the tumor tends to move along with the anterior mitral leaflet and enters the left ventricle. When it reaches its maximum excursion, its further movement is suddenly stopped. This results in a sound, which has similar characteristics as the S3[85] (Figs. 6.38A and B). *The sound tends to occur sometimes slightly after the rapid filling wave peak. It often is followed by a low medium frequency diastolic murmur due to the mitral obstruction. In addition, the elevated left atrial pressure produces a loud banging M1, which may be actually palpable (Fig. 6.39).* Also, one will be able to note the presence of a systolic murmur of mitral regurgitation.

Summation Gallop

When the atrial contraction happens to occur during the RFP for any reason, then the energy acquired by the moving column of blood becomes

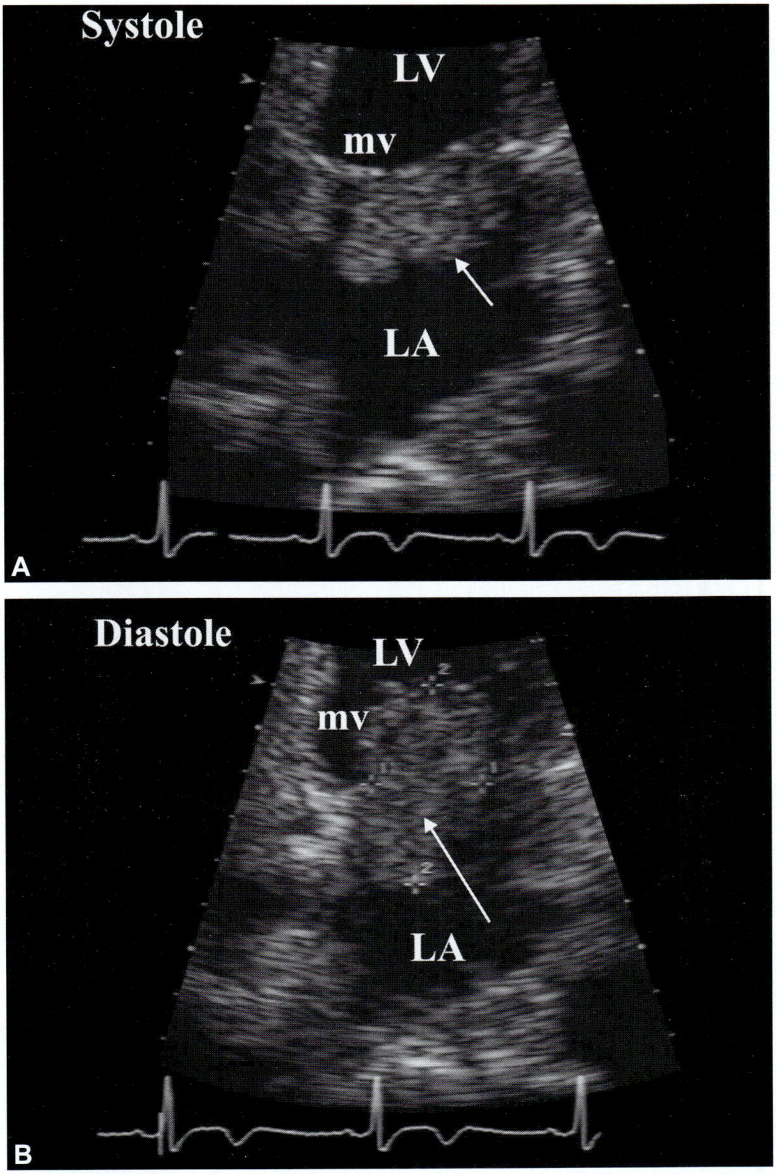

Figs. 6.38A and B: Stop frames from the two-dimensional echocardiogram taken at the left parasternal long axis from a patient with left atrial myxoma. During ***systole*** the dense echogenic mass representing the tumor in the ***left atrium*** is seen just at the edge of the closed mitral valve ***(mv).*** The tumor mass is seen to protrude into the ***left ventricle*** in diastole when the ***mv*** opens.

augmented. In such situations, the deceleration that follows, due to the normal transition from the period of rapid expansion to the slow expansion may be sufficient to generate an S3. *This requires a normal atrial contraction and abnormal timing of the atrial depolarization in relationship to the ventricular*

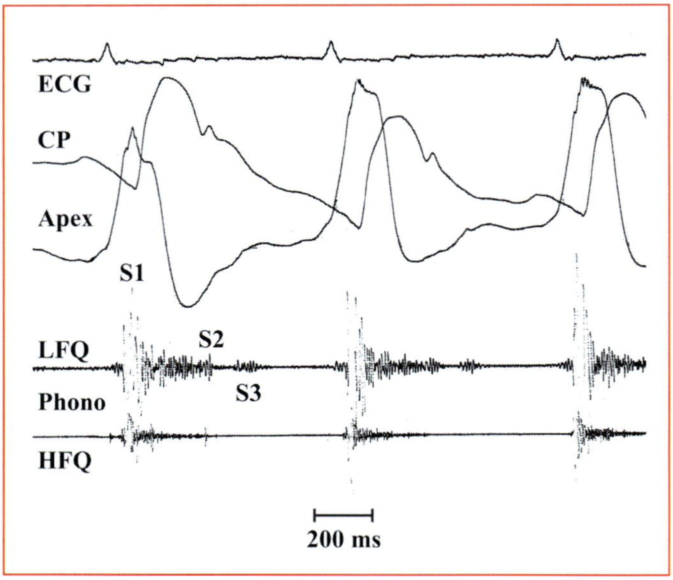

Fig. 6.39: Phono recording taken at the lower left sternal border area from a patient with left atrial myxoma along with the ***Apex*** and ***carotid pulse*** recordings. The tumor plop sound ***(third heart sound)*** is seen in the ***low frequency*** range. Also seen in the Phono are the loud first heart sound (S1) and the systolic mitral regurgitation murmur.

depolarization. This can occur in the presence of mild sinus tachycardia with shortening of diastole resulting in atrial contraction to occur at the time of the RFP. This can also occur when the PR interval is long enough (first-degree AV block) that the atrial contraction occurs early in diastole. It can also occur if the atrial contraction and the ventricular contraction are dissociated as in AV dissociation for instance caused by complete AV block, or in patients whose ventricles are paced by an electronic pacemaker and who have an underlying undisturbed regular atrial rhythm. The augmentation can occur only whenever the atrial contraction occurs during the RFP. Therefore in AV dissociation this is likely to occur only intermittently.

When an S3 is made louder by the fortuitous occurrence of atrial contraction at the time of the RFP, it is termed a ***summation sound or gallop.*** When this occurs in the presence of mild sinus tachycardia, application of carotid sinus pressure by slowing the sinus rate may be able to dissociate the atrial contraction from occurring at the time of the RFP thereby abolishing the summation effect.

Summation gallop itself may not signify a pathological state particularly if seen only during mild sinus tachycardia. Significance of summation gallop sound will depend on the clinical circumstance under which it develops.[76]

If either the S3 or the S4 are pathological and the sound is made louder by the timing of the atrial contraction at the time of the RFP, then the resulting sound is sometimes termed ***"augmented gallops".***[86]

CLINICAL FEATURES OF S3

Third heart sound is a sound that occurs at the end of the RFP of diastole at pressures, which are generally low. Therefore the S3 is a ***low frequency*** sound or a thud similar to the sound caused by a small lead ball falling on a cushioned floor. It occurs at the peak of the RFP and is therefore separated from the S2 by the combined duration of the isovolumic relaxation and the period of rapid inflow. The former is approximately between 60 and 100 ms. The latter lasts on an average for 100 ms. The S3 therefore occurs at a fair distance after S2. ***This creates a cadence Lubb ....dup....bum.***

The left-sided S3 is obviously best audible over the apex area, which is usually formed by the left ventricle. It is best elicited by auscultation with the bell, which picks up the low frequencies. Third heart sound is also somewhat affected by proximity. Often S3 may be best heard only when the patient is turned to the left lateral position and auscultated over the area of the apical impulse. *It is usually uncommon to have S3 when the apex beat is not palpable. Rarely it may be audible in the absence of a palpable apex beat, e.g. in acute myocardial infarction, in severe cardiomyopathy with severe reduction in the LV ejection fraction and in constrictive pericarditis.*

If the apex beat were to hide behind the ribs during certain phase of respiration, then the S3 may also become soft or inaudible at that time. It may become audible only when the apex beat becomes palpable between the ribs namely in the intercostal space. The phase of respiration that this may happen may vary from patient to patient. Although the LV filling becomes relatively more on expiration, the usual left-sided S3 does not always increase on expiration. If the proximity effect is better on inspiration, it may become better audible only on inspiration. When loud, S3 may be audible even at the base. Third heart sound generally will tend to disappear or become softer in the standing position due to decreased venous return.

Right-sided S3 generally is best heard over the xiphoid area and over the lower sternal region. It usually will increase on inspiration in its intensity or loudness (Fig. 6.40).

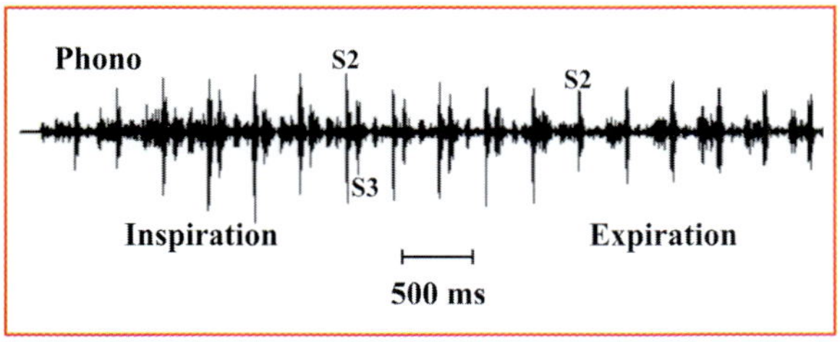

Fig. 6.40: Digital display of a magnetic audio recording taken at the xiphoid area of the sternum from a patient with severe pulmonary hypertension secondary to scleroderma with right ventricular decompensation. During Inspiration (identified by the noise in the base line) a third heart sound ***(S3)*** is seen clearly which is not seen during expiration confirming the right-sided origin of the sound.

Physiologic S3 and Pathologic S3 are very similar in all respects with regard to the auscultatory features. Therefore, the distinction is only made by the associated features. Generally, the S1 intensity is good in physiologic S3 and the apical impulse will be normal and not sustained on palpation.

CLINICAL ASSESSMENT OF S3

Third heart sound should be looked for in situations where it is expected to be heard such as in children, pregnant women, rapid circulatory states, in patients when the apical impulse is felt to be abnormal and sustained, or hyperdynamic as in ventricular volume overload, in patients with signs and symptoms of peripheral or systemic congestion with elevated jugular venous pressure. Since it is a ***low frequency*** sound, it must be searched for ***with the bell*** of the stethoscope. Patient should be turned to the left lateral position and the apical impulse located and the area of the palpable apex beat must be auscultated. *The presence of S3 is identified by its typical cadence namely One.....two....bum, Lubb.....dup....bum.*

In mitral regurgitation and other similar ventricular volume overload states, if S3 is heard, it will often have some duration and sounds more like a short low medium frequency murmur. The presence of S3 in these conditions often would indicate that the lesion causing the volume overload is significant. In mitral regurgitation for instance the presence of S3 would only be heard when the degree of regurgitation is moderately severe or severe. If the degree of regurgitation is not significant and a definite S3 is present, then it must mean coexisting LV dysfunction. If tricuspid regurgitation is considered either on the basis of an elevated venous pressure with jugular contour showing a large prominently rising ***v wave*** with a ***y descent*** or by detecting the murmur, then a right-sided S3 should be looked for. A right-sided S3 classically is heard maximally over the xiphoid and the lower sternal area and increases typically on inspiration.

Third Heart Sound Persisting on Standing

Third heart sound generally disappears or gets softer on standing. Most physiologic S3, S3 associated with ventricular volume overload and even the usual heart failure S3 generally follow this rule. *However, if it persists and continues to be well heard it must indicate an unusual situation where a high v wave pressure in the atrium is associated with significant decrease in compliance. This may occur for instance in constrictive pericarditis and/or severe cardiomyopathy* (*see* Fig. 6.37).

Second heart sound and third heart Sound versus wide split S2:

1. Third heart sound is separated far enough from the S2; therefore it is unusual for it to be mistaken for a wide split S2. In addition, when the S2 is widely split, both components of S2 are sharper and of higher

frequencies. They also tend to be similar to each other. This is unlike the S3, which has a much lower frequency, and often better heard with the bell.
2. The maximum loudness of left-sided S3 is over the area of a palpable LV apex beat. Split S2 when wide is better heard often over the second, third and sometimes over the fourth left intercostal space at the left sternal border.
3. Third heart sound tends to get softer and usually would tend to disappear also on standing.

Third Heart Sound Differentiation from OS

A late occurring OS may sometimes be mistaken for an S3.

Distinguishing features between S3 and OS are as follows:

1. *Third heart sound is of low frequency and heard best over the apex whereas the OS is of high frequency and often heard best between the apex and the lower left sternal border.*
2. *The S1 is often loud and may be palpable in the presence of a good OS. It is unusual to have a palpable S1 with an S3.*
3. *If a clear-cut "triple sound or trill" is identified, then the presence of OS is confirmed.*
4. *On standing, S3 will become softer or often disappear whereas the OS if still audible will be found to come later.*
5. *If audible on standing and does not change much in timing, consider unusual S3 such as a pericardial knock, or that caused by a severe cardiomyopathy.*

Very rarely, one may encounter the presence of both an S3 and an OS. This may occur in the presence of significant mitral regurgitation in rheumatic mitral disease, which is characterized by a shortened and severely restricted posterior mitral leaflet together with a freely mobile anterior leaflet. The severe mitral regurgitation may bring out the S3 and the freely mobile anterior leaflet may be part of the causation of the OS.[87]

Third Heart Sound Differentiation from Tumor Plop

Tumor plop sounds like an S3. However, it is associated with a loud banging M1, which may be palpable. In addition, there often will be low medium frequency diastolic murmur following the sound due to the mitral obstruction.

Intermittent S3

Third heart sound, in fact when heard, often is actually intermittent and occasionally varies with different phases of respiration. **The most common cause for this is the effect of proximity.** Depending on the location of the apex beat and whether it hides intermittently behind the ribs may determine when it may be heard best.

When there is AV dissociation as in complete AV block or patient with a permanent ventricular demand single chamber electronic pacemaker, one may hear an S3 whenever the dissociated atrial contraction occurs during the RFP of diastole. Such *AV dissociation will also be expected to affect the intensity of S1* and will produce variable softer and louder intensity of M1. *If atrial contraction were to occur in the RFP and produce an S3 effect, then the S1 immediately following the S3 will be soft. This unique situation with varying S1 intensity and intermittent S3 is likely to occur only with the presence of AV dissociation.*

FOURTH HEART SOUND (S4)

Mechanism of Formation of the S4

The atrium normally contracts at the end of diastole and gives an extra stretch to the ventricles. When the ventricular compliance is significantly reduced due to factors such as hypertrophy, ischemia, infarction, fibrosis or infiltrates, then this evokes a more vigorous contraction from the atrium. This augments ventricular filling at the end of diastole and helps in its expansion.[88] The increased force of atrial contraction also raises the atrial *a wave* pressure peak. This augmented pressure head tends to accelerate the diastolic inflow at the end of diastole. Since the ventricular compliance is reduced, the accelerated inflow at this phase of diastole is decelerated fairly rapidly. This of course will depend on the extent of reduction in the compliance. This sudden deceleration of the column of blood entering the ventricle at end-diastole leads to dissipation of energy, which results in the production of the sound (Fig. 6.41). The sound forms inside the ventricle and the entire hemic mass, the mitral structures and the underlying ventricular myocardium participate in its production. The sound is sometimes referred to as atrial gallop and can be simply termed as S4. The sound being generated at low pressures of diastole has low frequency very similar to the S3. However, the timing is different. It is closer to S1.

The cadence therefore is different, and is as follows:

S4..S1.....S2........Ha..ha.....tu........

The prerequisites for S4 formation:

1. *Reduced ventricular compliance*
2. *Healthy atrium*
3. *Regular sinus rhythm*
4. *Absence of AV valve obstruction.*

The ***causes of reduced compliance*** are already discussed in relation to S3. These causes are: *completeness of relaxation, chamber size, thickness of the wall, composition of the wall* (inflammation, infiltrate, ischemia or infarction, scars, etc.), pericardium and RV volume/pressure in the case of the left ventricle.

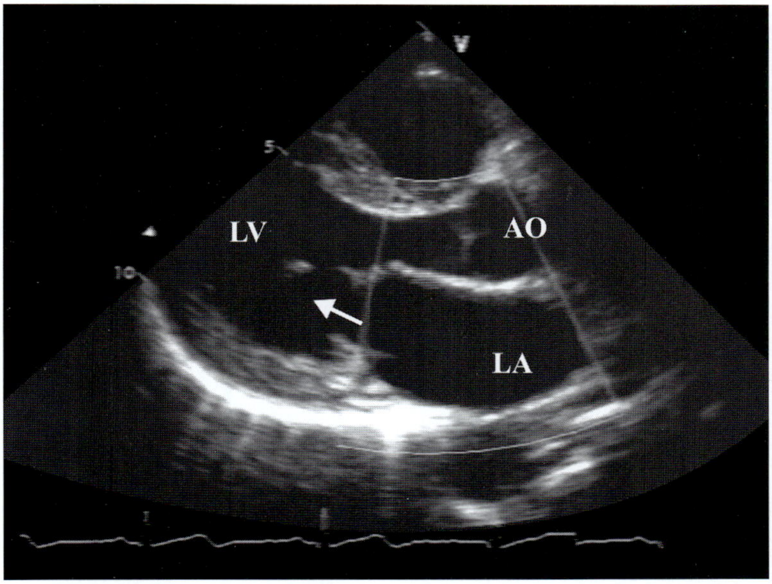

Fig. 6.41: Stop frame during end-diastole from a two-dimensional echocardiogram of a patient taken in the parasternal long axis. The moving column of blood (arrow) from the left atrium (LA) into the left ventricle (LV) is shown. Strong atrial contraction during this phase augmenting the ventricular filling, which could be decelerated abruptly if the ventricular compliance is reduced for any reason producing a fourth heart sound.

While the small size of the ventricle in children offers resistance to rapid inflow in early diastole, once the ventricle has begun to expand by the on rushing flow, then by the end of diastole the size may no longer be restrictive to filling. This explains the usual absence of S4 in children. This is best appreciated by the analogy of blowing into a balloon to expand the same. The resistance is maximal when the size is smallest namely when one first begins to blow into a balloon. Once the balloon is partially expanded, it is easier to inflate it further.

On the other hand with increasing age, the ventricle does become more stiff due to various factors including age-related hypertrophy as well as due to acquired diseases including ischemic heart disease even if asymptomatic. Thus, S4 is often heard in the older subjects (above the age of 60 years) even in the absence of clear clinical heart disease.[89] Hypertension is the most common cause of hypertrophy in the elderly. However, in the elderly, there could also be atrial disease as well as sinus node dysfunction with development of atrial arrhythmias such as atrial fibrillation. ***Therefore, S4 may not be always present in everyone in this age group.*** Calcific aortic stenosis is more common in the elderly over the age of 65 and yet not everyone with significant stenosis (outflow gradient >74 mm Hg) with resultant marked hypertrophy will have a definite S4.

Significant aortic stenosis in the younger age group, on the other hand, will have a loud S4 since the hypertrophy associated with such outflow obstruction will not only result in marked decrease in compliance of the ventricle but also the left atrium is more than likely to be healthy and normal to help generate a strong contraction. When a vigorous left atrial contraction occurs in such situation then the expansion of the ventricle at that time will raise its wall tension enough to become palpable at the apex. The palpable expansion of the apical impulse resulting from such a strong atrial contraction is referred to as the atrial kick[88] (Fig. 6.42). *It must be understood that the sound itself never ever becomes loud enough to be palpable.* The atrial kick has the same significance as the S4.

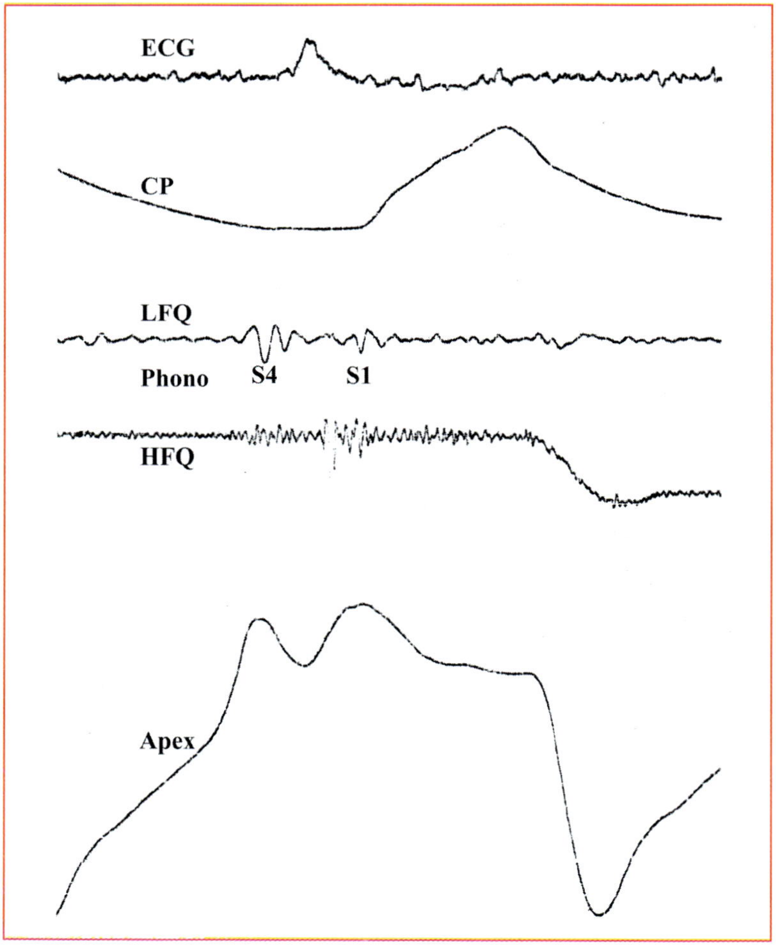

Fig. 6.42: Phono recording from a patient with significant aortic valvular stenosis taken from the apex area along with the Apex and ***carotid pulse*** tracings. The Phono shows a low frequency fourth heart sound (S4) at the time of the augmented A wave in the ***Apex*** recording.

The presence of S4 in hypertrophic ventricle with outflow tract obstruction usually indicates significant stenosis or obstruction whether right sided or left sided (pulmonary or aortic stenosis).[90] Fourth heart sound in the presence of systemic hypertension would imply significant decrease in compliance due to hypertensive heart disease. The associated pathologic changes may be significant hypertrophy, focal fibrosis and/or associated coronary heart disease. In the absence of significant LV outflow obstruction such as aortic stenosis or significant hypertension, a loud S4 at the LV apex area may be indicative of a cardiomyopathy (e.g. hypertrophic cardiomyopathy,[91] occasionally other myocardial diseases) or ischemic heart disease[66,92-94] (Figs. 6.43 and 6.44).

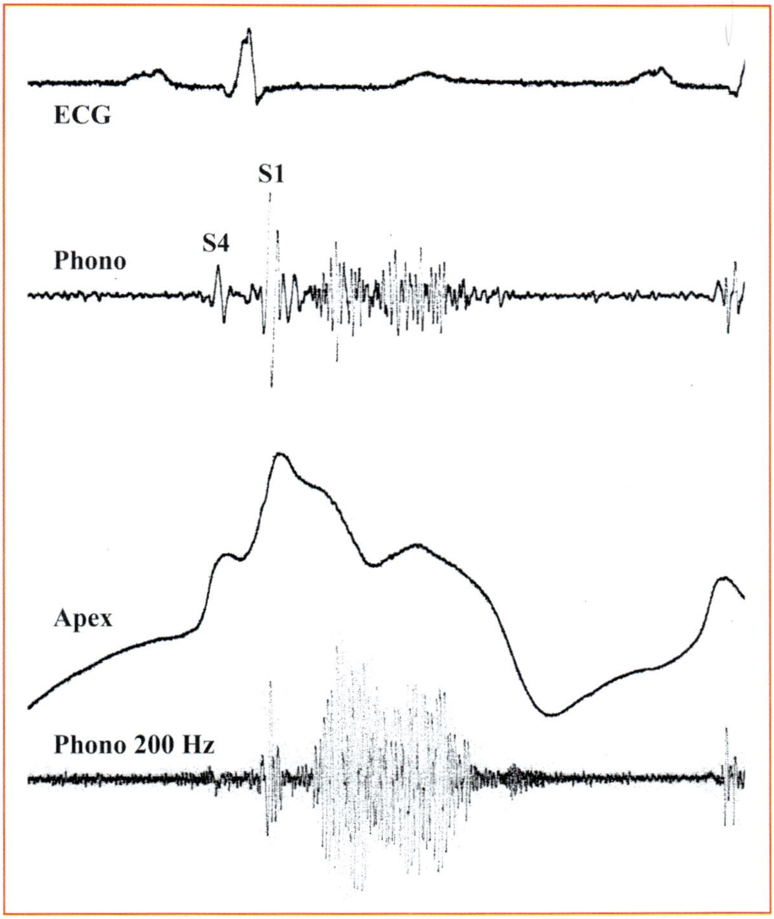

Fig. 6.43: Phono recording from a patient with hypertrophic cardiomyopathy with significant left ventricular outflow tract obstruction taken from the apex area along with the ***Apex*** tracing. The Phono shows a low frequency fourth heart sound (S4) at the time of the ***atrial kick*** in the ***Apex*** recording. Note also the systolic ejection murmur of the subaortic stenosis.

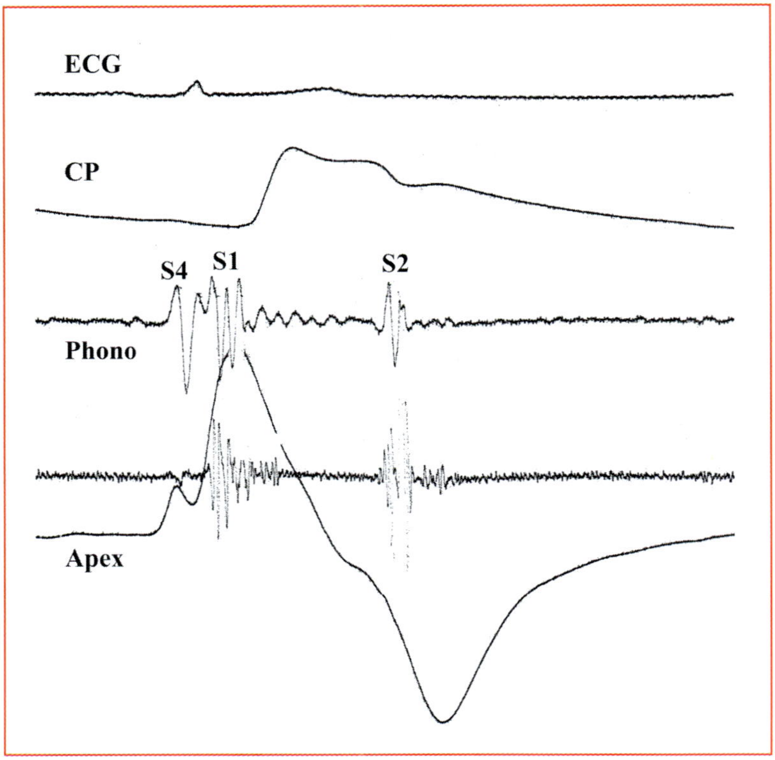

Fig. 6.44: Phono recording from a patient with ischemic heart disease taken from the apex area along with the ***Apex*** and ***carotid pulse*** tracings. The Phono shows a low frequency fourth heart sound (S4) at the time of the augmented A wave in the ***Apex*** recording.

Ventricular volume overload usually causes dilatation of the ventricle and therefore is accompanied by better ventricular compliance. Thus S4 is not a feature of volume overload states such as mitral regurgitation. ***Acute mitral regurgitation*** such as due to ruptured chordae tendineae either spontaneous or secondary to infective endocarditis is however an exception where an S4 may be heard.[95] In acute mitral regurgitation, both the left atrium and the left ventricle are often presented with significant volume due to the regurgitation and yet they have not had time to develop secondary dilatation. *The lack of significant dilatation of the left ventricle means relatively decreased LV compliance* and raised LV diastolic pressures. Sometimes the levels of the LV diastolic pressures and the left atrial pressures are very high and may produce pulmonary edema. When left atrial pressure is elevated but not to the degree of causing pulmonary edema then the extra stretch provided by the volume may evoke a powerful Starling effect from the left atrium. This in the presence of a relatively less compliant left ventricle produces an S4.

Constrictive pericarditis does not allow expansion of the ventricle beyond the early RFP and therefore S4 is not a feature of this condition.

CLINICAL ASSESSMENT OF S4

Left-sided S4 is best audible close to the LV apex area. Often when the S4 is loud, it may be heard over a wide area of the precordium. ***Right-sided S4*** is best audible over the xiphoid area and the lower sternal region. It is detected by its increase in intensity on inspiration or audibility only on inspiration. The jugular contour is also likely to show a prominent rise before the usual systolic ***x′ descent.*** Left-sided S4 may also be somewhat better heard with the patient in the left lateral decubitus position, although when loud enough it does become audible in the usual supine position and medial to the apex. Occasionally, left-sided S4 may be accompanied by a palpable atrial kick of the apical impulse.[93] Rarely, with significant RV hypertrophy as in pulmonary hypertension, the right-sided S4 may be accompanied by similar right atrial kick, which may be palpated by the subxiphoid palpation of the right ventricle on deep inspiration.

Fourth heart sound being a low frequency sound is best elicited by listening with the bell of the stethoscope with just light pressure to make an air seal. Firm pressure with the chest piece of the stethoscope may sometime eliminate the transmission of such low frequencies by tautening the skin thus making the S4 soft or altogether disappear. Fourth heart sound is also affected by venous return and atrial filling. Thus on standing when the venous return falls and the atrial filling diminishes, then S4 will either become soft or disappear. The increased sympathetic activity associated with diminished venous return may speed up the heart rate and shorten the PR interval and thus may also make the S4 come closer to S1 and actually merge with the latter.

In hypertrophic cardiomyopathy, the compliance is markedly decreased and this often evokes a loud S4.[91] When there is significant associated LV outflow obstruction in this disorder, the strong atrial contraction may also generate a palpable atrial kick. These patients are generally younger and often have hypertrophied but otherwise healthy left atria early in the course of their disease process.

Fourth heart sound also is usually sensitive to changes in venous return and filling of the heart. Maneuvers, which reduce venous return such as standing posture, will tend to decrease the intensity or abolish the S4 altogether. Rapid volume expansion, cold pressor test and isometric hand grip will accentuate the S4.[93] Isometric hand grip tends to raise the heart rate, cardiac output and the blood pressure.[96,97] It also can raise the peripheral resistance.

If S4 does not disappear on standing, then one must consider the presence of significant decrease in compliance as seen in patients with markedly hypertrophied hearts. Fourth heart sound–first heart sound interval is not only determined by the PR interval but also to a certain extent on the degree of decrease in compliance or the severity of the underlying disease. When the decreased compliance is significant as in markedly hypertrophied ventricle, the resultant S4 tends to be well separated from S1.[93,98] Thus in such patients with significant decrease in compliance S4 may still be heard on standing.

Fourth Heart Sound (S4) Differentiation from the Split S1

1. S4 sounds different from the M1 component that follows it since it contains much lower frequency ranges and therefore heard better with the bell. This is therefore unlike the M1-A1 split where both components are more or less similar in frequencies and more often in the higher ranges. Thus the split S1 is heard just as well with the diaphragm.
2. The lower frequency S4 may be abolished or made softer by firm pressure with the chest piece (the bell) whereas the split S1 is not likely to be affected by such a pressure.
3. Decreasing venous return by standing the patient will only lengthen the isovolumic contraction phase which separates the M1 from A1 by decreasing the rate of rise of ventricular pressure which will accompany reduced ventricular filling. Thus the split is usually better separated on standing. On the other hand, the decreased atrial filling due to reduced venous return and the slight shortening of PR associated with increase in heart rate secondary to sympathetic stimulation will make the S4 softer and make it come closer to M1 making the separation less distinct.

Gallop Rhythm

In the presence of tachycardia, diastole is somewhat shortened and when an S3 is heard then it is often called the protodiastolic gallop, the S3 gallop or also sometimes referred to as the ventricular diastolic gallop. The cadence or the rhythm of the S1 and S2 followed by S3 simulates the sounds of a horse in gallop: ***one ....tu.....bum.....one ....tu....bum....one....tu....bum***

This is usually heard in patients with significant heart failure and decreased cardiac output. Occasionally in some patients with LV dysfunction, the pathophysiologic changes may provide the prerequisites for both an S3 and an S4. If the heart rate is fast, then both sounds may in fact merge with each other causing a summation or ***summation gallop.*** It will be difficult to distinguish this as such at these fast heart rates and may be simply detected as a gallop rhythm. However, when the heart rate is only mildly fast and both sounds may be easily audible in diastole. This is called the ***double gallop*** or the quadruple rhythm or gallop. This will have a cadence of both S4 and S3 together namely: ***ha...ha .....tu......bum...ha...ha.....tu......bum.***

Treatment of the heart failure and clearance of the symptoms and signs of failure may be accompanied by an S3 either becoming softer or totally inaudible. This usually indicates falling left atrial pressure as well as improvement in LV function. At this time an S4 may become audible even if it was not present initially. This means that the left atrium is no longer overstretched or dilated but the LV compliance is still abnormal thereby evoking a good atrial contraction. Such a sequence usually indicates good prognosis.

S3 and S4 and Left Ventricular Dysfunction

One recent study evaluating the sensitivity and the specificity of the presence of phonocardiographically detected S3 and/or S4 for detecting LV dysfunction as measured by LV diastolic pressures, LV ejection fraction and the B-type natriuretic peptide concluded as expected that the phonocardiographic S3 and S4 are not sensitive markers of LV dysfunction and that the phonocardiographic S3 was more specific for LV dysfunction than the phonocardiographic S4.[99] Over the years, significant clinical experience has been accumulated as to the significance of these sounds when they are audible. When one takes proper account of the mechanisms behind the production of these sounds, it becomes obvious as to their significance when they are detected at the bedside. Thus, S4 when clinically audible is relatable only to a strong atrial contraction of a healthy atrium in the presence of decreased LV compliance. The latter could result from a variety of pathologic processes not all of which would necessarily entail LV systolic dysfunction. Thus it is not expected to be very specific for LV systolic dysfunction. Since an S3 can be physiologic as well as pathologic, the clinical group of patients being evaluated is also an important determinant of whether it is going to correlate clinically to significant LV dysfunction. Therefore, the presence or otherwise of these sounds on auscultation will become relevant only when taken in conjunction with the clinical context. Finally, it is important to realize that studies merely based on phonocardiographic recordings of low frequency vibrations could lead to misleading information, because they may not be audible.

REFERENCES

1. Dock W. The forces needed to evoke sounds from cardiac tissues and the attenuation of heart sounds. Circulation. 1959;19:376.
2. Rushmer RF. Cardiovascular Dynamics, 3rd edition. Philadelphia: WB Saunders; 1970.
3. Leon DF, Shaver JA. Physiologic principles of heart sounds and murmurs. Monograph 46. New York: American Heart Association, Inc.; 1975. p. 1.

4. Leatham A. Splitting of the first and second heart sounds. Lancet. 1954;267: 607-14.
5. Shah PM, Mori M, Maccanon DM, et al. Hemodynamic correlates of the various components of the first hear sound. Circ Res. 1963;12:386-92.
6. Sakamoto T, Kusukawa R, Maccanon DM, et al. Hemodynamic determinants of the amplitude of the first heart sound. Circ Res. 1965;16:45-57.
7. Luisada AA, Shah PM. Controversial and changing aspects of ausculation. I. Areas of ausculation: a new concept. II. Normal and abnormal first and second sounds. Am J Cardiol. 1963;11:774-89.
8. Piemme TE, Barnett GO, Dexter L. Relationship of heart sounds to acceleration of blood flow. Circ Res. 1966;18:303-15.
9. Thompson ME, Shaver JA, Heidenreich FP, et al. Sound, pressure and motion correlates in mitral stenosis. Am J Med. 1970;49:436-50.
10. Laniado S, Yellin EL, Miller H, et al. Temporal relation of the first heart sound to closure of the mitral valve. Circulation. 1973;47:1006-14.
11. Lakier JB, Fritz VU, Pocock WA, et al. Mitral components of the first heart sound. Br Heart J. 1972;34:160-6.
12. Shah PM. Hemodynamic determinants of the first heart sound. Monograph 46. New York: American Heart Association, Inc.; 1975. p. 2.
13. O'Toole JD, Reddy SP, Curtiss EI, et al. The contribution of tricuspid valve closure to the first heart sound. An intracardiac micromanometer study. Circulation. 1976;53:752-8.
14. Kincaid-Smith P, Barlow J. The atrial sound and the atrial component of the first heart sound. Br Heart J. 1959;21:470-8.
15. Waider W, Craige E. First heart sound and ejection sounds. Echocardiographic and Phonocardiographic correlation with valvular events. Am J Cardiol. 1975; 35:346.
16. Constant J. Bedside Cardiology, 2nd edition. Boston: Little Brown and Company; 1976.
17. Luisada AA. "Tricuspid" component of the first heart sound. American Heart Association Monograph 46, 1975:19-26.
18. Shaver JA, Griff W, Leonard JJ. Ejection sounds of left sided origin. American Heart Association Monograph 46, 1975:27-34.
19. Shah PM, Kramer DH, Gramiak R. Influence of the timing of atrial systole on mitral valve closure and on the first heart sound in man. Am J Cardiol. 1970;26:231-7.
20. Thompson ME, Shaver JA, Leon DF, et al. Pathodynamics of the first heart sound. Am Heart Assoc Monogr. 1975;46:8-18.
21. Reddy PS, Leon DF, Krishnaswami V, et al. Syndrome of Acute Aortic Regurgitation. Am Heart Assoc Monogr. 1975;46:166-74.
22. Wigle ED, Labrosse CJ. Sudden, severe aortic insufficiency. Circulation. 1965; 32:708-20.
23. Meadows WR, Vanpraagh S, Indreika M, et al. Premature mitral valve closure: a hemodynamic explanation for absence of the first sound in aortic insufficiency. Circulation. 1963;28:251-8.
24. Fontana ME, Wooley CF. Sail sound in Ebstein's anomaly of the tricuspid valve. Circulation. 1972;46:155-64.
25. Mills PG, Brodie B, McLaurin L, et al. Echocardiographic and hemodynamic relationships of ejection sounds. Circulation. 1977;56:430-6.

26. Hancock EW. The ejection sound in aortic stenosis. Am J Med. 1966;40:569.
27. Martin CE, Shaver JA, O'Toole JD, et al. Ejection sounds of right sided origin. Am Heart Assoc Monogr. 1975;46:35-44.
28. Hultgren HN, Reeve R, Cohn K, et al. The ejection click of valvular pulmonic stenosis. Circulation. 1969;40:631-40.
29. Shaver JA, Nadolny RA, O'Toole JD, et al. Sound pressure correlates of the second heart sound. An intracardiac sound study. Circulation. 1974;49:316-25.
30. Shaver JA, O'Toole JD, Curtiss EI, et al. Second heart sound: the role of altered greater and lesser circulation. Am Heart Assoc Monogr 1975;46:58-67.
31. Curtiss EI, Matthews RG, Shaver JA. Mechanism of normal splitting of the second heart sound. Circulation. 1975;51:157-64.
32. Curtiss EI, Shaver JA, Reddy PS, et al. Newer concepts in physiologic splitting of the second heart sound. Am Heart Assoc Monogr. 1975;46:68-73.
33. Adolf RJ. Second heart sound. the role of altered electromechanical events. Am Heart Assoc Monogr. 1975;46:45-57.
34. Hultgren HN, Craige E, Fujii J, et al. Left bundle branch block and mechanical events of the cardiac cycle. Am J Cardiol. 1983;52:755-62.
35. Shaver JA, O'Toole JD. The second heart sound: newer concepts. Part I: normal and wide physiological splitting. Mod Concepts Cardiovasc Dis. 1977;46:7-12.
36. Shaver JA, O'Toole JD. The second heart sound: newer concepts. Part II: paradoxical splitting and narrow physiological splitting. Mod Concepts Cardiovasc Dis. 1977;46:13-16.
37. Wood P. The Eisenmenger syndrome or pulmonary hypertension with reversed central shunt. Br Heart J. 1963;2:701.
38. Luisada AA. The second heart sound in normal and abnormal conditions. Am J Cardiol. 1971;28:150-61.
39. Ranganathan N, Sivaciyan V. Abnormalities in jugular venous flow velocity in pulmonary hypertension. Am J Cardiol. 1989;63:719-24.
40. Shapiro S, Clark TJ, Goodwin JF. Delayed closure of the pulmonary valve in obliterative pulmonary hypertension. Lancet. 1965;2:1207-11.
41. Perloff JK. Auscultatory and phonocardiographic manifestations of pulmonary hypertension. Prog Cardiovasc Dis. 1967;9:303.
42. Perloff JK. The Clinical Recognition of Congenital Heart Disease, 5th edition. Philadelphia: W.B. Saunders; 1979. pp.81:279.
43. Logue RB, Woodfin B, Cobbs BW, et al. The second heart sound in pulmonary embolism and pulmonary hypertension. Trans Am Clin Climatol Assoc. 1967;78:38-50.
44. Schrire V, Vogelpoel L. The role of the dilated pulmonary artery in abnormal splitting of the second heart sound. Am Heart J. 1962;63:501-7.
45. Perloff JK, Harvey WP. Mechanisms of fixed splitting of the second heart sound. Circulation. 1958;18:998-1009.
46. Aygen MM, Braunwald E. The splitting of the second heart sound in normal subjects and in patients with congenital heart disease. Circulation. 1962;25:328-45.
47. Kalke BR, Carlson RG, Ferlic RM, et al. Partial anomalous pulmonary venous connections. Am J Cardiol. 1967;20:91-101.
48. Frye RL, Marshall HW, Kincaid OW, et al. Anomalous pulmonary venous drainage of the right lung into the inferior vena cava. Br Heart J. 1962;24:696-702.
49. Wood P. An appreciation of mitral stenosis. I. Clinical features. Br Med J. 1954;1:1051.

50. Wood P. An appreciation of mitral stenosis. II. Investigations and results. Br Med J. 1954;1:1113-24.
51. Margolies A, Wolferth CC. The opening snap (claquement d'ouverture de la mitrale) in mitral stenosis. Its characteristics, mechanism of production and diagnostic importance. Am Heart J. 1932;7:443.
52. Perloff JK. The physiologic mechanisms of cardiac and vascular physical signs. J Am Coll Cardiol. 1983;1:184-98.
53. Wooley CF, Klassen KP, Leighton RF, et al. Left atrial and left ventricular sound and pressure in mitral stenosis. Circulation. 1968;38:295.
54. Perloff JK, Harvey WP. Auscultatory and phonocardiographic manifestations of pure mitral regurgitation. Prog Cardiovasc Dis. 1962;5:172-94.
55. Neil P, Mounsey P. Auscultation in patent ductus arteriosus with description of two fistulae simulating patent ductus. Br Heart J. 1958;20:51.
56. Tavel ME. Opening snaps: mitral and tricuspid. Am Heart Assoc Monogr. 1975;46:85-91.
57. Henderson Y. Diastolic relaxation. Physiol Rev. 1923;3:165-208.
58. Zile MR, Brutsaert DL. New concepts in diastolic dysfunction and diastolic heart failure: Part I: diagnosis, prognosis, and measurements of diastolic function. Circulation. 2002;105:1387-93.
59. Zile MR, Brutsaert DL. New concepts in diastolic dysfunction and diastolic heart failure: Part II: causal mechanisms and treatment. Circulation. 2002;105:1503-8.
60. Hein S, Arnon E, Kostin S, et al. Progression from compensated hypertrophy to failure in the pressure-overloaded human heart: structural deterioration and compensatory mechanisms. Circulation. 2003;107:984-91.
61. Leite-Moreira AF, Correia-Pinto J, Gillebert TC. Afterload induced changes in myocardial relaxation: a mechanism for diastolic dysfunction. Cardiovasc Res. 1999;43:344-53.
62. Brutsaert DL, Rademakers FE, Sys SU. Triple control of relaxation: implications in cardiac disease. Circulation. 1984;69:190-6.
63. Zile MR, Gaasch WH. Load-dependent left ventricular relaxation in conscious dogs. Am J Physiol. 1991;261:H691-9.
64. Zile MR, Blaustein AS, Gaasch WH. The effect of acute alterations in left ventricular afterload and beta-adrenergic tone on indices of early diastolic filling rate. Circ Res. 1989;65:406-16.
65. Ariel Y, Gaasch WH, Bogen DK, et al. Load-dependent relaxation with late systolic volume steps: servo-pump studies in the intact canine heart. Circulation. 1987;75:1287-94.
66. Ranganathan N, Juma Z, Sivaciyan V. The apical impulse in coronary heart disease. Clin Cardiol. 1985;8:20-33.
67. Papapietro SE, Coghlan HC, Zissermann D, et al. Impaired maximal rate of left ventricular relaxation in patients with coronary artery disease and left ventricular dysfunction. Circulation. 1979;59:984-91.
68. Gamble WH, Shaver JA, Alvares RF, et al. A critical appraisal of diastolic time intervals as a measure of relaxation in left ventricular hypertrophy. Circulation. 1983;68:76-87.
69. Gaasch WH, Levine HJ, Quinones MA, et al. Left ventricular compliance: mechanisms and clinical implications. Am J Cardiol. 1976;38:645-53.
70. Levine HJ, Gaasch WH. Diastolic compliance of the left ventricle. I: causes of a noncompliant ventricular chamber. Mod Concepts Cardiovasc Dis. 1978;47:95-8.

71. Levine HJ, Gaasch WH. Diastolic compliance of the left ventricle. II: chamber and muscle stiffness, the volume/mass ratio and clinical implications. Mod Concepts Cardiovasc Dis. 1978;47:99-102.
72. Zile MR, Baicu CF, Gaasch WH. Diastolic heart failure—abnormalities in active relaxation and passive stiffness of the left ventricle. N Engl J Med. 2004;350: 1953-9.
73. Grossman W, McLaurin LP. Diastolic properties of the left ventricle. Ann Intern Med. 1976;84:316-26.
74. McLaurin LP, Rolett EL, Grossman W. Impaired left ventricular relaxation during pacing-induced ischemia. Am J Cardiol. 1973;32:751-7.
75. Van de Werf F, Boel A, Geboers J, et al. Diastolic properties of the left ventricle in normal adults and in patients with third heart sounds. Circulation. 1984;69:1070.
76. Shah PM, Jackson D. Third heart sound and summation gallop. Am Heart Assoc Monogr. 1975;46:79.
77. Drzewiecki GM, Wasicko MJ, Li JK. Diastolic mechanics and the origin of the third heart sound. Ann Biomed Eng. 1991;19:651-67.
78. Glower DD, Murrah RL, Olsen CO, et al. Mechanical correlates of the third heart sound. J Am Coll Cardiol. 1992;19:450-7.
79. Downes TR, Dunson W, Stewart K, et al. Mechanism of physiologic and pathologic S3 gallop sounds. J Am Soc Echocardiogr. 1992;5:211-8.
80. Tribouilloy CM, Enriquez-Sarano M, Mohty D, et al. Pathophysiologic determinants of third heart sounds: a prospective clinical and Doppler echocardiographic study. Am J Med. 2001;111:96-102.
81. Van de Werf F, Minten J, Carmiliet P, et al. The genesis of the third and fourth heart sounds. A pressure flow study in dogs. J Clin invest. 1984;73:1400-07.
82. Reddy PS, Meno F, Curtiss EI, et al. The genesis of gallop sounds: investigation by quantitative phono- and apexcardiography. Circulation. 1981;63:922-33.
83. Feruglio GA, Sreenivasan A. Intracardiac phonocardiogram in thirty cases of atrial septal defect. Circulation. 1959;20:1087-94.
84. Tyberg TI, Goodyer AV, Langou RA. Genesis of pericardial knock in constrictive pericarditis. Am J Cardiol. 1980;46:570-5.
85. Bass NM, Sharratt GP. Left atrial myxoma diagnosed by echocardiography, with observations on tumour movement. Br Heart J. 1973;35:1332-5.
86. Grayzel J. Gallop rhythm of the heart. I. Atrial gallop, ventricular gallop and systolic sounds. Am J Med. 1960;28:578-92.
87. Nixon PG, Wooler GH, Radigan LR. Mitral incompetence caused by disease of the mural cusp. Circulation. 1959;19:839-44.
88. Gibson TC, Madry R, Grossman W, et al. The A wave of the apexcardiogram and left ventricular diastolic stiffness. Circulation. 1974;49:441-6.
89. Spodick DH, Quarry VM. Prevalence of the fourth heart sound by phonocardiography in the absence of cardiac disease. Am Heart J. 1974;87:11-4.
90. Goldblatt A, Aygen MM, Braunwald E. Hemodynamic-phonocardiographic correlations of the fourth heart sound in aortic stenosis. Circulation. 1962;26:92-8.
91. Braunwald E, Morrow AG, Cornell WP, et al. Idiopathic hypertrophic subaortic stenosis. Clinical, hemodynamic and angiographic manifestations. Am J Med. 1960;29:924.
92. Benchimol A, Dimond EG. The apex cardiogram in ischaemic heart disease. Br Heart J. 1962;24:581-94.
93. Craige E. The fourth heart sound. Am Heart Assoc Monogr. 1975;46:74.

94. Adolph RJ. The fourth heart sound. Chest. 1999;115:1480-1.
95. Cohen LS, Mason DT, Braunwald E. Significance of an atrial gallop sound in mitral regurgitation. A clue to the diagnosis of ruptured chordae tendineae. Circulation. 1967;35:112-8.
96. Cohn PF, Thompson P, Strauss W, et al. Diastolic heart sounds during static (handgrip) exercise in patients with chest pain. Circulation. 1973;47:1217-21.
97. Grossman W, McLaurin LP, Saltz SB, et al. Changes in the inotropic state of the left ventricle during isometric exercise. Br Heart J. 1973; 35:697-704.
98. Duchosal P. A study of gallop rhythm by a combination of phonocardiographic and electrocardiographic methods. Am Heart J. 1932;7:613.
99. Marcus GM, Gerber IL, McKeown BH, et al. Association between phonocardiographic third and fourth heart sounds and objective measures of left ventricular function. JAMA. 2005;293:2238-44.

Chapter 7

Heart Murmurs (Part I)

Snapshot

- Principles Governing Murmur Formation
- Hemodynamic Factors and Cardiac Murmurs
- Frequencies of Murmurs
- The Grading of the Murmurs
- Systolic Murmurs
- Ejection Murmurs
- Regurgitant Systolic Murmurs
- Mitral Regurgitation
- Tricuspid Regurgitation
- Ventricular Septal Defect (VSD)
- Clinical Assessment of Systolic Murmurs

PRINCIPLES GOVERNING MURMUR FORMATION

In the cardiovascular system, the blood essentially flows through cylindrical tubes (blood vessels) and the cardiac chambers. It is common experience that water flow through a normal garden hose, which is unkinked or uncoiled with an open end (without a constricting nozzle at the end) is essentially noiseless. The flow through such a garden hose can be described as "laminar" and is defined by determinants of ***Poiseuille's law.*** The pressure head is directly proportional to the length of the pipe, to the velocity of flow, to the viscosity of the liquid and is inversely related to the fourth power of the radius.[1] The term ***"laminar"*** comes from the fact that if you inject dye to observe the nature of the stream in a transparent tube, it will have a parabolic shape, the particles in the central axis of the tube move faster than those near the wall each succeeding layer distributing itself as a series of laminae. Closest to the wall, the particles may almost be motionless. If the garden hose is suddenly partially kinked or its open end is partially pinched, the pressure proximal to the end will rise and the flow coming out will be under this higher pressure head with greater velocity and also will lead to production of noise. The flow at the point of this constriction is no longer laminar and is ***"turbulent".*** When turbulent flow is observed by injection of dye, the particles will be seen to have many different randomly distributed directions in addition to the general direction of flow.

With the advent of two-dimensional (2D) echocardiography and the application of Doppler techniques together with color coded flow mapping, one can easily appreciate the difference between the normal smooth undisturbed laminar flow through the heart versus a disturbed and abnormal turbulent flow. In this technique of color coding of flow, the smooth laminar flow toward the interrogating ultrasound probe is usually depicted by the color "red" whereas similar flow but opposite in direction to the probe is depicted by the color "blue". On the monitoring screen, the probe location is usually displayed at the top of the screen. Looking at the image of the heart's chambers and their anatomy as revealed through the various views, one can easily appreciate the directional flow through the chambers as depicted by the simultaneous color display (Figs. 7.1A and B). However, whenever the color flow depicts a mixture of colors or a mosaic pattern, we know that the flow is no longer the normal laminar flow but turbulent implying that the red cells that are bouncing off the ultrasound beam are moving in various random directions. If a patient with mitral regurgitation is observed by this technique, the regurgitant stream will appear in the left atrium (LA) during systole and will have a mixture of colors (Fig. 7.2). Similarly, the aortic outflow jet in a patient with aortic stenosis will demonstrate the characteristic pattern of turbulence. In fact, whenever a significant cardiac murmur is noted, one can always demonstrate turbulent flow associated with it by color flow mapping. The amount and extent of turbulence may vary according to the underlying abnormality and its severity. *Thus turbulent flow is an important cause of cardiovascular murmurs.*[1–4]

The factors governing turbulent flow were described by Osborne Reynolds (1883). *The critical point where laminar flow turns into turbulent flow seems to be dependent on the diameter of the tube, mean velocity of flow, the density of the liquid and its viscosity.*[1] The greater the velocity of flow the greater will be the resulting turbulence. Cardiac lesions such as narrowed outflow tracts from the ventricles as seen in aortic or pulmonary stenosis will be expected to have a high velocity of flow under high systolic pressures and therefore will be expected to produce turbulence. Similarly obstructive lesions to inflow such as mitral stenosis will cause turbulent flow through the mitral valve. The velocity of flow will be greater than what is normally seen through normal mitral valves due to the elevated left atrial pressures caused by the mitral stenosis. In addition, the entire systemic venous return flows through the mitral valve indiastole. This also means that a large volume of flow is subjected to turbulence. In regurgitant lesions, by virtue of the fact that

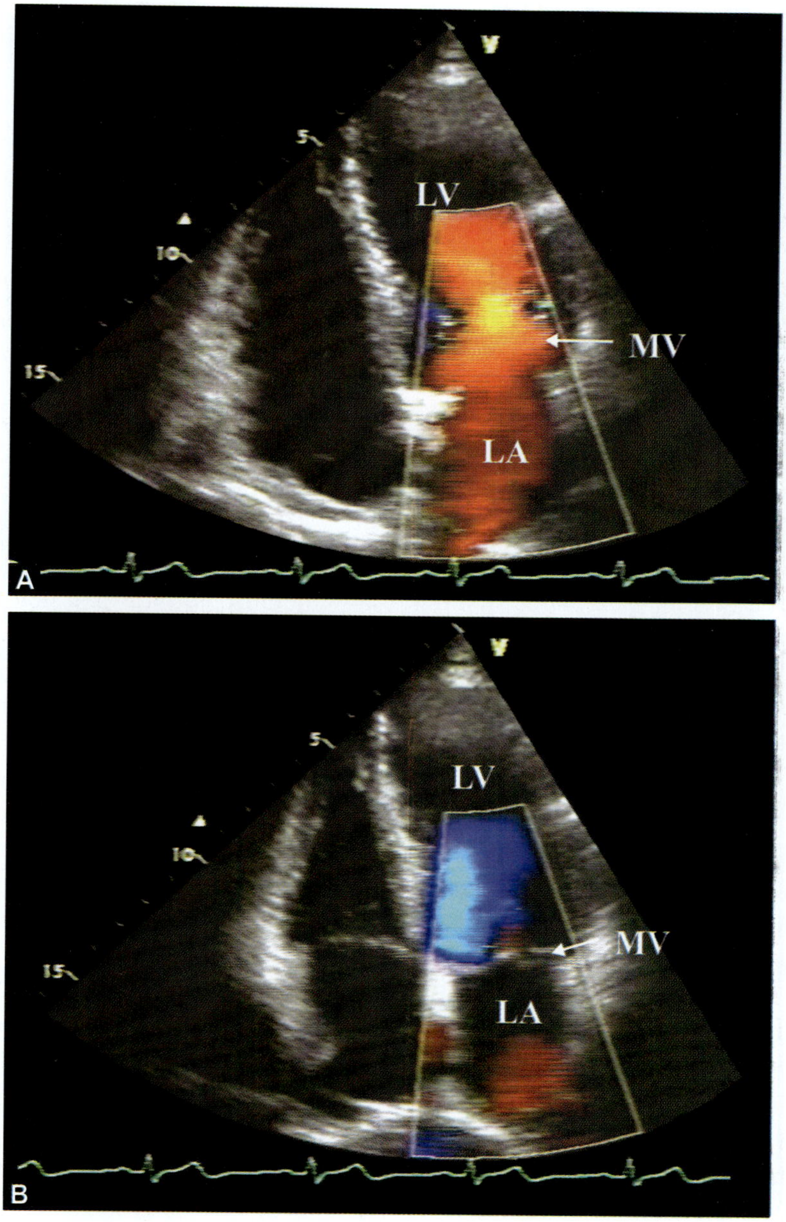

Figs. 7.1A and B: Two-dimensional echocardiographic images with Doppler color flow mapping from a normal subject in the apical four-chamber view taken in diastole (A) and systole (B). The normal mitral inflow in diastole from the left atrium (LA) into the left ventricle (LV) through the open mitral valve (MV), is laminar and appears smooth shown in red indicating the direction of flow that is toward the probe facing the apex of the left ventricle located at the top of the screen. The systolic flow out through the left ventricular outflow tract is in a smooth blue color indicating that it is laminar but with a direction away from the probe (apex).

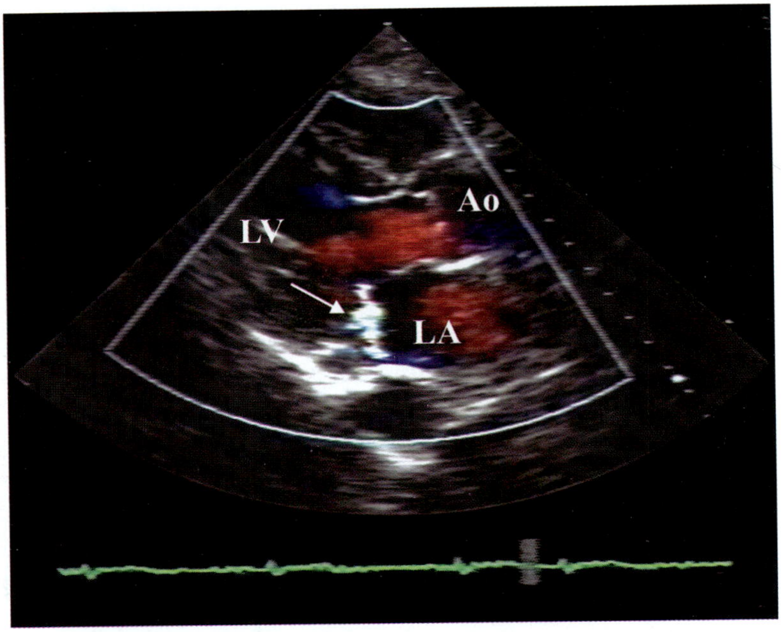

Fig. 7.2: Two-dimensional echocardiographic image and Doppler color flow mapping from a patient with mitral regurgitation taken in the parasternal long axis. The arrow points to the regurgitation jet in the left atrium that is seen to have a mosaic appearance due to a mixture of colors depicting that the red cells are moving in different directions with varying velocities due to a turbulent flow.

the flow occurs in a reverse direction and from a high pressure chamber to a low pressure chamber (e.g. mitral regurgitation, flow occurring from the left ventricle to the LA), the velocity will also be high due to a higher pressure head and will contribute to the resulting turbulence.

Given all the necessary conditions, turbulence is more likely to occur in a larger than a smaller vessel. Turbulence is also related to the density of the liquid being directly related to it whereas it is inversely related to its viscosity. It is well known that in anemia the viscosity of blood is low and therefore the resulting Reynolds number from ***Reynolds formula*** will be high. (Reynolds formula is $Re = VD/v$, where V is the mean velocity of flow, D is the diameter of the tube, v is the fraction expressing the density of liquid over viscosity of the liquid.)[1] The volume of flow usually does not enter into the formula of Reynolds; increased volume of flow is often associated also with increased velocity in general. Tortuosity and irregularities of vessels will also be expected to cause more turbulence.

Although turbulence is an important cause of cardiovascular murmurs, sometimes turbulent flow within the heart or the blood vessels may be noted and yet there may be no associated murmur with it. This has become more and more evident since color flow mapping techniques have become available. This should be evidence of the fact that perhaps there are other factors such as production of eddies or vortices or resonance of structures needed besides turbulence. Eddies most certainly must occur around the edge of the cardiac valves. In addition, in situations where blood flows at high velocity but through narrow vessels, e.g. arteriovenous fistula or persistent ductus, large eddies are likely to be created as the jet from the narrowed orifice enters a wider area of vessel. These may also contribute to the murmurs in these conditions.[1,4]

In addition, the sounds generated by turbulence need to be in the audible range of frequencies and also have enough energy to overcome the muffling effect of the surrounding anatomic structures and body tissues as well as loss due to conduction through the body surface before they can become audible.[2] *The latter may be an important reason why in a number of instances valvular regurgitation and associated turbulent flow could be demonstrated by color flow mapping and yet auscultation may not reveal a corresponding murmur.*

HEMODYNAMIC FACTORS AND CARDIAC MURMURS

The timing and the character or the quality of the murmurs as determined by the predominant frequencies will depend on the underlying abnormality and the resulting turbulence and the hemodynamic factors associated with the turbulence. The loudness or intensity is also to a certain extent determined by the degree of the underlying disturbance in flow. The timing of the murmurs can thus be related to systole, diastole or both. This will obviously depend on the lesion (e.g. aortic stenosis that will cause turbulent flow in systole and therefore a systolic murmur whereas mitral stenosis will cause a diastolic turbulence and diastolic murmur). The character of the resulting murmur as determined by its predominant frequencies depends to a large extent on the pressure gradients as well as the volume of flow involved in the resulting turbulence.

FREQUENCIES OF MURMURS

Most cardiovascular murmurs show a frequency range extending from almost 0 to 700 Hz (cycles per second). The louder the murmur the wider will be the spectrum of frequencies that are recordable. The musical term "pitch" refers to what one hears. High pitch as when a soprano in an opera makes a note usually reflects high frequency, whereas the low pitch of a man's voice in an opera indicates lower frequency. *The frequencies of murmurs that are clinically important generally relate to both the pressure gradients involved in the production of the turbulent flow as well as the actual volume or amount of flow involved.* Turbulent flow differs from laminar flow in the relationship between the pressure gradient and velocity of flow. Turbulent flow requires a larger pressure gradient than the equivalent laminar flow. Because of random directions more energy is also required to maintain flow necessitating higher pressure gradient.[1]

It is generally observed that ***when the pressure gradients are high*** and produce turbulence, the resulting murmur often tends to be ***predominantly high in frequency,*** e.g. mitral regurgitation where the turbulence due to the regurgitation occurs under high pressure difference between the LV and the LA. In a normotensive patient this may be as high as 100 mm Hg. The murmur of mitral regurgitation is often blowing in character like the noise caused by blowing through a hollow reed. When the regurgitation is mild it often is almost all high in frequency. When the mitral regurgitation is severe and large in volume then the murmur may assume lower and medium frequencies and begins to sound harsher. In mitral stenosis, the narrowed mitral orifice causes a turbulent mitral inflow into the LV. The flow occurs under a higher diastolic pressure gradient between the LA and the LV. Normally the left atrial pressure ***v wave*** (approximately 12–15 mm Hg) provides the pressure difference during the beginning of diastole, i.e. during the rapid filling phase. In mitral stenosis, the left atrial pressure may be elevated to twice the normal level or more (25–35 mm Hg). The pressure gradient may also tend to persist throughout diastole. The pressure gradient although persistent is still in the lower ranges (10–20 mm Hg). Thus the turbulent flow occurs under low pressure gradients. However the entire stroke volume of the LV must go through the mitral orifice in diastole. Therefore, there is a large volume of flow associated with the turbulence. Because of these two factors, the mitral stenosis murmur tends to be low and medium in frequencies and is described as resembling the rumble of distant thundering clouds. In aortic stenosis, the outflow obstruction will raise the left ventricular systolic pressure in order to maintain forward stroke output. This pressure gradient between the LV and the aorta (AO) will depend on the severity of the obstruction. In addition, the entire systemic output must go through the aortic valve. Thus the murmur of aortic stenosis must have mixed frequencies (low and high) because of both flow and pressure gradients contributing to the turbulence.

Thus the general relationship between the murmur frequencies and the pressure gradients and flow can be stated as follows: *The greater is the pressure gradient the higher is the frequency of the murmur. The greater is the flow on the other hand the lower is the frequency ("more flow"-"more low").* The two heads of the stethoscope are selectively designed to capture the higher and the lower frequency ranges of sounds and murmurs. The high frequency and blowing type murmurs are better brought out by the use of the diaphragm and the lower frequency murmurs are better defined by the use of the bell. An experienced auscultator may define the characteristics of the murmur irrespective of the chest piece used, as long as the murmur is loud enough. Faint low frequency rumbles are however best identified by the use of the bell.

THE GRADING OF THE MURMURS

The murmurs are also graded as to their loudness using the same system as described in relation to the heart sounds.[5] ***Palpable murmurs*** are described as having a ***thrill.*** Thrills, like murmurs, have duration as opposed to sounds, which are transients. Thrills give a feeling to the hand as when one feels the purring of a cat. When a murmur is not immediately audible, the moment one begins to auscultate and one has to tune in to detect the presence of the murmur by eliminating mentally the room noise, then the grade of the murmur is Grade I. Grade I murmurs are not generally appreciated by the beginners in auscultation. Grade II murmur does not require this tuning in process. It is immediately audible the moment one begins to listen. Grade III murmur is the loudest murmur audible but however not associated with a palpable thrill. When a murmur is audible and associated with a thrill it must be between grade IV and VI. Grade IV murmur requires full contact of the chest wall with the chest piece of the stethoscope for its detection. Grade V murmur requires only a partial contact like the edge of the chest piece for its detection. Grade VI murmur on the other hand is audible even when the chest piece is held slightly but completely off the chest.

SYSTOLIC MURMURS

Cardiac murmurs heard during systole ***("systolic murmurs")*** have been traditionally classified in different ways by terms descriptive of some of the features of the murmurs. Some are defined by the timing of the murmurs in relation to the duration of systole from the first to the second heart sound, some are defined by their quality or character and some defined according to their assumed shape. When it is confined to part of the duration of systole, it has been called early systolic, mid-systolic or late systolic depending on which part of systole it is heard. When it lasts throughout systole, it is described as holosystolic or pansystolic.[6,7] While pansystolic murmurs are often caused by regurgitation, regurgitant lesion can also produce murmurs confined to only part of systole for instance late systole. When described according to the quality or character, terms such as harsh or blowing are used. These terms in general describe the pre-dominant pitch or frequency of the murmur whether medium or high. The character or the pre-dominant frequency of the murmur relates to the pressure gradients and the flow involved in the turbulence. However, it does not help to define the origin of the murmur. Term such as "diamond shaped or kite shaped systolic murmur" when used assumes a certain shape of the murmur that is hardly definable by auscultation. It would require a phonocardiogram to confirm. Even when defined as such on a phonocardiogram, it does not relate to the origin or the cause of the murmur.

Systolic murmurs arise generally either due to turbulent flow across the ventricular outflow tract during ejection or from regurgitation of blood (i.e. flow in reverse direction) from the ventricle into a low pressure chamber like the atrium as in mitral or tricuspid regurgitation or through a communication in the ventricular septum from the LV into the right heart. Ejection of blood through the ventricular outflow tract is a normal function of the heart. On the other hand, the occurrence of regurgitation of blood from the ventricle in a reverse direction is always abnormal. The factors governing ejection of blood across the ventricular outflow tract and the abnormalities that may lead to turbulent flow and cause systolic murmurs of ejection are therefore different from those that are associated with regurgitation.[8]

The murmurs of ejection origin have also certain characteristic features that are not shared by the murmurs of regurgitant origin. Since this distinction has direct practical clinical application, systolic murmurs will be discussed under the following two major categories:

1. Ejection murmurs
2. Regurgitant murmurs.

EJECTION MURMURS

Normal Physiology of Ventricular Ejection

In addition to the inherent contractility of the ventricular myocardium and the heart rate at which the ventricle performs its pumping function, the major determinant of its stroke output is the end-diastolic volume, which is essentially the pre-load. The end-diastolic pressure achieved prior to the onset of systolic contraction will primarily depend on the diastolic function reflecting of course both ventricular relaxation and compliance. These have been discussed in relation to the third heart sound (S3) and fourth heart sound (S4). Once systole is set in motion by electrical depolarization of the ventricular myocardium, the excitation-contraction coupling leads to actin-myosin bridge formation. As the ventricular contraction proceeds, more and more of the myofibrils are recruited into contraction resulting in rise of the ventricular pressure. The force exerted by the contracting ventricle on the blood mass it contains imparts energy to it. Once the inertial resistance offered by the blood mass is overcome, the blood mass begins to accelerate and move toward the low pressure area of the mitral region where it gets decelerated due to the closure of the mitral valve. The energy dissipated when deceleration occurs results in the production of the mitral component (M1).

After this event, continued ventricular contraction during the isovolumic phase (extending from the time of mitral valve closure to the time when the aortic valve opens) produces further rise in the ventricular pressure. When the ventricular pressure exceeds the aortic pressure, the aortic valve opens and ejection begins. By this time the blood mass has gained significant momentum that aids its forward movement. The forces that operate to oppose this forward flow have been termed the impedance, which has been previously discussed, in the previous chapter under second heart sound (S2). These include the vascular capacity, the viscosity of the blood and the resistance of the systemic arterial and the pulmonary vascular beds. To this, one can also add the proximal aortic and pulmonary artery distensibility or compliance. The momentum gained by the blood mass will keep it moving forward into the AO and the pulmonary artery even during the later part of systole when the ventricular pressure begins to fall below that of the AO and the pulmonary artery respectively.[9] However with the falling ventricular pressure, the opposing impedance will prevent further forward flow. The blood mass close to the aortic and the pulmonary valves will suddenly tend to reverse its flow direction toward the ventricle, which presents a low pressure area due to the falling ventricular pressure. This will close the aortic and the pulmonary valves. Deceleration of the column of blood in the AO against the closed aortic valve generates the aortic component (A2) and similar deceleration against the pulmonary valve results in pulmonary component (P2). Since the impedance in the pulmonary circuitis lower, this deceleration occurs later. These have been discussed previously under S2.

During ejection phase, the left ventricular pressure remains slightly higher than the aortic pressure in the early to mid-part of systole. This pressure gradient, which has been measured by catheter tip micro sensors, has been termed ***the impulse gradient*** (Fig. 7.3). The peak flow acceleration and peak impulse gradients occur very early in systole.[9] The aortic flow velocity peaks slightly later with slow return to zero flow at the end of ejection. A smaller right-sided impulse gradient has also been shown between the right ventricle and the pulmonary artery.[9]

With exercise, the cardiac output is increased due to the increased venous return. There is a significant increase in heart rate in untrained individuals and the stroke output may or may not be increased. With trained athletes, the heart rate increases slowly. The increased cardiac output is achieved by the increased stroke volume. With exercise, the ejection time shortens particularly when the heart rate increases. The stroke output whether increased or normal is accomplished over shorter ejection time. This has been shown to be accompanied by an increase in the impulse gradient and increase in flow acceleration.[9]

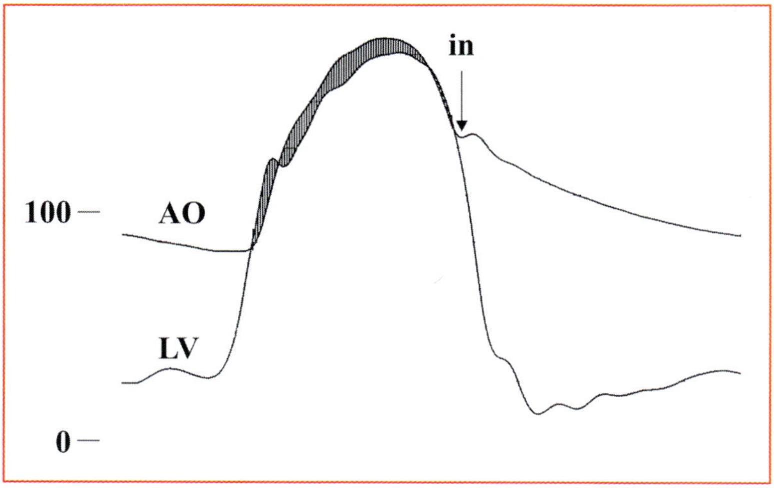

Fig. 7.3: Simultaneous recording of the left ventricular (LV) and the aortic (AO) pressures through catheters placed in the LV and AO respectively showing a small but discernible pressure gradient, "the impulse gradient" between the LV and the AO.

The flow through normal ventricular outflow tracts and the semilunar valves is still smooth and laminar in most instances. *Conditions, which lead to increase in the velocity of flow or actual increase in volume of flow, particularly in the presence of anatomic abnormalities of the outflow tract, are all likely to result in turbulent flow.*

Formation of Ejection Murmurs

Turbulent flow during ejection leading to the formation of ejection murmurs can be expected to occur under the following circumstances:

1. Increased velocity of ejection of either normal or increased stroke volume of blood across normal aortic and/or pulmonary valves and the respective outflow tracts
2. *Ejection of a large stroke volume of blood across a normal aortic and/or the pulmonary valves and the respective outflow tracts*
3. *Ejection of blood across roughened or stenosed aortic and/or pulmonary valves or their respective outflow tracts.*

Characteristics of Ejection Murmurs

1. *Ejection murmurs are often harsh and have pre-dominant medium and low frequencies:* Since the entire stroke output of the ventricle flows through the outflow tract and will be involved in any turbulence during ejection, the ejection murmurs will tend to have a lot of medium and low frequency components caused primarily by flow. If the stroke volume is actually

increased for some reason, then this effect will be enhanced. The predominant low and medium frequency will make the ejection murmurs sound harsh in quality.

2. ***The ejection murmurs have a characteristic cadence or rhythm***: The ejection phase begins as soon as the isovolumic phase of contraction ends. The first heart sound (S1) with its M1 and aortic components just precede ejection and ejection murmurs therefore begin with the S1.[10] The physiology of ejection is such that there is an initial phase of acceleration with build-up of momentum. When there is no fixed outflow obstruction or stenosis, this reaches a peak in early to mid-systole and begins to decline after. The flow velocity also reaches a peak in early to mid-systole and gradually returns to zero flow in late systole. Reflecting this, the ejection murmur also increases in intensity to reach a peak and there after declines in late systole and ends before the S2 (Fig. 7.4). ***The murmur has thus a crescendo decrescendo character.***[8] Depending on the side of origin whether it is left-sided or right-sided, the murmur will end before the A2 or the P2. *The S1, the peak of the crescendo followed by a pause before S2, make a cadence or rhythm:*

S1.... peak ...S2
Da.....Ha ....Da

When there is significant fixed obstruction or stenosis in the outflow tract, the ventricular pressure will be increased to overcome the stenosis. The systolic pressure gradient between the ventricle and the AO or the pulmonary artery depending on the side involved in the obstruction, will reflect its severity. The pressure gradient will rise with the onset of ejection becoming maximal in mid-systole. It will decrease later in systole with falling ventricular pressure. The more severe the stenosis the greater is this pressure gradient. In severe stenosis, the pressure gradient

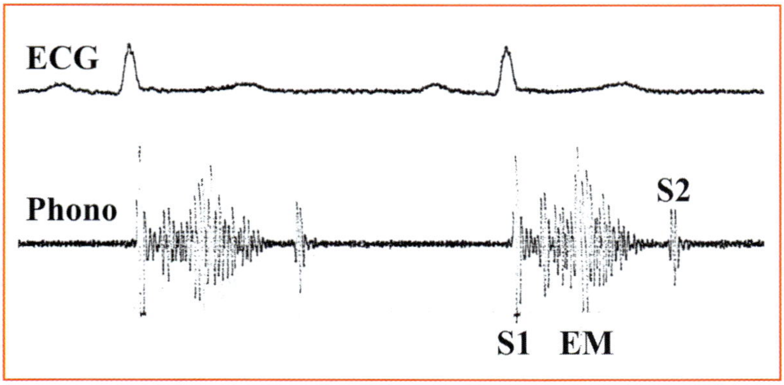

Fig. 7.4: Phonocardiographic recording from the apex area of a patient with an ejection murmur. Note that the murmur starts with the first heart sound and reaches a peak in mid-systole and gradually tapers and ends before the second heart sound, thus showing a crescendo and decrescendo effect.

may be in excess of 75 mm Hg. The stroke volume in the presence of outflow tract obstruction is ejected over a longer period. The flow velocity increases gradually and reaches a peak in mid-systole and the murmur also becomes somewhat longer and achieves the peak intensity in mid-systole. Following the peak it decreases in intensity still retaining the crescendo decrescendo character and eventually fades out before the S2. Thus, a pause is often recognizable between the end of the murmur and the S2. In addition to the low and medium frequencies produced by the flow, the higher pressure gradient in severe stenosis will contribute to some of the higher frequencies of the murmur.

3. *Ejection murmur tends to accentuate in its intensity or loudness after long diastolic intervals*: Long diastolic period occurs for instance following pre-mature ventricular beat due to the compensatory pause. *The ejection murmur during the beat after the compensatory pause has a louder intensity than the regular sinus beat before it* (Fig. 7.5). The reason for this is that the post-ectopic beat has a stronger contraction and increased stroke output. The compensatory pause allows longer diastolic filling time thus increasing the volume and providing a Starling effect on contractility. This helps also in enhancing the stroke output of the post-ectopic beat. In addition, during the long pause, the aortic diastolic pressure continues to fall and the post-ectopic beat thus has less afterload or impedance to ejection. The third reason for the augmented contractility is the post-extrasystolic potentiation that a pre-mature depolarization provides. This is probably due to availability of extra calcium within the myocardium for the contractile process. Any early or pre-mature depolarization will cause this (*see* Chapter 2). Similar phenomenon can also be observed ***during atrial fibrillation*** where the diastolic intervals naturally vary. *The ejection murmur will not only vary in intensity but it will also be noted to be louder following long diastoles.*[11]

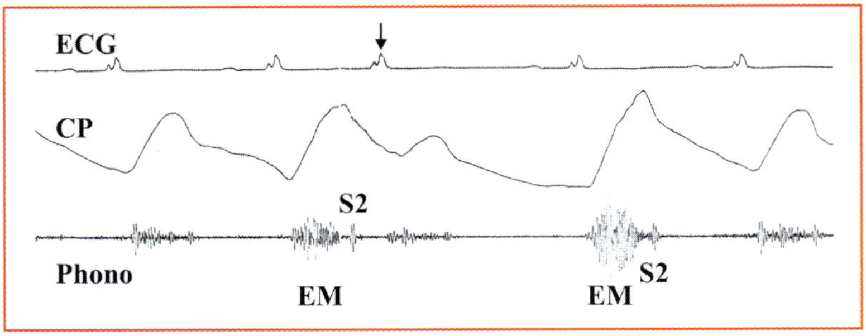

Fig. 7.5: Simultaneous recordings of phonocardiogram (Phono), electrocardiogram (ECG) and the carotid pulse, from a patient with a systolic murmur. The ECG shows the presence of a premature ventricular beat (arrow). Note the murmur has greater amplitude in the beat following the ectopic (premature) beat compared to the sinus beat before it. This confirms that the systolic murmur is an ejection murmur.

Anatomic Differences Between the Left and the Right Ventricular Outflow Tract

Since ejection murmurs are caused by turbulent flow accompanying ejection of blood through the ventricular outflow tract, the anatomy of the outflow tracts needs to be understood. The outflow tract of both ventricles is formed not only by the respective semilunar valve (the aortic and the pulmonary valves) but also by the structures just above and below the valve itself. The supravalvular portion of the outflow tract consists of the aortic root on the left side and the pulmonary artery on the right side.

The left ventricular outflow tract below the semilunar aortic valve has essentially two boundaries. The sub-aortic ventricular septum is on the anteromedial side whereas on the lateral side is the anterior mitral leaflet. This is due to the fact that the anterior mitral leaflet shares its attachment to the aortic root with the aortic valve (Fig. 7.6A). The anatomic organization is different of course on the right side where the pulmonary valve shares no such common attachment with the tricuspid valve tricuspid valve ring. The latter fully occupies the entire circumference of the right atrioventricular (AV) ring. The pulmonary valve is separated from the inflow tract by the infundibular chamber or tract. The infundibulum is separated from the main body of the right ventricular by the crista supraventricularis muscle (Fig. 7.6B).

These anatomic differences are important with regard to abnormalities or lesions, which may contribute to the turbulent flow and the production of ejection murmurs from the left and the right sides of the heart.

Causes of Ejection Murmurs

Rapid Circulatory States

Rapid circulatory states such as in young children, anemia and thyrotoxicosis are often associated with systolic ejection murmurs although the aortic and the pulmonary valves and the outflow tracts are often entirely normal. In these conditions, the increased velocity of flow contributes to the increased turbulence. The murmur will often have peaks in early to mid-systole. Occasionally, the normal flow through a normal pulmonary outflow tract in children may be associated with some turbulence, which may be shown to be associated with an ejection murmur, which may be recordable in the pulmonary outflow tract with intracardiac phonocatheters. These pulmonary ejection murmurs may be more easily audible in some subjects than others due to either *thin body build or decreased anteroposterior diameter of the chest, which* may help to bring the heart to a closer proximity of the chest wall. *In some adults, with loss of the normal thoracic kyphosis and with a straight back, similarly closer proximity of the heart to the chest wall may contribute to the audible ejection murmurs that are pre-sumably pulmonary in origin since they are often of maximal loudness in the second left interspace.*[12]

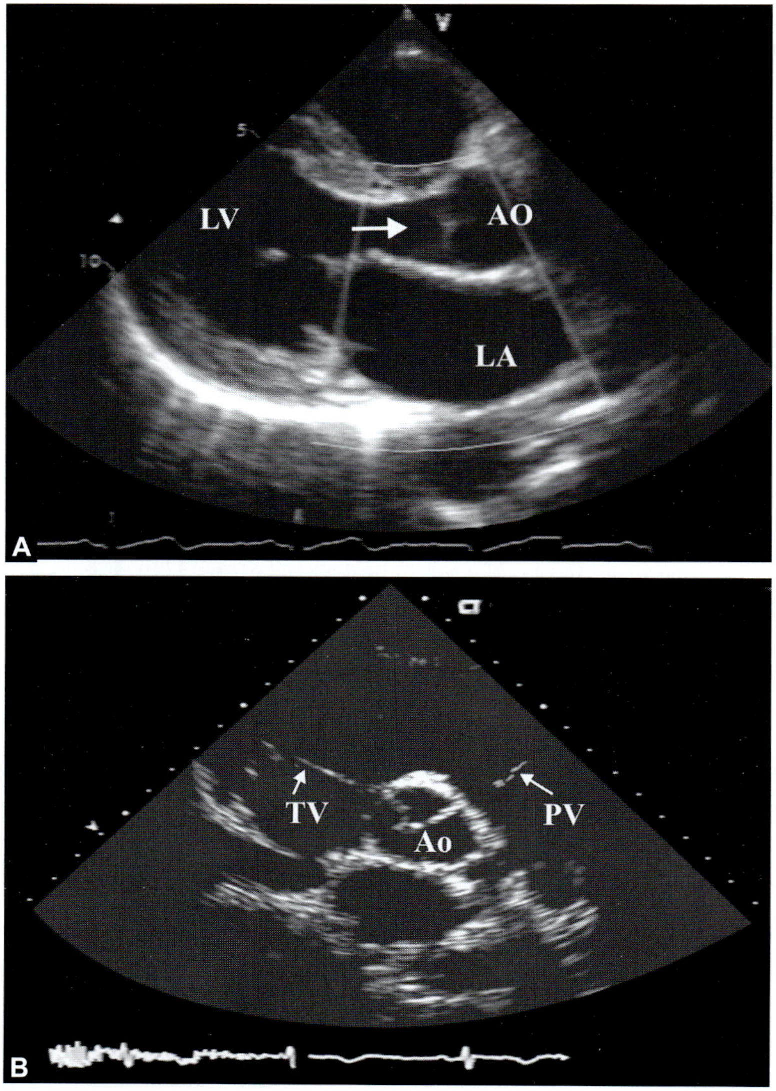

Figs. 7.6A and B: Two-dimensional echocardiographic images in the parasternal view. (A) shows the long axis of the left ventricle (LV). The transducer on the anterior chest wall is shown at the top of the image. The LV outflow tract (the arrow) is between the interventricular septum anteriorly and the anterior mitral leaflet posteriorly that has a common attachment to the aortic root. (B) shows the short axis view at the aortic level. The pulmonary valve is separated from the tricuspid valve by the right ventricular outflow tract anterior to the aortic root.

In some young children, the ejection murmur may be somewhat vibratory in quality like twanging a string. This is often due to pure or uniform frequencies in the medium range. It has been called the ***Still's murmur*** after Still who described it first.[13] The mechanism may actually involve some structures in the heart such as congenital longitudinal intracardiac bands in the ventricle actually vibrating. The rapid circulatory state may be a contributory factor.[14,15]

Ejection of a Large Stroke Volume

Ejection of a large stroke volume as may be found in bradycardia, complete AV block and secondary to conditions such as aortic regurgitation (where the blood flowing backward into the LV from the AO as well as the normal mitral inflow are received by the ventricle in diastole and ejected during systole) are all known to cause ejection systolic murmurs of left-sided origin. In atrial septal defect, the RV receives extra volume of blood because of the left-to-right shunt across the interatrial septum in addition to the usual systemic venous return. This increases the right ventricular stroke volume. Often the main pulmonary artery is also dilated due to the large volume of blood that it receives. Both these factors contribute to the pulmonary ejection murmur in this condition.[16]

Abnormalities of the Outflow Tract Structures or the Semilunar Valves without Stenosis

Aortic valve may be ***bicuspid*** congenitally. This may lead to ejection of an eccentric jet into the proximal AO. Since the bicuspid valves are structurally inadequate for perfect competence of the valve, it may be accompanied by aortic regurgitation. The bicuspid aortic valve may also become calcific in the elderly. Even the normal aortic valve may also become ***thickened and sclerosed*** and occasionally even calcified in the elderly. But the cusp opening may be still good with very little stenosis if any. The intima of the aortic root may also be abnormally thickened or roughened with atherosclerotic plaques. In addition, the AO or the proximal aortic root may be dilated or aneurysmal particularly in the presence of hypertensive and/or atherosclerotic disease. The orientation of the normal interventricular septum is usually along the axis of left ventricular cavity. This can sometimes be easily visualized on a 2D echocardiographic image. Occasionally, the interventricular septum may be somewhat angulated and the proximal portion of the septum may be hypertrophied focally. In some of these patients, ***the septum may be sigmoid in shape.***[17] The outflow tract is therefore oriented slightly off in axis to the direction of the longitudinal axis of the left ventricular cavity (Figs. 7.7A and B). This often would result in turbulence in flow, which can be seen on the color Doppler mapping of the aortic outflow in such patients. Under all these circumstances, aortic ejection murmurs are often common. In fact, for these various reasons, ejection murmur is fairly common above the age of 50 years (Fig. 7.8).

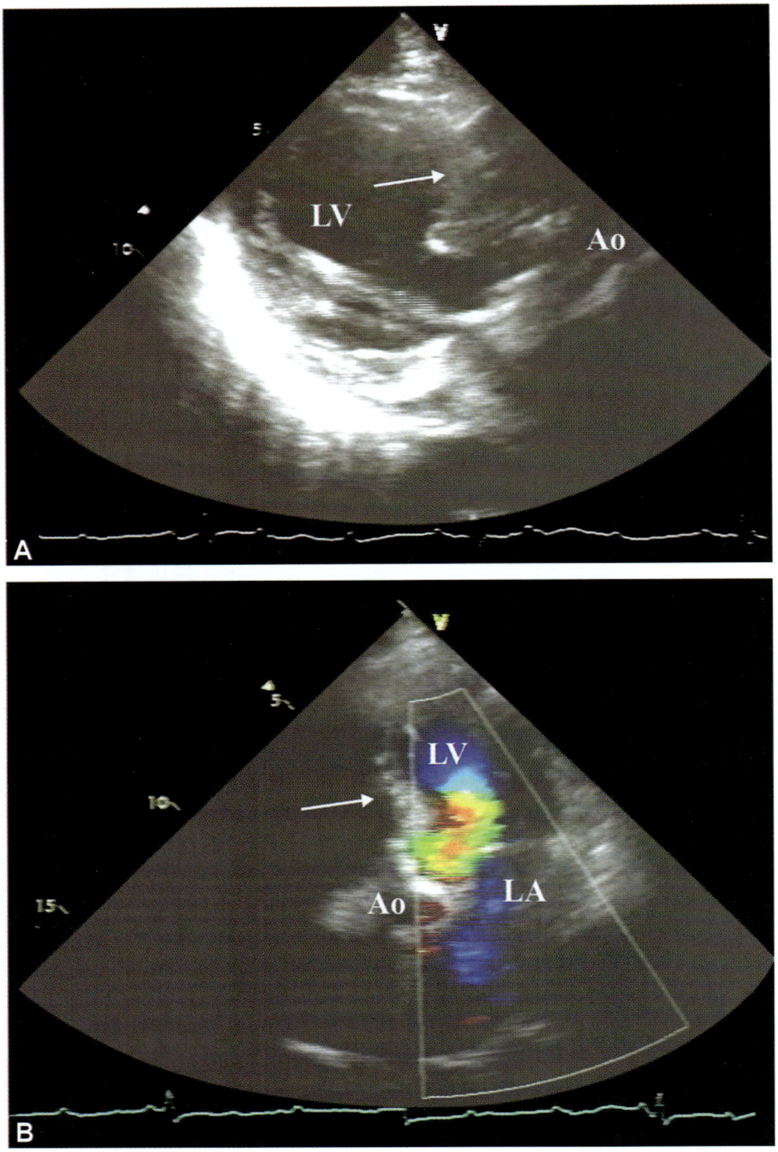

Figs. 7.7A and B: (A) Two-dimensional echocardiographic image in the parasternal long axis showing the interventricular septum (arrow) to be sigmoid in shape. (B) The color flow image shows turbulent flow across the left ventricular outflow shown in the apical four-chamber view.

Outflow Tract Obstruction

Left Ventricular

Aortic valve stenosis: Isolated aortic valve stenosis is often congenital in origin even in the elderly due to calcification of an abnormal often bicuspid

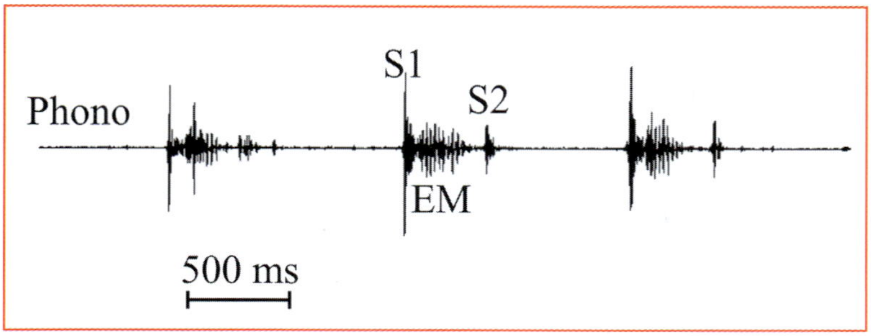

Fig. 7.8: Digital display of a magnetic audio recording from an elderly patient taken at the apex area showing a typical ejection systolic murmur beginning with the first heart sound and ending with a pause before the second heart sound.

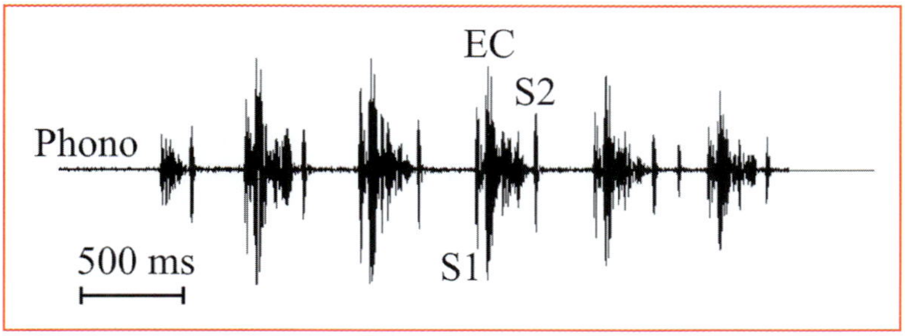

Fig. 7.9: Digital display of a magnetic audio recording from a patient with congenital aortic stenosis taken at the apex area showing a high frequency sharp ejection click closely following the first heart sound at the onset of the ejection murmur.

aortic valve. This may typically lead to symptoms in the sixth or the seventh decade in men. Bicuspid aortic valve may be associated with stenosis or obstruction even in the younger age group. Aortic stenosis may result occasionally due to rheumatic heart disease. In this instance it often is associated with aortic regurgitation and/or mitral valve disease.[18,19] Rarely degenerative changes of the cusps occurring with old age may eventually lead to stenosis in the eighth decade.

The ejection murmur of aortic valve stenosis is no different in quality or even loudness from those caused by other causes listed above where there is no structural abnormality of the outflow tract. When the valve is still mobile, one may hear an aortic ejection click before the onset of the murmur (Fig. 7.9). The presence of the aortic ejection click may sometimes be surmised by the presence of a clicking S1 with the onset of the murmur.

The murmur may be audible all along the true aortic sash area extending from the second right interspace along the left sternal border to the left ventricular apex. The murmur may also be transmitted to the neck. However, the murmur is usually loudest at the second right interspace but may be equally loud at the apex. In some elderly patients, the murmur may be loudest only

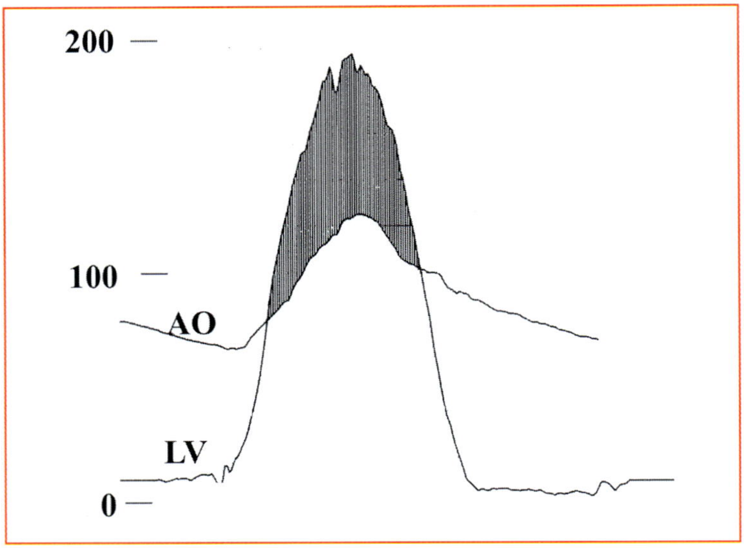

Fig. 7.10: Recording of simultaneous left ventricular (LV) and aortic (AO) pressure curves from a patient with severe aortic stenosis. It can be seen that the significantly high peak LV systolic pressure will necessarily take a long time to fall below that of the aorta, thereby delaying the occurrence of the aortic component.

at the apex. If the stenosis is severe, the murmur will be often longer and will have a delayed peak. *The murmur of aortic stenosis is occasionally quite high frequency and even musical and cooing in quality at the apex while it retains the harshness at the base. While the reason for this is not necessarily clear, it may be partly due to the fact that the higher frequencies of the turbulence tend to be transmitted upstream more selectively (Gallavardin phenomenon).*[20]

In severe stenosis, the left ventricular pressure is significantly high and takes a long time to fall below that of the AO (Fig. 7.10). The A2 will be significantly delayed and there will be a reversed sequence. The P2 will be buried in the end of the murmur and the only component that may be audible will be A2. The latter however will be soft. *If in the presence of a long and loud systolic murmur, a soft S2, which is softer than the murmur, is heard it would mean that the murmur has ended before the S2. This will be a clue to the fact that the murmur is in fact ejection in type (Fig. 7.11).* Occasionally, one may also hear an S4 just before the onset of the murmur. This will reflect the severity as well since S4 will only occur when the stenosis is severe enough to evoke significant left ventricular hypertrophy thereby causing decreased ventricular compliance.[18,21,22]

Sub-valvular Aortic Obstruction

Sub-valvular aortic stenosis can be of ***two types***:

1. Fixed (membranous)
2. Dynamic (hypertrophic)

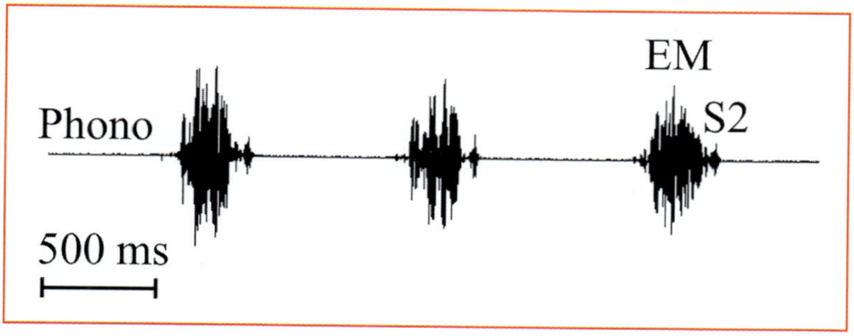

Fig. 7.11: Digital display of a magnetic audio recording from a patient with severe aortic stenosis taken from the apex area showing a large amplitude (loud) systolic murmur followed by a distinct but significantly lower amplitude (soft) second heart sound (S2). Since the S2 is still clearly audible, it must mean that the murmur ends before S2 and therefore must be an ejection murmur.

Membranous: The sub-valvular aortic outflow may be the seat of obstruction congenitally due to a membrane stretching from the anterior mitral leaflet to the interventricular septum. Rarely there could be abnormal attachments of parts of the anterior mitral leaflet or its chordae leading to narrowing of the outflow tract.[19] The membrane is usually made of thick fibrous structure with a stenosed or narrow orifice. *Often the aortic outflow jet from the sub-valvular obstruction will over time cause structural damage to the aortic cusps resulting in some degree of aortic regurgitation. The abnormal tissue from the anterior mitral leaflet rarely can encroach into the mitral orifice leading to some interference with mitral inflow in diastole.*

Hypertrophic: The second cause of sub-aortic obstruction is usually in association with hypertrophic cardiomyopathy. In this condition, there is often severe hypertrophy of the LV particularly involving the interventricular septum. The cavity is small and the ventricle contracts powerfully and ejects blood very rapidly. The obstruction is dynamic[23] and is due to the sudden anterior movement of the anterior mitral leaflet from its closed posterior position. This ***systolic anterior motion ("SAM")*** of the mitral leaflet causes abnormal apposition of the anterior mitral leaflet with the hypertrophic and bulging interventricular septum in the middle of systole causing the outflow obstruction. *The reason for this sudden anterior movement of the anterior mitral leaflet is the rapid and powerful ejection that is characteristic of this disorder. This leads to the development of a negative pressure or suction-like effect (Venturi effect) on the mitral leaflet as the blood is being ejected very rapidly out of the LV (Figs. 7.12A to D).*[23-30] The latter mechanism has been questioned by some and the SAM has been attributed to pushing or pulling of the miral valve by the anatomic distortion aggravated by vigorous contraction in these patients with marked hypertrophy of the left ventricular walls associated with small cavity.[28]

If the septal hypertrophy is severe, the obstruction may be present at rest. Occasionally, the obstruction may not be evident at rest and may only be brought out under certain conditions. *These include interventions or maneuvers that decrease the ventricular size thus increasing the septal-mitral contact*. This can be achieved by assumption of a standing position, which will decrease the venous return. The smaller ventricular size aids the septal-mitral apposition or contact during systole. ***Obstruction can also be augmented by***

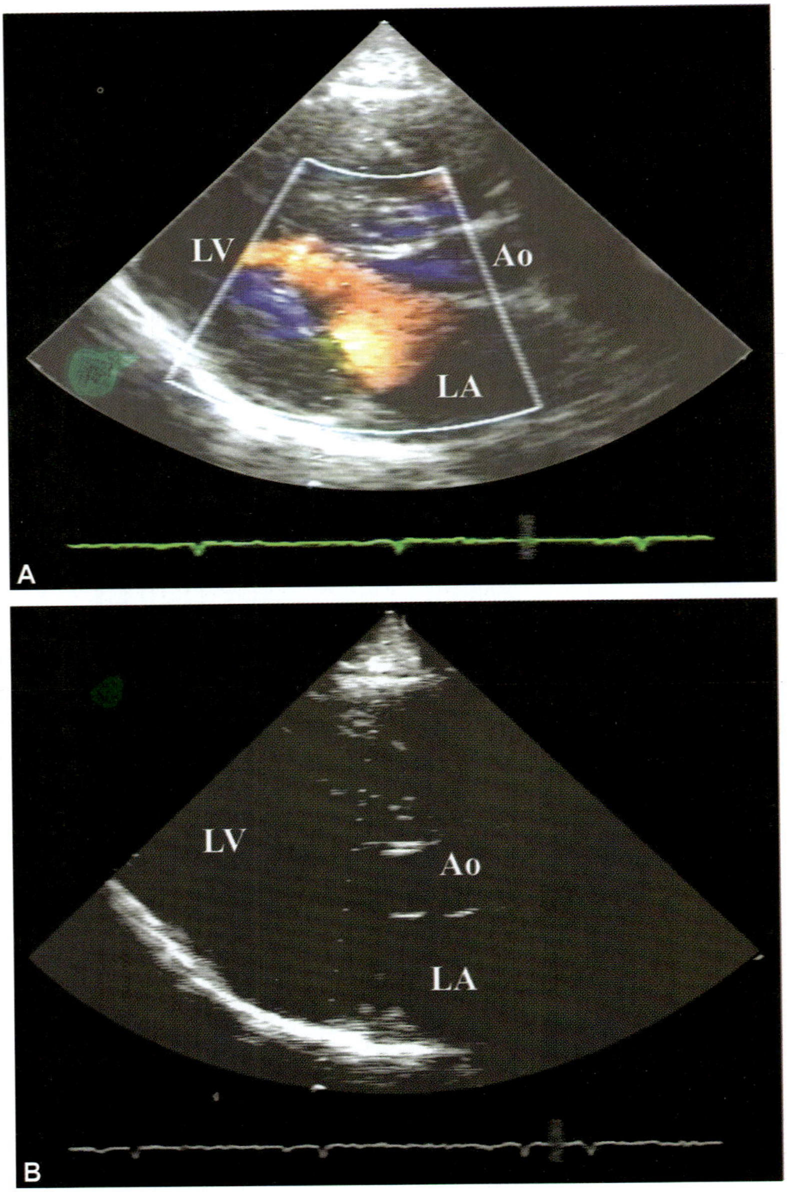

Figs. 7.12A and B

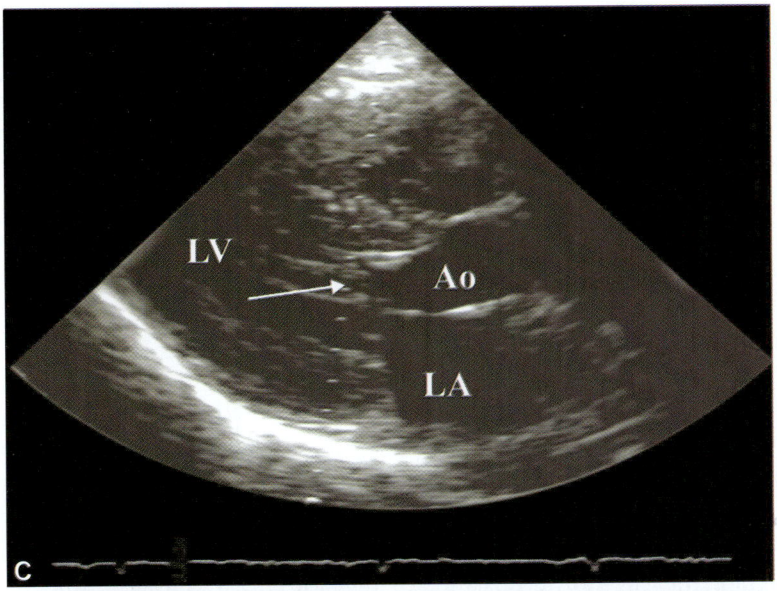

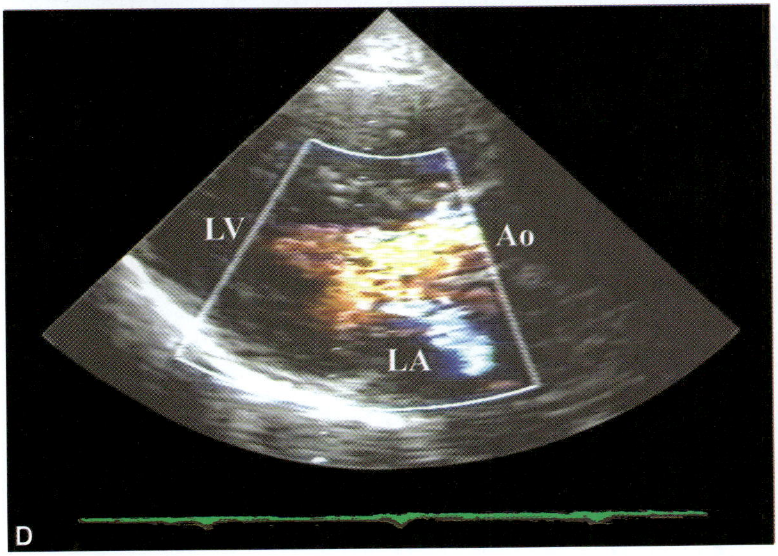

Figs. 7.12A to D: Two-dimensional echocardiographic images in the parasternal view from a patient with hypertrophic obstructive cardiomyopathy with severe sub-aortic obstruction. The diastolic frame (A) showing the open mitral valve allowing the inflow from the left atrium into the left ventricle. The interventricular septum in continuity with the anterior wall of the aorta as well as the posterior left ventricular free wall are markedly hypertrophied. Stop frame at the onset of systole (B) showing the mitral valve in the closed position. The left ventricle contracts powerfully and causes rapid ejection. This rapid ejection out of the left ventricle causes suction-like effect on the anterior leaflet leading to it being pulled forward and anteriorly (the arrow). This systolic anterior motion of the anterior mitral leaflet and the resulting contact with the interventricular septum causes obstruction to the left ventricular outflow in mid-systole (C). This leads to turbulent outflow as well as some mitral regurgitation seen in the Doppler color flow (D).

inotropic stimuli (including the pharmacological agents such as isoproterenol or digoxin), which increase the contractile force. The increased inotropic effect caused by exercise can also augment the obstruction. When there is inotropic stimulation, the increased contractile force favors the development of the Venturi effect on the mitral leaflet more readily (Figs. 7.13A and B). *Finally, the obstruction can also be made worse by lowering the peripheral resistance as caused by peripheral arterial dilatation.* This includes pharmacological agents that lower the blood pressure by dilating the peripheral vessels. *The pressure distending the aortic root acts on the mitral leaflet opposing the Venturi effect of the rapidly moving outflow. When the aortic pressure is lowered by peripheral arterial dilatation, the mitral-septal contact becomes more pronounced.* The pressure gradient across the left ventricular outflow tract will thus be increased by amyl nitrite inhalation, which causes peripheral arterial dilatation. Raising the blood pressure by peripheral vasoconstriction will do the opposite and help to prevent the systolic anterior motion of the anterior mitral leaflet (Fig. 7.13C).[18,23,31]

When the sub-aortic obstruction develops in mid-systole due to the systolic anterior motion of the anterior mitral leaflet, the mitral valve does

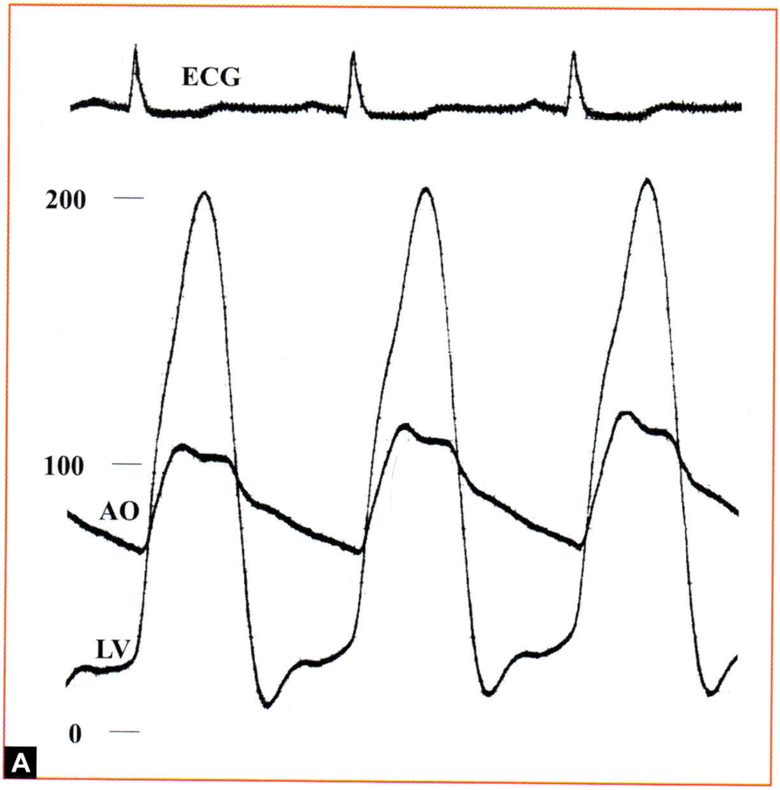

Fig. 7.13A

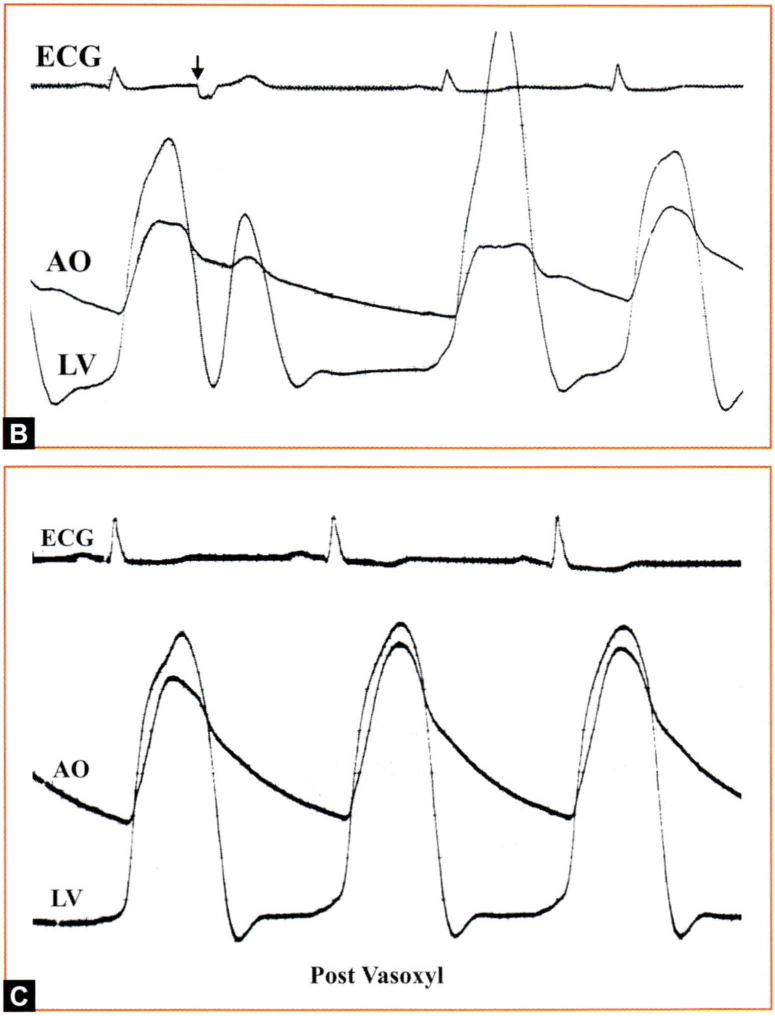

Figs. 7.13A to C: Simultaneous recordings of the electrocardiogram, the left ventricular (LV) and the aortic (AO) pressure curves obtained at cardiac catheterization from a patient with hypertrophic obstructive cardiomyopathy. (A) shows the measurements at rest indicating the presence of a systolic pressure gradient across the left ventricular outflow tract. The rise of the AO curve is relatively rapid distinguishing this from the valvular form of aortic stenosis. (B) shows recordings made during mechanically induced premature ventricular contractions. The systolic pressure gradient between the LV and the AO at rest gets accentuated in the beat following the premature ventricular contraction (the arrow). This is due to the effect of the post-extrasystolic potentiation of the ventricular contractility. (C) shows the abolition of the resting systolic pressure gradient after the administration of a peripheral arterial vasoconstricting agent, Vasoxyl.

become incompetent.[29] The outflow obstruction at this point favors mitral regurgitation as well. The degree of mitral regurgitation is variable. Generally, it is mild and does not contribute much to the characteristics of the murmur.

The murmur of hypertrophic sub-aortic stenosis shares all features of the ejection murmur described above. The murmur is generally maximally loud at the apex. The murmur also tends to be somewhat longer but nevertheless ends before A2. The murmur intensity or loudness is variable and this usually depends to a large extent on the degree and severity of the obstruction. The murmur may be absent at rest and may be only brought out by maneuvers that produce one or more of the following namely decrease in ventricular size, increase in contractility or decrease in the peripheral resistance. *The simplest maneuver that will bring on the murmur or accentuate the loudness of the murmur is making the patient stand suddenly from a supine position.* This will decrease the venous return thereby decreasing the left ventricular volume. Standing also causes a slight fall in arterial pressure causing sympathetic stimulation and increase in heart rate. The sub-aortic obstruction will get worse and this will accentuate the murmur intensity. An opposite maneuver will be to make the patient squat. ***During squatting,*** the venous return increases from the periphery due to increased abdominal pressure and compression of the veins in the lower extremities. This will help to increase the ventricular size. In addition, the arteries in the lower extremities get compressed, thus increasing the arterial resistance and the blood pressure. This will also cause a decrease in heart rate. The combined effects of these changes ***will reduce the intensity of the ejection murmur (Fig. 7.14A).*** Similarly, other maneuvers can also be used to change the hemodynamicstatus either to augment obstruction or decrease the obstruction.[18,23,31,32] During the strain phase of the Valsalva maneuver, the decreased venous return and increase in heart rate will accentuate the murmur.[33] The Mueller maneuver will produce the opposite effect. Inhalation of amyl nitrite will increase the murmur intensity since the powerful arterial dilatation it causes will drop the aortic pressure and increase the degree of obstruction. The tachycardia and the sympathetic stimulation, which accompany the drop in blood pressure, also will help augment the obstruction.

When the obstruction is severe at rest, the A2 will be significantly delayed resulting in a reversed sequence of S2. The P2 may be buried in the end of the murmur and the only component audible will then be a delayed A2. Occasionally the reversed sequence with a paradoxical split on expiration may also be audible. The decreased left ventricular compliance due to abnormal hypertrophy will often evoke an S4, which may be heard and will precede the onset of the ejection murmur[18] (Fig. 7.14B).

Proximal Septal Hypertrophy with Angulated Septum Causing Mild Outflow Obstruction

Occasionally in patients with an angulated septum or when ***the septum*** is somewhat ***sigmoid*** in shape, the most proximal portion of the septum may

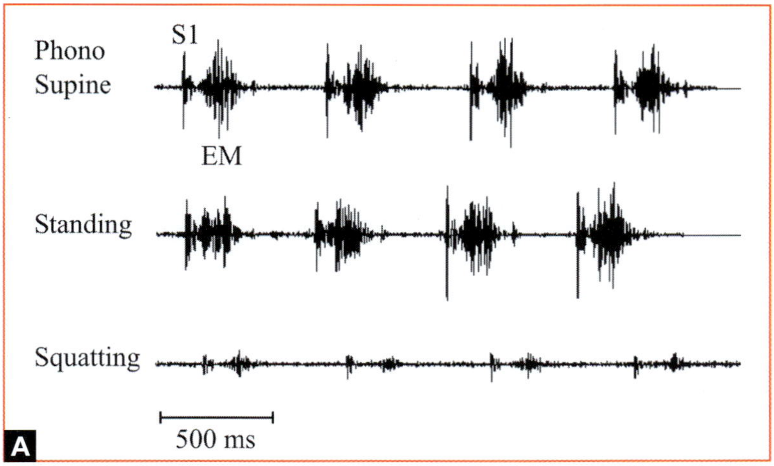

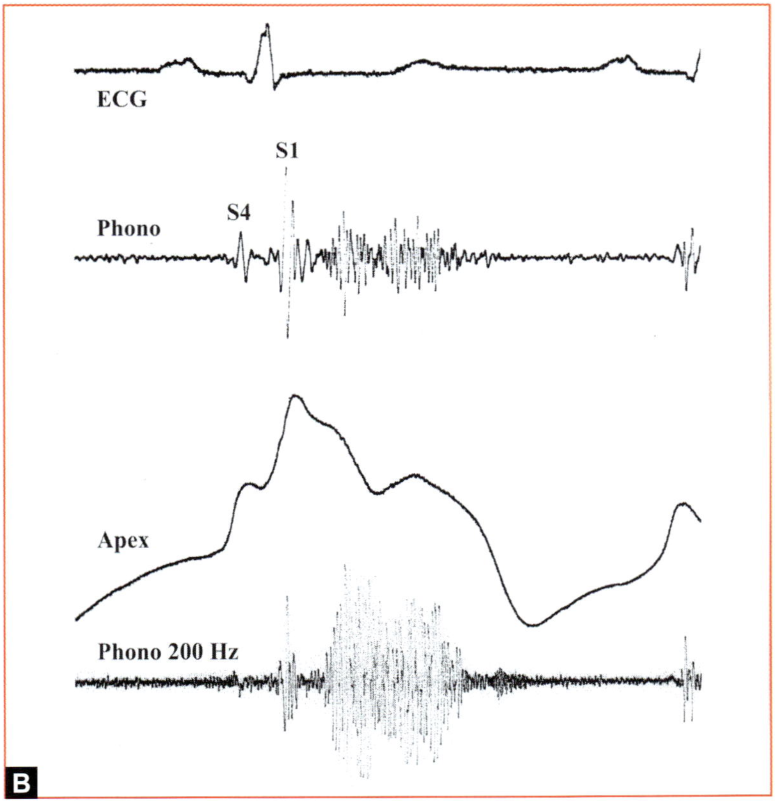

Figs. 7.14A and B: (A) Digital display of a magnetic audio recording from a patient with hypertrophic sub-aortic stenosis taken from the apex area demonstrating the effects of the changing postures on the intensity of the ejection murmur. The murmur gets slightly accentuated on standing and significantly diminished in intensity on squatting compared to the supine position. (B) Simultaneous recordings of electrocardiogram, phonocardiogram and apexcardiogram from a patient with hypertrophic cardiomyopathy with obstruction taken from the apex area demonstrating the typical long ejection murmur. There is a fourth heart sound with a corresponding atrial kick on the apexcardiogram.

be hypertrophied due to coexisting hypertension or coexisting mild to moderate aortic valvular stenosis. This may actually cause some mild degrees of outflow obstruction in the sub-aortic region and ***generate pressure gradients*** *that* ***on Doppler flow mapping may be late peaked*** as in hypertrophic cardiomyopathy.[17] The 2D images however will be marked by the absence of any systolic anterior motion of the anterior mitral leaflet.[34] The murmur will be typically ejection and behaves more like the murmur of aortic valvular stenosis. The features of classic hypertrophic obstructive cardiomyopathy mentioned above will be absent since the underlying pathology is totally different.

Supravalvular Stenosis

Supravalvular aortic stenosis is often congenital and affects the AO above the sinuses of Valsalva. The obstruction may be caused by focal stenosis, by a membrane or due to diffuse hypoplasia of the ascending AO. Occasionally, the supravalvular aortic stenosis is associated with hypercalcemia, mental retardation and typical facial features as well as abnormal dentition. Rarely, stenosis of the pulmonary arteries may coexist. The post-stenotic segment of the AO is not usually dilated.

In supravalvular stenosis, the murmur is often maximal at the suprasternal notch. The high velocity jet from the supravalvular stenosis tends to be preferentially directed to the right innominate artery, making the murmur more prominent over the right side. In many of these patients, the right carotid and the right arm vessels are more prominent than the left. Often the arterial pressure in the right arm is higher than in the left.[35-38] The preferential direction of the high velocity jet toward the right innominate artery has been attributed to a Coandă effect.[39]

Right Ventricular

Pulmonary Valvular Stenosis

Pulmonary valvular stenosis is often congenital and the cusps are often fused and shaped like a fish mouth and the valve may become domed during ejection. There is often some post-stenotic dilatation of the main pulmonaryartery as well as the left pulmonary artery. Rarely the cusps may be thickened and fused and show abnormal myxomatous degeneration. Due to low pressures on the right side, pulmonary valve stenosis never becomes progressively worse or calcified even with increasing age. The pulmonary stenosis can be associated with other congenital defects, in particular a ventricular septal defect (VSD).

When the ventricular septum is intact, the ejection murmur of pulmonary stenosis is no different in quality or even loudness from other ejection murmurs. The murmur is generally audible over the second and third left interspace close to the sternal border and when louder it may be heard over the lower sternal border region as well. *The location of maximal loudness however is usually the second left interspace. The murmur may be equally loud in the third left interspace particularly if there has been secondary infundibular hypertrophy (Figs. 7.15A and B)*. The murmur also tends to get louder on inspiration although this may be difficult to appreciate. Often one can hear the characteristic pulmonary ejection click at the onset of the murmur. *The pulmonary ejection click typically gets softer on inspiration and gets louder on expiration.* Occasionally, the click may actually be the predominant feature and may be heard as a clicking S1.

When ***pulmonary stenosis is mild or moderate*** in severity, the murmur will be noted to be followed by a ***widely split S2.*** When the pulmonary stenosis is significant or ***severe, the murmur gets quite long and has a late peak*** and may then go past the A2, which may be buried in the end of the murmur. The soft S2 heard after the long murmur will be the delayed P2.[40]

When the ventricular septum is intact, severe pulmonary stenosis will evoke a strong right atrial contraction. The decreased compliance caused by the hypertrophied RV is the cause of this strong atrial contraction, which may produce ***a right-sided S4,*** which is usually accentuated with inspiration. The effect of this may be visible in the jugular *a wave* as well, which may become ***prominent (Fig. 7.16).*** These *signs* will tend to be ***absent in*** the presence of a ***VSD*** despite severe pulmonary stenosis.[40,41]

Pulmonary stenosis in the presence of a VSD is the important component of the tetralogy of Fallot.

Sub-valvular Pulmonary Stenosis

The sub-valvular area on the pulmonary side is the infundibulum. This may be the seat of a congenital localized narrowing at the entrance of the outflow tract beyond which the infundibulum may be dilated. Occasionally, the stenosis may result from the hypertrophied crista supraventricularis muscle. In rare instances the stenosis can be sub-infundibular. Sub-valvular stenosis is often associated with a VSD.[40] *The maximal loudness of the murmur in infundibular stenosis is often found at the third left interspace although occasionally it can be the fourth left interspace. Pulmonary ejection click of course will be absent in infundibular stenosis.* The lesion may be associated with a VSD as seen in tetralogy of Fallot.

Supravalvular Pulmonary Stenosis

The site of stenosis is either in the pulmonary trunk, its bifurcation or the branches. Rarely, a supravalvular membrane may be the site of stenosis. The murmur is often systolic ejection in type. The obstruction is usually associated with a systolic gradient across the stenotic segment and will be expected

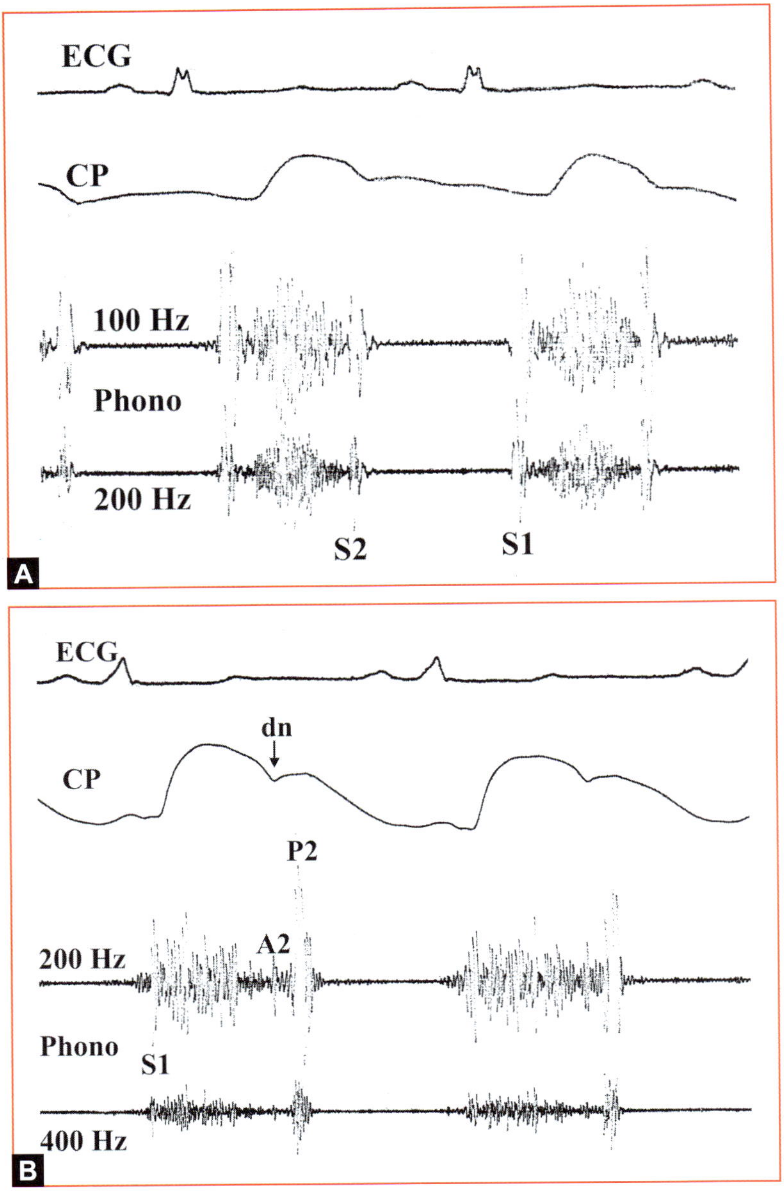

Figs. 7.15A and B: (A) Simultaneous recordings of electrocardiogram (ECG), the carotid pulse (CP) and the phonocardiogram (Phono) from a patient with pulmonary stenosis taken from the second left interspace close to the sternal border, showing the ejection systolic murmur. The murmur appears to go all the way to the S2 that is essentially the aortic component (A2) but it ends however before the pulmonary component (P2). The P2 being soft and not easily audible is not seen on the Phono tracing. (B) Simultaneous recordings of ECG, the CP and the Phono from a patient with atrial septal defect secundum taken at the second to third left interspace. A split second heart sound follows the ejection murmur. The A2, which usually occurs at the time of the incisura of the aortic pressure curve, is seen to occur slightly before the dicrotic notch due to the transmission delay of the CP. The P2 has greater intensity and is well separated from the A2.

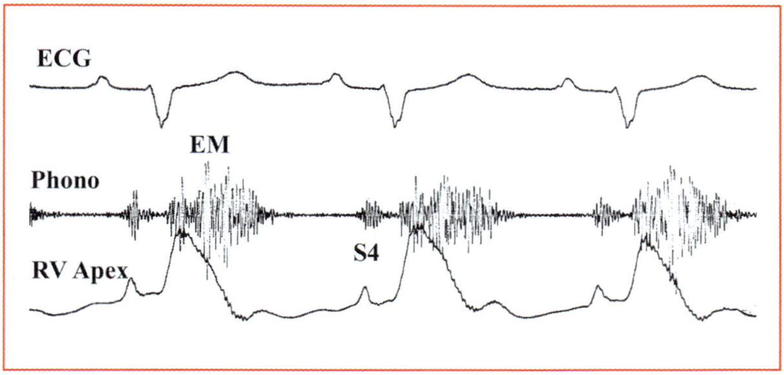

Fig. 7.16: Simultaneous recordings of electrocardiogram, the phonocardiogram (Phono) and the right ventricular impulse (RV apex) from a patient with severe pulmonary stenosis with intact interventricular septum taken at the third left interspace at the left sternal border. The prominent fourth heart sound on the Phono corresponds to the A wave of the RV apex recording indicating it is probably right-sided in origin. The ejection systolic murmur is quite long in duration.

to cause a rise in the systolic pressure in the proximal segment. *The murmurs may be at the base but also may be heard peripherally over the chest.* Rarely, there may be a gradient even in diastole and this may be associated with some turbulent flow persisting into diastole. This will be accompanied by a longer duration of the systolic murmur, which may spill, into diastole ***making the murmur continuous.***[40] Neither the intensity nor the timing of the pulmonary component of S2 is affected in supravalvular pulmonary artery stenosis. The S2 split is often entirely normal.

REGURGITANT SYSTOLIC MURMURS

Regurgitation usually implies blood flow in the reverse direction across the cardiac chambers usually from a high pressure chamber into a low pressure chamber. Regurgitation ***during systole*** can occur under the following conditions:

1. ***When the mitral valve is incompetent,*** reverse flow can occur from the high pressure LV into the low pressure LA.
2. ***When the tricuspid valve is incompetent,*** reverse flow can occur from the high pressure RV into the low pressure right atrium.
3. ***In VSD,*** the reverse flow can occur from the high pressure LV into the low pressure RV across the septal defect.
4. ***In persistent ductus arteriosus,*** the reverse flow can occur from the high pressure AO into the low pressure pulmonary artery through the ductus. In this condition, however, the reverse flow in systole can also continue into the diastole as long as the pulmonary resistance is lower than the systemic resistance.

The characteristics of regurgitant systolic murmurs are as follows:

1. The high pressure gradient that is usually present in most regurgitant lesions mentioned above will imply that *regurgitant systolic murmurs will have pre-dominantly high frequency* and this will make the murmurs sound more blowing in quality.[42] They can be imitated by long whispering "hoo", "haaa" or saying long "shoo".
2. *The regurgitant murmur could acquire lower and medium frequencies and sounds harsher if the degree of regurgitation is severe* resulting in large amount of backward flow.
3. Since the pressure gradient often persists between the chambers well into the isovolumic relaxation phase and beyond, the murmur often will not end before the S2 and will often spill over into the very early part of diastole. *Thus, there is generally no pause between the end of the murmur and the S2*. The audibility of S2 with a regurgitant murmur however is mainly related to the relative loudness of the murmur and the S2. The S2 may be audible if the grade of the murmur is softer than the grade of the S2. If the murmur is louder than the S2, then the murmur lasting all the way to the S2 will engulf the S2. This will result in S2 not being heard separately.
4. *Regurgitant murmurs unlike ejection murmurs usually do not change in intensity significantly following sudden long diastole* as may happen following the compensatory pause after a pre-mature or ectopic beat or during varying cycle lengths in atrial fibrillation.[43] The mechanisms involved in post-extrasystolic potentiation were discussed under ejection murmurs. *Regurgitant lesions imply that there are two outlets for the blood to flow during systole*. For instance, in the case of mitral regurgitation, one outlet is the AO and the other is through the regurgitant or incompetent mitral valve into the LA. The extra volume of blood received by the ventricle during the long diastolic interval by the Starling mechanism will increase the contractility of the ventricle. This will be further aided by the extrasystolic potentiation from the pre-mature depolarization. During the long diastolic pause, the aortic pressure will continue to fall and this will result in decrease in afterload when the ventricle will begin to eject. The more complete emptying of the ventricle will result in larger amount of forward flow into the AO due to the fall in afterload accompanying the falling aortic pressure during the pause. This usually means that the volume of blood going in the reverse direction would remain relatively the same keeping the regurgitant flow and the resulting murmur the same.

MITRAL REGURGITATION

Normal Mitral Valve and Function

The mitral valve apparatus is a complex unit which comprises of the annulus, the anterior and the posterior mitral leaflets, the chordae tendineae, the papillary muscles and the underlying left ventricular wall.[44-47] The annulus shares a common attachment to the aortic root anteriorly. The posterior annulus is a large fibromuscular structure. The commissural areas can be easily defined by the recognition of the fan-shaped chordae "the commissural chordae". These arise as single stems and branch like the struts of a fan to insert into the free margins of the leaflet tissue at the commissures (Fig. 7.17A). Although both the commissural area have equal amount of valvular tissue, the posteromedial commissural chordae have a wider spread making this region more vulnerable for mitral regurgitation. The posterior leaflet, which covers a larger annular circumference, is usually divided into three scallops, the middle one being the largest with two smaller scallops on either side near the commissures. Fan-shaped chords also insert into the clefts in between the scallops of the posterior leaflet (Fig. 7.17B). The anterior leaflet is generally however larger than the middle scallop of the posterior leaflet. The distal third of the leaflet surface is rough to palpation and receives the insertion of chordae on the ventricular aspect. The rough zone of both the anterior and the posterior leaflets receives insertion of chordae. Typically each rough zone chord divides into three branches, the first branch inserts into the free margin, the second branch inserts beyond the free margin at the line of closure (the proximal edge of the rough zone) and the third branch in between the two (Fig. 7.17C). Two of the rough zone chordae to the anterior leaflet are by far the thickest and these arise from the tips of the papillary muscles and insert between the four and five o'clock position on the posteromedial side and between seven and eight o'clock position on the anterolateral side. These are the strut chordae (Fig. 7.17D). Avulsion or rupture of these would result in severe mitral regurgitation.

The chordae passing to the anterolateral commissure and the adjoining half of the anterior and the posterior leaflets arise from the anterolateral papillary muscle group. The chordae passing to the posteromedial commissure and the adjoining half of the anterior and the posterior leaflets arise from the posteromedial papillary muscle group. In all, there are 25 chordae that insert into the mitral valve: 9 into the anterior leaflet, 14 into the posterior leaflet and 2 into the commissures.[47]

There are two groups of papillary muscles in the LV, the anterolateral and the posteromedial. Each group supplies one-half of the chordae to one-half of both leaflets. Each group of papillary muscle may have one or two distinct "bellies" of muscle occasionally more than two especially in the posteromedial group. The Left ventricular papillary muscle groups may have varying morphologic features. They may be free and finger-like, very much tethered to the underlying sub-endocardium of the ventricular wall or have an intermediate morphology. The arterial supply for the anterolateral papillary muscle arises from the anterior descending, one of the diagonal branches or the marginal branches of the circumflex. The posteromedial group derives its blood supply from the right coronary or the circumflex branch of the left coronary artery. The arterial vasculature of the papillary muscles is often related to the morphologic feature. The finger-like papillary muscle has a central artery, which arises at its base from one of the epicardial arteries. This vessel is often terminal and has very few vascular connections to the extrapapillary sub-endocardial network (Fig. 7.17E). The tethered type of papillary muscle often has a segmental type of distribution of the long penetrating intramyocardial vessels. The mixed or the intermediate type has a mixed

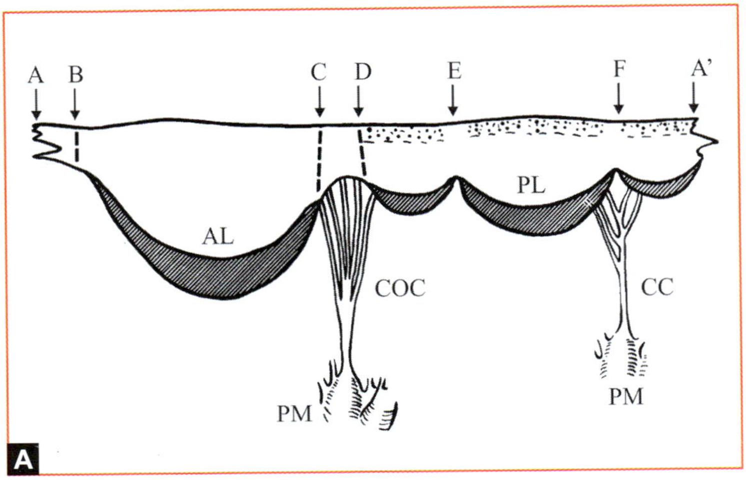

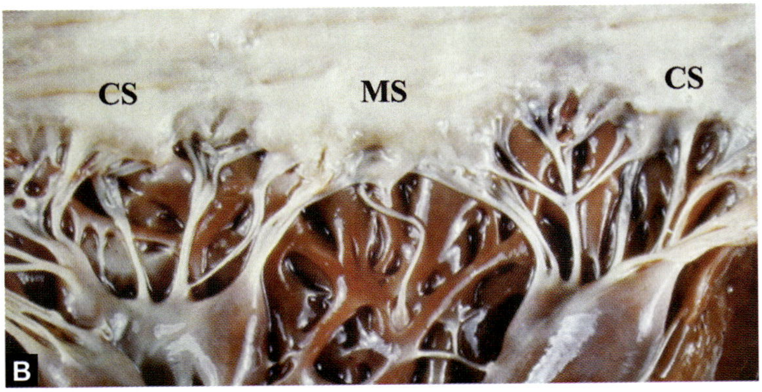

Figs. 7.17A and B: (A) The diagrammatic representation of the mitral valve (MV) cut open to show the atrial surface of the anterior leaflet (AL) on the right and the posterior leaflet (PL) on the left side. The commissural chordae, which are fan-shaped charade, insert and define the commissural areas between the AL and the PL. C-D is the posteromedial commissural area whereas A-B is the anterolateral commissural area. The distal third of the leaflets is thick and rough and receives insertion of chordae on the ventricular surfaces. The proximal two-thirds of the leaflet are clear and membranous. The PL is usually a tri-scalloped structure. Fan-shaped chords called the cleft chordae insert and define the clefts between the individual scallops of the PL. Source: Modified and reproduced from Ranganathan N, Lam JH, Wigle ED, Silver MD. Morphology of the human mitral valve. II. The value leaflets. Circulation. 1970;41:459-67; with kind permission from Lippincott Williams and Wilkins). (B) The MV cut open to show the atrial surface of the normal triscalloped PL. The middle scallop is usually the largest with the two respective commissural scallops on either side of it. The fan-shaped chordae insert into the clefts between the individual scallops.

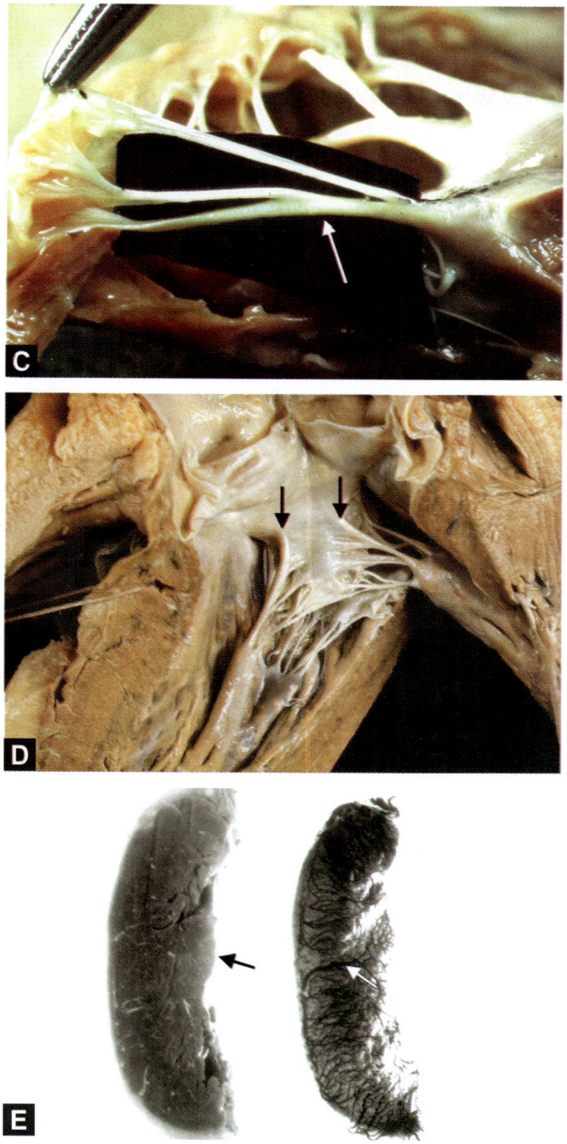

Figs. 7.17C to E: (C) shows a typical rough zone chordae with its three branches, the first inserting into the free margin of the leaflet, the second inserting into the proximal edge of the rough zone and the third in between the two on the ventricular aspect of the mitral leaflet. (D) shows the anterior mitral leaflet and its attachment to the aortic root. The arrows indicate the two strut chordae arising from the tips of the papillary muscles and inserting on the rough zone of the ventricular surface of the anterior mitral leaflet. (E) shows the excised left ventricular wall obtained at necropsy demonstrating a free finger-like morphology of the papillary muscle (the right half) and its arterial supply (on the left half) demonstrated by contrast injection into the coronary vessels with stereo-radiography prior to the section. The finger-like papillary muscle has arterial supply through a central artery with very few vascular connections to the extrapapillary sub-endocardial network.

type arterial vasculature.[46] The arterial vasculature has a bearing on the incidence of papillary muscle dysfunction in ischemic heart disease.

When the LV contracts and raises the pressure during systole above that of the LA, the mitral valve leaflets come together and close the orifice. After the valve closure the continued rise in pressure from the ventricular contraction will open the aortic valve once the pressure exceeds the aortic pressure. *With the onset of ejection the ventricle will begin to decrease in volume and size. During most of ejection, the ventricular pressure remains fairly high. The chordae tendineae have fixed lengths and they cannot shorten to keep the leaflets together. The closed mitral valve leaflets will evert and prolapse into the LA under the high pressure but for the synchronous and effective contraction of the papillary muscles and the underlying left ventricular myocardium. The muscular fibers in the annulus do contract to help reduce the annular width toward the end of systole as well thereby maintaining a competent valve (Fig. 7.18).*

Causes of Mitral Regurgitation

The mitral regurgitation therefore can arise from anatomic and/or functional defect from any one of the components of its complex anatomy.[48] The lesion may result from a congenital or an acquired cause. The process may be

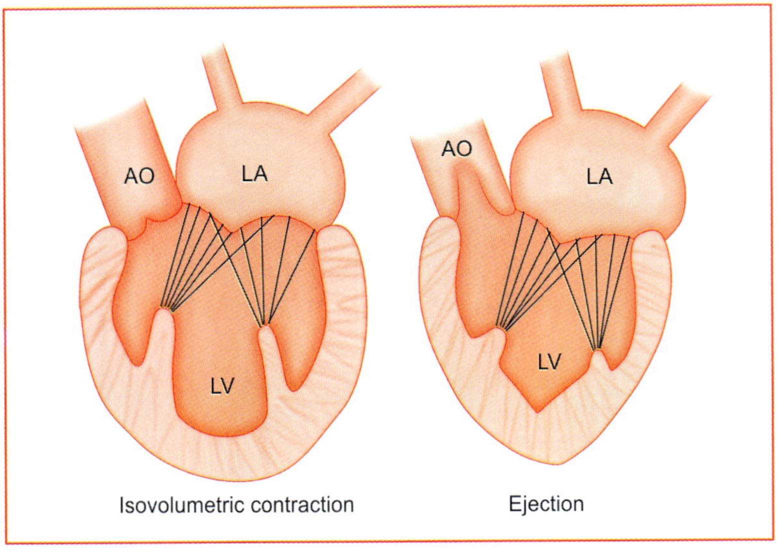

Fig. 7.18: Diagrammatic representation of the normal spatial relationship between the mitral valve and the left ventricular cavity. This relationship seen at the onset of systole at the isovolumic phase is maintained during the remainder of systole during the ejection phase despite the rising intraventricular pressure and decreasing size of the left ventricular cavity, by the contracting papillary muscles and the underlying left ventricular wall that prevents eversion of the mitral leaflets into the left atrium keeping the mitral valve competent.

genetic, inflammatory, infective, traumatic, ischemic, degenerative or neoplastic in nature. As often is the case, more than one component of the structures may be involved. Rarely mitral regurgitation may also be induced iatrogenically during surgical commissurotomy or balloon techniques of mitral valvuloplasty for relief of mitral stenosis.

Annular Abnormalities

The annulus may become idiopathically dilated or calcified and therefore may not function normally. Dilated annulus making the orifice larger allows poor apposition of the leaflets. This is compounded by the fact that it also contracts poorly. Calcification on the other hand interferes with the normal annular contraction.

Leaflet and Chordal Abnormalities

The leaflet may be congenitally cleft and this abnormality may be seen in association with ostium primum atrial septal defect.[40] The leaflets may also be congenitally large and redundant and may show overhanging hooded or prolapsed appearance due to myxomatous degeneration.[49,50] The chordae may also be excessively lengthened as well showing some thickening. The chordae could rupture spontaneously if the elastic fibers are significantly destroyed due to myxomatous degeneration. The leaflets on the other hand may be contracted and scarred due to repeated inflammation as may happen with rheumatic involvement. It may eventually show areas of calcification. The chordae that are scarred and shortened will prevent proper leaflet closure. In addition, the commissures may be fused resulting in varying degrees of stenosis. In infective endocarditis, the infective process could cause destructive lesions in the leaflets or the chordae besides formation of vegetation. The latter may interfere with proper leaflet apposition particularly when large. The chordae could rupture as a result of the infective process.[51] In congenitally corrected transposition of the great vessels that is a rare congenital defect, the left AV valve that has the morphology similar to that of the tricuspid valve of the normal heart, may show downward displacement as inEbstein's anomaly. With this malformation, part of the arterial ventricle gets atrialized and thin and the valve is often incompetent resulting in "mitralregurgitation."[52]

Papillary Muscle and Left Ventricular Wall Pathology

In ischemic heart disease, the papillary muscles may not contract properly due to ischemia with or without concurrent necrosis that may also involve the underlying myocardium.[53-56] The papillary muscles may show scarring due to ischemic damage. When ischemic necrosis occurs involving the papillary muscles sometimes this could lead to avulsion of the chordal origin from the necrotic muscle.[57,58] Papillary muscle could also rupture due to its involvement in the acute infarction.[59] In late stages of infarction with development of aneurysm of the underlying myocardium, the papillary muscles may be displaced and the distortion may make the valve incompetent.[55] Similar disturbance in function could occur in other myocardial diseases like dilated cardiomyopathy.

Atrial Myxoma

Rarely a left atrial myxoma, which is considered a benign tumor usually, attached to the atrial septum by a stalk, could be large enough to prolapse into the LV during diastole. With the onset of systole, the tumor may move back into the LA but in the process may obstruct proper leaflet apposition and cause mitral regurgitation.[60]

The severity of the mitral regurgitation may depend on the extent of the lesions and the functional derangement as well as the acuteness of the process. Long-standing mitral regurgitation would result in left atrial and left ventricular dilatation, which will further cause stretching of the annulus making the mitral regurgitation worse. Thus ***"mitral regurgitation begets more mitral regurgitation".***

Pathophysiology of Mitral Regurgitation

Chronic Mitral Regurgitation

Mitral regurgitation is ***a volume overload state for the LV*** since during diastole the ventricle receives not only the normal pulmonary venous return but also the extra volume of blood, which went into the LA during systole. This volume overload when significant would result in left ventricular dilatation and enlargement. The LV dilatation is accompanied initially by a better compliance of the LV, which helps to maintain relatively normal left ventricular diastolic pressures ***(pre a wave)*** despite the large volume of blood, which enters the LV during diastole. *The LA will also become enlarged when the regurgitation is significant and chronic in duration. The left atrial enlargement is accompanied by increased compliance of the LA that helps to maintain a low v wave pressure in the LA during systole despite increased volume it receives due to the regurgitation (Figs. 7.19A and B). In addition, the LV has an advantage during systole since it has two outlets for emptying namely the AO as well as the LA. The two outlet system allows a supernormal emptying (ejection fraction) when the ventricular function is normal and preserved and a near normal ejection fraction when the LV actually develops some dysfunction.[61-63]*

In late stages however, the increased size of the LV will lead to increased wall tension stimulating hypertrophy. The hypertrophy is often eccentric rather than concentric.[64] This will reduce the left ventricular compliance.

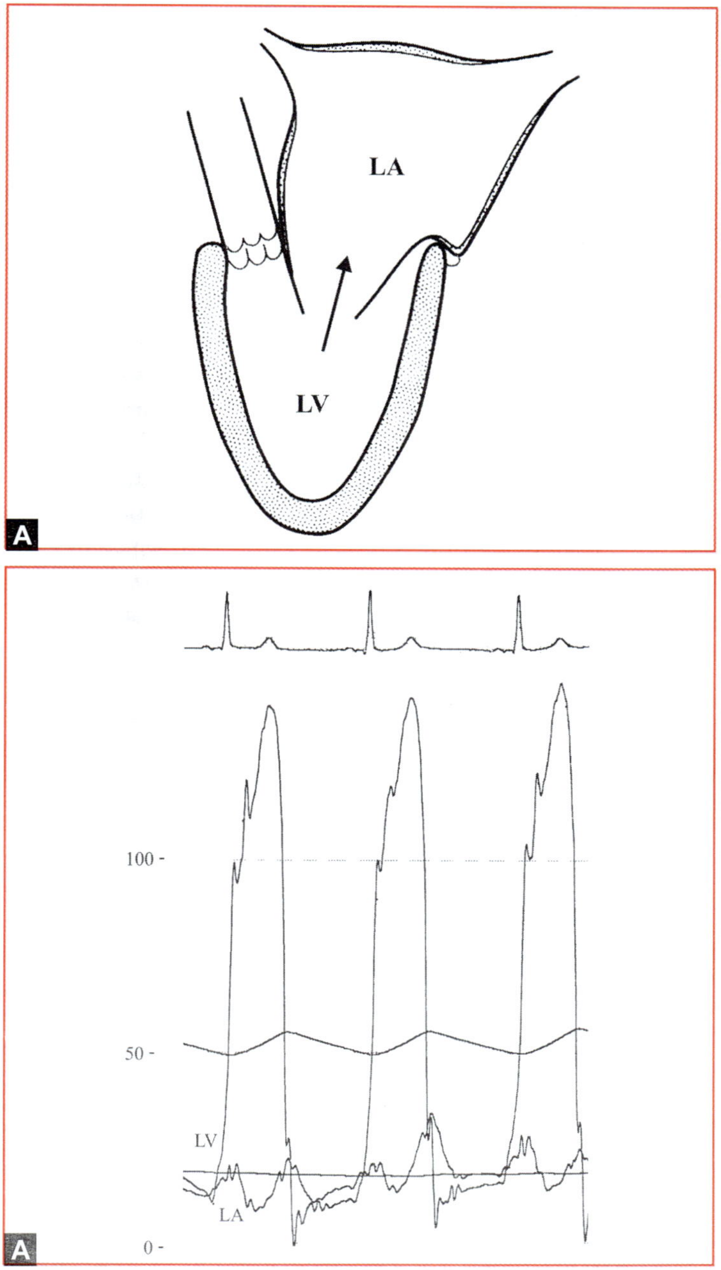

Figs. 7.19A and B: (A) Diagrammatic representation of the left atrium (LA) and the left ventricle (LV) in chronic severe mitral regurgitation. The volume overload leads to enlargement and dilatation of the LV and the LA. The LV however has a systolic advantage since it has two outlets. (B) Simultaneous recordings of the electrocardiogram, the left ventricular (LV) and the left atrial (LA) pressure curves from a patient with chronic severe mitral regurgitation showing only a mild elevation of the left atrial v wave. The pressure difference between the LV and the LA is seen to persist throughout systole.

In addition, sub-endocardial ischemia and fibrosis may develop that will further depress the compliance and begin to raise the ***"pre a wave pressure".*** Since the latter forms the baseline filling pressure over which the ***a*** and ***v waves*** build up occur (very similar to what has been shown and discussed in relation to the right-sided pressures under jugular venous pulsations—*see* Chapter 4), the raised ***pre a wave*** pressure will further raise the ***v wave*** pressure height in the LA. The upper normal left ventricular diastolic pressure for the end of diastole ***(post a wave)*** is usually between 12 and 15 mm Hg whereas the upper normal left ventricular ***pre a wave*** pressure is between 5 and 8 mm Hg. The normal ***v wave*** in the LA may be between 12 and 18 mm Hg. In chronic mitral regurgitation even when the regurgitation is severe, the left atrial ***v wave*** height may only be mild to moderately elevated (20–35 mm Hg.) This would mean a persistent pressure difference between the LV and the LA throughout systole making the regurgitant flow to last until the very end of systole and well into the isovolumic relaxation phase (*see* Fig. 7.19B). The murmur therefore usually lasts for the whole of systole (thus termed pansystolic) and thus all the way to the S2. In addition, the gradient remains relatively large and constant from the beginning of systole to its end giving rise to a plateau high frequency murmur.

Acute Mitral Regurgitation

If the mitral regurgitation is severe and acute in onset as with ruptured chordae, then there may *not be enough time to develop compensatory dilatation of either the LA or the LV (Fig. 7.20A). The large volume of regurgitant blood entering a relatively stiff and non-dilated LA will result in steep rise in the v wave pressure in the LA (sometimes as high as 50–70 mm Hg) (Fig. 7.20B).*[65,66] The entry of large volume of blood during diastole into a non-dilated LV will tend to raise the diastolic filling pressures in the LV. The raised ***pre a wave*** pressure may further add to the ***v wave*** height. *The high v wave build up in the LA during systole would mean a decreased and rapidly falling pressure difference between the LV and the LA toward the later part of systole. This will in turn limit the regurgitant flow during later part of systole making the regurgitant flow and the murmur decrescendo. In addition, the excess flow would cause lower and medium frequencies making the murmur sound harsher.*

Characteristics of Mitral Regurgitation Murmurs

1. *Mitral regurgitation murmur shares all the features listed previously for all regurgitation murmurs. In general, it is high in frequency and blowing in quality, usually will last all the way to S2 and may even spill slightly beyond S2 (Fig. 7.21).*

2. *It may be harsh and have low and medium frequencies if the regurgitation is severe.*
3. *Mitral regurgitation murmurs will be expected to change very little in loudness following sudden long diastole as may happen in atrial fibrillation or following an ectopic beat (Fig. 7.22).*
4. *Mitral regurgitation murmurs may have different shapes depending on the etiology (Fig. 7.23). It is often pansystolic in relatively fixed orifice regurgitation as with rheumatic involvement. It may be confined to mid- and late-systole when due to papillary muscle dysfunction or caused by prolapsed myxomatous mitral leaflets and chordae (Fig. 7.24). In these conditions it may also increase in intensity toward the end of systole, i.e. crescendo to the S2. With prolapsed myxomatous mitral leaflets and chordae the mid-late systolic murmur may start with a mid-systolic click or clicks. In addition in this disorder, the murmur may be shown to start earlier in systole and also increase in intensity with maneuvers that decrease the ventricular size such as standing. With squatting, that will cause increased venous return and therefore increase the ventricular size, the click will start later and the murmur may either disappear or decrease in intensity.*[49,67–69] *Rarely mitral regurgitation may be confined to early and mid-systole, start with S1 and become decrescendo. This is characteristically associated with acute and severe mitral regurgitation caused by ruptured chordae. Because of the excess flow the murmur will also be harsh due to a lot of low and medium frequencies.*[65]
5. *Irrespective of the etiology, the mitral regurgitation murmur is maximal in loudness at the apex. The murmur may be equally louder slightly lateral to the apex.*

Severity of Mitral Regurgitation

1. The loudness of the mitral regurgitation murmur does not always correlate with the severity of the regurgitation. ***If the murmur is harsher*** and has a lot of low and medium frequencies it usually indicates ***a lot of flow*** and therefore will imply significant regurgitation.
2. If the murmur, on the other hand, is all pure high frequency and confined only to late systole, then it must indicate a high pressure difference between the LV and the LA and therefore only mild regurgitation.
3. When the mitral regurgitation is severe, the volume overload on the LV will be high resulting in an enlarged LV. This may be reflected in a displaced hyperdynamic wide area left ventricular apical impulse. In addition, the hyperdynamic LV will have rapid ejection. This will make the A2 occur early resulting in a ***wide split S2.*** Thus a wide split S2 in the presence of mitral regurgitation is a sign of severe regurgitation if the wide split is not caused by P2 delay.
4. In addition, severe regurgitation due to the volume load effect will have a torrential inflow through the mitral valve during diastole. This will set up

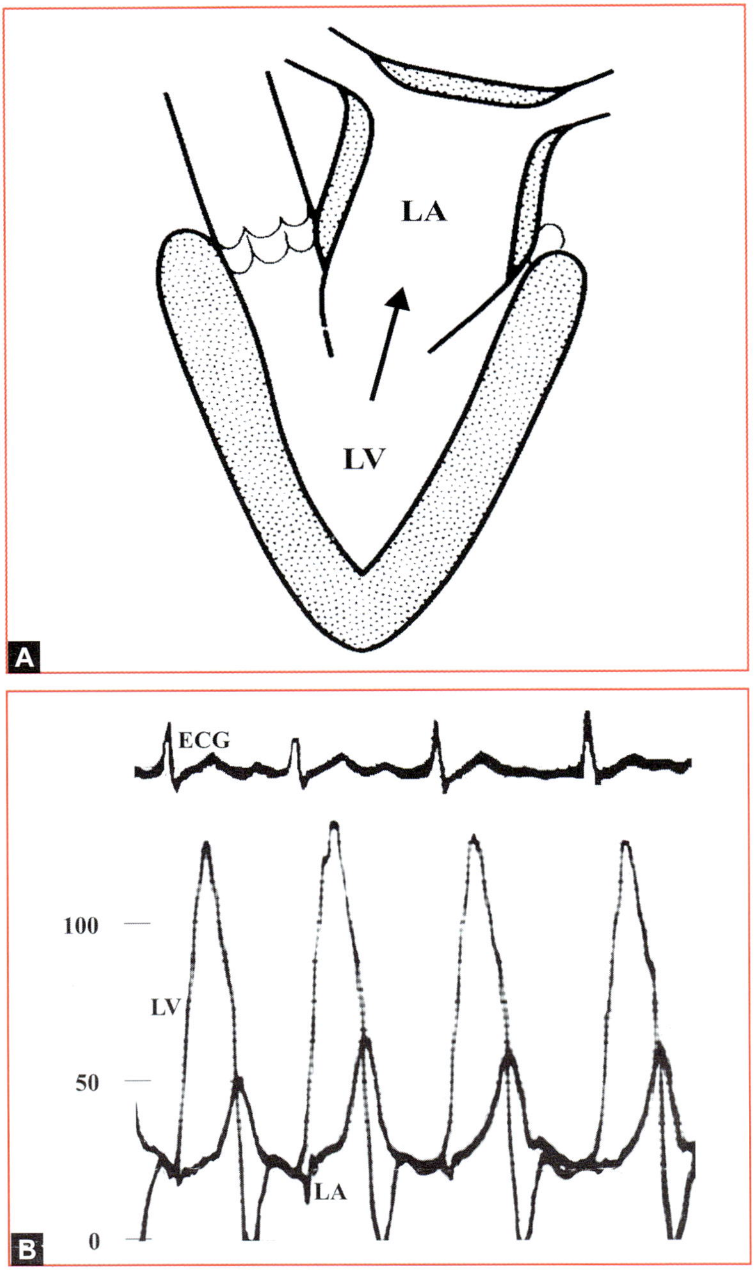

Figs. 7.20A and B: (A) Diagrammatic representation of the left atrium (LA) and the left ventricle (LV) in acute severe mitral regurgitation. The LV and the LA do not have time to develop compensatory dilatation. The relatively normal sized LA receiving a large regurgitant volume in systole builds up a high pressure. (B) Simultaneous recordings of the electrocardiogram, the left ventricular (LV) and the left atrial (LA) pressure curves from a patient with acute severe mitral regurgitation showing a high v wave measuring up to 50 mm Hg. The pressure difference between the LV and the LA is seen to fall toward the later part of systole, which will in turn limit the regurgitation during this phase.

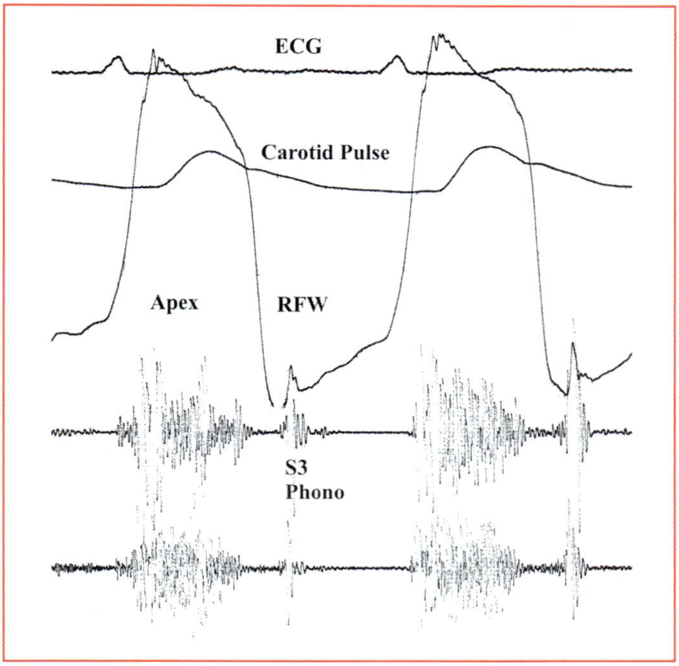

Fig. 7.21: Simultaneous recordings of electrocardiogram, the carotid pulse, the apex-cardiogram (Apex) and phonocardiogram (Phono) from a patient with severe mitral regurgitation taken at the apex area. The systolic murmur is seen to last all the way to the second heart sound. The Apex shows an exaggerated rapid filling wave with a corresponding third heard sound on the Phono.

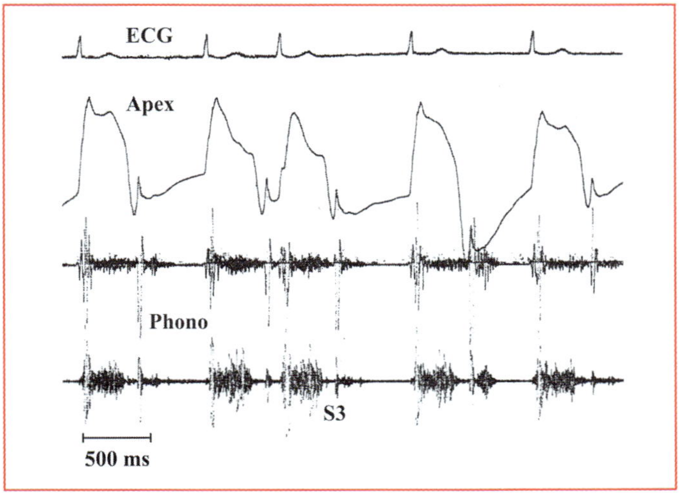

Fig. 7.22: Simultaneous recordings of the electrocardiogram, the apexcardiogram (Apex) and the Phono from a patient with mitral regurgitation and atrial fibrillation. Note that the changing diastolic durations and the varying filling do not affect the intensity of the systolic regurgitant murmur. The presence of the third heart sound would indicate that the regurgitation must be significant.

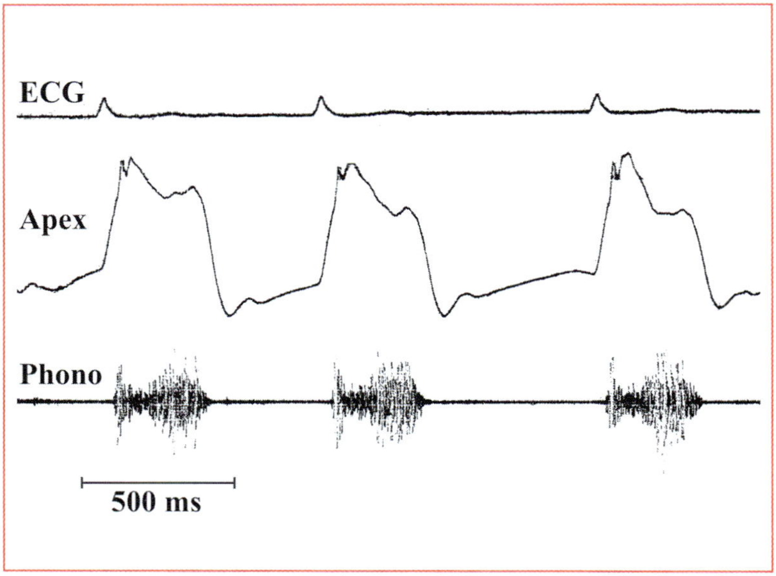

Fig. 7.23: Simultaneous recordings of the electrocardiogram, the apexcardiogram (Apex) and the phonocardiogram (Phono) from a patient with mitral regurgitation secondary to prolapsed myxomatous mitral valves taken from the apex area showing accentuation in intensity of the murmur in late systole.

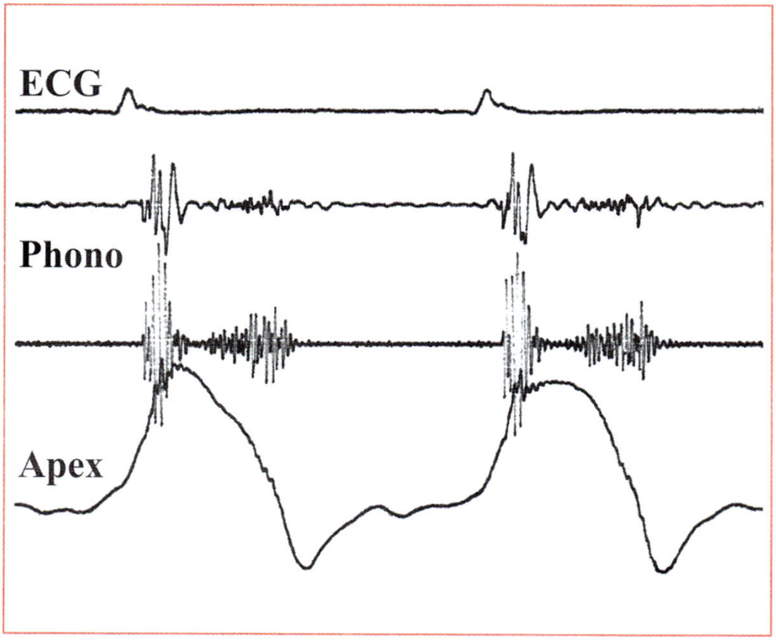

Fig. 7.24: Simultaneous recordings of the electrocardiogram, the apexcardiogram (Apex) and the phonocardiogram (Phono) from a patient with ischemic heart disease and papillary muscle dysfunction. The regurgitant murmur is late systolic in timing and appears to peak toward the end of systole.

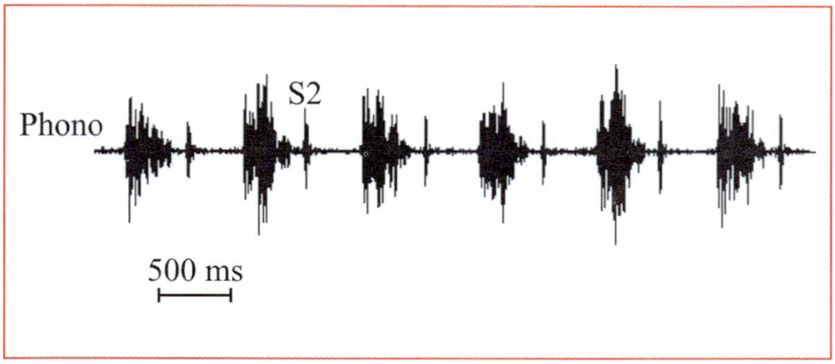

Fig. 7.25: Digital display of a magnetic audio recording from a patient with acute severe mitral regurgitation secondary to ruptured chordae taken from the apex area. The murmur diminishes in intensity toward the later part of systole (decrescendo shape).

the necessary conditions for the production of an ***S3 or a mid-diastolic inflow rumble.*** The presence of an S3 or an inflow rumble at the apex will therefore be a sign of significant mitral regurgitation as well.

5. As mentioned previously, a ***harsh decrescendo mitral regurgitation murmur*** is usually indicative of severe regurgitation since the decrescendo effect is caused by early build-up of a very high ***v wave*** pressure in the LA due to a severe degree of regurgitation, thus decreasing the gradient in late systole (Fig. 7.25).
6. *Severe mitral regurgitation may also cause symptoms and signs of high left atrial pressure such as nocturnal dyspnea, orthopnea, and pulmonary congestion both clinically and radiologically.*
7. The elevated left atrial pressure indirectly may also raise the pulmonary artery pressures causing ***signs of pulmonary hypertension.*** The latter may be evidenced by the presence of elevated venous pressure with or without abnormal jugular contours, loud and/or palpable P2, sustained right ventricular impulse as judged by sub-xiphoid palpation.

Specific Etiologic Types of Mitral Regurgitation

Rheumatic Mitral Regurgitation

In acute rheumatic fever the inflammatory process may affect the leaflets or the chordae and the valve may become incompetent with somewhat rolled up edges of the leaflets without any significant stenosis. With chronic rheumatic involvement the mitral valve pre-dominantly becomes stenotic due to commissural fusion. When the leaflets are significantly tethered and in particular contracted, then mitral regurgitation could result. The pathologic changes will often be such that the orifice is not only stenosed but also fails to close completely so as to cause regurgitation. Calcification of the leaflets may occur but is not a pre-requisite for regurgitation. Rarely the posterior leaflet may be more involved and significantly retracted and contracted resulting in pre-dominant or pure regurgitation alone. Occasionally after mitral stenosis is either surgically corrected by open or closed commissurotomy or by the modern balloon valvuloplasty one may have some iatrogenic mitral regurgitation. This may be caused by unintended non-commissural tears. In long standing cases, marked left atrial enlargement eventually will result in the development of atrial fibrillation. The underlying rheumatic process may also involve the atrium and the conduction system including the sinoatrial node, which also pre-disposes partly to the development of atrial fibrillation.

Mitral regurgitation due to rheumatic process has pathophysiologic changes described under chronic mitral regurgitation. The murmur is often typical high frequency and blowing with maximal loudness at the apex. It often begins with S1 and will generally last all the way to S2. The S1 intensity may be normal if the ventricular function is not impaired and the mitral regurgitation is not severe. If diminished, it must indicate that one or both factors may be operative. The associated findings of stenosis such as a loud S1, an opening snap or the mitral diastolic murmur may or may not be present. If the regurgitation is severe however a short mid-diastolic rumble may be heard indicative of the large volume load causing excess mitral inflow.

Mitral Regurgitation Secondary to the Prolapsed Mitral Leaflets

The most common cause of isolated mitral regurgitation (i.e. without mitral stenosis) particularly in the developed countries would appear to be non-rheumatic in etiology. Myxomatous degeneration leads the list under the non-rheumatic causes.[51,63,70] Myxomatous degeneration of the mitral leaflets and chordae may be isolated and idiopathic, and rarely familial. It can also occur as part of other inherited connective tissue defect such as the Marfan's syndrome. The disorder may be associated with mitral regurgitation in all age groups and often somewhat more common in the female gender.[49,69,71-77] The posterior mitral leaflet is more commonly affected. The involved scallops of the posterior leaflet become markedly hooded and redundant. The chordae often are thickened and elongated as well. Often the annulus is also involved in the process and shows dilatation. The condition results in prolapse of the hooded and redundant leaflets during systole. This may be identified on a 2D echocardiographic imaging or a left ventricular angiogram easily.

The onset of prolapse typically is quite early in systole in the excessively redundant valves. This is clearly different from some bulging of the normal mitral leaflets at end systole, which may be seen in any 2D echo imaging. *The maximal prolapse with the abnormal redundant leaflets and chordae will occur at a critical ventricular dimension.[77] The critical dimension is relatable to the leaflet and chordal redundancy or length since chordae have fixed lengths and they cannot shorten during systole.* When the ventricular dimension diminishes during systole, the chordal length may become disproportionately longer at certain time during systole when the leaflets could no longer be maintained together and the involved leaflet or the parts of the leaflet will bulge or prolapse into the LA (Fig. 7.26). The S1 intensity is often well preserved since the mitral leaflet coaptation is intact initially and the column of blood will be able to decelerate against the closed valve as in the normals. However, as systole proceeds, the leaflets may become prolapsed once the critical dimension is reached that is dependent as mentioned on the redundancy of the leaflet and chordae. The column of blood will not only be ejected through the AO but part of the blood mass will also continue to move behind the bulging leaflets toward the low pressure LA. When the prolapse reaches the maximum limit as determined by the ventricular dimension achieved, there will be a sudden deceleration of the column of blood against the prolapsed leaflet or scallops. This may be associated with an audible clicking sound during middle of systole termed ***the non-ejection click (Fig. 7.27A).*** Sometimes there could be multiple clicks. The latter may represent minute variations in time of maximal prolapse of the different portions of the leaflet (Fig. 7.27B). The timing of the clicks may vary in systole. They can also be made to come earlier or later by maneuvers that alter the venous return and thereby the ventricular size. For instance, standing the patient suddenly by decreasing the venous return will make the heart small and bring the maximal prolapse early and thereby make the click come earlier. Squatting by increasing the venous return and the ventricular size will make the click occur later. Mitral leaflets may lose coaptation once prolapse begins to occur and this will result in the onset of mitral regurgitation in early or mid-systole. The regurgitation may become more in late systole when the ventricle reaches the maximum shortening and causes maximal prolapse. Thus the click in mid-systole may be followed by a late systolic regurgitant high frequency murmur (Figs. 7.27C and 7.28). The auscultatory features associated with the prolapsed mital valve leaflets may vary. Occasionally, the patient may only have a non-ejection click. The murmur of mitral regurgitation may be intermittent. In some the click is followed by the typical late systolic murmur. In others the regurgitation may start quite early in systole and last throughout systole and cause a pansystolic murmur. The non-ejection click may then be conspicuously absent. In some patients the mitral regurgitation murmur associated with the prolapsed leaflets may have a peculiar loud ***honking or whooping*** quality. Occasionally, the patients themselves may be aware of the loud systolic honk or the whoop. Sometimes they may be audible from a distance.

The disorder when it occurs in the idiopathic form may be characterized by symptoms, which have no particular relationship to the degree or severity of the mitral regurgitation. The patients may present for reason of chest pains, palpitations or abnormal T waves in the electrocardiogram (ECG), arrhythmias or simply on account of the characteristic auscultatory features. They may exhibit certain skeletal abnormalities such as scoliosis, significant laxity of joints and a high arched palate. In some patients with chest pain in this condition abnormal lactate uptake has been demonstrated and in some coronary spasm has also been shown. Some patients may have transient embolic symptoms due to platelet thrombi forming between the hooded leaflets and the left atrial wall underneath it. Rarely infective endocarditis may develop. In view of the variety of symptoms that they may present with, the disorder is often described as ***idiopathic prolapsed mitral leaflet syndrome.*** The mitral regurgitation is usually mild or mild to moderate in most patients. However, it can become more severe and cause acute symptoms of high left atrial pressure such as sudden pulmonary edema, orthopnea or paroxysmal nocturnal dyspnea. The reason for such deterioration is usually ruptured chordae either due to spontaneous rupture or secondary to infective endocarditis.

Occasionally, papillary muscle dysfunction can be associated with prolapse of the leaflets but careful assessment of the leaflet and chordal morphology on the 2D echo image as well as the assessment of the mitral annular dimension will help to identify secondary prolapse as a result of papillary muscle dysfunction as opposed to the prolapse due to chordal leaflet pathology. Rarely coronary disease can exist with the prolapsed and abnormal

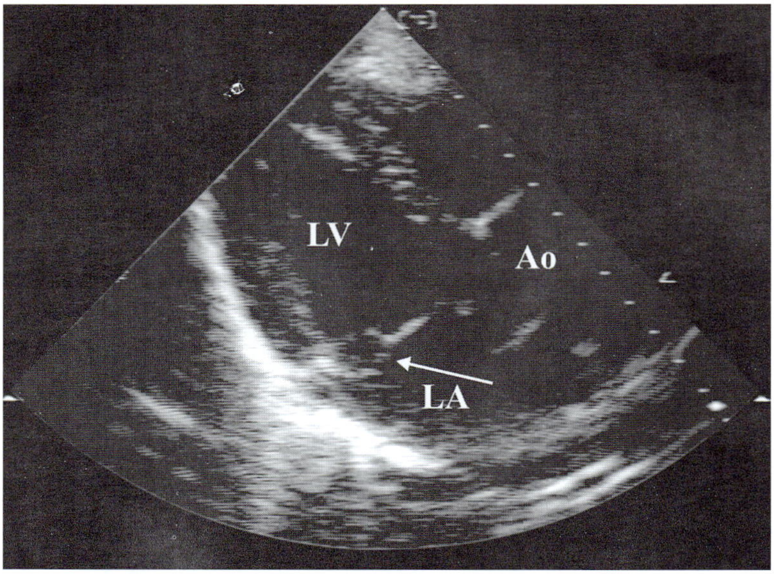

Fig. 7.26: Two-dimensional echocardiographic image of the left ventricle, the aorta and the left atrium (LA), in the parasternal long axis from a patient with redundant myxomatous posterior mitral leaflet scallops with prolapse and mitral regurgitation. Stop frame taken relatively early in systole shows the bulging posterior mitral leaflet (arrow) prolapsing into the LA.

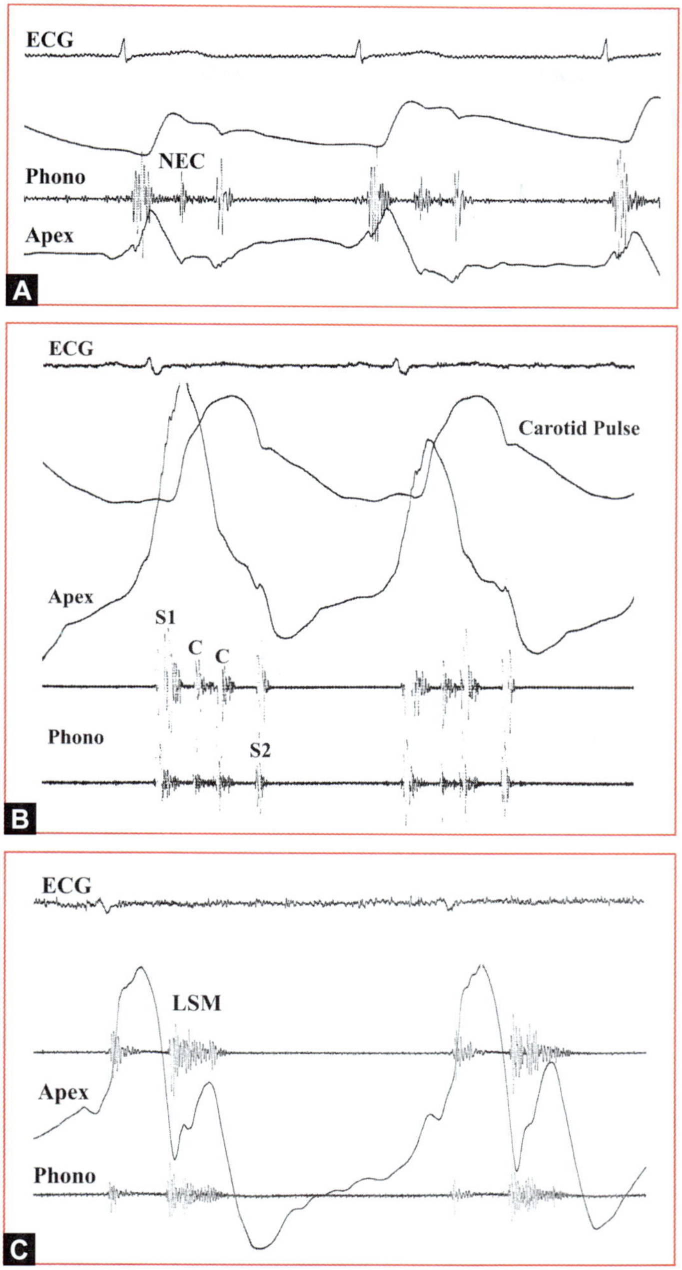

Figs. 7.27A to C: (A) Simultaneous recordings of the electrocardiogram (ECG), the carotid pulse (CP), the apexcardiogram (Apex) and the phonocardiogram (Phono) from a patient with prolapsed mitral valve (MV) syndrome taken from the apex area showing a mid-systolic non-ejection click (NEC). (B) Simultaneous recordings of the ECG, the CP, the apexcardiogram (Apex) and the Phono from a patient with prolapsed MV syndrome taken from the apex area showing two clicks (C) in systole. (C) Simultaneous recordings of the ECG, the apexcardiogram (Apex) and the Phono from a patient with prolapsed MV syndrome taken from the apex area showing a systolic murmur confined to late systole.

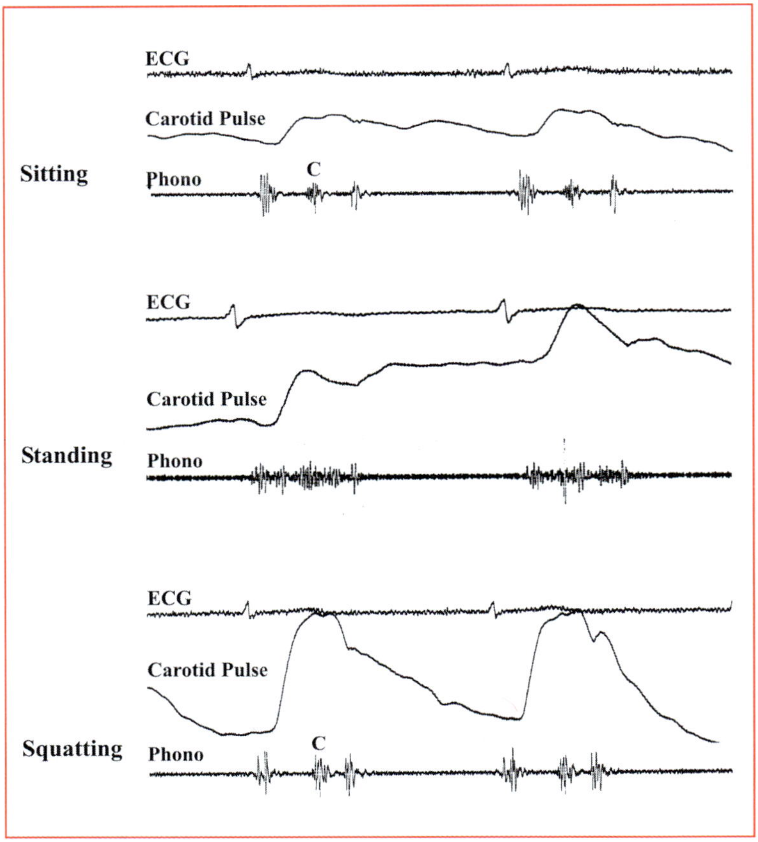

Fig. 7.28: Simultaneous recordings of the electrocardiogram, the carotid pulse and the phonocardiogram (Phono) from a patient with prolapsed mitral valve syndrome taken from the apex area demonstrating the effect of changing postures on the auscultatory findings. The systolic click (C) is seen to occur earlier in systole in the sitting position compared to the squatting position. While on standing the click is replaced by a pansystolic mitral regurgitation murmur.

mitral leaflets in the same patient. Coexistence with hypertrophic obstructive cardiomyopathy has also been described. In some rare patients with hypertrophic obstructive cardiomyopathy, loud mid-systolic non-ejection clicks may be heard.[78] Our observation in one such patient revealed the coexistence of abnormal prolapsed and redundant mitral leaflet at surgery for relief of the severe outflow obstruction.

Mitral Regurgitation Secondary to Papillary Muscle Dysfunction

In ischemic heart disease, mitral regurgitation may be noted to develop during an active episode of angina and *the murmur may be noted to be typically late systolic and often crescendo to the S2. It is often high in frequency.*[79] The murmur may actually disappear when the angina is relieved by nitroglycerin or rest. However, if one were to selectively damage the papillary muscle belly alone without affecting the underlying left ventricular myocardium as can be done in experimental animal models, mitral regurgitation does not always develop.[53] The reason for this is that a scarred or fibrosed papillary muscle alone may not lead to any failure in maintaining mitral leaflet coaptation as long as the left ventricular contraction is preserved at the base of the papillary muscles. The contraction at the base pulling on the scarred papillary muscles can effectively maintain the mitral leaflets together. This observation has therefore led to the concept that *mitral regurgitation due to papillary muscle dysfunction usually implies that the left ventricular myocardium underneath the papillary muscles must also be involved in the dysfunction.*[54] Hypokinesis of the sub-papillary myocardium can result in impaired lateral shortening in the interpapillary muscle distance between the papillary muscles as shown by cardiac magnetic resonance imaging in humans.[80] The loss of lateral shortening can tether the leaflet edges preventing proper closure. *This does not exclude the possibility of mitral regurgitation from a markedly contracted and scarred papillary muscle* that can effectively keep the leaflets retracted or pulled down on the affected side thereby preventing proper coaptation of the two leaflets during systole.[55,56]

The arterial vasculature of the papillary muscles has been shown to be related to the morphology of the papillary muscle itself. The free and finger-like papillary muscles would appear to be more vulnerable in ischemic disease due to the less prominent collateral connection to the extrapapillary sub-endocardial network in this morphologic type. It is reasonable to expect that acute coronary occlusion can result in necrosis of the papillary muscle and the underlying left ventricular wall.[46] Due to the fact that the posteromedial commissural area is wider than the anterolateral commissural area, ischemia and/or infarction involving the posteromedial group of the papillary muscles would likely produce mitral regurgitation more easily than those involving the anterolateral group. In fact, mitral regurgitation is more often clinically encountered in inferior and posterior infarction than the anterior infarction.[81,82] *Acute necrosis of the papillary muscles may leave the origins of the main stems of the rough zone chordae quite vulnerable for avulsion. Papillary muscles being the most terminal regions of the sub-endocardial circulation may suffer necrosis even though the clinical picture of the patient may be interpreted as simply acute coronary insufficiency and not necessarily acute myocardial infarction.* Depending on the location and number of chords avulsed one may develop fair degree of mitral regurgitation. For instance the mitral regurgitation can be very severe when the anterior leaflet strut chord is avulsed due to necrosis of the papillary muscle.[45,50] In addition, in acute myocardial infarction, *rarely the papillary muscle head could actually rupture causing wide open and severe mitral regurgitation and pulmonary edema.*[59]

In late stages of myocardial infarction, the underlying myocardium may become ***aneurysmal and the LV*** may become dilated. This may ***displace the papillary muscle*** base downward and produce ***distortion*** of the mitral apparatus. This will effectively interfere with proper leaflet apposition and result in mitral regurgitation.

Papillary muscle dysfunction may occur in anomalous origin of the left coronary artery from the pulmonary artery. This congenital lesion can result in ischemia and infarction of the anterolateral wall and the anterolateral papillary muscle.[40] When the high pulmonary artery pressures of the newborn fall after a few weeks of birth, the low pressure left coronary artery offers a path of least resistance through intercoronary anastomotic connections for the blood from the AO to reach the pulmonary artery. Once this retrograde flow is established, the capillary bed of the left coronary artery is bypassed and the myocardium supplied by it becomes ischemic. The symptoms characteristically start a few months after birth reflecting the lag period before retrograde flow will become established.

Papillary muscle dysfunction can also occur in myocardial diseases of other etiology besides the ischemic heart disease.[81] It can for instance occur in ***dilated cardiomyopathy.***

Clinical Features of Papillary Muscle Dysfunction

The degree or severity of mitral regurgitation in papillary muscle dysfunction is somewhat variable.[55,56,83] It can vary in severity from mild to severe depending on the underlying pathology. The murmur more typically is late systolic and crescendo to the S2. Such is the case with active ischemia. If pathologic alterations are such as to cause disruption of chordal support then the regurgitation will more than likely be pansystolic and severe depending on the extent and location of such disruption. If the pathology is such as to cause distortion of the mitral apparatus as in ventricular aneurysm then the regurgitation murmur will also be pansystolic and the severity may be variable. Mitral regurgitation with a severely scarred and retracted papillary muscle may begin early in systole and could be pansystolic or may decrease toward the end of systole.

Mitral regurgitation murmurs of papillary muscle dysfunction are like other mitral regurgitation murmurs maximal in intensity or loudness at the apex. Papillary muscle dysfunction due to active ischemia often results in a soft blowing high frequency late systolic murmur (*see* Fig. 7.24). Occasionally, the papillary muscle dysfunction due to ischemia may be associated with ***mid-systolic or non-ejection click or sound.*** The non-ejection sound or click probably arises from a similar mechanism as described with prolapsed leaflet. The ischemic papillary muscle by failure of its contraction may allow the leaflets to bulge into the LA due to rising ventricular pressure of systole. The column of blood may move with the bulging leaflets or scallops as well.

When the anatomic length of the chordal-leaflet unit is maximally taut during mid-systole, the moving column of blood underneath will suddenly become decelerated resulting in dissipation of energy and the production of the mid-systolic sound or click. The latter may occur without any significant mitral regurgitation. This click may not be as sharp and high frequency as heard in mitral leaflet prolapse.

When acute chordal avulsion has taken place due to necrosis of the papillary muscles, the resulting regurgitation murmur could be quite loud and have a fair bit of medium and low frequencies due to the large flow. On the other hand, *when acute rupture of the papillary muscle head complicates myocardial infarction, the mitral regurgitation could be quite severe and yet in some of these patients the regurgitation murmur may not be very loud and sometimes very faint or silent. This may be due to a wide open mitral valve with coexisting left ventricular dysfunction due to the myocardial infarction.*[82,84,85]

Mitral Regurgitation Secondary to Ruptured Chordae

There are approximately 25 chordae in the human mitral valve. Excepting the fan-shaped chordae that insert into the commissures between the leaflets and into the clefts between the scallops of the posterior leaflet, the most of the remainder of the chords are primarily those that insert into the distal rough zone of the leaflets. These arise as main stems from the papillary muscles and each main stem divides into three branches with the first branch inserting into the line of leaflet closure, the second into the free edge of the leaflets and the third in between the two. Two of the rough zone chords of the anterior leaflet are particularly large and thick and are termed the strut chordae.[47] *Chordae tendineae may rupture either spontaneously or due to trauma or because of infective endocarditis.*[82] *While infective endocarditis may affect any part of the leaflet and therefore cause rupture of any part of the chordae and their branches, spontaneous rupture will generally affect the main stem of the chordae.* Spontaneous rupture could occur if the tensile strength of the chordae is weakened due to elastic tissue loss as may happen in myxomatous degeneration or due to idiopathic reasons.[86] In fact, in patients with prolapsed mitral leaflet, chronic mild degree of mitral regurgitation may become suddenly severe due to the development of ruptured chordae. Rarely, chordal origins from the papillary muscle may avulse due to necrosis of the papillary muscle. This may happen with underlying ischemic heart disease. This may also lead to sudden severe mitral regurgitation.

In a series of 27 consecutive patients studied by us with ruptured chordae over a period of 10 years, nine presented with the acute onset of severe mitral regurgitation with no known previous mitral regurgitation while 18 had sudden deterioration of chronic mild mitral regurgitation. The majority of the patients were male (23 of 27 and varied in age between 37 and 75 years) (Table 7.1). Both groups of patients had symptoms secondary to high left

Table 7.1: Severe mitral regurgitation secondary to ruptured chordae.

Etiology	*Acute 9 pts*	*Acute on chronic 18 pts*
Idiopathic	4	2
Avulsion secondary to papillary muscle necrosis	2	1
Myxomatous degeneration	3	12
Infective endocarditis	0	3

atrial pressures causing orthopnea, pulmonary congestion and/or pulmonary edema as well as nocturnal dyspnea. The majority of the patients had mitral regurgitation murmurs, grade IV or more in intensity. Third heart sound gallop was noted in most of them while an S4 gallop was noted in about seven patients (three in the acute group and four in the acute on chronic group). Accentuated and loud P2 was noted in half of all patients indicating pulmonary hypertension. Hemodynamic measurements confirmed evidence of pulmonary hypertension as well as very high ***v wave*** pressures in the pulmonary capillary wedge reflecting high left atrial pressures. The presence of pulmonary edema was however uncommon in isolated posterior leaflet rough zone chordal rupture (1 of 17 patients). It was more common with anterior leaflet strut chordal rupture and or when both leaflets had rough zone chordae rupture. Atrial fibrillation was noted in a few of the patients. Despite similarities in clinical symptoms and signs, the pathology of the ruptured chordae in the two groups was somewhat different. *Myxomatous degeneration was the most common cause in those with acute on chronic mitral regurgitation while this was rare in acute mitral regurgitation.* (In the acute group the etiology was idiopathic in four, avulsion of chordae secondary to papillary muscle necrosis in two and myxomatous degeneration in three. On the other hand, in those with acute on chronic mitral regurgitation, 12 of 23 had myxomatous degeneration, infective endocarditis was the cause in three, papillary muscle necrosis causing avulsion in one and idiopathic in two) (Figs. 7.29A and B).[58]

The location and type of chordal rupture also had a bearing on the etiology of the rupture. The anterior leaflet chordal rupture was mostly idiopathic or due to papillary muscle necrosis whereas the majority of posterior leaflet chordal rupture appeared to be secondary to myxomatous degeneration (13 of 17 patients).[58]

Clinical Features of Mitral Regurgitation Secondary to Ruptured Chordae

1. Typically the pathophysiology is alluded to under acute mitral regurgitation. The excess flow into the LA gives rise to a harsh murmur due to

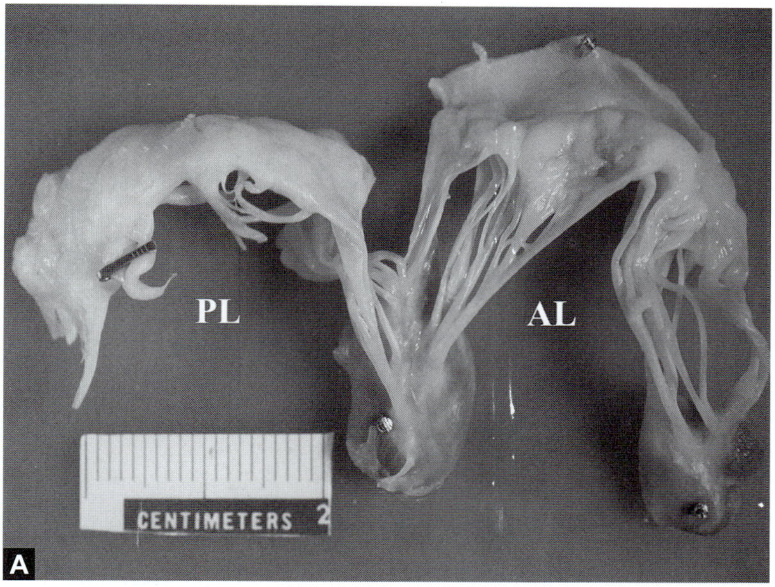

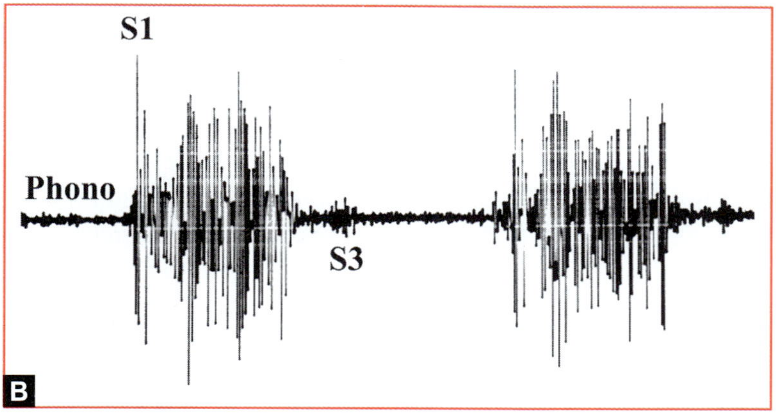

Figs. 7.29A and B: (A) Excised mitral valve from a patient with myxomatous prolapsed posterior leaflet (PL), who had acute on chronic mitral regurgitation secondary to ruptured chordae. The clip around it shows the ruptured rough zone chordae of the PL. (B) Phono recording taken at the apex area from the patient with acute on chronic mitral regurgitation whose excised mitral valve is shown in (A). The regurgitation murmur is followed by a third heart sound.

a lot of low and medium frequencies. *The murmur also tends to become decrescendo due to high v wave build up in the LA, which would limit the regurgitation in late systole (see Fig. 7.25).*

2. ***The maximal intensity of the murmur is at the apex.*** In addition, the murmur may be transmitted either to the base or to the back. The posterior leaflet chordal rupture has been considered to cause radiation of the murmur to the base more readily than toward the back. The anteriorly

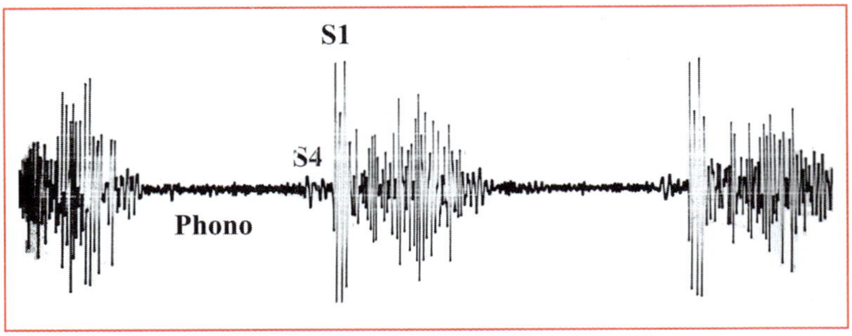

Fig. 7.30: Phono recording taken at the apex area from a patient with acute severe mitral regurgitation showing a fourth heart sound indicating that the left ventricle that is not very much dilated offers resistance to filling.

directed jet of mitral regurgitation is presumed to be conducted toward the AO and therefore to the base. The reverse is postulated for anterior leaflet chordal rupture with radiation of the murmur toward the back.[81] This however was not always the case in our experience.

3. On account of the severe mitral regurgitation, the apex may become more hyperdynamic. The P2 may become loud due to the development of pulmonary hypertension.
4. The S2 may be widely split due to the early occurrence of A2.
5. In addition, there will often be an S3 due to excess mitral inflow that the volume overload state produces. The S3 may sound like a short mid-diastolic murmur.
6. If the patient remains in sinus rhythm, which is more often the case due to shorter duration of the severe mitral regurgitation, an S4 may also be heard (Fig. 7.30).[87] This is due to the fact that the LA is still healthy and the relatively less dilated LV will be somewhat non-compliant offering resistance to filling in diastole.
7. Unlike papillary muscle rupture the murmurs of ruptured chordae are never silent and they are often fairly loud grades III-IV or more. Since they are harsh and decrescendo they are likely mistaken for ejection murmurs. Occasionally, the fact that they do not intensify following long diastoles may have to be used for their differentiation and recognition.

TRICUSPID REGURGITATION

Tricuspid Valve Anatomy and Function

Tricuspid valve anatomy differs from that of the mitral valve in some respects. It has three leaflets namely the anterior, the posterior and the septal leaflet. The leaflets vary in size and in most normals the anterior leaflet is the largest. *All three leaflets and the commissures in between them are inserted into the tricuspid valve ring or the annulus, which forms part of the entire circumference of the right AV groove.*[88] Medially it is attached to the central cardiac skeleton. Thus the tricuspid valve has no common attachment to the pulmonary valve like the mitral valve does to the aortic root. The pulmonary valve is separated from the inflow by an outflow tract or the infundibulum. This arrangement has a bearing on the function of the tricuspid valve. This means that *any degree of right ventricular dilatation can lead to stretching of the tricuspid annulus resulting in valvular incompetence*. The chordal arrangement of the tricuspid valve is similar to the mitral valve except in general the chordae are often somewhat thinner and one does not find chordae similar to the strut chordae of the mitral anterior leaflet.

The competence of the tricuspid valve is maintained during ventricular systole by the contracting papillary muscles and the underlying right ventricular myocardium pulling on the chordae to keep the leaflets together in apposition very similar to the mitral valve.

Causes of Tricuspid Regurgitation

Tricuspid regurgitation can arise from anatomic and/or functional defect of any of the components of its complex anatomy. The etiologic factors may be congenital or acquired. The pathologic process can be genetic, inflammatory, infective, traumatic, degenerative or neoplastic. Sometimes more than one component of the valve structures may be involved.[89,90]

Annular Abnormalities

The annulus may become idiopathically dilated or calcified and therefore may not function normally. Dilated annulus with voluminous leaflets may be part of cardiac involvement of connective tissue diseases such as Marfan and Ehlers–Danlos syndromes. *Dilatation of the annulus secondary to* right ventricular *dilatation is another important cause, which can either induce tricuspid regurgitation or worsen the degree of pre-existing tricuspid regurgitation.* Right ventricle will generally dilate secondary to volume overload especially when it is significant and long-standing. This can occur for instance in ***atrial septal defect*** that brings in extra volume of blood due to the left-to-right shunt at the atrial level. Right ventricle will also dilate in the *late stages of chronic pressure overload as in pulmonary hypertension* or significant pulmonary stenosis. Acute dilatation of the RV may also occur when there is a sudden and significant rise in pulmonary artery pressures as may happen with acute pulmonary embolism. Under all these circumstances annular dilatation will eventually lead to the development of tricuspid regurgitation. No matter how tricuspid regurgitation is produced initially, the resulting right ventricular dilatation will only lead to increase in the degree of regurgitation due to annular stretch. This will be particularly more so in the presence of pulmonary hypertension since RV does not usually tolerate raised pulmonary pressures.

Leaflet and Chordal Abnormalities

The leaflet may be congenitally cleft and this may be an associated feature of endocardial cushion defect. One or more of the leaflets may be large in particular the anterior leaflet and the whole *leaflet insertion may be displaced downward resulting in atrialization of the part of the base of the RV. This congenital abnormality of the tricuspid valve is called Ebstein's anomaly.*[40,91] The tricuspid valve in this disorder is often incompetent.

The tricuspid leaflets and chordae may also be large and redundant, hooded and prolapsed due to myxomatous degeneration. This may occur in association with similar mitral valve abnormality. The disorder may also occur as part of other connective tissue defect as in Marfan's syndrome. Leaflets and chordae may be scarred and contracted with some commissural fusion in rheumatic involvement. This is quite rare and usually will occur only with associated mitral and aortic valve involvement. The leaflets may also be involved in carcinoid syndrome with fibrous carcinoid plaques deposited on the ventricular surfaces of the leaflets making them adhere to the underlying right ventricular wall thereby making the valve incompetent.[92] Infective endocarditis can also cause destructive lesions of leaflet and chordae as well as cause vegetations. *Tricuspid valve endocarditis and pulmonary valve endocarditis are well recognized complications of intravenous drug abuse.* While chordal rupture could occur as a result of endocarditis, spontaneous rupture of tricuspid valve chordae is extremely rare.

Papillary Muscle and Right Ventricular Wall Pathology

In contrast to the LV, infarction of the RV is less common. It may however occur in about 10% of patients with acute inferior myocardial infarction. In that setting acute right ventricular dysfunction may compromise cardiac output and contribute to low output state or cardiogenic shock. Some patients who haverecovered from this may have residual chronic RV dysfunction contributing to tricuspid regurgitation.[90] Ischemia of the right ventricular is extremely rare and not usually a cause of tricuspid regurgitation.

Atrial Myxoma

Right atrial myxoma is even more uncommon than left atrial myxoma. When it does occur it can present with both tricuspid obstruction as well as interfere with proper leaflet closure and therefore produce tricuspid regurgitation.

Others

Transvenous pacemaker wires inserted across the tricuspid valve will often interfere with proper valve closure and invariably produce tricuspid regurgitation. However, the degree of tricuspid regurgitation is generally no more than mild to moderate in most instances.

Pathophysiology of Tricuspid Regurgitation

Tricuspid Regurgitation Secondary to Pulmonary Hypertension

From the foregoing consideration, it will be apparent that *tricuspid regurgitation may either occur with normal right ventricular systolic pressures or elevated right ventricular systolic pressures.* Chronic pulmonary hypertension regardless of etiology will have an element of reactive vasospasm initially in the pulmonary arterial bed. With persistence of the high pressures, intimal damage will ensue and lead to obstructive changes due to thrombosis. In addition there will be smooth muscle proliferation in the media and replacement fibrosis. These secondary changes lead to reduction of the total cross sectional area of the pulmonary vascular bed. This will aggravate the pulmonary hypertension and make this more irreversible.[93-99] *The etiologic factors that can cause pulmonary hypertension are as follows:*

a. *Left-sided pathology, which raises the left atrial pressures as with mitral obstruction (like mitral stenosis, left atrial myxoma, or cor triatriatum)* or mitral regurgitation or left ventricular failure. In these situations, the raised left atrial pressure is passively transmitted to the pulmonary arteries through the pulmonary capillary bed. Rarely the problem may be one of obstruction to pulmonary venous drainage as in ***pulmonary veno-occlusive disease.***

b. ***Large intracardiac left-to-right shunts*** such as through a VSD, atrial septal defect or persistent ductus. Initially the high pulmonary pressures may be secondary to large flow alone *(hyperkinetic pulmonary hypertension). When reactive and obstructive changes develop in the pulmonary arterial bed,* the pulmonary pressures will rise significantly and may reach systemic levels. This will lead to reversal of the left-to-right shunt causing right-to-left shunt. This will result in central cyanosis and the clinical disorder is termed ***Eisenmenger's syndrome.***[98]

c. Pulmonary arterial obstruction in particular ***pulmonary thromboembolism.***

d. ***Pulmonary disease:*** Pulmonary hypertension may develop in certain long-standing diseases of the lungs particularly those that lead to reduction of the total cross-sectional area of the pulmonary bed due to structural changes in the parenchyma that involve the vessels as well. The ensuing pulmonary hypertension and its effects on the right heart constitute the condition ***cor pulmonale. The hypoxia may trigger pulmonary vasospasm*** and directly raise the pulmonary pressures. This may be an important mechanism of pulmonary hypertension in chronic obstructive pulmonary disease, restrictive lung disease and various forms of interstitial pulmonary fibrosis. In addition, a direct effect of the tobacco smoke on the intrapulmonary vessels has also been implicated causing abnormal production of mediators that control vasoconstriction, vasodilatation and vascular cell proliferation, leading to abnormal vascular remodeling and aberrant vascular physiology. These changes are similar to those seen in other forms of pulmonary hypertension. The vessels themselves may become distorted, occluded and entrapped in replacement fibrosis as may occur with various forms of ***interstitial pulmonary fibrosis.*** In addition, the vessels may be involved in a ***vasculitis.*** This may be an important mechanism in some disorders such as collagen vascular disease (e.g. progressive systemic sclerosis, lupus erythematosus and rheumatoid arthritis).

e. ***Hypoventilatory disorders:*** When hypoxia is associated with respiratory acidosis as may happen with alveolar hypoventilation, pulmonary artery pressures tend to rise significantly. This situation may occur in various hypoventilatory disorders (***Pickwickian's syndrome*** where marked obesity plays a prominent role, *sleep apnea, neuromuscular disorders such as myasthenia, chest wall abnormalities as in kyphoscoliosis).*

f. ***Primary pulmonary hypertension:*** This is rare but tends to be seen in women of childbearing age. In this disorder, pathologic changes develop in the pulmonary arterial bed for some unknown reasons. The intimal fibrosis may have an onion-skin appearance. The medial hypertrophy may be accompanied by fibrinoid necrosis and formation of plexiform lesions, which are not usually seen in other forms of pulmonary hypertension.

In all these situations, the tricuspid valve itself is anatomically normal and the regurgitation is caused by right ventricular dilatation. The latter will stretch the tricuspid annulus and cause tricuspid regurgitation. The latter sets in late stages when right ventricular hypertrophy is no longer able to compensate for ***the pressure load.*** The high pressure tricuspid regurgitation is often less well tolerated by the RV. The right ventricular hypertrophy would usually precede the development of the tricuspid regurgitation and the right ventricular diastolic pressures in particular the ***pre a wave*** pressure would be elevated. This will lead to significant elevation of the right atrial and jugular venous pressures. *The raised venous pressure would cause systemic venous congestion resulting in abdominal distension, hepatomegaly and peripheral edema. The jugular venous contour will be abnormal reflecting the tricuspid regurgitation showing large amplitude v wave with a y descent. The normal dominant x′ descent will be absent* due to the regurgitation raising the right atrial pressure during systole. The contour is often visible from a distance. The right ventricular dysfunction will often cause low output symptoms such as fatigue and tiredness.

Tricuspid Regurgitation with Normal Pulmonary Artery Pressures

In contrast to tricuspid regurgitation in the presence of pulmonary hypertension, tricuspid regurgitation with normal right ventricular systolic pressure is usually due to some primary tricuspid valve abnormality. In addition, the tricuspid regurgitation associated with normal pulmonary pressures may be well tolerated. The problem being primarily valvular in origin, the RV will have a primary volume load. The resulting compensatory dilatation will help maintain good right ventricular compliance for a long time especially when the lesion producing the tricuspid regurgitation is chronic. This will maintain relatively normal right ventricular diastolic pressures. The resulting venous pressure elevation will therefore be somewhat minimized. Finally, secondary right ventricular hypertrophy will develop in late stages, which may reduce the compliance leading to elevation of the right ventricular diastolic pressures. The latter may cause further rise in the venous pressures. The signs of systemic congestion may therefore be less pronounced andappear later in the course.

Acute Tricuspid Regurgitation

This may be seen as part of the clinical presentation of patients with *acute pulmonary embolism, post-right ventricular infarction or secondary to tricuspid valve endocarditis.*[100] In acute pulmonary embolism alone, the tricuspid regurgitation will beassociated with pulmonary hypertension. The right ventricular diastolic pressures will be elevated due to right ventricular dysfunction as well as due to the acuteness of the disorder that does not allow time for compensatory right ventricular dilatation. The clinical picture however will be dominated by the underlying condition and not by the tricuspid regurgitation.

Characteristics of Tricuspid Regurgitation Murmurs

1. Tricuspid regurgitation murmur shares all the features listed under the general characteristics of regurgitant murmurs. In general, it is ***high in frequency and blowing in quality*** and usually lasts all the way to S2.
2. The frequency will tend to be higher in the presence of pulmonary hypertension. In the initial stages of decompensation the murmur may be intermittent and audible only on inspiration. In some patients, the murmur may have a whoop or honking character. When decompensation becomes more pronounced, the regurgitation murmur may be audible throughout the phases of respiration. The coexistent right ventricular dysfunction and consequent decrease in cardiac output will lead to some decrease in the right ventricular systolic pressures (to about 50 mm Hg). But the pressure is still high enough to contribute to the high frequencies.

3. Tricuspid regurgitation murmurs may have some *low and medium frequencies when the regurgitation is severe.*
4. Tricuspid regurgitation murmurs will also *not change in intensity or loudness following sudden long diastoles as in atrial fibrillation or following an ectopic beat.*
5. Irrespective of the etiology, tricuspid regurgitation murmurs are *maximal in loudness over the xiphoid area and over the lower sternal region.* In addition, typically tricuspid regurgitation murmur will *accentuate in intensity or loudness on inspiration (Carvallo's sign).*[6] They may be heard over the apex area if the RV is enlarged or dilated and has taken over the apex area.
6. Tricuspid regurgitation murmurs may have different shapes depending on the etiology. In general, it will be pansystolic when there is annular dilatation primary or secondary as well as when the orifice is fixed as in rheumatic involvement. It may be late systolic if caused by prolapsed myxomatous leaflets and chordae. The murmur may also begin with a mid-systolic click in some of these patients. However, the findings may be compounded by the coexistence of mitral prolapse. In the presence of Ebstein's anomaly, the murmur may be preceded by a somewhat delayed and loud T1.

   The murmur may vary in length, early systolic to being holosystolic or pansystolic. When the regurgitation is associated with normal right ventricular pressures, the murmur is often soft and short with low medium frequencies and confined to early half of systole.[100] The intensity often diminishes toward the end of systole since the right atrial ***v wave*** and the rising right ventricular systolic pressure tend to equalize toward the end of ejection. This will cause the regurgitant flow to diminish in later systole. The inadequacy of the right ventricular function may also produce a poor inspiratory increase in its stroke volume. This may therefore result in a poor inspiratory increase in the intensity of the murmur. In rheumatic involvement of the tricuspid valve, which is quite rare, there may be associated features of loud T1 and even tricuspid opening snap. Right atrial myxoma producing tricuspid regurgitation will be associated with loud tricuspid component of S1, which may accentuate with inspiration. In addition, there may be a loud sound in diastole mimicking an S3, which is due to the tumor plop. Also, this would be followed by a diastolic rumble due to the tricuspid obstruction that often would occur with the right atrial myxoma. Transvenous pacemakers may cause squeaky type tricuspid regurgitation murmur, which may accentuate with inspiration.
7. If the regurgitation is significant and severe, then the excess diastolic inflow from the right atrium may result in a *right-sided S3 or short mid-diastolic low frequency murmur or rumble.* Both of these will be audible

best over the xiphoid area or the lower sternal region and ***will accentuate in intensity on inspiration.***

8. ***The audibility of tricuspid regurgitation murmur is often variable.*** Sometimes significant tricuspid regurgitation may be present on the Doppler and yet the associated murmur may be absent. This is more likely when the right ventricular systolic pressures are normal. Jugular venous pulse contour may sometimes be characteristic of tricuspid regurgitation and yet the murmur may be inconspicuous. While the ***x′ descent*** may be visible with mild and occasionally mild to moderate tricuspid regurgitation on the Doppler, significant tricuspid regurgitation will usually lead to the loss of the normal ***x′ descent*** in the jugulars. In addition, the typical fast rising large amplitude ***v wave*** followed by the *y descent* will reveal the tricuspid regurgitation. *In Ebstein's anomaly, the huge right atrium due to partial atrialization of the RV and the resultant high capacitance effect of the right atrium may sometimes hide the presence of tricuspid regurgitation in the jugulars and the jugular pulsations may in fact be quite unimpressive in such patients.*

VENTRICULAR SEPTAL DEFECT (VSD)

Defect in the interventricular septum can be either ***congenital or acquired.*** Congenital defects may involve either the ***membranous or the muscular*** portion of the interventricular septum. The defect in the membranous ventricular septum is by far the commonest.[40,101-106] It is located usually below the aortic valve close to the commissure between the right coronary and the non-coronary cusps. The outer edge of the defect may involve the adjoining portion of the muscular septum. For this reason, the defect is usually termed ***perimembranous.*** Occasionally, the membranous portion of the septum can be aneurysmal and the defect may be located in the wall of the aneurysmal bulge. The aneurysm can cause some obstruction to the right ventricular outflow as well.

The muscular septum consists of three portions as viewed from the right ventricular side namely the inlet, the trabecular and the outlet portions.[106] The ***defects in the muscular septum*** in turn may involve the inlet, the trabecular or the outlet portion of the septum respectively. The defect can be either single or multiple. In addition, the size of these defects may also vary. ***Doubly committed*** sub-arterial VSDs are located in the outlet portion of the septum and they are bordered by a fibrous continuity of the aortic and the pulmonary valves. These defects are more common in Asian patients.

The ***acquired form*** of VSD usually occurs as a result of *septal rupture complicating acute myocardial infarction.*[107-110] Septal rupture complicating anterior myocardial infarction usually involves the apical region of the muscular septum whereas those that complicate inferoposterior infarction usually involve the posterobasal portion of the muscular septum. The latter is less common.

Congenital Ventricular Septal Defects

1. *The degree of left-to-right shunt through a congenital ventricular septal defect is dependent on essentially the size of the defect and on the pulmonary vascular resistance.*[102,104,105] The larger the size the larger will be the flow as long as the pulmonary vascular resistance is not high. The ***pulmonary vascular resistance is initially high in the newborn*** due to the muscular nature of the pulmonary vasculature. This usually takes a few weeks to regress. Thus the ***murmur of the VSD may not be apparent at birth*** and may become audible only a few weeks after birth.
2. If the defect is large enough then there could be a large left-to-right shunt causing excess pulmonary flow. Contrary to what may seem logical to a beginner, despite the fact that the shunt through a VSD occurs from the LV to the RV, the volume overload is presented to the LA and the LV and not to the RV. The shunt occurs during systole due to the higher left ventricular pressure. The contracting RV is in no position to accept the shunted volume, since the RV is also contracting and emptying at the same time. Therefore, the left-to-right shunt goes through the defect and directly into the pulmonary artery. The excess pulmonary flow due to the shunt is eventually returned through the pulmonary veins to the LA. This will lead to left atrial and left ventricular enlargement since these two chambers receive the extra volume of blood. The volume overload of the LV may result in ***congestive heart failure during the first year of life.*** However, ***spontaneous improvement may often occur due to reduction in size of the defects*** with the normal growth of the heart or the ***development of increased pulmonary vascular resistance*** or occasionally due to development of infundibular hypertrophy that may also reduce the left-to-right shunt because of the ***acquired infundibular stenosis.***
3. ***Spontaneous closure*** of VSDs is fairly common during infancy and early childhood years ***(up to 45% of cases).***[40] Occasionally, spontaneous closure may occur even in older children and young adults. Even large defects causing excess pulmonary flow with flow-related pulmonary hypertension are known to undergo spontaneous closure. Several factors may play a role in spontaneous closure. These include appositions of the margins of defects, endocardial proliferation, adherence of the septal leaflet of tricuspid valve or prolapse of the aortic cusp through the defect. The prolapsed aortic cusp may be associated however with varying degrees of aortic regurgitation.
4. Large VSDs causing excess left-to-right shunt in the early childhood may either decrease in size, undergo spontaneous closure or may develop increased pulmonary vascular resistance due to intrinsic changes in the vascular bed brought about by the excess flow and pressure ***(Eisenmenger reaction).***[98] When the pulmonary vascular resistance is

high, this will not only limit the left-to-right shunt but eventually can lead to reversal of shunt and development of cyanosis. The fact that the process can be prevented by timely surgical closure of large VSDs with increasing pulmonary vascular resistance at a stage when there is still significant left-to-right shunt would suggest that the pulmonary vascular damage is to an extent dependent on the excess flow.

5. *Ventricular septal defects, which are small or medium in size and associated with normal pulmonary vascular resistance and that do not undergo spontaneous closure, will persist through the adult years.* These will produce the typical VSD murmurs due to flow through the defect. However, they often will not cause large enough left-to-right shunt to produce either left ventricular volume load or raise the pulmonary pressures. However, the normal left-sided pressures together with normal pulmonary pressures will give a large pressure gradient driving the left to right flow through the defect. These will therefore result in a high velocity flow jet, which can be picked up by using Doppler echocardiography. The only important risk however is the risk of infective endocarditis. The high velocity jet may damage the endocardium on the right ventricular side of the defect near the septal leaflet of the tricuspid valve, which may become the nidus of infection when there is a bacteremia. The risk of endocarditis is always a possibility in all VSDs.
6. ***The clinical spectrum of the small, moderate and large isolated VSDs*** described above had been classified based on physiology into two types: ***restrictive*** and ***non-restrictive.*** The term ***restrictive*** is applied when the resistance that limits the left-to-right shunt is at the site of the defect alone. It means therefore that the right ventricular pressure is either normal or if elevated it is still less than that of the LV in the absence of right ventricular outflow obstruction. When the left-to-right shunt is not limited at the site of the defect, the term ***non-restrictive*** is applied. This means equal right ventricular and left ventricular systolic pressures in the absence of right ventricular outflow obstruction. It implies therefore equal pulmonary and aortic systolic pressures and the amount of left-to-right shunt is determined essentially by the pulmonary vascular resistance.[111]

The hemodynamic severity has been classified into four grades based on the ratio of right ventricular to left ventricular systolic pressures and the ratio of pulmonary flow (QP) to systemic flow (QS) determined at cardiac catheterization.[112] The grades of hemodynamic severity are as follows:

Small: when the ratio of pulmonary to aortic systolic pressure is <0.3 and the QP/QS ratio is <1.4.

Moderate: when the ratio of pulmonary to AO systolic pressures is >0.3 and the QP/QS ratio is in the range of 1.4–2.2.

Large: when the systolic pressure ratio is >0.3 and the QP/QS ratio is >2.2; and

Eisenmenger: when the systolic pressure ratio is close to 1 and the QP/QS ratio is <1.5 and the net intracardiac shunt is right to left.

Septal Rupture Secondary to Myocardial Infarction

This complication used to occur in approximately 1–2% of patients with myocardial infarction before thrombolytic era. In the current era of routine thrombolytic therapy, its frequency has fallen to about 0.2%.[108] It accounts for about 5% of all deaths from myocardial infarction. The septal rupture is usually associated with the first myocardial infarction and will generally occur ***within the first week after the infarct.*** It is more common with anterior myocardial infarction than with the inferior infarct. Rupture may be simple or complex and serpigenous. The ECG may show right bundle branch block or complete AV block. The onset is recognizable with the ***detection of a new murmur.*** The left ventricular volume load due to the shunt will not be well tolerated by the already compromised LV secondary to the myocardial infarction. Eventually this may lead to the development of congestive cardiac failure within a few hours to a few days. The outcome is poor when associated with cardiogenic shock (usually in the context of a large infarct), when there is significant right ventricular dysfunction or when the rupture involves the posterior septum.

General Characteristics of the VSD Murmur

1. Ventricular septal defect is a regurgitant lesion since the blood flows through the defect from the high pressure chamber LV into the low pressure chamber RV. The flow through the defect is turbulent due to the high pressure difference. *The high pressure gradient would produce a high frequency systolic murmur, which is plateau, and will last throughout systole.*[113,114] The murmur will last until the S2. The holo- or pansystolic murmur will sound very much like a mitral regurgitation murmur due to the pre-dominant high frequencies.
2. The VSD murmur also will *not be expected to change significantly in intensity during sudden long diastoles such as following a post-extrasystolic pause or during atrial fibrillation.* The LV has two outlets for systole when there is a VSD namely the normal AO and the right heart through the septal defect. Although the long diastole allows greater filling of the LV and increases the force of contraction both by a Starling's mechanism as well as through post-extrasystolic potentiation, the larger volume gets ejected more easily through the aorta due to fall in the aortic diastolic pressures during the pause. Thus, the flow through the defect will not increase and the murmur will remain essentially unchanged.

3. *The maximal loudness of the murmur in most VSDs is the lower left sternal border area in the third and the fourth left interspace (Fig. 7.31).*

Variations in Clinical and Auscultatory Features in Ventricular Septal Defects

Sub-pulmonic VSD

When the defect is sub-pulmonic, the LV ejects blood directly into the pulmonary artery through the defect. The resulting ***murmur*** will therefore be ***maximally heard at the second left interspace.*** The murmur may have some crescendo character possibly due to decrease in size of the defect by the late contraction of the infundibulum causing perhaps increased velocity of flow.[115] Often the S2 would also be widely split. Aortic regurgitation also tends to develop in these patients due to prolapse of the right coronary cusp of the aortic valve. The latter might help to reduce the size of the defect. *The long systolic murmur that is crescendo to the A2 followed by diastolic murmur of aortic regurgitation heard over the second left interspace may be mistaken for a continuous murmur of persistent ductus arteriosus.*

Large VSD

When the VSD is large and allows significant left-to-right shunt, the resulting left ventricular volume load will produce an enlarged LV. The apical

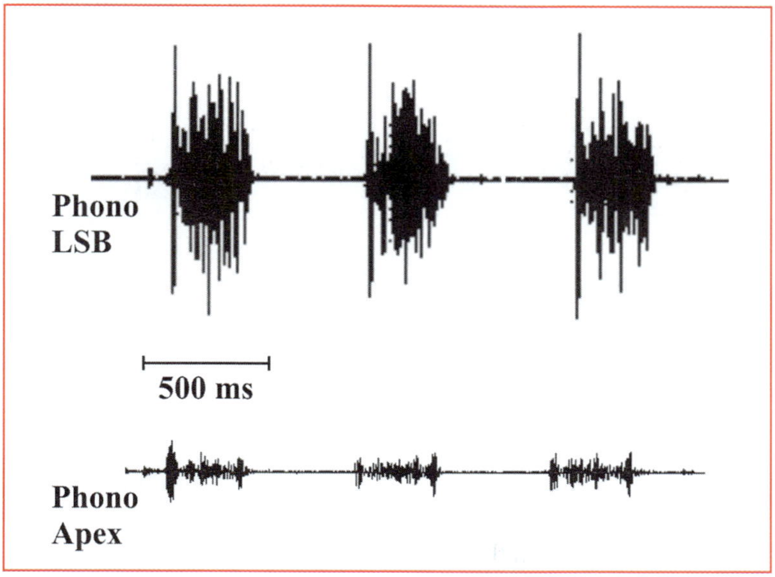

Fig. 7.31: Digital display of magnetic audio recordings from a patient with congenital ventricular septal defect showing the maximal loudness of the murmur at the lower left sternal border area (shown at the top) and not at the apex area (shown at the bottom).

impulse may demonstrate a wide area hyperdynamic impulse with good medial retraction. The excess pulmonary flow received by the LA will have to go through the mitral valve in diastole and the rapid and large volume inflow may cause a short mid-diastolic flow rumble (like an S3 with a duration) at the apex.

Small Muscular VSD

When the VSD is small and affects the muscular portion of the septum, ***the murmur may be pre-dominantly early systolic*** since during end systole the defect itself may be fully closed secondary to the ventricular contraction. Similarly, when the defect begins to undergo spontaneous closure in early childhood, the murmur may become shorter and pre-dominantly early systolic since in later part of systole the defect may be in fact closed. In both these instances however the murmur will still retain the high frequencies due to the high pressure gradient between the LV and the right side.[40]

VSD Murmurs and Vasoactive Agents

Ventricular septal defect murmurs can be influenced by vasoactive agents as well as by other maneuvers, which alter the systemic pressures. *Vasopressor agents by increasing the systemic arterial pressures will increase the left to right pressure difference and cause the murmur to become loud.* If the VSD is small and/or in the process of closing and has a short early systolic high frequency murmur, the murmur may be noted to become longer and pansystolic and louder indicating that the defect is not fully anatomically closed. *Squatting by raising the aortic pressure could cause similar change in the intensity of the murmur.* Amyl nitrite inhalation by reducing the systemic arterial pressure will reduce the left-to-right shunt through the defect and therefore diminish the loudness of a VSD murmur. In the presence of a vasoreactive pulmonary hypertension, amyl nitrite inhalation could cause a more significant fall in the pulmonary artery pressures and the intensity of the murmur may remain unchanged or increase somewhat.

Ventricular Septal Defect Eisenmenger

When the VSD develops Eisenmenger reaction (pulmonary vascular disease) and increased pulmonary vascular resistance, the murmur will become shorter with increasing right ventricular systolic pressures.[98] Eventually when the pulmonary pressures are equal to systemic levels, there is no pressure difference as such between the LV and the RV. The VSD murmur is no longer heard and isreplaced by an ejection murmur due to ejection of blood into a dilated pulmonary artery. *The right-to-left shunt occurs pre-dominantly during the isovolumic relaxation phase of the cardiac cycle.* Simultaneous left ventricular and right ventricular pressure recordings would demonstrate that the *pulmonary hypertensive RV has a slower rate of fall of pressure during the phase of isovolumic relaxation.* This presumably reflects the presence of diastolic dysfunction in the RV. The pressure on the right ventricular side falls more slowly as a result of this, compared to the left side. This creates enough pressure difference to cause a right-to-left shunt. Injection of agitated saline containing micro bubbles of air into a systemic vein during Doppler echocardiography can be shown to cross over to the left heart only during the phase of isovolumic relaxation. It must also be pointed out that *right-to-left shunt never produces any turbulence to cause murmurs.*

The other signs of pulmonary hypertension may also be present such as a sub-xiphoid right ventricular impulse. The P2 may be loud and palpable. The S2 split at this stage is not present resulting in a single S2. There may also be a pulmonary ejection sound. Rarely the ***pulmonary valve may be regurgitant*** secondary to the high pulmonary artery pressures. This may cause an early diastolic blowing murmur, which starts with a loud P2. This murmur is termed the ***Graham Steell murmur.*** This is often loudest at the second left interspace.[116]

Ventricular Septal Defect with Pulmonary Stenosis

The combination of a VSD with pulmonary stenosis is an important feature of classic tetralogy of Fallot where these two components are the major determinants of the clinical features and presentation. The other two components of the Tetralogy namely the straddling or overriding AO and right ventricular hypertrophy have very little bearing on the clinical features. *The spectrum of clinical findings that can occur will depend on the size of the VSD and the severity of the pulmonary stenosis* and the specific combinations of the two lesions.[117,118]

Large VSD with Severe Pulmonary Stenosis

With a large VSD in the presence of severe pulmonary stenosis, the right ventricular pressures will rise secondary to the obstruction to systemic levels but not higher due to the large size of the VSD. There will be less blood ejected into the pulmonary artery due to the obstruction and the venous blood from the RV may be directly ejected into the AO. This is the case with ***classic cyanotic form of tetralogy.*** The pulmonary stenosis can be either at the valve or, as is the case, more often at the infundibular level. The AO would receive a large volume of blood from the RV and may become dilated. *The VSD will not have significant left-to-right shunt due to the raised right ventricular pressures and the VSD murmur will be replaced by a pulmonary ejection murmur. The murmur however may be shorter and softer when the obstruction is severe* since pulmonary blood flow will be significantly diminished. The dilated AO may be associated with an aortic ejection sound. The S2 is usually single since the P2 is often inaudible. The RV of the newborn is usually able to withstand the systemic pressures and seldom will show dilatation or failure with secondary tricuspid regurgitation. The jugular venous pulse will also show a relatively normal contour for the same reason. When the obstruction is very severe as in pulmonary atresia then there will be no blood reaching through to the pulmonary trunk. There will be compensatory bronchial collaterals, which may supply the lungs. They may produce continuous murmurs. The cyanosis may be present at birthunlike classic Tetralogy where the cyanosis may be noted only weeks or months after birth.

Large VSD with Mild Pulmonary Stenosis

When the VSD is large but the pulmonary stenosis is mild then the clinical features may be like that of an isolated large VSD (sometimes called acyanotic form of tetralogy). The large left-to-right shunt through the defect will cause pre-dominant left ventricular volume load. The systolic murmurs may be due to both the VSD and the pulmonary stenosis. The ejection murmur of pulmonary stenosis may be audible over the third left interspace since the stenosis may be infundibular. *The S2 split may be somewhat wide and this is not usually the case in isolated VSD.* The pulmonary stenosis may increase due to hypertrophy of the crista supraventricularis causing some infundibular stenosis as well. As the degree of resistance at the site of stenosis keeps increasing then the left-to-right shunt will diminish and the VSD murmur may shorten and eventually be replaced by an ejection murmur of pulmonary stenosis.

Small VSD with Severe Pulmonary Stenosis

The VSD may be small initially or a large VSD may have been partially closed by the septal leaflet of the tricuspid valve. In the presence of a small defect and severe pulmonary stenosis, the right ventricular pressures can rise above the systemic level since the RV will not have a direct access to the AO. The clinical features will therefore resemble more closely pulmonary stenosis with an intact ventricular septum. The murmur will be essentially that of pulmonary stenosis namely ejection in type since the high right ventricular pressure will not allow any left-to-right shunt. The stenosis is generally infundibular in the presence of a VSD and the murmur will be maximal in loudness in the third and the fourth left interspaces.

Small VSD with Mild Pulmonary Stenosis

The defect will allow very little volume overload of the LV and the right-sided pressures would be only minimally elevated. The murmur is however predominantly due to the VSD and will be pansystolic and regurgitant in type.

Total Absence of Ventricular Septum

This congenital anomaly implies that there is a single ventricle. The most common type is morphologically a LV with a small remnant of the right ventricular infundibulum forming the outflow into the AO. The great vessels are invariably transposed meaning that the AO is anterior and somewhat to the right of the posterior pulmonary artery. The anomaly may or may not be associated with pulmonary stenosis. Both AV valves are present generally and properly related.

When there is no pulmonary stenosis, the blood from both atria stream through the ventricle without too much mixing. Pulmonary blood flow is increased and the cyanosis is minimal. The increased pulmonary flow would cause volume load on the LA and the single ventricle. Sometimes there may be an element of sub-aortic obstruction at the level of the infundibulum. Ejection murmurs may be heard, and may be best heard at the lower left sternal border and the apex. The S2 is usually loud and single from both components being loud. Aortic component is accentuated due to the anterior position of the AO. Pulmonary hypertension, which is usually present, would increase the P2. The increased flow through the mitral valve may cause a short mid-diastolic flow murmur.

But when there is pulmonary stenosis or when the pulmonary vascular resistance is increased there would be greater mixing and the pulmonary flow would be reduced with increased cyanosis. The loudness and length of the ejection murmur of the pulmonary stenosis would vary inversely with the severity of the stenosis. The S2 would be single and would be due to the A2 component.

Post-Myocardial Infarction Septal Rupture

In the acquired septal rupture secondary to acute myocardial infarction the murmur may be audible, near the apex particularly when the septal rupture is in the apical portion of the septum. *However, the maximal loudness may be demonstrated to be medial to the apex. This is different from papillary muscle rupture causing mitral regurgitation murmur, which has maximal loudness at the apex and immediately lateral to the apex (Fig. 7.32).*

CLINICAL ASSESSMENT OF SYSTOLIC MURMURS

Clinical history when obtained and properly interpreted will often give direction to what the various possibilities are, that need to be considered in the differential diagnosis. Then a more focused physical examination can be performed taking into account all the possibilities that are being considered, paying careful attention to the features of the venous pulse, the arterial

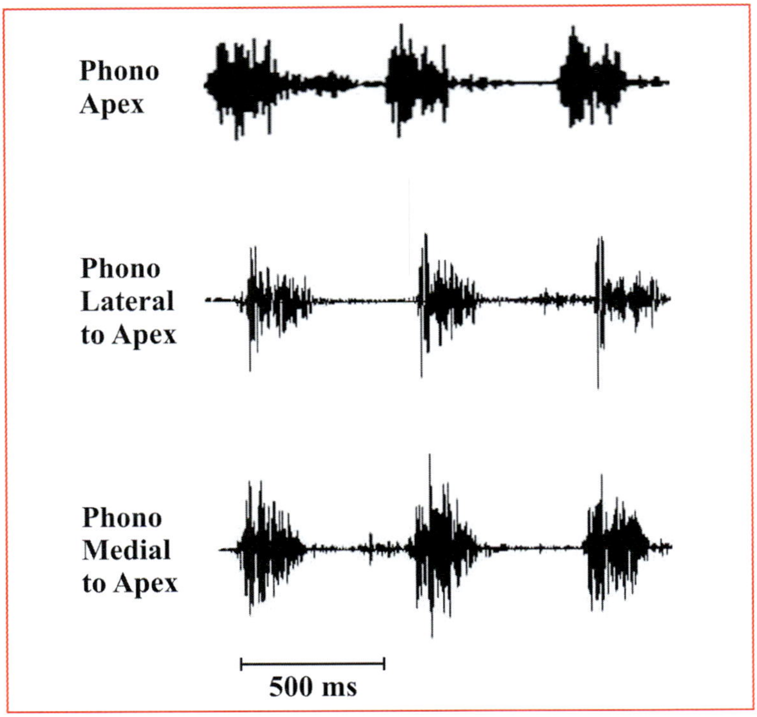

Fig. 7.32: Digital display of magnetic audio recordings taken at the apex (top), lateral to the apex (middle) and medial to the apex (bottom) from a patient with septal rupture complicating acute myocardial infarction. The maximal loudness of the murmur is at the apex and medial to the apex. The murmur is less intense lateral to the apex.

pulse and the pre-cordial pulsations including the apical impulse. Each one of these must be evaluated in relation to the various possible diagnoses entertained. If one trains oneself to do such a focused examination often by the time one is ready to auscultate the diagnosis is generally obvious. Auscultation then becomes confirmatory of what one suspects the diagnosis to be. For instance in the case of a 65-year-old man presenting with exertional dyspnea and angina, differential diagnosis must include among other things aortic valve disease. A slow rate of rise of the carotid pulse (CP) with normal or low amplitude will point to aortic stenosis whereas a large amplitude CP with normal or fast rate of rise together with bounding peripheral pulses and a hyperdynamic wide area left ventricular apical impulse will suggest the presence of aortic regurgitation. On the other hand, a fast rising CP with normal amplitude and normal peripheral pulses and a wide area hyperdynamic left ventricular impulse would suggest a lesion such as mitral regurgitation. In such a situation one looks for the murmur of mitral regurgitation on auscultation and one also will look for the auscultatory signs to assess its severity.

Sometimes however asymptomatic patients may be referred for evaluation of heart murmurs. *Often when a patient is referred for heart murmur evaluation, it will invariably be for a systolic murmur since systolic murmurs are generally more easily detected.* The clinical assessment of systolic murmurs even in asymptomatic patient still includes the careful assessment of the venous pulse, the arterial pulses and the pre-cordial pulsations and the evaluation of the clues that these can provide in terms of the cause of the systolic murmurs. The auscultatory assessment comes next.

The Auscultatory Assessment of Systolic Murmurs

Auscultatory assessment of systolic murmurs presupposes that the heart sounds had been auscultated, identified and characterized including the normal S1 and S2 as well as any extra sounds that may be recognized such as the S4, S3, opening snap, ejection clicks as well as non-ejection click or clicks. Next the systolic murmur itself is auscultated noting its character, its pre-dominant frequencies whether low, medium (harsh) or high frequencies (blowing), its length, the location of its maximal loudness as well as all the locations where it is heard. The following points will be of help in its analysis.

1. *Attempt should be made to determine whether the murmur is ejection or regurgitant in type. If the S2 is present, one should listen for the cadence of the ejection murmur, namely da ...ha.. da, formed by the S1, the peak of the crescendo of the ejection murmur and then the S2*. If a typical cadence of an ejection murmur is recognized then the problem becomes easy.
2. ***Mere audibility of S2 does not mean a murmur is ejection in type*** indicating a pause between the end of the murmur and the S2. *This sign is only helpful when the relative grade of loudness of the murmur and that of the S2 are considered together. When the murmur is louder than the S2, then audibility of S2 will mean that there is a distinct pause between the end of the murmur and the S2, therefore the murmur must be ejection in type*. In the converse situation where the murmur is softer than the S2, the S2 may be audible and the murmur could be regurgitant. In such a situation more importance needs to be paid to the pre-dominant frequencies of the murmur namely whether it is harsh and low, medium or blowing and high in frequency. The former of course is more characteristic of an ejection murmur, while the latter favors a regurgitant murmur. *In general radiation of the murmurs has no diagnostic value in terms of its origins.* While mitral regurgitation murmurs generally may be transmitted to the axilla and posteriorly and the aortic ejection murmurs may be transmitted to the carotids, exceptions to these occur more often than not to make this a useful distinguishing feature.

3. When S2 is not heard then the cadence of the ejection murmur will not exist and this method of recognition will no longer be possible. When ejection murmurs are long and have delayed peak it may cause some confusion. This may happen for instance with significant pulmonary valvular or infundibular stenosis murmurs. These murmurs may go past the A2 and if the P2 is soft, the S2 may not be clearly audible. Then other methods such as the effect of sudden long diastole may have to be looked for. One should attempt to observe for any sudden change in rhythm of the heart such as due to a pre-mature beat. Sometimes turning the patient to the left lateral decubitus position may bring out a pre-mature beat. Occasionally patients may have spontaneous extra-systoles or could be in atrial fibrillation with changing RR intervals and therefore changing durations of diastoles. If any of these is present, *one needs to pay attention to the effect of the long diastolic pause on the loudness of the murmur*. Sometimes, this may occur even before one is ready to look for it. It is important to make use of the situation as and when it presents when listening to a systolic murmur. *Sudden long diastolic pause accentuates the intensity of the ejection murmurs* for reasons that have been dealt with at length in the previous sections.
4. Once the murmur is characterized as an ejection in type, then all causes of ejection murmurs need to be considered. These include increased ejection velocity of either normal or increased stroke volume, ejection of increased stroke volume through normal outflow tracts as well as ejection through roughened or stenosed outflow tracts. The length of the murmur often helps since *short ejection murmurs are not usually associated with any significant stenosis. Next location of maximal loudness* whether it is second left interspace, third left interspace, lower left sternal border area, apex area or second right interspace becomes an important consideration. *Pulmonary ejection murmurs are often maximally loud at the second left interspace whereas the aortic ejection murmurs are best heard at the apex and occasionally at the apex and the second right interspace. Hypertrophic obstructive cardiomyopathy usually has murmur intensity maximal at the left sternal border and the apex. The infundibular pulmonary stenosis murmurs usually have maximal intensity over the third left interspace.*
5. *When right-sided ejection murmurs are considered, the effect of inspiration* on the intensity of the murmur also needs to be assessed since these murmurs typically get louder on inspiration. *In addition one needs to pay attention to whether or not an ejection click is present. If an ejection click is detected then attempt should be made to decide whether it has the characteristics of a pulmonary ejection click, which typically softens or disappears on inspiration. If a left-sided ejection murmur is detected,*

one needs to look for aortic ejection click. When outflow tract obstruction is being considered, the presence of ejection click of course would indicate stenosis at the valvular level of the outflow tract.

6. In addition, evaluation of left-sided ejection murmurs requires the assessment of *the effects of changing posture such as standing and squatting on the intensity of the murmurs*. These are obviously important in confirming or ruling out hypertrophic obstructive cardiomyopathy, which is an important cause of a left-sided ejection murmur. The dynamic obstruction in this disorder gets worse on standing due to decrease in heart size caused by decreased venous return. The murmur therefore gets louder. On squatting, reverse will happen. The murmur will get softer or disappear. The aortic ejection murmurs of all other causes will either not change or actually diminish in intensity due to the decreased stroke output caused by the decreased venous return due to standing.
7. *If the murmur is considered regurgitant and the murmur is pansystolic, then the location of maximal loudness becomes important in the differential diagnosis. Mitral regurgitation murmurs are typically maximal in intensity at the apex and slightly lateral to the apex whereas the maximal loudness of a VSD murmur is at the lower left sternal border area and medial to the apex. The tricuspid regurgitation murmur is maximally loud over the lower sternum and the xiphoid area. In addition, tricuspid regurgitation murmur may be noted to increase on inspiration*. Abnormal jugular contours (large amplitude ***v wave*** with a ***y descent***) characteristic of tricuspid regurgitation and a sub-xiphoid right ventricular impulse are additional features, which will favor tricuspid regurgitation. Sometimes, an enlarged RV may take over the normal apex area and the murmur of tricuspid regurgitation may be heard also fairly well at the apex. The character of the apical impulse may reveal this to be right ventricular with a lateral retraction. Both mitral regurgitation as well as VSD when significant will cause left ventricular volume overload and therefore would be associated with a wide area hyperdynamic left ventricular impulse. Both may produce an S3 or a short mid-diastolic flow rumble at the apex reflecting the increased mitral inflow. A wide split S2 if present may reflect severe mitral regurgitation. This is not a feature in VSD. Loud M1 and an opening snap when detected will point to a rheumatic etiology for the mitral regurgitation. If the murmur is mid-late systolic and crescendo to S2 or preceded by the presence of non-ejection mid-late systolic click or clicks, it will suggest the presence of mitral prolapse as a cause of the mitral regurgitation murmur.
8. ***Then the effect of change in posture*** becomes important since mitral regurgitation murmurs from prolapsed and redundant mitral valve leaflets

become longer and louder on standing with decrease in venous return and decreased heart size. The opposite will happen with squatting. The papillary muscle dysfunction murmurs usually do not behave this way. In fact they may increase in intensity with squatting if there is significant rise in blood pressure. Ventricular septal defect murmurs may also tend to increase in intensity on squatting if there is a significant rise in blood pressure.

9. Occasionally, both an ejection murmur and a regurgitant murmur may be present in the same patient as in some instances of aortic stenosis and mitral regurgitation. The recognition of the presence of both murmurs may sometime be easy. The aortic stenosis ejection murmur may be maximally loud at the second right interspace and may have all the characteristics of an ejection murmur and its typical cadence. The mitral regurgitation murmur may be maximally loud at the apex and may have all the features of the mitral regurgitation murmur, with typical blowing quality and high frequency, lasting all the way to S2. At other times however, the recognition may not be so easy due to the well-known *Gallavardin phenomenon whereby the high frequency components of an aortic ejection murmur may be selectively transmitted upstream and therefore to the apex. If this should happen, there may be only one lesion for instance aortic stenosis and yet one may mistake it for two lesions namely both aortic stenosis and mitral regurgitation.* The best way to be sure, of the presence of both lesions and two different murmurs, will be identification of two different responses of the murmurs to sudden change in rhythm producing a long diastole. If the patient were in atrial fibrillation it would then become easier. Then one can assess the effect of the long pause on the intensity of the murmur in both locations namely the second right interspace and the apex area. If they behave differently namely if the murmur at the second right interspace gets louder and the one at the apex does not change much, then one can be certain of the presence of both the ejection and the regurgitant murmurs.

10. ***Similar problem may arise with acute severe mitral regurgitation.*** In this instance, the murmur will have often a lot of low and medium frequencies and may sound harsher in quality. The murmur may end before S2 being ***decrescendo secondary to early build-up of a high*** left atrial ***v wave pressure.*** In addition, the murmur may be heard over a wide area including the base of the heart. A hyperdynamic left ventricular apical impulse and a fast rising CP with normal amplitude and an S3 (or its equivalent short mid-diastolic flow murmur) may bear clues to the presence of significant mitral regurgitation. If the patient were to have pre-mature beats, the behavior of the murmur following the post-ectopic pause will show that it is not an ejection murmur.

11. If the murmur cannot be categorized accurately as to whether it is ejection or regurgitant in type, then it is best described by its pre-dominant frequencies as to whether it is harsh and low medium in frequencies (meaning ejection in quality) or it is high in frequency and blowing (meaning regurgitant in quality). It gives a reference point to work with in trying to arrive at its cause. It needs to be considered obviously in relation to all the findings on examination. Again the length of the murmur, the location of maximal loudness, the effect of inspiration and the effect of changing postures namely the effect of standing and squatting all need to be determined and used in a similar fashion as described previously.

REFERENCES

1. McDonald DA. Blood Flow in Arteries. London: Edward Arnold Publishers Ltd; 1960.
2. McKusick VA. Cardiovascular Sound in Health and Disease. Baltimore: Williams and Wilkins; 1958.
3. Rushmer RF. Cardiovascular Dynamics. Philadelphia: WB Saunders, Co; 1970.
4. Bruns DL. A general theory of the causes of murmurs in the cardiovascular system. Am J Med. 1959;27:360-74.
5. Constant J, Lippschutz EJ. Diagramming and grading heart sounds and murmurs. Am Heart J. 1965;70:326-32.
6. Perloff JK. The physiologic mechanisms of cardiac and vascular physical signs. J Am Coll Cardiol. 1983;1(1):184-98.
7. Lembo NJ, Dell'Italia LJ, Crawford MH, et al. Bedside diagnosis of systolic murmurs. New Engl J Med. 1988;318:1572-8.
8. Leatham A. Systolic murmurs. Circulation. 1958;17(4, Part 1):601-11.
9. Murgo JP, Altobelli SA, Dorethy JF, et al. Normal ventricular ejection dynamics in man during rest and exercise. In: Leon DF, Shaver JA (Eds). Physiologic Principles of Heart Sounds and Murmurs. New York: American Heart Association; 1975. p. 92.
10. Constant J. Bedside Cardiology, 2nd edition. Boston: Little, Brown and Company; 1976.
11. Henke RP, March HW, Hultgren HN. An aid to identification of the murmur of aortic stenosis with atypical localization. Am Heart J. 1960;60:354-63.
12. Deleon AC, Jr, Perloff JK, Twigg H, et al. The straight back syndrome: clinical cardiovascular manifestations. Circulation. 1965;32:193-203.
13. Still GF. Common disorders and diseases of childhood. London: Frowde, Hodder and Stoughton; 1909.
14. Joffe HS. Genesis of Still's innocent systolic murmur. Br Heart J. 1992;67:206.
15. Donnerstein RL, Thomsen VS. Hemodynamic and anatomic factors affecting the frequency content of Still's innocent murmur. Am J Cardiol. 1994;74(5): 508-10.
16. Leatham A, Gray I. Auscultatory and phonocardiographic signs of atrial septal defect. Br Heart J. 1956;18(2):193-208.
17. Dalldorf FG, Willis PW 4th. Angled aorta ("sigmoid septum") as a cause of hypertrophic subaortic stenosis. Hum Pathol. 1985;16:457-62.

18. Paley HW. Left ventricular outflow tract obstruction heart sounds and murmurs. Am Heart Assoc Monogr. 1975;46:107-17.
19. Edwards JE. Pathology of left ventricular outflow tract obstruction. Circulation. 1965;31:586.
20. Gallavardin L, Pauper-Ravault. Le souffle' duretrecissement aortique puet changer de timbre et devenir dans sa propagation apexienne. Lyon Med. 1925: 523.
21. Bonner AJ, Jr, Sacks HN, Tavel ME. Assessing the severity of aortic stenosis by phonocardiography and external carotid pulse recordings. Circulation. 1973;48 (2):247-52.
22. Braunwald E, Roberts WC, Goldblatt A, et al. Aortic stenosis: physiological, pathological, and clinical concepts. Combined Clinical Staff Conference at the National Institutes of Health. Ann Intern Med. 1963;58:494-522.
23. Glancy DL, Shepherd RL, Beiser D, et al. The dynamic nature of left ventricular outflow obstruction in idiopathic hypertrophic subaortic stenosis. Ann Intern Med. 1971;75(4):589-93.
24. Ross J Jr, Braunwald E, Gault JH, et al. The mechanism of intra-ventricular pressure gradient in idiopathic hypertrophic subaortic stenosis. Circulation. 1966;34:558.
25. Murgo JP, Alter BR, Dorethy JF, et al. Dynamics of left ventricular ejection in obstructive and nonobstructive hypertrophic cardiomyopathy. J Clin Invest. 1980;66(6):1369-82.
26. Braunwald E, Morrow AG, Cornell WP, et al. Idiopathic hypertrophic subaortic stenosis. Clinical, hemodynamic and angiographic manifestations. Am J Med. 1960;29:924.
27. Shah PM, Gramiak R, Adelman AG, et al. Role of echocardiography in diagnostic and hemodynamic assessment of hypertrophic subaortic stenosis. Circulation. 1971;44(5):891-8.
28. Sherrid MV, Gunsburg DZ, Moldenhauer S, et al. Systolic anterior motion begins at low left ventricular outflow tract velocity in obstructive hypertrophic cardiomyopathy. J Am Coll Cardiol. 2000;36(4):1344-54.
29. Wigle ED, Adelman AG, Auger P, et al. Mitral regurgitation in muscular subaortic stenosis. Am J Cardiol. 1969;24(5):698-706.
30. Braunwald E, Seidman CE, Sigwart U. Contemporary evaluation and management of hypertrophic cardiomyopathy. Circulation. 2002;106(11):1312-6.
31. Mason DT, Braunwald E, Ross J, Jr. Effects of changes in body position on the severity of obstruction to left ventricular outflow in idiopathic hypertrophic subaortic stenosis. Circulation. 1966;33(3):374-82.
32. Grewe K, Crawford MH, O'Rourke RA. Differentiation of cardiac murmurs by dynamic auscultation. Curr Probl Cardiol. 1988;13(10):669-721.
33. Nishimura RA, Tajik AJ. The Valsalva maneuver and response revisited. Mayo Clin Proc. 1986;61(3):211-7.
34. Iida K, Sugishita Y, Ajisaka R, et al. Sigmoid septum causing left ventricular outflow tract obstruction: a case report. J Cardiogr. 1986;16:237-47.
35. Logan WF, Jones EW, Walker E, et al. Familial supravalvar aortic stenosis. Br Heart J. 1965;27:547-59.
36. Beuren AJ, Schulze C, Eberle P, et al. The syndrome of supravalvular aortic stenosis, peripheral pulmonary stenosis, mental retardation and similar facial appearance. Am J Cardiol. 1964;13:471-83.

37. Wooley CF, Hosier DM, Booth RW, et al. Supravalvular aortic stenosis. Clinical experiences with four patients including familial occurrence. Am J Med. 1961; 31:717-25.
38. Goldstein RE, Epstein SE. Mechanism of elevated innominate artery pressures in supravalvular aortic stenosis. Circulation. 1970;42(1):23-9.
39. French JW, Guntheroth WG. An explanation of asymmetric upper extremity blood pressures in supravalvular aortic stenosis: the effect. Circulation. 1970;42 (1):31-6.
40. Perloff JK. The clinical Recognition of Congenital Heart Disease. Philadelphia: WB Saunders; 1979. p. 81.
41. Perloff JK. Recognition and Differential Diagnosis of Pulmonary Stenosis. Segal BL (Ed). Philadelphia: FA Davis Co; 1963.
42. Perloff JK, Harvey WP. Auscultatory and phonocardiographic manifestations of pure mitral regurgitation. Prog Cardiovasc Dis. 1962;5:172-94.
43. Karliner JS, O'Rourke RA, Kearney DJ, et al. Haemodynamic explanation of why the murmur of mitral regurgitation in independent of cycle length. Br Heart J. 1973;35(4):397-401.
44. Ranganathan N, Lam JH, Wigle ED, et al. Morphology of the human mitral valve. II. The value leaflets. Circulation. 1970;41(3):459-67.
45. Ranganathan N, Silver MD, Wigle ED. Recent Advances in the knowledge of the anatomy of the mitral valve. In: Kalmanson D (Ed). Publishing Sciences Group Inc; 1976.
46. Ranganathan N, Burch GE. Gross morphology and arterial supply of the papillary muscles of the left ventricle of man. Am Heart J. 1969;77(4):506-16.
47. Lam JH, Ranganathan N, Wigle ED, et al. Morphology of the human mitral valve. I. Chordae tendineae: a new classification. Circulation. 1970;41(3): 449-58.
48. Perloff JK, Roberts WC. The mitral apparatus. Functional anatomy of mitral regurgitation. Circulation. 1972;46(2):227-39.
49. Fontana ME, Sparks EA, Boudoulas H, et al. Mitral valve prolapse and the mitral valve prolapse syndrome. Curr Probl Cardiol. 1991;16(5):309-75.
50. Ranganathan N, Silver MD, Robinson TI, et al. Angiographic-morphologic correlation in patients with severe mitral regurgitation due to prolapse of the posterior mitral valve leaflet. Circulation. 1973;48(3):514-8.
51. Selzer A, Katayama F. Mitral regurgitation: clinical patterns, pathophysiology and natural history. Medicine (Baltimore). 1972;51(5):337-66.
52. Rotem CE, Hultgren HN. Corrected transposition of the great vessels without associated defects. Am Heart J. 1965;70:305-18.
53. Tsakiris AG, Rastelli GC, Amorim Dde S, et al. Effect of experimental papillary muscle damage on mitral valve closure in intact anesthetized dogs. Mayo Clin Proc. 1970;45(4):275-85.
54. Mittal AK, Langston M, Jr, Cohn KE, et al. Combined papillary muscle and left ventricular wall dysfunction as a cause of mitral regurgitation. An experimental study. Circulation. 1971;44(2):174-80.
55. Phillips JH, Burch GE, Depasquale NP. The syndrome of papillary muscle dysfunction. Its clinical recognition. Ann Intern Med. 1963;59:508-20.
56. Shelburne JC, Rubinstein D, Gorlin R. A reappraisal of papillary muscle dysfunction; correlative clinical and angiographic study. Am J Med. 1969;46(6): 862-71.
57. Cuasay RS, Morse DP, Spagna P, et al. Massive mitral regurgitation from chordal rupture and coronary artery disease. Ann Thorac Surg. 1978;25(5):438-43.

58. Ranganathan N, Silver MD, Freeman M, et al. Clinico-pathologic Correlations in Acute and Acute on Chronic Mitral Regurgitation. XII Inter-American Congress of Cardiology, Vancouver, June 16–21, 1985.
59. Clements SD, Jr, Story WE, Hurst JW, et al. Ruptured papillary muscle, a complication of myocardial infarction: clinical presentation, diagnosis, and treatment. Clin Cardiol. 1985;8(2):93-103.
60. Bass NM, Sharratt GP. Left atrial myxoma diagnosed by echocardiography, with observations on tumour movement. Br Heart J. 1973;35(12):1332-5.
61. Carabello BA. Progress in mitral and aortic regurgitation. Prog Cardiovasc Dis. 2001;43(6):457-75.
62. Bonow RO, Carabello BA, Chatterjee K, et al. ACC/AHA guidelines for the management of patients with valvular heart disease. A report of the American College of Cardiology/American Heart Association. Task Force on Practice Guidelines (Committee on Management of Patients With Valvular Heart Disease). J Am Coll Cardiol. 1998;32:1486-588.
63. Carabello BA. Mitral valve regurgitation. Curr Probl Cardiol. 1998;23(4):202-41.
64. Carabello BA. Concentric versus eccentric remodeling. J Card Fail. 2002;8 (6 Suppl):S258-63.
65. Ronan JA, Jr, Steelman RB, DeLeon AC, Jr, et al. The clinical diagnosis of acute severe mitral insufficiency. Am J Cardiol. 1971;27(3):284-90.
66. Sutton GC, Craige E. Clinical signs of severe acute mitral regurgitation. Am J Cardiol. 1967;20(1):141-4.
67. Barlow JB, Pocock WA. The significance of late systolic murmurs and mid-late systolic clicks. Md State Med J. 1963;12:76-7.
68. Fontana ME, Pence HL, Leighton RF, et al. The varying clinical spectrum of the systolic click-late systolic murmur syndrome. Circulation. 1970;41(5):807-16.
69. Ranganathan N, Silver MD, Robinson TI, et al. Idiopathic prolapsed mitral leaflet syndrome angiographic clinical correlations. Circulation. 1976;54:707-15.
70. Waller BF, Morrow AG, Maron BJ, et al. Etiology of clinically isolated, severe, chronic, pure mitral regurgitation: analysis of 97 patients over 30 years of age having mitral valve replacement. Am Heart J. 1982;104(2 Pt 1):276-88.
71. Barlow J, Pocock WA, Marchand P, et al. The significance of late systolic murmurs. Am Heart J. 1963;66:443-52.
72. Ronan JA, Perloff JK, Harvey WP. Systolic clicks and the late systolic murmur; intracardiac phonocardiographic evidence of their mitral valve origin. Am Heart J. 1965;70:319-25.
73. Wigle ED, Rakowski H, Ranganathan N, et al. Mitral valve prolapse. Annu Rev Med. 1976;27:165-80.
74. Criley JM, Lewis KB, Humphries JO, et al. Prolapse of the mitral valve: clinical and cine-angiocardiographic findings. Br Heart J. 1966;28(4):488-96.
75. Leon DF, Leonard JJ, Kroetz FW, et al. Late systolic murmurs, clicks, and whoops arising from the mitral valve. A transseptal intracardiac phonocardiographic analysis. Am Heart J. 1966;72(3):325-36.
76. Hancock EW, Cohn K. The syndrome associated with midsystolic click and late systolic murmur. Am J Med. 1966;41(2):183-96.
77. Fontana ME, Kissel GL, Criley M. Functional anatomy of mitral valve prolapse. Am Heart Assoc Monogr. 1975;46:126.
78. Luisada AA, Leon F, Singhal A, et al. Various types of systolic clicks in patients with muscular subaortic stenosis. Jpn Heart J. 1985;26:133-43.

79. Holmes AM, Logan WF, Winterbottom T. Transient systolic murmurs in angina pectoris. Am Heart J. 1968;76(5):680-4.
80. Kalra K, Wang Q, McIver BV, et al. Temporal changes in interpapillary muscle dynamics as an active indicator of mitral valve and left ventricular interaction in ischemic mitral regurgitation. J Am Coll Cardiol. 2014;64(18):1867-79.
81. Sanders CA, Armstrong PW, Willerson JT, et al. Etiology and differential diagnosis of acute mitral regurgitation. Prog Cardiovasc Dis. 1971;14(2):129-52.
82. DePace NL, Nestico PF, Morganroth J. Acute severe mitral regurgitation. Pathophysiology, clinical recognition, and management. Am J Med. 1985;78(2): 293-306.
83. Tavel ME, Campbell RW, Zimmer JF. Late systolic murmurs and mitral regurgitation. Am J Cardiol. 1965;15:719-25.
84. Forrester JS, Diamond G, Freedman S, et al. Silent mitral insufficiency in acute myocardial infarction. Circulation. 1971;44(5):877-83.
85. Nishimura RA, Schaff HV, Shub C, et al. Papillary muscle rupture complicating acute myocardial infarction: analysis of 17 patients. Am J Cardiol. 1983; 51(3):373-7.
86. Caulfield JB, Page DL, Kastor JA, et at. Connective tissue abnormalities in spontaneous rupture of chordae tendineae. Arch Pathol. 1971;91(6):537-41.
87. Cohen LS. Atypical and acute mitral regurgitation. Am Heart Assoc Monogr. 1975;46:122-5.
88. Silver MD, Lam JH, Ranganathan N, et al. Morphology of the human tricuspid valve. Circulation. 1971;43(3):333-48.
89. Wooley CF. The spectrum of tricuspid regurgitation. Am Heart Assoc Monogr. 1975;46:139-48.
90. Ewy GA. Tricuspid Valve Disease, 3rd edition. Alpert JS, Dalen JE, Rahimtoola SH (Eds). Philadelphia: Lippincott Williams and Wilkins; 2000.
91. Gotzsche H, Falholt W. Ebstein's anomaly of the tricuspid valve; a review of the literature and report of 6 new cases. Am Heart J. 1954;47(4):587-603.
92. Roberts WC. A unique heart disease associated with a unique cancer: carcinoid heart disease. Am J Cardiol. 1997;80:251-6.
93. Rubin LJ. Primary pulmonary hypertension. New Engl J Med. 1997;336:111-7.
94. Dartevelle P, Fadel E, Mussot S, Chapelier A, Herve P, de Perrot M, et al. Chronic thromboembolic pulmonary hypertension. Eur Respir J. 2004;23(4):637-48.
95. Wright JL, Levy RD, Churg A. Pulmonary hypertension in chronic obstructive pulmonary disease: current theories of pathogenesis and their implications for treatment. Thorax. 2005;60(7):605-9.
96. Keogh AM, McNeil KD, Williams T, et al. Pulmonary arterial hypertension: a new era in management. Med J Aust. 2003;178(11):564-7.
97. Palevsky HI, Fishman AP. Chronic cor pulmonale. Etiology and management. JAMA. 1990;263(17):2347-53.
98. Wood P. The Eisenmenger syndrome or pulmonary hypertension with reversed central shunt. Br Heart J. 1963;2:701.
99. Wood P. Pulmonary hypertension. Br Med Bull. 1952;8:348.
100. Rios JC, Massumi RA, Breesmen WT, et al. Auscultatory features of acute tricuspid regurgitation. Am J Cardiol. 1969;23(1):4-11.
101. Becu LM, Burchell HB, Dushane JW, et al. Anatomic and pathologic studies in ventricular septal defect. Circulation. 1956;14(3):349-64.
102. Blount SG, Jr, Mueller H, McCord MC. Ventricular septal defect Clinical and hemodynamic patterns. Am J Med. 1955;18:871.

103. Beck W, Schrire V, Vogelpoel L, et al. Hemodynamic effects of amyl nitrite and phenylephrine on the normal human circulation and their relation to changes in cardiac murmurs. Am J Cardiol. 1961;8:341-9.
104. Bloomfield DK. The natural history of ventricular septal defect in patients surviving infancy. Circulation. 1964;29:914-55.
105. Schrire V, Vogelpoel L, Beck W, et al. Ventricular septal defect: the clinical spectrum. Br Heart J. 1965;27(6):813-28.
106. Anderson RH, Becker AE, Lucchese E. Morphology of Congenital Heart Disease. Baltimore: University Park Press; 1983.
107. Topaz O, Taylor AL. Interventricular septal rupture complicating acute myocardial infarction: from pathophysiologic features to the role of invasive and noninvasive diagnostic modalities in current management. Am J Med. 1992;93:683-8.
108. Birnbaum Y, Fishbein MC, Blanche C, et al. Ventricular septal rupture after acute myocardial infarction. N Engl J Med. 2002;347(18):1426-32.
109. Crenshaw BS, Granger CB, Birnbaum Y, et al. Risk factors, angiographic patterns, and outcomes in patients with ventricular septal defect complicating acute myocardial infarction. GUSTO-I (Global Utilization of Streptokinase and TPA for Occluded Coronary Arteries) Trial Investigators. Circulation. 2000;101(1):27-32.
110. Figueras J, Cortadellas J, Soler-Soler J. Comparison of ventricular septal and left ventricular free wall rupture in acute myocardial infarction. Am J Cardiol. 1998;81(4):495-7.
111. Perloff JK. The Clinical Recognition of Congenital Heart Disease. Philadelphia: WB Saunders; 2001.
112. Therrien J, Dore A, Gersony W, et al. CCS Consensus Conference 2001 update: recommendations for the management of adults with congenital heart disease. Part I. Can J Cardiol. 2001;17(9):940-59.
113. Leatham A, Segal B. Auscultatory and phonocardiographic signs of ventricular septal defect with left to-right shunt. Circulation. 1962;25:318-27.
114. Hollman A, Morgan JJ, Goodwin JF, et al. Auscultatory and phonocardiographic findings in ventricular septal defect. A study of 93 surgically treated patients. Circulation. 1963;28:94-100.
115. Farru O, Duffau G, Rodriguez R. Auscultatory and phonocardiographic characteristics of supracristal ventricular septal defect. Br Heart J. 1971;33(2):238-45.
116. Perloff JK. Auscultatory and phonocardiographic manifestations of pulmonary hypertension. Prog Cardiovasc Dis. 1967;9: 303.
117. Perloff JK. Ventricular septal defect with pulmonary stenosis. In: The Clinical Recognition of Congenital Heart Disease. Philadelphia: WB Saunders Co; 1970. pp. 349-91.
118. McCord MC, Van Elk J, Blount SG Jr. Tetrology of Fallot. Clinical and hemodynamic spectrum of combined pulmonary stenosis and ventricular septal defect. Circulation. 1957;16:736.

Chapter

8 Heart Murmurs (Part II)

Snapshot

DIASTOLIC MURMURS

Diastolic murmurs can be caused by turbulent flow through the atrioventricular valves (the mitral and the tricuspid valves) or turbulence caused by regurgitation of blood through the semilunar valves (the aortic and the pulmonary valves). We will first discuss diastolic murmurs arising from turbulent flow through the atrioventricular valves.

DIASTOLIC MURMURS OF MITRAL ORIGIN

Turbulent flow across the mitral valve capable of producing a diastolic murmur can occur under the following conditions:

1. *When there is increased pressure in the left atrium due to obstruction at the valve*
2. *When there is excessive volume of flow during diastole through the mitral valve with or without elevated left atrial pressure*
3. *Normal or increased mitral inflow velocity through a somewhat abnormal mitral valve*

4. *Normal mitral inflow through a functionally stenotic mitral orifice in the absence of organic valvular disease.*

Mitral Obstruction Secondary to Mitral Valvular Stenosis

Mitral valvular obstruction may occur on account of congenitally stenosed valve or ***acquired*** stenosis such as caused by ***rheumatic*** heart disease where the leaflets get tethered and the commissures become fused due to the rheumatic process.[1-4] ***Congenital*** mitral stenosis is ***rare*** and when it occurs in combination with an atrial septal defect the condition goes by the name of ***Lutembacher's syndrome.***[5-7] Rarely the obstruction may be caused by a left atrial tumor such as an atrial myxoma.[8,9] ***Atrial myxoma*** is a benign tumor with myxoid matrix of gelatinous consistency. It may be associated with constitutional symptoms such as fever and systemic inflammatory signs such as elevated sedimentation rate. The myxoma is usually attached by a stalk to the inter-atrial septum and may prolapse into the ventricle in early diastole when the valve opens and cause obstruction to the mitral inflow.

In the normal heart, the ***v wave*** pressure that is built up in the left atrium at the end of systole provides the gradient in early diastole for the diastolic flow to occur through the mitral valve. At this time, the left ventricular pressure is close to zero. During the rapid filling phase of diastole there is a fall in the left atrial pressure and a rise in the left ventricular diastolic pressure due to emptying of the left atrium and filling of the left ventricle, respectively. When there is any significant obstruction to flow at the mitral valve, the left atrial pressure will be elevated due to the obstruction and the flow through the valve in diastole will occur under a higher ***v wave*** pressure gradient. The more severe the obstruction or the stenosis the more persistent will be the elevation in the left atrial pressure. The pressure gradient between the left atrium and the left ventricle will tend to persist throughout diastole. The diastolic flow occurring under a higher and a persistent pressure gradient will contribute to a turbulent flow, which may persist throughout diastole. The normal left atrial ***v wave*** pressure is usually about 12–15 mm Hg. When there is significant mitral stenosis, the ***v wave*** pressure may be elevated up to 25–30 mm Hg (Fig. 8.1). *However, the pressure gradient noted even with severe mitral stenosis is still fairly low in terms of the absolute mmHg elevation. On the other hand, the volume of flow through the mitral valve is always significant since the entire stroke volume of the heart will have to go through the mitral valve in diastole. Thus, a large volume going through the mitral valve under relatively low levels of pressure will be expected to give rise to turbulence, which will produce predominantly low-frequency murmur.* In fact, the low pitch of the mitral stenosis murmur gives its characteristic rumbling quality on auscultation. The loudness of the murmur produced by the turbulence will

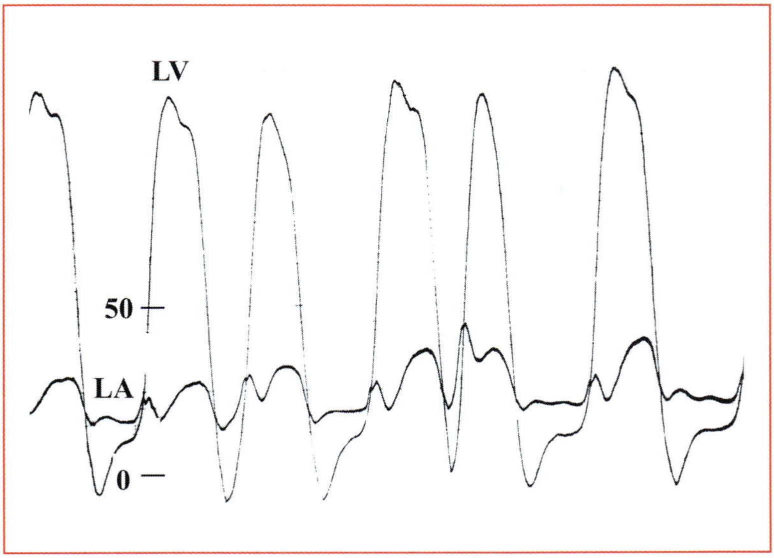

Fig. 8.1: Simultaneous recording of the left ventricular (LV) and the left atrial (LA) pressure curves obtained at cardiac catheterization from a patient with significant mitral stenosis. The rhythm is atrial fibrillation with varying diastolic intervals. A significant and persistent gradient throughout diastole is noted between the LA and the LV pressures even when the diastole is relatively long (e.g. following the fifth beat).

depend on the adequacy of the cardiac output, whereas the length will depend more on the length of time the pressure gradient persists in diastole. The latter will tend to last throughout diastole when the stenosis is severe.[1,3,10-13]

Characteristics of Mitral Stenosis Murmurs

1. The mitral diastolic murmur of mitral stenosis will be expected to begin in diastole after the mitral valve opens and the rapid filling phase of diastole begins. The murmur is low pitched and often very well ***localized to the apex.*** The murmur may be so localized that unless one auscultates at the apex it may be missed. The best way to hear the murmur is to have the patient turn to the left lateral decubitus position and locate the left ventricular apex and use the bell to listen. *The murmur has a rumbling quality and sounds like a distant roar of a thunder. The loud S1 and the opening snap following the S2, which are invariably present in classical mitral stenosis, give the background for auscultation. Together they make a cadence:*
   One ....Two ...ta r r r r r r r r
2. The loudness of the murmur has no relationship to the severity of the stenosis. *The loudness of the murmur may be related to the adequacy of the cardiac output.*

In severe pulmonary hypertension secondary to the mitral stenosis, the high pulmonary vascular resistance is usually associated with decreased cardiac output. In such patients with severe mitral stenosis and low output symptoms, the murmur may be soft and rarely may be even inaudible. Occasionally, in over diuresed patients and decreased intravascular volume the murmur may be soft despite significant stenosis. When the cardiac output is increased by slight exercise such as walking for a few minutes, the murmur may be brought out more clearly

3. *The length of the murmur has an important relationship to the severity of the mitral stenosis.* If the stenosis is severe and is associated with a persistent diastolic gradient, the murmur will last throughout diastole until the beginning of next systole (Fig. 8.2). In atrial fibrillation, the varying diastolic pauses allow good opportunity to assess the length of the murmur in relation to the long pauses of diastole
4. The diastolic murmur of mitral stenosis will often have a ***pre-systolic crescendo*** to the loud M1 (Fig. 8.2).[14,15] Occasionally, one may hear only the pre-systolic murmur (Fig. 8.3). If this were the case then it usually means that the mitral stenosis is mild. The pre-systolic murmur tends to have ***some higher frequencies*** in that one can easily hear this with the chest piece of the stethoscope unlike the diastolic rumble. Generally, the presystolic murmur is not heard when the valve is heavily calcified and rigid.

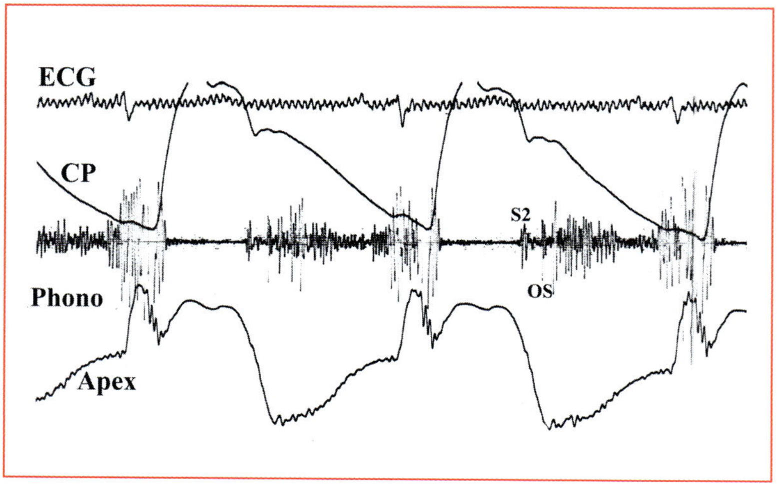

Fig. 8.2: Simultaneous recording of the ECG, the carotid pulse (CP), the apexcardiogram (Apex) and phonocardiogram (Phono) taken at the apex area from a patient with severe mitral stenosis. The Phono recording shows the full-length diastolic murmur, which begins immediately following the opening snap (OS). The low-frequency murmur is initially loud and diminishes slightly later to become accentuated with a crescendo shape ending with a loud intensity first heart sound (S1). The systole is free of murmur.

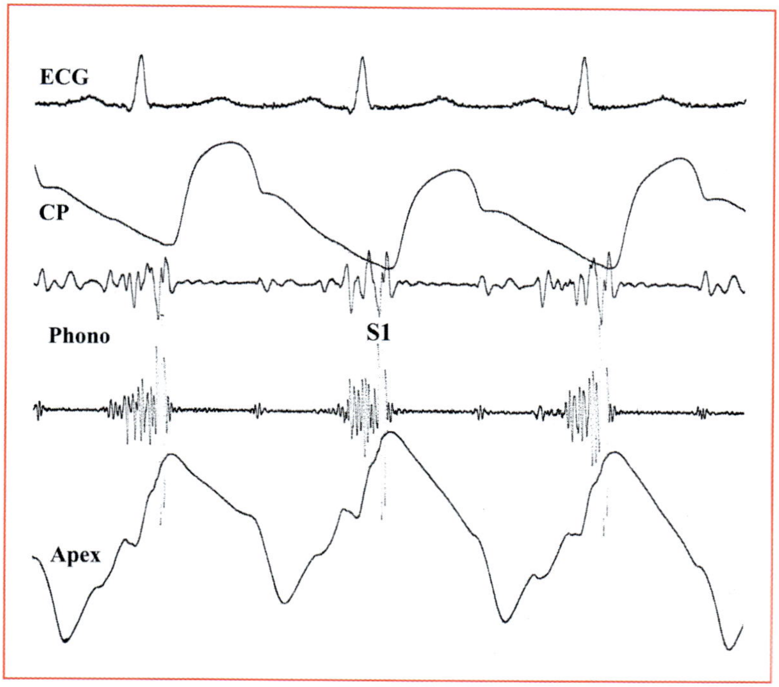

Fig. 8.3: Simultaneous recording of the ECG, the carotid pulse (CP), the apexcardiogram (Apex) and phonocardiogram (Phono) taken at the apex area from a patient with mild mitral stenosis. The Phono shows predominantly a pre-systolic murmur increasing in intensity ending with a large amplitude first heart sound (S1). Note that the murmur has predominantly high frequency.

The left ventricle begins to contract at the end of diastole. When the left ventricular pressure exceeds the left atrial pressure the mitral valve will close. The column of blood contained in the left ventricle being moved by the contracting left ventricle will be suddenly decelerated against the closed mitral valve causing the loud M1. The loudness of M1 stems from the high dP/dt of the left ventricle at the time of closure of the mitral valve as a result of the elevated left atrial pressure. This has been discussed previously in relation to the S1.

Although with sinus rhythm and preserved atrial contraction and relaxation one should expect a crescendo-decrescendo murmur with the increasing flow velocity associated with atrial contraction and decreasing flow velocity during atrial relaxation only the crescendo pre-systolic murmur is characteristic of mitral stenosis. Very rarely when the PR interval is prolonged one may observe and record a crescendo-decrescendo murmur. Simultaneous recording of the left ventricular and left atrial pressures will show that *the pre-systolic crescendo effect actually occurs at a time when the gradient is diminishing with the rising left ventricular pressure due to its contraction just before the crossover point of the pressures.*[4] In addition, the pre-systolic crescendo of the diastolic murmur can be *recognized in shorter diastoles during atrial fibrillation.*[15] This would suggest that the increased volume and velocity of flow during ***a wave*** rise in the left atrial pressure due to atrial systole in sinus rhythm alone is not adequate to explain its mechanism. *Doppler measurements of mitral flow velocity at the time of diminishing pressure gradient at the end of diastole show that the flow velocity decreases and the slope of deceleration appears to be more steep with the crescendo effect seen on the murmur. It is conceivable that the rising left ventricular pressure caused by its contraction and its increasing dP/dt not only decelerates the mitral flow but also produces increased turbulence, resulting in the increased intensity of the murmur.*[16]

Mitral Obstruction Secondary to Left Atrial Myxoma

This benign tumor is usually attached by a stalk to the interatrial septum. If it is large enough it will obstruct mitral inflow during diastole and cause turbulence of mitral inflow giving rise to the diastolic murmur.[8,9] It has been previously discussed in the context of the tumor plop sound, how the tumor by elevating the left atrial ***v wave*** helps to initiate a rapid expansion in the rapid filling phase. The tumor prolapses into the left ventricle when the mitral valve opens. When it reaches its maximum excursion its further movement is suddenly stopped. This gives rise to a filling sound, which is a loud S3 like sound called the tumor plop. The tumor plop sound occurs shortly after the rapid filling wave peak. It is followed by a low-pitched diastolic rumble. The length of the murmur again will correspond to the duration of the diastolic gradient. Since the tumor will prevent proper leaflet apposition, there will be always some mitral regurgitation. This is usually not severe. The elevated left atrial pressure increases the M1 intensity. *The loud S1, the S2 and the tumor plop sound followed by the low-pitched diastolic murmur as well as the high-frequency blowing systolic regurgitation murmur are very characteristic of this condition (Fig. 8.4).*

Excess Diastolic Mitral Inflow

The entire stroke volume of the heart usually goes through the mitral valve during diastole except when there is an atrial septal defect. In certain conditions, however, there may not be increased forward output through the aorta, but nevertheless, there may be more than normal pulmonary venous inflow, which may go through the mitral valve in diastole. These conditions are associated with volume overload of the left atrium and the left ventricle as may be seen in mitral regurgitation, ventricular septal defect and persistent ductus arteriosus.[10,17,18] In mitral regurgitation, the mitral inflow will have to include not only the volume that went back into the left atrium due to the systolic regurgitation but also the normal pulmonary venous return. In ventricular

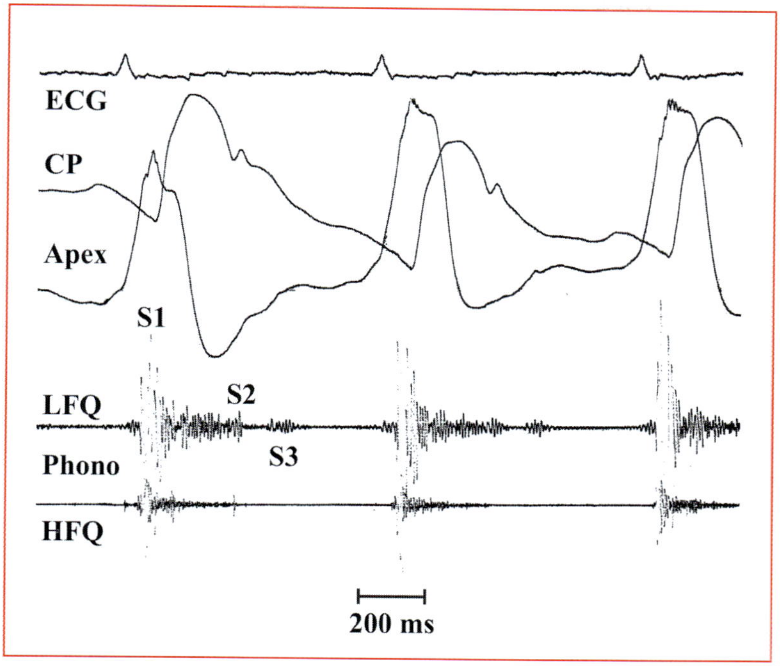

Fig. 8.4: Simultaneous recording of the ECG, the carotid pulse (CP), the apexcardiogram (Apex) and phonocardiogram (Phono) taken from the apex area from a patient with a left atrial myxoma. The Phono shows the characteristic features of a loud first heart sound (S1), a regurgitant systolic murmur followed by a tumor plop sound at the time of a third heart sound (S3).

septal defect and persistent ductus arteriosus, the excess pulmonary flow due to the left-to-right shunt is added onto the normal pulmonary venous return. In these two conditions with left-to-right shunt, the left atrial ***v wave*** pressure may still be normal as long as the left ventricular diastolic function is preserved and its ***pre a wave*** pressure remains normal (approximately 5 mm Hg). In mitral regurgitation, however, the ***v wave*** pressure in the left atrium may be somewhat elevated secondary to the systolic regurgitation. The degree of elevation of the left atrial ***v wave*** pressure will depend not only on the severity of the mitral regurgitation but also on its duration and the left atrial compliance or distensibility. Thus, the increased mitral inflow during diastole in the above conditions may or may not be accompanied by increased ***v wave*** pressure gradient during early diastole. Nevertheless, the excess flow in diastole through the mitral valve will produce enough turbulence to generate mid-diastolic low-frequency murmurs.[15] The normal semiclosure movement of the mitral valve leaflets after the full opening in early diastole that can be easily appreciated in two-dimensional echocardiographic images, further helps to increase the turbulence by slightly narrowing the functional orifice.

When there is high cardiac output as may occur in anemia, thyrotoxicosis, pregnancy and others, there will be obligatory increase in mitral inflow along with increased velocity of flow. In children, the increased sympathetic tone will also be accompanied by increased velocity of flow through the heart. In children, pregnant women, anemia and other high output states, it is not uncommon to have physiologic S3 and this has been discussed previously. Occasionally, there may be some turbulence caused by the excessive and/or rapid inflow to produce short mid-diastolic flow murmurs in these states.

In patients with complete atrioventricular block (where atrial depolarizations of sinus nodal origin fail to conduct to the ventricle), when the independent atrial contraction happens to occur during the rapid filling phase of diastole, a short mid-diastolic flow murmur may also be noted to occur. The mechanism of origin of these intermittent mid-diastolic flow murmurs (sometimes called the ***Rytand murmur***) is also similar.[19,20]

Flow Through Abnormal but Non-Stenotic Mitral Valve

In acute rheumatic fever the mitral valve structures may be acutely inflamed with some thickening and edema. The involvement of the mitral structures in the acute rheumatic process may be accompanied by mid-diastolic murmurs presumably caused by some turbulence of flow during the rapid filling phase. These murmurs are typically low pitched and of short duration in mid-diastole. At this stage of the rheumatic process, the mitral valve is far from being stenosed. Often there may be at least moderate degree of mitral regurgitation. The latter will also contribute to the increased mitral inflow during diastole. The presence of this murmur is good evidence of ***active carditis in rheumatic fever.*** It is called the ***Carey Coombs murmur.***[21]

Flow Through Functionally Stenotic Mitral Valve

In ***aortic regurgitation,*** often the regurgitant jet is directed toward the anterior mitral leaflet. In fact, the anterior mitral leaflet may be shown to exhibit some fine fluttering in diastole due to this jet hitting it. This can be seen particularly well on the M-mode of the echocardiogram. When the aortic regurgitation is significant and directed toward the anterior mitral leaflet, it may actually prevent the latter from opening well during diastole. The semiclosed mitral valve can also be well seen on the two-dimensional echocardiogram well separated from the ventricular septum. In such patients, the diastolic inflow through the mitral valve will be accompanied by turbulence. The left atrial ***v wave*** pressure may not be elevated however. The turbulent mitral inflow due to the ***functional stenosis*** caused by the aortic regurgitation may be accompanied by ***a low-frequency diastolic murmur.*** The murmur will sound quite similar to the diastolic rumble of mitral stenosis and is best heard at the apex. This goes by the name of ***Austin Flint murmur.***[4,22–26] The Austin Flint murmur as a sign of severe aortic regurgitation can in fact be proven by improving forward flow through the aorta by arterial dilator such as amyl nitrite, thereby diminishing the degree of aortic regurgitation. Amyl nitrite is usually administered as a vapor through inhalation. It causes profound arterial and arteriolar dilatation. It has a very short half-life in the body and is usually eliminated by the lungs. The profound arterial and arteriolar dilatation causes the systemic arterial pressure to fall. This leads to sympathetic stimulation and tachycardia. The sympathetic stimulation often will cause venoconstriction and increase the venous return. This will lead to increased cardiac output. Amyl nitrite differs from nitroglycerin in this respect. The latter causes less dramatic fall in blood pressure and the sympathetic stimulation is less profound. In addition, nitroglycerin lasts slightly longer in the body, which leads to significant venodilatation. This results in decreased venous return and decreased cardiac output. The decreased venous return is an important hemodynamic effect, which helps to reduce the heart size, and by diminishing the size of the heart it reduces the wall tension, thereby reducing the oxygen demand. This is one of the important effects of nitroglycerin for the improvement of ischemia in addition to its effect on direct coronary vasodilatation and peripheral arterial bed. When Amyl nitrite is administered in aortic regurgitation, the resulting peripheral arterial and arteriolar dilatation would improve forward runoff, thereby decreasing the degree of aortic regurgitation. When the aortic regurgitation is reduced, there will be less restriction on the mitral anterior leaflet. *Austin Flint murmur will disappear on amyl nitrite inhalation* despite the fact that the actual volume of flow through the mitral valve is increased due to the increased venous return and cardiac output. Amyl nitrite will have an opposite effect on organic mitral stenosis murmur since the increased flow through the mitral valve will actually increase the intensity of the murmur. In fact, this was the method used often at the bedside to distinguish Austin Flint murmur and true mitral stenosis before the advent of two-dimensional echocardiography. It is still a useful bedside method.[27]

DIASTOLIC MURMURS OF TRICUSPID ORIGIN

Turbulent flow across the tricuspid valve capable of producing a diastolic murmur can occur under the following conditions:

1. *When there is increased pressure in the right atrium due to obstruction at the valve*
2. *Normal or increased tricuspid inflow velocity through abnormal non-stenotic tricuspid valve*
3. *When there is excessive volume of flow during diastole through the tricuspid valve with or without elevated right atrial pressure.*

Tricuspid Obstruction Secondary to Tricuspid Valve Stenosis

Tricuspid Stenosis due to rheumatic heart disease is quite rare and it is usually associated with mitral stenosis and aortic valve disease. The right atrial and the jugular venous pressures will be elevated. The latter may show a large amplitude ***a wave*** followed by the ***x′ descent*** in patients with sinus rhythm. *Generally, the pressure gradient in patients with sinus rhythm is usually noted at the end of diastole (presystole).* In patients with atrial fibrillation, the gradient may be observed in mid-diastole. The entire stroke volume of the heart goes through the tricuspid valve as well similar to the mitral valve at fairly low pressure gradients. The murmur therefore is low pitched and generally reflects the diastolic gradient.[28–33]

Characteristics of Tricuspid Stenosis Murmur

1. *In patients with sinus rhythm, the murmur is only presystolic but with a crescendo-decrescendo effect* due to atrial contraction augmenting flow velocity followed by atrial relaxation diminishing the velocity. In patients with atrial fibrillation, the murmur will tend to be more mid diastolic and low pitched.
2. The tricuspid component of S1 may be loud and there may be a tricuspid opening snap but both may be difficult to recognize due to a loud M1 and mitral opening snap secondary to associated mitral stenosis.
3. *The maximal loudness of the murmur will be at the lower sternal region and the murmur may be shown to augment in intensity on inspiration and also by turning the patient to the right lateral decubitus.*[29]

Tricuspid Obstruction Secondary to Right Atrial Myxoma

The mechanism of tricuspid valve obstruction secondary to a right atrial myxoma is similar to what has been described under mitral obstruction secondary to a left atrial myxoma. The right atrial pressure will be elevated raising the jugular venous pressure. The myxoma will cause obstruction to the tricuspid inflow and also interfere with the apposition of the leaflets and therefore cause tricuspid regurgitation. The elevated right atrial pressure will cause a diastolic gradient and contribute to the diastolic turbulence and murmur. The jugular venous pulse may show both X' and Y descents. The loud T1 will be the reason for a loud S1 and will be shown to increase in intensity on inspiration. There may be a loud tumor plop sound corresponding to the timing of an S3, which will be followed by a low-pitched diastolic murmur. The latter again will be best heard over the lower left sternal area and may also augment in intensity on inspiration.[34,35]

Flow Through Abnormal but Non-Stenotic Tricuspid Valve

Tricuspid valve may be ***congenitally abnormal as in Ebstein's anomaly.*** In certain ***acquired*** disorders such as the ***carcinoid*** syndrome, the tricuspid valve leaflets may show abnormal thickening and fibrosis. The tricuspid valve will often be regurgitant in these conditions. The tricuspid inflow under these conditions will often be associated with a low-pitched diastolic murmur as well.[36,37]

Excess Diastolic Tricuspid Inflow

Excess volume of tricuspid inflow will be expected in certain situations where there is right atrial and right ventricular volume overload. These include atrial septal defect with a left-to-right shunt and tricuspid regurgitation. In atrial septal defect when there is a significant left-to-right shunt, the shunt flow added onto the normal venous return will cause both right atrial and right ventricular volume overload. In significant tricuspid regurgitation of whatever etiology, tricuspid inflow will be increased in the same way the mitral regurgitation increases mitral inflow. In both these conditions, the right atrial pressure may or may not be elevated. Nevertheless, one can expect a tricuspid inflow rumble. In fact, the presence of such a rumble in atrial septal defect is a sign of a significant left-to-right shunt. In tricuspid regurgitation, there may be a right-sided S3 and occasionally it may have enough duration to it simulating a low-pitched diastolic murmur.[38-40]

SEMILUNAR VALVE REGURGITATION

Regurgitation of blood (backward flow) through the semilunar valves, namely the aortic and the pulmonary valves during diastole can cause turbulence and lead to the production of diastolic murmurs.

We will discuss aortic regurgitation first.

AORTIC REGURGITATION

Causes of Aortic Regurgitation

Aortic Regurgitation can result either from intrinsic ***valvular*** pathology ***or*** arise from ***aortic root dilatation.***[31,41-43]

Valvular Causes

Valvular abnormalities that can result in aortic regurgitation can either be ***congenital or acquired.*** Congenitally, the aortic valve cusps may have ***fenestrations, which*** may result in regurgitation particularly when there is associated systemic hypertension. Occasionally, the aortic valve may be ***bicuspid.*** In fact, this abnormality is often the most common congenital anomaly of the heart occurring in about 1% of the population. The bicuspid valve is often eccentric with unequal cusps and generally tends to be insufficient.[44] Aortic valve cusps sometime develop ***prolapse in*** the presence of a congenital ***perimembranous ventricular septal defect.*** While this may help in the spontaneous closure of the defect it can result in varying degrees of aortic regurgitation.[38]

The aortic valve may be involved in ***rheumatic*** heart disease and the valve can become both stenotic and regurgitant due to commissural fusion and thickening and scarring of the cusps. In the elderly, the aortic valve may become ***calcific*** and these will be more commonly associated with some degree of regurgitation. Rarely the aortic valve cusps may have ***myxomatous infiltration, which*** may make the cusps somewhat large and allow them to prolapse into the left ventricle. These changes generally, however, occur in individuals with Marfan's syndrome, who may also have aortic root disease and dilatation. Infective ***endocarditis*** can occur on the aortic valve and this may cause aortic regurgitation to become clinically evident for the first time. Formations of vegetations may interfere with apposition of the cusps. In addition, infective destruction or perforations in the cusps could occur. It can also aggravate and worsen the degree of pre-existing aortic regurgitation. The cusps may become thickened and develop sclerotic changes with aging. In the presence of associated hypertension, may lead to some aortic regurgitation. Rarely blunt chest ***trauma*** can result in a tear of the aortic valve cusps and lead to aortic regurgitation.

Aortic Root Disease

Aorta and the aortic root may be involved in disease process, which may lead to significant dilatation of the aortic root.[42,43] The latter will stretch the aortic valve ring and make the cusps incompetent. The list of entities that can result in such a process include congenital ***aneurysm of the sinus of Valsalva, syphilitic aortitis*** that is now quite uncommon, ***cystic medial necrosis with and without overt Marfan's*** syndrome, ***spondylitis,*** rheumatoid arthritis, ***Paget's disease, osteogenesis imperfecta*** and hypertensive ***atherosclerotic aneurysm*** of the ascending aorta. The pathology will vary according to the disease entity involved. In many of these entities, the elastic tissue in the media of the aorta gets destroyed and this leads to expansion of the aorta. For instance, in the atherosclerotic aneurysm it has been shown that the media gets infiltrated with macrophages that elaborate metalloproteinases leading to the destruction of the elastic tissue. Occasionally, the aortic medial disease may make the aorta ***vulnerable for dissection*** particularly in the presence of ***hypertension.*** In this instance, ***the intima may tear*** on account of the hemodynamic stress and the tear can extend and dissect through the media of the aorta. The dissection ***will result in two lumens in the aorta*** one being the true lumen the other being a false lumen. When the dissection occurs in the ascending aorta and extends into the aortic root, the aortic valve cusps will lose support and this will cause aortic regurgitation.

Pathophysiology of Chronic Aortic Regurgitation

The aortic valve closes at the end of systole when the left ventricular pressure begins to decline due to relaxation and falls below that of the aorta. The falling left ventricular pressure provides a low pressure area and the column of blood at the aortic root close to the aortic valve will tend to reverse the forward direction of flow and move toward the aortic valve. In the process, it will be decelerated against the closed aortic valve and the dissipation of the energy of the moving column of blood will cause the A2. If the aortic valve is not competent for any reason, then there will be backward flow of blood from the aorta to the left ventricle in diastole, which will start at the time of A2. ***This backward flow will occur under relatively high pressure gradient*** since the aortic diastolic pressure is significantly high soon after the closure of the aortic valve, whereas the left ventricular pressure would have fallen close to zero at the onset of diastole. The high pressure gradient will cause turbulence that will result in ***predominantly a high-frequency blowing type murmur (Fig. 8.5).*** Following the rapid filling phase of diastole, the left ventricular diastolic pressure will begin to rise and there will be a further rise in diastolic pressure of the left ventricle at the end of diastole due to atrial contraction augmenting filling. At the same time, the aortic diastolic pressure will gradually fall due to the peripheral runoff. Thus, the diastolic pressure gradient between the aorta and the left ventricle will be maximal at the beginning of diastole and will tend to fall gradually during diastole reaching the minimal level toward the end of diastole. Thus, the ***decreasing diastolic gradient*** will have an effect on the diastolic murmur, which often will exhibit a ***decrescendo*** character starting at A2. During the rapid filling phase of diastole, the left ventricular pressure falls to zero and then rises. Thus, the pressure gradient between the aorta and the left ventricle may have an initial increase followed by a decrease. This transitory change in the pressure gradients may have an initial crescendo effect on the murmur followed by the typical decrescendo murmur.

The filling of the left ventricle during diastole will be augmented due to both the regurgitant volume of blood from the aorta and the normal pulmonary venous return through the mitral inflow. The left ventricle will enlarge due to the volume overload effect. The extent of rise in the filling pressure of the left ventricle will depend both on the severity of the regurgitation as well as on the compliance or distensibility of the left ventricle. In ***chronic aortic regurgitation,*** the left ventricle ***initially*** undergoes ***dilatation*** and its ***compliance is generally preserved.*** This will help to keep the rise in the diastolic

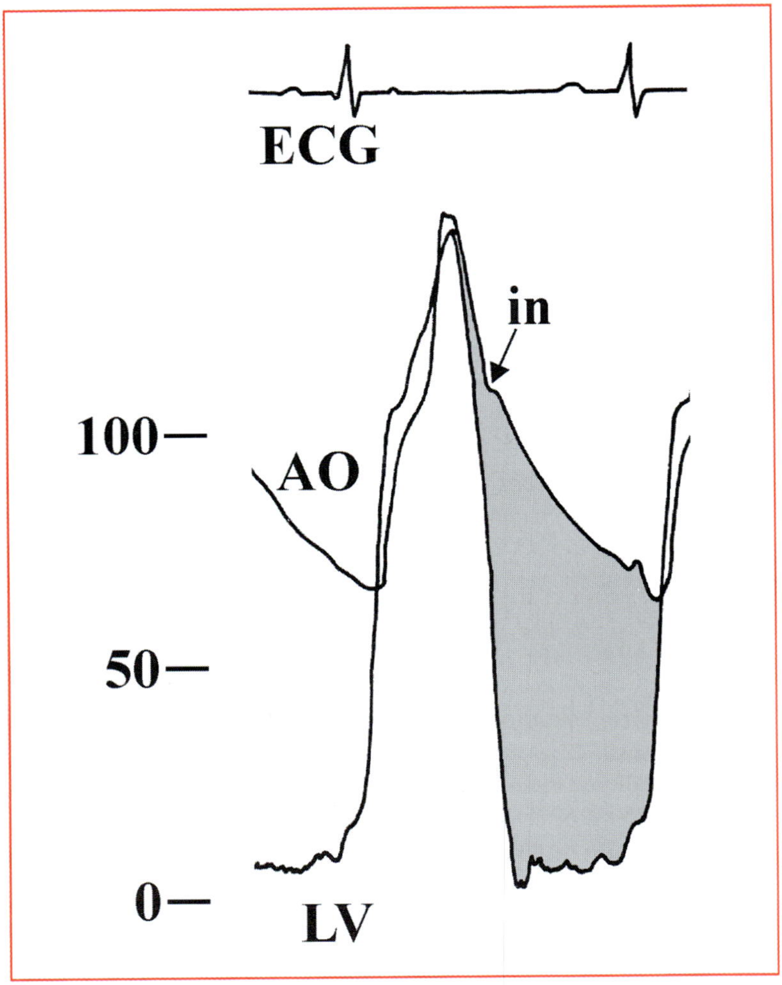

Fig. 8.5: Simultaneous recordings of the ECG, the left ventricular (LV) and the aortic (AO) pressure curves from a patient with chronic aortic regurgitation. There is a high pressure gradient between the AO and the LV during diastole (shaded area). The gradient is the highest initially at the incisura (In) falling off gradually during the remainder of the diastole.

left ventricular pressure to a minimal degree.[42,45,46] On the other hand, the increased dimension of the left ventricle due to dilatation will increase the ventricular wall tension. This will be understandable since the wall tension is directly proportional to the radius by the ***Laplace formula. The increased wall tension*** will ***increase the myocardial oxygen demand.*** This is one of the reasons that patients with aortic regurgitation may experience symptoms of exertional angina. The increase in the left ventricular wall tension is also a ***stimulus for secondary myocardial hypertrophy.*** In long-standing aortic regurgitation of more than moderate degree, therefore, the left ventricle will undergo secondary hypertrophy.[47] Thus in chronic severe aortic regurgitation, the left ventricle is not only dilated and enlarged but also significantly hypertrophied. The markedly hypertrophied and enlarged heart in aortic regurgitation is sometimes massive and referred to by the term ***"cor bovinum".*** The increased wall thickness will help to reduce the wall tension slightly. The hypertrophic process is eccentric and is associated with replication of sarcomeres in series together with elongation of myofibers. The ratio of wall thickness to the radius of the cavity is maintained.[48] This is unlike the concentric hypertrophy that occurs in pressure overload states such as aortic stenosis, where the sarcomeres increase in parallel, and the ratio of wall thickness to the radius of the cavity is increased.[49] The hypertrophy will, however, tend to make the left ventricle more stiff and its ***compliance will become eventually diminished.*** This will result in further elevation of the left ventricular diastolic pressure. The increased left ventricular diastolic pressure will tend to interfere with sub-endocardial coronary perfusion. Since normal coronary flow occurs mostly in diastole, and since the arterial diastolic pressures are often low in significant aortic regurgitation due to compensatory peripheral vasodilatation, this will further compromise the coronary flow by reducing the coronary perfusion pressure. Although the reduced coronary reserve may not affect baseline left ventricular function, during periods of increased metabolic demands induced by stress, exercise and other activities may not be met by increased coronary flow. The increased myocardial oxygen demand together with ***decreased sub-endocardial perfusion*** will often result in some myocyte necrosis and replacement ***fibrosis.*** This will further depress the compliance of the left ventricle and cause ***additional rise in the left ventricular diastolic pressure.*** This will further adversely affect the systolic left ventricular function as well.[42,50-55]

Since the mitral valve is open in diastole, any elevation of the diastolic pressure before the ***a wave*** will lead to ***increased left atrial pressure.*** The elevated left atrial pressure will be transmitted to the pulmonary capillary bed and will cause symptoms of ***dyspnea.*** When the elevation of the left ventricular diastolic pressure is severe and associated with decreased left ventricular systolic function, the resulting high left atrial pressure will lead to aggravation of symptoms of dyspnea as well as cause orthopnea and paroxysmal nocturnal dyspnea.

Pathophysiology of Acute Severe Aortic Regurgitation

Unlike chronic aortic regurgitation, when the aortic regurgitation is ***severe and acute*** in onset as may happen with rapidly progressive aortic valve endocarditis with a virulent and destructive pathogen such as the *Staphylococcus aureus* or caused by a sudden rupture of a cusp or sudden disruption of a previously normal aortic valve prosthesis, the left ventricle will ***not have enough time to undergo compensatory dilatation.*** The severe regurgitation into the left ventricle is accommodated only with a significant elevation of the ***left ventricular diastolic pressure.*** The latter can rise to levels not only higher than the prevailing left atrial pressure in diastole but also ***typically reach levels close to the aortic diastolic pressure.*** In fact, often by the end of diastole the left ventricular diastolic pressure becomes equal to the aortic diastolic pressure. The large regurgitant volume of blood from the incompetent aortic valve together with the mitral inflow during the rapid filling phase of diastole often lead to abrupt and large rise in the left ventricular diastolic pressure. The latter will have a significant deceleration effect on both the regurgitant column and the mitral inflow column of blood. This may result in the production of an S3. In addition, the rapidly rising left ventricular diastolic pressure when it exceeds the left atrial pressure in mid-diastole will tend to ***close the mitral valve prematurely (Fig. 8.6).*** The premature closure of the mitral valve can be seen quite easily in M-mode recordings of the echocardiograms. The premature mitral closure will make the ***S1 soft and almost inaudible.*** This has been discussed previously under S1.[56,57]

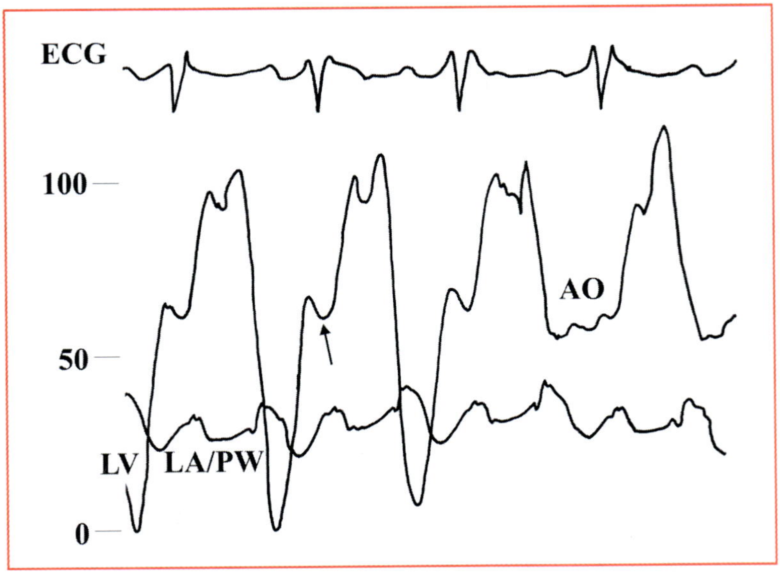

Fig. 8.6: Simultaneous recordings of the left ventricular (LV) and the indirect left atrial/pulmonary capillary wedge (LA/PW) pressures obtained at cardiac catheterization from a patient with acute severe aortic regurgitation secondary to infective endocarditis. The aortic (AO) pressure is recorded while pulling back the catheter from the LV. The severity of the AO regurgitation and its acuteness do not allow enough time for the LV to undergo compensatory dilatation, thereby making the LV non-compliant. The LV diastolic pressure rises quickly with early diastolic inflow exceeding the LA pressure and continues to rise and becomes equal at end-diastole to the diastolic AO pressure (arrow).

The *large volume of regurgitant aortic diastolic flow will give rise to predominantly low and medium frequency* aortic regurgitation murmur making it harsher in quality. In addition, the rapidly rising left ventricular diastolic pressure will limit the regurgitant flow by diminishing the pressure difference between the aorta and the left ventricle. This will make the murmur somewhat shorter. In the presence of a sinus tachycardia with the associated shortening of the diastole sometimes one could misinterpret the harsh diastolic murmur to be a systolic ejection murmur.

Auscultatory Features in Aortic Regurgitation

1. The high pressure gradient between the aorta and the left ventricle during diastole generally tends to give the aortic regurgitation murmur, ***the classic high-frequency blowing quality.*** The beginner may mistake the murmur for the breath sound. Thus, aortic regurgitation murmur is best auscultated for, with the breath held at the end of expiration preferably with the patient sitting up and leaning forward.
2. The aortic regurgitation murmur usually ***starts with the A2 and is often decrescendo in character.*** This follows the decreasing pressure gradient, which is maximal at the beginning of diastole and gradually diminishes toward the end of diastole. It usually can be mimicked by the following: ***Lubbb........Phoooooooooo.***
3. Occasionally, the initial crescendo effect of the increasing pressure gradient (during the rapid filling phase) may not be heard leaving a slight pause after A2. It may then sound like ***1................2-haaaaa.***
4. The murmur may have low and medium frequencies if the degree of regurgitation is moderate to severe. This is especially so in acute and severe aortic regurgitation where the murmur could sound somewhat harsh in quality (Fig. 8.7).
5. The aortic regurgitation murmur is generally ***heard over the "sash area"*** that extends from the second right interspace along the left sternal border to the apex.

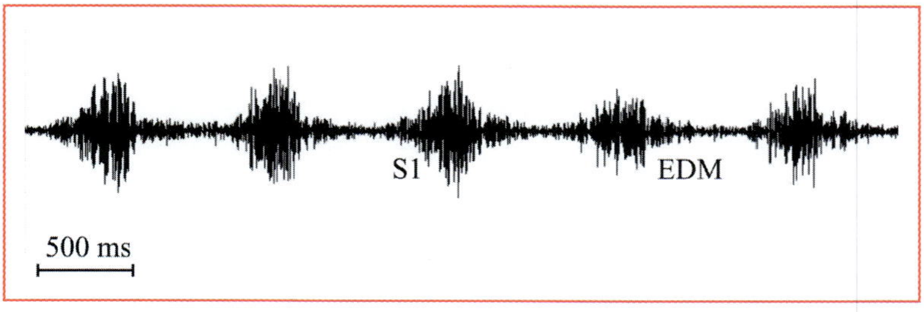

Fig. 8.7: Digital display of a magnetic audio recording from a patient with acute severe aortic regurgitation taken at the apex area. The first heart sound is very low in amplitude (soft). There is a systolic ejection murmur followed by a decrescendo high-frequency diastolic murmur of the aortic regurgitation.

6. The location of the maximal loudness can vary. It is generally along the left sternal border in most instances where valvular disease is the cause of the regurgitation. ***When the aortic root is dilated*** and the dilatation is the principal cause of the regurgitation the *murmur may tend to be equally loud or louder in the second and third right interspace compared to the left sternal border* area.
7. Rarely the aortic regurgitation murmur may only be heard best in certain unusual locations. When it is heard best in the left axillary area it goes by the name ***of Cole-Cecil murmur.***[58] This may also occur in short stocky type of individuals where the left ventricular apex is somewhat high in the axilla.
8. The aortic regurgitation murmur can ***occasionally sound quite musical and sound like dove cooing in quality.*** When this occurs, it is probably due to some aortic valve structure resonating and vibrating at a fixed frequency. This can be demonstrated on a phonocardiogram, which will show the even frequency (Fig. 8.8). In one study with dual echocardiography, the

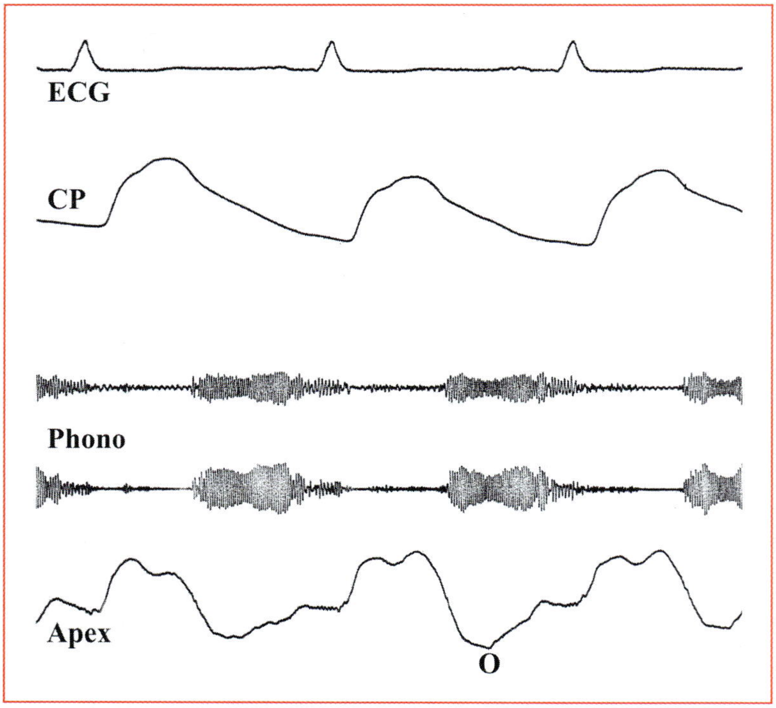

Fig. 8.8: Simultaneous recordings of the ECG, the carotid pulse (CP), the apexcardiogram (Apex) and the phonocardiogram (Phono) taken at the lower left sternal border area from a patient with significant aortic regurgitation and a dove cooing musical murmur. The Phono shows the even frequencies of the diastolic murmur characteristic of the musical quality. The aortic regurgitation murmur as expected precedes the O point of the Apex, which corresponds to the mitral valve opening.

murmur was associated with coarse fluttering of the posterior aortic wall. The onset and the end of the resonant vibrations of the posterior aortic wall corresponded to the opening and closing of the anterior mitral leaflet.[59]

9. The loudness of the aortic regurgitation murmur does not usually have much bearing on the severity of the regurgitation. Sometimes, severe aortic regurgitation may have soft murmurs.
10. When the regurgitation is significant (moderately severe or severe) and its jet is directed toward the anterior mitral leaflet then the mitral valve may be prevented from opening fully. This will then cause a functional mitral stenosis resulting in the production of a diastolic rumble at the apex. This is called *the Austin Flint rumble. It is usually mid-diastolic and has predominant low frequencies like the mitral stenosis rumble (Fig. 8.9).* The

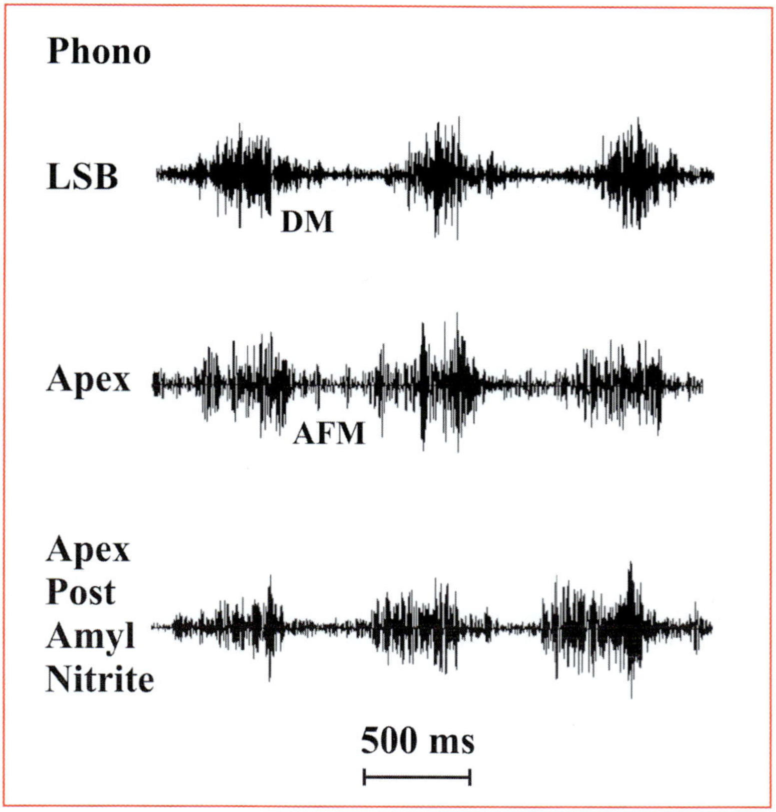

Fig. 8.9: Digital display of magnetic audio recordings taken from the left sternal border (LSB) area, the apex area (Apex) at rest and following amyl nitrite inhalation (Apex post amyl nitrite) from a patient with severe aortic regurgitation. The early diastolic decrescendo murmur of aortic regurgitation (DM) is seen to follow the systolic ejection murmur at the LSB. The diastolic murmur of Austin Flint (AFM) at the Apex noted at rest is not seen in the post-amyl nitrite recording.

presence of this murmur is indicative of significant aortic regurgitation and requires that the regurgitant jet be directed toward the mitral leaflets. When the jet is directed toward the interventricular septum as sometimes may happen, then the Austin Flint rumble will not be present despite severe degree of aortic regurgitation. The Austin Flint murmur characteristically starts during the rapid filling phase of mitral inflow. Therefore, *there is usually a pause between the S2 and the onset of the Austin Flint rumble*. The latter is maximally loud at the left ventricular apex area.[22-26,60]

11. The Austin Flint rumble needs to be distinguished from the *low-frequency components of the aortic regurgitation murmur.* The latter may sometimes be transmitted to the apex area. However, these low-frequency components of the aortic regurgitation murmur usually start with the ***A2 without any appreciable pause.***
12. Often when the aortic regurgitation is mild or faint, the intensity of the murmur can be increased by increasing the peripheral resistance. This can be done at the bedside by asking the patients to *squeeze their hands to clench their fingers and at the same time squat as well. This will tend to raise the blood pressure as well as the venous return and bring out the faint aortic regurgitation murmurs.*[61]
13. When aortic regurgitation is moderate to severe, there is an increased diastolic volume, which will have a Starling effect on the left ventricle. This will lead to rapid ejection of an increased stroke volume. This may result in an ejection murmur during systole. Sometimes, the ejection murmur can be quite loud.

PULMONARY REGURGITATION

Pulmonary valve regurgitation may occur either with pulmonary hypertension or with normal pulmonary artery pressures.

Pulmonary Hypertensive Pulmonary Regurgitation

When there is pulmonary hypertension of whatever cause, the pulmonary valves become easily incompetent. The reason for this is twofold. One is the ***elevated pulmonary diastolic pressure*** itself. The second reason is the ***pulmonary artery dilatation*** that eventually results from the high pulmonary pressures. The pulmonary valve ring gets stretched and the valve becomes easily regurgitant as a result of this.

Normotensive Pulmonary Regurgitation

Pulmonary valve can become incompetent in the presence of normal pulmonary artery pressures due to either valvular pathology or due to disease of the pulmonary artery. Congenitally, the pulmonary valve may be absent, malformed or have fenestrations. The pulmonary valve may become the seat of infective *endocarditis. This is most likely to be associated with intravenous drug abuse.* The pulmonary valve may also be made *iatrogenically incompetent following pulmonary valvotomy.* This is often seen in patients operated for Fallot's tetralogy. Occasionally, the valve cusps may be quite normal and there may be idiopathic dilatation of the pulmonary artery. The latter can stretch the valve ring and result in pulmonary valve regurgitation.

Pathophysiology of Pulmonary Regurgitation

Pulmonary regurgitation causes hemodynamic burden on the right ventricle similar to what happens on the left side in aortic regurgitation. The backward flow of blood into the right ventricle during diastole increases the right ventricular volume in diastole causing a right ventricular volume overload. As a result of this the right ventricle often enlarges and undergoes dilatation. The enlarged right ventricle can take over a large area anteriorly and sometimes form the apex beat.

The pressure difference under which the turbulent flow occurs as well as the degree of regurgitation will determine the pre-dominant frequency of the resulting murmur. The pressure difference is between the pulmonary diastolic pressure and the right ventricular diastolic pressure. This is maximal at S2 at the onset of diastole and diminishes gradually toward the end of diastole, giving a decrescendo feature.

When the pulmonary artery pressure is high as ***in pulmonary hypertension,*** then the actual pressure difference is significantly high and the resulting murmur will have predominantly ***high frequencies very similar to aortic regurgitation.***

When the pulmonary artery pressure is normal, however, then the murmur will be low in frequency due to turbulent flow occurring at low levels of pressure difference. Initially, the right ventricular pressure falls more rapidly during the rapid filling phase than the pulmonary artery pressure. Then it quickly rises giving a short crescendo-decrescendo shape to the gradient. The murmur will start after the P2 but will sound more like a rumble somewhat short in duration.

When the regurgitation is severe and long-standing, then secondary hypertrophy of the right ventricle can occur leading to somewhat decreased right ventricular compliance. This may lead to elevation of the right ventricular diastolic pressures. When the ***pre a wave*** pressure is elevated, it will result in elevation of the right atrial and jugular venous pressures. In addition, the decreased compliance can result in sudden deceleration of both the regurgitant column of blood and the tricuspid inflow at the end of the rapid filling phase. This can, therefore, result in the production of a right-sided S3. This is more likely to occur when there has been pre-existing right ventricular hypertrophy as in patients with tetralogy of Fallot who have undergone pulmonary valvotomy as part of the tetralogy correction.

Auscultatory Features of Pulmonary Regurgitation

1. In the presence of pulmonary hypertension, the pulmonary regurgitation murmur assumes a high-frequency decrescendo character. It will start with P2 and blowing and decrescendo in quality very similar to the aortic regurgitation murmur. The S2 split may be narrow or wide. The P2 may be even loud and palpable at the second left interspace. The murmur is best heard over the second, third and fourth left interspace and occasionally over the left sternal border area. The maximum loudness is often over the third left interspace. This murmur when heard in a patient with severe mitral stenosis and secondary pulmonary hypertension is referred to as the Graham Steell murmur.[1,62–66] Features are relatively the same, however, the pulmonary hypertension is caused. It is often indistinguishable from aortic regurgitation by the auscultatory features alone.
2. When the pulmonary artery pressures are normal, the turbulence occurring under low pressure gradients produces predominantly a low-frequency murmur.[67] It sounds like a rumble starting after a brief pause after A2. The S2 split may be variable and occasionally wide but generally physiologic. The maximal loudness is over the third and fourth left interspace at the left sternal border. The murmur often is short and somewhat decrescendo to the ear (Fig. 8.10). There may be an associated ejection systolic murmur when the right ventricular stroke volume is increased due to the volume overload effect. Both the systolic and the diastolic murmurs may be shown to increase in intensity on inspiration. There may be associated pulmonary ejection clicks.[68]

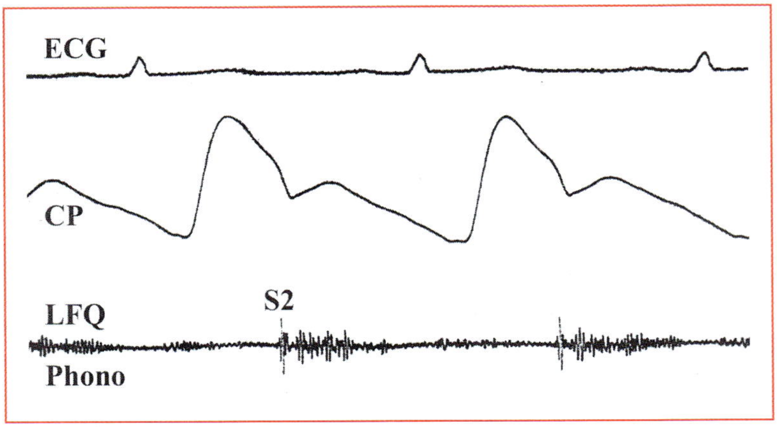

Fig. 8.10: Simultaneous recordings of the ECG, the carotid pulse (CP) and the phonocardiogram (Phono) taken in the low frequency (LFQ) range (50–100 Hz) over the third left interspace at the left sternal border from a patient with post-traumatic pulmonary regurgitation with normal pulmonary artery pressures. The murmur begins right after S2 and lasts through early diastole and is predominantly a low-frequency murmur.

CLINICAL ASSESSMENT OF DIASTOLIC MURMURS

Evaluation of Symptoms

Since ***diastolic murmurs*** are often not very loud and sometimes very highly localized as in mitral stenosis they ***could be missed easily.*** Therefore, it is not common for patients with diastolic murmurs to present merely as problem of diagnosis of the cause of the murmur. ***More than likely*** they often will ***be referred for other symptoms***. Carefully obtained clinical history and its proper interpretation often would give clues to what possibilities that need to be considered. Symptoms of *orthopnea and/or paroxysmal nocturnal dyspnea would imply high left atrial pressures.*[63] Orthopnea is due to the gravitational shift of intravascular volume from the lower extremities raising the central blood volume and therefore the filling pressures in the left atrium. The nocturnal dyspnea is due to the elevation of the left atrial pressure occurring after a few hours of sleep at night, which is caused by the redistribution of fluid volume in the body compartments. The extravascular fluid enters the vascular compartment during sleep and increases the blood volume and this leads to the rise of the left atrial pressure. The *classic paroxysmal nocturnal dyspnea, which occurs with left ventricular failure, is usually relieved with erect posture and does not occur more than once in a night.*[63] Patients with significant aortic regurgitation who develop symptoms of left ventricular decompensation may give this history. *In significant mitral stenosis, the left atrial pressure will remain high* and can cause orthopnea. However, *the nocturnal dyspnea will tend to be somewhat atypical* in that it will not easily clear up quickly on assuming an erect posture. Patients may also complain that they may be waking up dyspneic more than once during the night. Symptoms suggestive of acute pulmonary edema needing emergency attention can occur if atrial fibrillation should develop suddenly in a patient with significant mitral obstruction due to any cause.[1] It can also occur in severe aortic regurgitation. Low output symptoms such as fatigue and lassitude may be present in significant mitral stenosis. Syncopal episodes and presyncopal episodes may occur in mitral obstruction due to tumors such as atrial myxoma. Characteristically these may be positionally aggravated particularly in the left lateral decubitus position.[8] Systemic embolic episodes are characteristic for mitral stenosis with atrial fibrillation. This may occur to a lesser extent in atrial myxoma. Severe pulmonary hypertension of whatever cause will often produce symptoms of low output as well as episodes of syncope or presyncope that may be exertional due to the inability of these patients to increase their cardiac output with exercise as a result of the high pulmonary vascular resistance.[63]

Clues from the Arterial Pulse, the Pre-cordial Pulsations and the Venous Pulse

The clues that can be derived from the careful examination of the arterial pulse, venous pulse and the pre-cordial pulsations are many and these in turn can be used in conjunction with the auscultatory findings to confirm suspected lesions. Tight mitral obstruction and severe pulmonary hypertension are conditions that are characterized by low amplitude pulse due to low stroke volume. Aortic regurgitation, which usually is associated with large stroke volume, will be characterized by large amplitude pulsations both peripherally and in the carotids. The carotid artery pulsation may be visible from a distance ***(Corrigan's pulse).*** Jugular venous pressure and the pulse contour may give clue to the presence or absence of abnormal right heart hemodynamics. How various stages of pulmonary hypertension and the presence of significant tricuspid regurgitation affect the venous pulse contours had already been discussed in detail in Chapter 4. The assessment of what dominates the pre-cordial pulsation also will point to the appropriate lesions that can be suspected. *Left ventricular impulse is often normal in pure mitral stenosis. Hyperdynamic left ventricular impulse forming a wide area with rapid and large amplitude displacement together with marked precordial or sternal retraction is often characteristic of significant aortic regurgitation.* Right ventricular volume and/or pressure overload states may often be reflected by right ventricular impulse, which may be detected by sub-xiphoid palpation. Rarely, a large right ventricle due to significant volume overload as may be seen in atrial septal defect or pulmonary regurgitation may form the apex beat with characteristic lateral retraction.

The Auscultatory Assessment of Diastolic Murmurs

The auscultatory assessment of diastolic murmurs presupposes that the heart sounds had been assessed including the S1 and S2 and extra sounds such as opening snap, S4, S3 and ejection clicks had been identified and characterized.

Next the murmur itself is assessed with reference to the following:

1. *Its pre-dominant frequencies as to whether rumbling and low pitched or highpitched and blowing in character*
2. *Its timing in diastole as to whether it is early diastolic, mid-diastolic or presystolic*
3. *Its length in diastole is also assessed to determine whether it occupies most of diastole or only part of diastole*
4. *If it occupied only part of diastole, whether it occupies early to mid-diastole or mid and late diastole*
5. *Its audible shape as to whether it is decrescendo or crescendo*
6. *Its location of maximal loudness*
7. *Finally whether or not inspiratory increase in intensity or loudness is present.*

The presence of a loud S1 and an opening snap will be a clue to the presence of mitral stenosis and its characteristic murmur can then be looked for. Identification of a well localized long diastolic low pitched rumble over the apex beat will be confirmatory. The presence of a ***typical aortic ejection click*** may be a clue to the presence of an abnormal ***bicuspid aortic valve*** and the characteristic decrescendo blowing early diastolic murmur with the maximal intensity over the sash area will be confirmatory. The presence of a pulmonary ejection click, which becomes soft on inspiration and louder on expiration, may be a clue and point the cause of a low-pitched diastolic murmur over the second and third left interspace to be due to pulmonary regurgitation with normal pulmonary pressures. *A fixed split S2 associated with signs of a large right ventricle may identify an atrial septal defect as the cause of a low-pitched diastolic rumble with maximal loudness over the lower left sternum and over the xiphoid area secondary to tricuspid inflow.* Palpable loud P2 over the second left interspace and the associated early blowing diastolic murmur maximal over the second and third left interspace will point to the presence of pulmonary regurgitation associated with pulmonary hypertension. When the pre-cordial pulsations and the arterial pulse are diagnostic of significant aortic regurgitation, the presence of a mid-diastolic low pitched rumble over the left ventricular apex area will be suggestive of an ***Austin Flint rumble.*** The latter ***will indicate,*** in addition, the presence of ***severe degree of aortic regurgitation.***

When aortic regurgitation is detected and if the murmur is equally loud over the right of the sternum then, it will be a clue to the presence of aortic root disease as the cause of the aortic regurgitation. When mitral stenosis is diagnosed and confirmed by auscultation one should still look for the presence of aortic regurgitation since rheumatic heart disease often involves also the aortic valve. Its presence must be determined by auscultation.

CONTINUOUS MURMURS

A murmur is considered to be continuous when it bridges systole and diastole, extending past the S2. In other words, *a continuous murmur lasts through all of systole and goes beyond S2 into a significant portion of diastole* although it may fade away and become inaudible in later part of diastole. It is very rare that a continuous murmur will last throughout systole and extend into all of diastole.[69]

Continuous murmurs represent a continuous turbulent blood flow where the cause of the turbulence extends beyond systole into diastole. Thus, *continuous murmurs may be expected to occur:*

1. *When there is a communication between a high pressure vessel and a low pressure vessel or a chamber so that a persistent pressure gradient is present throughout systole and diastole allowing continuous shunting of blood with turbulent flow.*

2. *When there is marked increase in velocity of blood flow resulting in turbulence over a local area or region either for physiologic or pathologic reasons.*
3. *When there is a localized constriction in an artery with poor collateral flow to the distal segment resulting in a pressure gradient, which extends beyond systole into diastole.*[69,70]

Communications Between a High Pressure Vessel and a Low Pressure Vessel or Chamber

Arteriovenous shunt surgically produced in a patient requiring hemodialysis for renal failure, therapy is a good example of a high pressure vessel (artery) directly communicating with a low pressure vessel (vein). Such a shunt bypasses the intervening capillary bed. Occasionally, arteriovenous fistulous communications may be present congenitally or may form following some local trauma. In all these instances, the communication or the shunt allows a pressure gradient between the two vessels to persist throughout systole and diastole resulting in a turbulent flow. It is invariable that when such a shunt is open and functional, one will be able to hear a continuous murmur over the vein and its immediate tributaries receiving the flow. The murmur may be accompanied by a continuous thrill over the same area. *The frequency of the murmur will depend not only on the level of the pressure gradient but also on the amount of actual flow. If the communication is large and between large size vessels such as the aorta and the pulmonary artery, for instance, through a persistent ductus arteriosus, then the turbulence will be influenced by both the pressure gradient and the actual flow. The resulting murmur will have mixed frequencies including both the high and the low frequencies. In addition, the murmur may exhibit an accentuation in systole due to the higher pressure gradient.*[69,71]

The high pressure vessel is generally an artery where the pressure is relatively high both during systole and diastole. Around the heart, the high-pressure vessel could be the aorta or the coronary artery with a normal origin while the low pressure area could be the pulmonary artery, abnormal coronary artery arising from the pulmonary artery, the right atrium or the right ventricle.

Rarely in the presence of mitral obstruction associated with an atrial septal defect ***(Lutembacher's syndrome),*** the left atrial pressures may be significantly elevated compared to the right atrium, and the continuous flow through the atrial septal defect may produce a continuous murmur.[72] However, this is very rare. In certain pulmonary diseases, some bronchial artery collaterals to pulmonary artery branches may develop. The disorders where these may develop include bronchiectasis and sequestration of lung. Bronchopulmonary collaterals do develop more commonly in cyanotic congenital heart diseases with reduced pulmonary flow such as tetralogy of Fallot.[6]

The maximum loudness of the murmur is usually over the receiving vessel or chamber. In the case of the persistent ductus, it is over the pulmonary artery and on the surface of the chest this usually corresponds to the second left interspace. If the receiving chamber is the right ventricular outflow tract, then the maximum loudness of the murmur may be over the third and fourth left interspace, when it is the mid-right ventricle, the maximum loudness will be lower sternal and the xiphoid area. If the receiving chamber is the right atrium, then the maximal loudness will be the right sternal edge or to the right of the lower sternum.[70]

In the case of the ***aortopulmonary communications,*** the pulmonary vascular resistance may become significantly elevated resulting in elevated pulmonary artery pressures. If this should occur, then the shunt will diminish due to diminishing pressure gradient and the murmur will become short and eventually may disappear ***when the pulmonary pressures become systemic.*** In addition, the shunt flow may actually reverse in direction leading to the development of cyanosis. In persistent ductus arteriosus, since the ductus joins the aorta beyond the origin of the left sub-clavian artery, the lower limbs will tend to become cyanotic, whereas the head and face and the upper extremities will be spared ***(differential cyanosis).***[38]

The following is a partial list of communications, which may be listed according to the feeding vessel.

1. ***From the aorta:***
   a. *Persistent Ductus Arteriosus (PDA)*
   b. *Aortopulmonary window*
   c. *Congenital sinus of Valsalva aneurysm with fistulae.*
2. ***From the coronary artery:***
   a. *Coronary AV fistulae draining into the right atrium, right ventricle or the pulmonary artery*
   b. *Anomalous origin of the left coronary artery from the pulmonary artery.*
3. ***Other arteriovenous communications:***
   a. *Bronchopulmonary collaterals*
   b. *Chest wall arteries-pulmonary vessels.*

Increased Velocity of Blood Flow

Physiologic causes of rapid blood flow leading to continuous murmurs include ***cervical venous hum*** due to rapid venous inflow through the internal jugular vein,[73,74] and ***mammary souffle*** heard in pregnant women close to term or immediately post-partum during lactating period.[75] Increased blood flow locally leading to continuous murmurs can occur under a variety of pathologic causes, which include hemangiomas, neoplasms with hypervascularity such as a hepatic carcinoma and renal cell carcinoma. In general, these murmurs have more low frequency components due to large volume of blood flow. *The location of maximal loudness will be related to sites of vessels involved.*[69]

Arterial Obstruction

Most local obstruction in arteries normally only generate a systolic murmur due to the fact that the distal segment usually receives enough collateral flow which helps to maintain relatively the same diastolic pressure as in the segment proximal to the stenosed area. Thus, *arterial obstructions that are associated with continuous murmurs mean that the collateral flow to the distal segment is poor resulting in a persistent gradient, which extends from systole through to diastole.* Continuous murmurs due to localized obstructions of this nature are known to occur in aortic arch vessel occlusions, in Takayasu's disease, atherosclerotic disease of the carotid vessels, occasionally in coarctation of aorta, also in main pulmonary artery stenosis and peripheral pulmonary artery stenosis.

Certain specific lesions producing continuous murmurs will be discussed further.

PERSISTENT DUCTUS ARTERIOSUS

Ductus arteriosus is a vascular channel that is normally present in the fetus connecting the aorta just distal to the left sub-clavian artery to the pulmonary trunk near the origin of the left pulmonary artery. In the unaerated lungs of the fetus, the pulmonary capillaries are shut down. The pulmonary vascular resistance is equal to the systemic. The mixed venous and placental blood from the right ventricle passes through the ductus into the descending aorta. At the same time, part of the mixed venous and the placental blood goes through the foramen ovale to the left side and is pumped by the left ventricle into the ascending aorta supplying the head and the upper extremities. At birth the expansion of the lungs and alveolar oxygenation lead to rapid lowering of the pulmonary vascular resistance. *The ductus normally closes functionally during the first 24 hours after birth. It becomes anatomically closed within a few weeks after birth. Closure may be delayed in premature, as well as hypoxemic full-term infants.* The *left-to-right shunt through the ductus is dependent on the pulmonary vascular resistance.* The pulmonary vascular ***resistance*** tends to be ***low in the premature infant*** and the ***excessive flow*** through the ductus can ***cause congestive heart failure*** in the premature infant. In the ***hypoxemic infant,*** the pulmonary vascular ***resistance*** is usually ***high*** raising the pulmonary artery pressure. The ***ductus*** in this instance will therefore ***not cause a continuous murmur.***[76]

Occasionally, the ductus remains open in the infant and persist into adulthood. Maternal rubella in the first trimester has a close association with a persistent ductus. Persistent ductus can either occur alone or associated with other anomalies such as a ventricular septal defect or coarctation of the aorta. *The degree of left-to-right shunt will depend on both the pulmonary vascular resistance and the size of the ductus.* The left-to-right shunt through the persistent ductus will cause volume overload of the left atrium and the left ventricle leading to their enlargement. This will cause the apical impulse to be hyperdynamic and formed by the left ventricle. The arterial pulse will have large amplitude with a rapid rise and a wide pulse pressure. The aortic diastolic pressure will fall to lower levels because of the large communication to the pulmonary artery with significantly lower vascular resistance.[38,71]

Persistent ductus generally causes no symptoms after first year of life until perhaps the third decade. In the majority of patients, the persistent ductus is associated with pulmonary pressures at levels considerably lower than the systemic. In about ***5% of patients,*** the pulmonary vascular resistance may become significantly elevated leading to pulmonary hypertension with the ***Eisenmenger's syndrome.***[64] This tends to occur in the ***early adult life.*** The shunt will become right to left when the pulmonary vascular resistance is high. *Since the ductus joins the aorta distal to the left sub-clavian, the cyanosis associated with reverse shunt will affect the lower extremities and the differential cyanosis and clubbing may point to the diagnosis on mere inspection.*

Auscultatory Features in PDA

1. The flow to the pulmonary artery during early systole is usually from the right ventricle. But in late systole and in diastole, the flow through the ductus increases. The turbulent flow under significant pressure difference is produced in late systole and during diastole. *Therefore the typical ductus murmur is a continuous murmur, which increases in intensity around the second heart sound and fades away toward the end of diastole (Fig. 8.11).*[38,71]

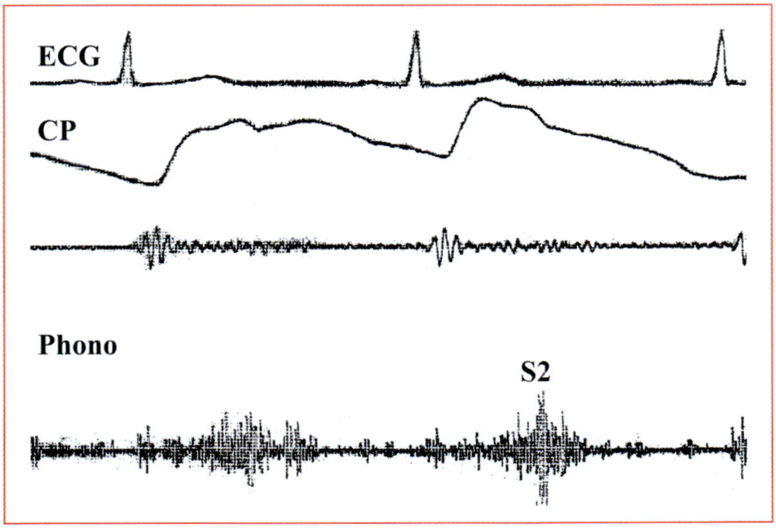

Fig. 8.11: Simultaneous recordings of the ECG, the carotid pulse and the phonocardiogram (Phono) taken over the second left interspace at the left sternal border from a patient with persistent ductus arteriosus. The Phono recording shows the murmur peaking around the second heart sound (S2).

2. When there is a large volume of flow, the ductus murmur is harsh and "machinery" like or "train in a tunnel" like and is associated with significant accentuation in later systole. They may also be associated with discrete ***"eddy" sounds, which may sometimes be like clicks or crackles.***[77]
3. When the ductus is small, the flow may occur under a high pressure gradient with a high velocity. This may give rise to a high-frequency continuous murmur.
4. The maximal loudness of the ductus murmur is usually over the second left interspace. The second best location for loudness is the first left interspace. This is an important differential point, which will help to distinguish persistent ductus from other causes of continuous murmurs.[60,71]
5. When the flow through the ductus is large enough to produce significant left ventricular enlargement, one may hear low-frequency short mid-diastolic rumble at the apex suggestive of increased mitral inflow.
6. *The S2 may be paradoxically split on inspiration when the left-to-right shunt is large* because of the reversed sequence caused by delayed A2. The A2 delay is best explained by the low systemic impedance consequent to a large communication (ductus), which exposes the entire pulmonary vascular bed to the aorta.
7. When pulmonary vascular resistance becomes elevated, initially the pulmonary diastolic pressures rise. This will abolish the diastolic pressure gradient between the aorta and the pulmonary artery abolishing the diastolic portion of the murmur. This will leave the ductus murmur pansystolic. Eventually when the pulmonary systolic pressures also become elevated, the murmur will become shorter and shorter in systole. Finally, other auscultatory signs of pulmonary hypertension may become evident. These will include pulmonary ejection sounds, loud P2, single or closely split S2 and occasionally pulmonary regurgitation murmurs (Graham Steell murmur).
8. *Since the pulmonary vascular resistance tends to be high in the neonatal period, a persistent ductus may only cause a systolic murmur initially and typical continuous murmur may only occur when the pulmonary vascular resistance falls to normal levels.*[38,76]

AORTOPULMONARY WINDOW

The defect is often rather large round or oval and is usually between the adjacent parts of the aortic root and the main pulmonary artery. It probably is due to gap in the development of the partition of the embryonic truncus arteriosus. The pathophysiology is very similar to the patent ductus. It is less common and tends to be associated with *higher incidence of pulmonary hypertension (Eisenmenger's syndrome).* The murmur may, therefore, not be continuous, and both the upper and the lower extremities will show cyanosis.

When the size of the defect is not large, then signs can be very similar to patent ductus. *However, the location of maximal loudness of the continuous murmur is lower and often over the second and third left interspace.*[38,78]

Sinus of Valsalva Aneurysm

Congenital aneurysms of sinus of Valsalva are due to focal defect in the media of the aortic sinus. They start as blind diverticulum, which may elongate and enlarge. They sometime can grow like a windsock. Eventually, they can rupture into the adjoining cardiac chamber. These aneurysms most often arise in the right coronary or the non-coronary sinus. They need to be distinguished from diffuse dilatation of the sinus as may occur in Marfan's syndrome. *Aneurysm involving the right coronary sinus communicates with the right ventricle and occasionally the right atrium. Aneurysms of the non-coronary sinus communicate with the right atrium.*

The pathophysiologic effects of these aneurysms depend on how rapidly the rupture (leading to fistula formation) occurs resulting in the left to right shunt, the amount of flow through the fistula and the chamber or chambers receiving the shunt.[38,79] If the communication develops gradually, the onset of symptoms will be insidious. If rupture occurs acutely, patient may present with sudden onset chest discomfort and dyspnea. Congestive heart failure may sub-sequently develop after a variable period of several hours to several days.[79] Right atrium and the right ventricle will become volume overloaded and enlarged if the rupture occurs into the right atrium. Right ventricle will show volume overload if rupture occurs into that chamber. Because of the left-to-right shunt at the right heart level, the pulmonary venous return will always be higher than normal leading to volume overload of the left atrium and the left ventricle. The arterial pulse will show rapid aortic runoff with wide pulse pressure, large amplitude and rapid upstroke. The jugular venous pressure will reflect the raised right ventricular ***pre a wave*** pressure and the contour will show equal ***x′ and y descents.*** If right ventricular failure occurs, tricuspid regurgitation may develop that may be reflected also in the jugulars. Rarely a large aneurysm bulging into the right ventricular outflow may cause signs of obstruction.

These congenital aneurysms may be well visualized in two-dimensional echocardiographic images with color flow Doppler mapping and their communication sites may be precisely defined.

Auscultatory Features

Once the communication is established, the congenital aneurysms of the sinus of Valsalva will lead to continuous murmurs. *The location of maximal loudness will depend on the chamber into which the left-to-right shunt drains.* If the communication is into the right atrium, the maximal loudness of the murmur is at the lower sternum and close to the right sternal edge and occasionally to the right of the sternal edge. Rupture into the right ventricle causes the murmur to be loudest at the lower left sternal border area and when it communicates into the right ventricular outflow tract then the murmur may be loudest at the left sternal edge but at a higher level (third left interspace). The murmur may be louder either in systole or diastole. Rarely right ventricular contraction may decrease the shunt in systole resulting in accentuation of the murmur in diastole. If the shunt is large then the murmur will have both high and low (mixed) frequencies. The low frequencies will arise from the large volume flow.

Coronary AV Fistulae

Coronary arteriovenous malformations are isolated congenital anomalies. They may arise from either the right or the left coronary artery and the majority of them drain into the right heart. The sites of drainage may be the right atrium, coronary sinus or the right ventricle. Rarely they may drain into the main pulmonary artery. The coronary artery that forms the fistula is often dilated and sometimes tortuous. Rarely, the fistulous coronary artery branch may steal flow from the normal coronary artery due to the lower pressure. Myocardial ischemia however is rare. *The left-to-right shunt generally is not very large and the diagnosis may be considered when the continuous murmur is fairly localized and the maximal loudness of the continuous murmur is at an atypical site. The location of maximal loudness will depend on the site of drainage of the fistula.* If the receiving chamber is the right atrium, then the maximal loudness is at the lower sternal area and often at the upper or lower right sternal border. When the fistula drains into the right ventricle the site of maximal loudness is over the xiphoid area or the lower sternum or the lower left sternal border area. When the fistula drains into the right ventricular outflow tract, the murmur is loudest at the third and the fourth left interspace. When it drains into the main pulmonary artery, then the murmur is loudest at the second and third left interspace. The murmur often tends to be soft. The murmur may have diastolic accentuation, since coronary flow occurs more during diastole than during systole. *Occasionally, systolic compression of the fistulous coronary by the contracting myocardium may significantly decrease the systolic portion of the continuous murmur.*[80]

Venous Hum

The venous hum is generally caused by rapid flow through the internal jugular and the sub-clavian veins, as they join the superior vena cava. It generally gives rise to a continuous roar and occasionally may have a whining quality. It is usually heard over the supraclavicular area between the clavicular and the sternal heads of the sternomastoid muscle. It tends to be louder on the right side. The bell of the stethoscope is most suited for listening for the venous hum, since it will provide the best air seal in this region. The murmur is often heard in young children and occasionally in pregnant women. The venous hum can be brought out even in the normal adult by causing slight angulation of the internal jugulars by turning the head to the opposite side and tilting it slightly upward. *Anemia and hyperthyroidism often lead to very rapid circulation and cause venous hums in the adults. In these instances, the venous hum may be audible without any need to turn the patient's head. The characteristic feature of the venous hum is that it can be temporarily abolished by digital pressure applied over the middle of the sternomastoid muscle so as to compress the internal jugular vein that runs underneath it.* The site of digital pressure must obviously be above the site of auscultation. Releasing the jugular compression will temporarily increase the intensity of the venous hum. The venous hum also tends to be louder in the sitting position and tends to disappear in the supine position. The diastolic component of the murmur is often louder. When the venous hum is very loud it may be transmitted to the infraclavicular area and may be mistaken for a persistent ductus arteriosus. Occasionally, the high-frequency components of the murmur may be selectively transmitted to the infraclavicular area and then it may be mistaken for aortic regurgitation murmur.[73,74]

Mammary Souffle

This is due to rapid and increased flow through the arteries in the breasts of pregnant women close to term or during lactation post-partum. The mammary arteries may be dilated. The murmur usually has a systolic accentuation and can be abolished by local pressure or pressure applied just lateral to the breast.[75]

CLINICAL ASSESSMENT OF CONTINUOUS MURMURS

A murmur must be considered continuous if it goes through S2 and extends into diastole. Most continuous murmurs do not extend throughout diastole. They generally fade away during later part of diastole. When a continuous murmur is heard, assessment of the following will be important in arriving at the probable cause of the murmur:

1. *The location of maximal loudness of the murmur*
2. *The location of the second best area of loudness of the murmur*
3. *The effect of internal jugular compression on the loudness of the murmur especially when the murmur is audible over the second and third interspace*
4. *Whether the murmur is harsh and has a lot of low frequencies*
5. *Signs pertaining to the arterial pulse, which may suggest early runoff as in aortic regurgitation with large amplitude bounding pulses*

6. *Signs of left ventricular volume overload as suggested by a wide area left ventricular apex beat, which is also hyperdynamic*
7. *Presence of mitral inflow rumble (low-pitched mid-diastolic murmur audible over a left ventricular apex area)*
8. *Abnormal jugular venous pressures and or contours*
9. *If S2 is split whether it is normal or wide and physiologic, fixed or reversed*
10. *Systemic signs such as cyanosis and its distribution.*

The three general causes of continuous murmurs need to be kept in mind in the differential diagnosis, namely:

1. *Communications between high pressure vessel and a low pressure vessel or chamber*
2. *Marked increase in localized flow*
3. *Localized arterial obstruction with poor collateralization to the distal segment.*

The radiation of the murmur as usual is not as ***important*** as ***the location of maximal loudness.*** In children and young adults with thin chest, loud venous hum could be heard over a large area of the chest due to wide area of transmission. The location of maximal loudness helps in identifying the receiving chamber (or vessel) in arteriovenous type communications. The most important lesion among these is a persistent ductus arteriosus.

The features that are worth noting about persistent ductus arteriosus are:

1. *The maximal loudness of the ductus murmur is over the second left interspace and the second best area of loudness for the ductus murmur is the first left interspace where it can be equally loud. If the murmur is equally loud over the third left interspace and not over the first left interspace, then communications of other types draining into the pulmonary artery or pulmonary outflow tracts should be considered and not a persistent ductus.*
2. *The ductus murmur increases in intensity around S2 and fades away in diastole.*
3. *When flow is large, the murmur is harsh.*
4. *One may often hear discrete crackling "eddy" sounds.*
5. *S2 may be paradoxically split.*

Other points to consider are as follows:

If internal jugular compression abolishes the murmur temporarily then a venous hum is suggested. When the maximal loudness is over the lower sternal and xiphoid area, then communications draining into mid right ventricle must be considered. When the maximal loudness is over the right sternal edge or right of the sternum, then right atrium is likely to be the receiving chamber. When the murmur is harsh in the presence of an abnormal arteriovenous communication, it usually indicates a significant shunt with a lot of flow. Presence of signs of an enlarged left ventricle with hyperdynamic impulse and a mitral inflow rumble would indicate excessive flow through the mitral valve. This would indicate also that the left-to-right shunt through the communication is significant.

Peripheral signs simulating aortic regurgitation such as those of large amplitude pulses with wide pulse pressure (bounding arterial pulses with early runoff) together with hyperdynamic and enlarged left ventricle could be produced in situations with severe anemia or arteriovenous communications, which are large with significant shunt. These signs are also exaggerated if aorta itself is involved in the communications such as through a persistent ductus arteriosus, aortopulmonary window and congenital sinus of Valsalva aneurysm with fistulae.

Abnormal jugular contours and elevated jugular venous pressure with acute onset of symptoms and signs of rapidly progressive congestive failure in the presence of a loud continuous murmur would point to a lesion such as ruptured sinus of Valsalva aneurysm communicating with the right atrium or the right ventricle.

Coronary arteriovenous fistulae may be considered when signs of a large left-to-right shunt are absent and the continuous ***murmur is localized to an atypical site.***

Localized arterial occlusions may be considered if arterial pulses are poorly felt or absent. This may affect the carotid vessels and vessels of the upper extremities in the case of Takayasu's disease.

PERICARDIAL FRICTION RUB

Acute pericarditis may occur as a result of infection of viral origin, secondary to underlying collagen vascular disease like rheumatoid arthritis and lupus erythematosus, secondary to trauma typically post-cardiac surgery, following acute myocardial infarction, in uremia and sometimes secondary to invasive tumors. In all these states, the cardiac motion against the inflamed pericardium with its two surfaces namely the visceral and the parietal will give rise to generation of friction noises, which is termed the pericardial friction rub. Often the diagnosis of acute pericarditis can be confirmed if a typical pericardial friction rub is heard. The rub could be transient and may be missed and sometimes absent due to accumulation of fluid between the two surfaces of the pericardium preventing friction. The pericardial effusion as a result of the inflammation may however be detected by echocardiography. The friction rub is also sometimes quite localized either over the lower sternal border area or the apex. Occasionally, it may be heard over a wide area of the precordium. Sometimes it may be audible only in certain positions of the patient.

The pericardial friction rub typically has three phases namely systolic (due to ventricular contraction), diastolic (due to ventricular relaxation and expansion during diastole) and atrial systolic (due to atrial contraction at the end of diastole). The noise is usually scratchy or squishy and will show the three phases. Occasionally, it may be harsh and have mixed frequencies and may simulate a murmur and may be difficult to distinguish particularly if the atrial systolic phase is absent. Systolic component is generally always present and may sometimes be the only component especially when the rhythm is atrial fibrillation. Pericardial friction rubs always tend to accentuate on inspiration, since the pericardium gets distorted and pulled by the inspiratory expansion of the lungs and the descent of the diaphragm. This sign therefore needs to be looked for whenever friction rub is suspected by careful auscultation during inspiration. The usual left-sided murmurs, on the other hand, will not increase on inspiration.[81-83]

INNOCENT MURMURS

The term innocent murmur is used when the conditions, which lead to the production of the murmur, is entirely benign to the exclusion of significant organic abnormalities. The turbulence, which accounts for these murmurs, are often due to normal or rapid flow and the murmur may be entirely systolic and occasionally continuous and very rarely mid-diastolic.

Systolic Murmurs

The systolic murmurs that may qualify under this category are ***ejection in type and they are often short in duration.*** They may be heard variably over the pre-cordium either at the second and third left interspace or over the lower left sternal border and at the apex area. They may occur in young children and young adolescents or in adults above the age of 50 years. In the former, it may arise from either the aortic or the pulmonary outflow tracts. In some young subjects with narrow anteroposterior diameter of the chest, the normal flow through the pulmonary outflow, which may be associated with some turbulence, may cause short ejection murmurs, which may be heard over the chest due to close proximity. In some children, they may be quite vibratory and humming as described by Still as ***"twanging string" murmur.*** It is usually ***best heard between the left sternal border and the apex.*** While they get accentuated by increased cardiac output, the frequency spectrum of these murmurs appear to be more related to the age of the patient and the left ventricular dimensions rather than to the flow velocities.[84] The vibratory nature of the murmur may actually be related to vibration of structures like some congenital intracardiac bands, which may stretch across the ventricular cavity unattached to the valves.[38,84-87]

In adults over the age of 50 years, benign ejection murmurs are again relatively common and may be due to some roughening or sclerosis of the aortic valve cusps, aortic root dilatation or distortion caused by atherosclerosis and hypertension and in some patients may also be due to an angulated septum (sigmoid septum) that may actually be seen on the two-dimensional echocardiographic images to be slightly hypertrophied at proximal level due to coexisting hypertension and lead to the production of outflow turbulence.[87,88]

The markers of the benign nature of these systolic murmurs are as follows:

1. *These are all ejection in type and generally short in duration with early peak.*
2. *The murmur may be musical and humming or vibratory that is hardly ever the case with organic semilunar valvular stenosis or obstructive outflow tracts.*
3. *The murmur will diminish in intensity on standing due to decrease in venous return and may actually disappear.*
4. *The murmur will also diminish in intensity during the strain phase of Valsalva maneuver.*
5. *The murmur will not be associated with ejection clicks.*

Continuous Murmurs

Continuous murmurs, which may be considered benign, are usually caused by excessive and rapid blood flow. ***Venous hum*** heard in children and adults with anemia and/or thyrotoxicosis and ***mammary souffle*** heard in the post-partum lactating women belong to this category. Venous hum can sometimes be loud and heard over a large area in the upper chest especially in children. It often is a low pitched roar. Occasionally, it may sound high in frequency particularly in the presence of anemia. It usually can be abolished temporarily by occluding digital pressure over the internal jugular vein. Mammary souffle also can be abolished by local pressure applied just lateral to the breast.[73-75]

Mid-Diastolic Murmurs

In some young adults and children, the physiologic S3 may have some vibrations, which may have some duration to it and may sound like a short rumble but it has the same significance as the physiologic S3.[87]

REFERENCES

1. Wood P. An appreciation of mitral stenosis: I clinical features. Brit Med J. 1954; 1:1051.
2. Wood P. An appreciation of mitral stenosis: II investigations and results. Brit Med J. 1954;1:1113.
3. Craige E. Phonocardiographic studies in mitral stenosis. N Engl J Med. 1957; 257:650.
4. Criley JM, Chambers RD, Blaufuss AH, et al. Mitral Stenosis: Mechanico-Acoustical Events. Monograph. American Heat Association Inc; 1975. p. 46.
5. Lutembacher R. De la stenose mitrale avec communication interauriculaire. Arch Mal Coeur. 1916;9:237.
6. Perloff JK. The Clinical Recognition of Congenital Heart Disease, 5th edition. Philadelphia: WB Saunders; 2003.
7. Angelino PF, Garbagni R, Tartara D. The Lutembacher syndrome: clinical and hemodynamic observations before and after surgery. Arch Mal Coeur Vaiss. 1961;54:511-24.

8. Nasser WK, Davis RH, Dillon JC, et al. Atrial myxoma. I. Clinical and pathologic features in nine cases. Am Heart J. 1972;83:694-704.
9. Nasser WK, Davis RH, Dillon JC, et al. Atrial myxoma. II. Phonocardiographic, echocardiographic, hemodynamic, and angiographic features in nine cases. Am Heart J. 1972;83:810-23.
10. Fortuin NJ, Craige E. Echocardiographic studies of genesis of mitral diastolic murmurs. Br Heart J. 1973;35:75-81.
11. Otto CM. Mitral Stenosis, 2nd edition. Philadelphia: WB Saunders; 2004.
12. Rahimtoola SH, Durairaj A, Mehra A, et al. Current evaluation and management of patients with mitral stenosis. Circulation. 2002;106:1183-8.
13. Wooley CF, Klassen KP, Leighton RF, et al. Left atrial and left ventricular sound and pressure in mitral stenosis. Circulation. 1968;38:295.
14. Criley JM, Feldman IM, Meredith T. Mitral valve closure and the crescendo pre-systolic murmur. Am J Med. 1971;51:456-65.
15. Criley JM, Hermer AJ. The crescendo pre-systolic murmur with atrial fibrillation. N Engl J Med. 1971;285:1284.
16. Hada Y, Amano K, Yamaguchi T, et al. Non-invasive study of the pre-systolic component of the first heart sound in mitral stenosis. J Am Coll Cardiol. 1986;7:43-50.
17. Perloff JK. The physiologic mechanisms of cardiac and vascular physical signs. J Am Coll Cardiol. 1983;1:184-98.
18. Perloff JK, Harvey WP. Auscultatory and phonocardiographic manifestations of pure mitral regurgitation. Prog Cardiovasc Dis. 1962;5:172-94.
19. Ayers CR, Boineau JP, Spach MS. Congenital complete heart block in children. Am Heart J. 1966;72:381-90.
20. Rytand DA. Auricular diastolic murmur with heart block in elderly patients. Am Heart J. 1946;32:579.
21. Coombs CF. Rheumatic myocarditis. Quarterly J Med. 1908;2:26.
22. Flint A. On cardiac murmurs. Am J Med Sci. 1862;44:29.
23. Landzberg JS, Pflugfelder PW, Cassidy MM, et al. Etiology of the Austin Flint murmur. J Am Coll Cardiol. 1992;20:408-13.
24. Reddy PS, Curtiss EI, Salerni R, et al. Sound pressure correlates of the Austin Flint murmur. An intracardiac sound study. Circulation. 1976;53:210-7.
25. O'Brien KP, Cohen LS. Hemodynamic and phonocardiographic correlates of the Austin Flint murmur. Am Heart J. 1969;77:603-9.
26. Fortuin NJ, Craige E. On the mechanism of the Austin Flint murmur. Circulation. 1972;45:558-70.
27. De Leon AC, Harvey PW. Pharmacological agents and auscultation. Mod Concepts Cardiov Dis. 1975;44:23-8.
28. Bousvaros GA, Stubington D. Some Auscultatory and Phonocardiographic Features of Tricuspid Stenosis. Circulation. 1964;29:26-33.
29. Leake H. Rheumatic tricuspid stenosis. Acta Med Scand. 1958;161:109.
30. Wooley CF, Fontana ME, Kilman JW, Ryan JM. Tricuspid stenosis. Atrial systolic murmur, tricuspid opening snap, and right atrial pressure pulse. Am J Med. 1985;78:375-84.
31. Carabello BA, Crawford FA Jr. Valvular heart disease. N Engl J Med. 1997;337:32-41.
32. el-Sherif N. Rheumatic tricuspid stenosis. A haemodynamic correlation. Br Heart J. 1971;33:16-31.
33. Ewy GA. Tricuspid Valve Disease, 3rd edition. Philadelphia: Lippincott Williams and Wilkins; 2000.

34. Ashman H, Zaroff LI, Baronofsky I. Right atrial myxoma. Diagnosis during life: successful surgical removal. Am J Med. 1960;28:487-96.
35. Waxler EB, Kawai N, Kasparian H. Right atrial myxoma: echocardiographic, phonocardiographic, and hemodynamic signs. Am Heart J. 1972;83:251-7.
36. Gotzsche H, Falholt W. Ebstein's anomaly of the tricuspid valve; a review of the literature and report of 6 new cases. Am Heart J. 1954;47:587-603.
37. Roberts WC. A Unique Heart Disesae Associated with a Unique Cancer: Carcinoid Heart Disease. Am J Cardiol. 1997;80:251-6.
38. Perloff JK. The Clinical Recognition of Congenital Heart Disease. Philadelphia: WB Saunders; 1979-81.
39. Wooley CF. The spectrum of tricuspid regurgitation. Am Heart Assoc Monogr. 1975;46:139-148.
40. Leatham A, Gray IR. Auscultatory and phonocardiographic signs of atrial septal defect. Brit Heart J. 1956;18:193.
41. Olson LJ, Subramanian R, Edwards WD. Surgical pathology of pure aortic insufficiency: a study of 225 cases. Mayo Clin Proc. 1984;59:835-41.
42. Carabello BA. Progress in mitral and aortic regurgitation. Prog Cardiovasc Dis. 2001;43:457-75.
43. Rahimtoola SH. Aortic regurgitation. In: Rahimtoola SH (Ed). Valvular Heart Disease. Philadelphia: Current Medicine; 1997.
44. Fedak PW, Verma S, David TE, et al. Clinical and pathophysiological implications of a bicuspid aortic valve. Circulation. 2002; 106:900-4.
45. Bonow RO, Carabello B, de Leon AC, Jr, et al. Guidelines for the management of patients with valvular heart disease: executive summary. A report of the American College of Cardiology/American Heart Association Task Force on Practice Guidelines (Committee on Management of Patients with Valvular Heart Disease). Circulation. 1998;98:1949-84.
46. Bonow RO. Chronic Aortic Regurgitation, 3rd edition. Philadelphia: Lippincott Williams & Wilkins; 2000.
47. Fielitz J, Hein S, Mitrovic V, et al. Activation of the cardiac renin-angiotensin system and increased myocardial collagen expression in human aortic valve disease. J Am Coll Cardiol. 2001;37:1443-9.
48. Gaasch WH, Carroll JD, Levine HJ, et al. Chronic aortic regurgitation: prognostic value of left ventricular end-systolic dimension and end-diastolic radius/thickness ratio. J Am Coll Cardiol. 1983;1:775-82.
49. Carabello BA. Concentric versus eccentric remodeling. J Card Fail. 2002;8:S258-63.
50. Borer JS, Truter S, Herrold EM, et al. Myocardial fibrosis in chronic aortic regurgitation: molecular and cellular responses to volume overload. Circulation. 2002;105:1837-42.
51. Bonow RO. Chronic aortic regurgitation. Role of medical therapy and optimal timing for surgery. Cardiol Clin. 1998;16:449-61.
52. Otto CM. Aortic Regurgitation, 2nd edition. Philadelphia: WB Saunders; 2004.
53. Vatner SF, Shannon R, Hittinger L. Reduced sub-endocardial coronary reserve. A potential mechanism for impaired diastolic function in the hypertrophied and failing heart. Circulation. 1990;81:III8-14.
54. Vatner SF, Hittinger L. Coronary vascular mechanisms involved in decompensation from hypertrophy to heart failure. J Am Coll Cardiol. 1993;22:34A-40A.
55. Hittinger L, Mirsky I, Shen YT, et al. Hemodynamic mechanisms responsible for reduced sub-endocardial coronary reserve in dogs with severe left ventricular hypertrophy. Circulation. 1995;92:978-86.

56. Reddy PS, Leon DF, Krishnaswami V, et al. Syndrome of Acute Aortic Regurgitation; 1975.
57. Wigle ED, Labrosse CJ. Sudden, severe aortic insufficiency. Circulation. 1965; 32:708-20.
58. Cole R, Cecil AB. The axillary diastolic murmur in aortic insufficiency. Bull Johns Hopkins Hosp. 1908;19:353.
59. Kohno K, Hiroki T, Arakawa K. Aortic regurgitation with dove-coo murmur with special references to the mechanism of its generation using dual echocardiography. Jpn Heart J. 1981;22:861-9.
60. Constant J. Bedside Cardiology, 2nd edition. Boston: Little, Brown and Company; 1976.
61. McCraw DB, Siegel W, Stonecipher HK, et al. Response of heart murmur intensity to isometric (handgrip) exercise. Br Heart J. 1972;34:605-10.
62. Steell G. The murmur of high pressure in the pulmonary artery. Med Chronicle. 1888;9:182.
63. Wood P. Diseases of the Heart and Circulation, 2nd edition. Philadelphia: JB Lippincott Co; 1956.
64. Wood P. The Eisenmenger syndrome or pulmonary hypertension with reversed central shunt. Br Heart J. 1963;2:701.
65. Perloff JK. Auscultatory and phonocardiographic manifestations of pulmonary hypertension. Prog cardiovasc Dis. 1967;9:303.
66. Grossman W, Braunwald E. Pulmonary hypertension. In: Philadelphia: WB Saunders Co; 1988.
67. Bousvaros GA, Deuchar DC. The mumur of pulmonary regurgitation which is not associated with pulmonary hypertension. Lancet. 1961;2:962-4.
68. Hultgren HN, Reeve R, Cohn K, et al. The ejection click of valvular pulmonic stenosis. Circulation. 1969;40:631-40.
69. Myers JD. The mechanisms and significances of continuous murmurs. Am Heart Assoc Monogr. 1975;46.
70. Huffman T, Leighton RF, Goodwin RS, et al. Continuous murmurs associated with shunts in the acyanotic adult: an anatomic classification. Am J Med. 1970; 49:160-9.
71. Gibson GA. Persistence of the arterial duct and its diagnosis. Edinburgh Med J. 1900;8:1.
72. Ross J Jr, Braunwald E, Mason DT, et al. Inter-atrial communication and left atrial hypertension. A cause of continuous murmur. Circulation. 1963;28:853.
73. Cutforth R, Wiseman J, Sutherland RD. The genesis of the cervical venous hum. Am Heart J. 1970;80:488-92.
74. Jones FL, Jr. Frequency, characteristics and importance of the cervical venous hum in adults. N Engl J Med. 1962;267:658-60.
75. Tabatznik B, Randall TW, Hersch C. The mammary souffle of pregnancy and lactation. Circulation. 1960;22:1069-73.
76. Zuberbuhler JR, Lenox CC, Park SC, et al. Continuous murmurs in the Newborn. Am Heart Assoc Monogr. 1975;46.
77. Hubbard TF, Neis DD. The sounds at the base of the heart in cases of patent ductus arteriosus. Am Heart J. 1960;59:807-15.
78. Morrow AG, Greenfield LJ, Braunwald E. Congenital aortopulmonary septal defect. Clinical and hemodynamic findings, surgical technic, and results of operative correction. Circulation. 1962;25:463-76.
79. Morgan JR, Rogers AK, Fosburg RG. Ruptured aneurysms of the sinus of Valsalva. Chest. 1972;61:640-3.

80. Morgan JR, Forker AD, O'Sullivan MJ Jr, et al. Coronary arterial fistulas: seven cases with unusual features. Am J Cardiol. 1972;30:432-6.
81. Harvey WP. Auscultatory findings in diseases of the pericardium. Am J Cardiol. 1961;7:15-20.
82. Spodick DH. Pericardial friction. Characteristics of pericardial rubs in fifty consecutive, prospectively stuied patients. N Engl J Med. 1968;278:1204-7.
83. Spodick DH. Pericardial rub. Prospective, Multiple observer investigation of pericardial friction in 100 patients. Am J Cardiol. 1975;35:357-62.
84. Donnerstein RL, Thomsen VS. Hemodynamic and anatomic factors affecting the frequency content of Still's innocent murmur. Am J Cardiol. 1994;74:508-10.
85. Still GF. Common disorders and diseases of childhood. London: Frowde, Hodder and Stoughton; 1909.
86. Joffe HS. Genesis of Still's innocent systolic murmur. Br Heart J. 1992;67:206.
87. Tavel ME. Innocent Murmurs. Am Heart Assoc Monogr. 1975;46.
88. Dalldorf FG, Willis PW 4th. Angled aorta ("sigmoid septum") as a cause of hypertrophic sub-aortic stenosis. Hum Pathol. 1985;16:457-62.

Chapter

9 Elements of Auscultation

Snapshot

- The Stethoscope
- The Methodical Way of Auscultation

In order to get the most and useful information, auscultation of the heart should be focused and done in a methodical way and not just carried out in a haphazard manner. Generally by the time one is ready to auscultate, the diagnostic possibilities must have been narrowed down considerably. This is of course achieved by the continuous synthesis of the analysis of what has been detected by examination of the venous pulse, the arterial pulse and the precordial pulsations in relation to the patient's presenting symptoms and the possibilities suggested by them. Thus, an experienced clinician must know what to expect on auscultation or what to listen for before auscultation is even begun. Thus, auscultation is used to confirm or rule out diagnoses that are already being considered. *Only a few conditions are diagnosed by auscultation alone.* For instance, auscultation may be the only way to diagnose the presence of mild mitral regurgitation due to prolapsed mitral valve leaflets, or mild pulmonary valvular stenosis with the typical pulmonary ejection click. In certain conditions, auscultation may not add much to the diagnosis, which is already suspected for instance chronic stable angina with no prior infarction.

THE STETHOSCOPE

Use of an optimum and well-designed stethoscope is important for proper auscultation, as is the auscultator's head that fits in between the two earpieces. Generally, the frequency range of heart sounds does not extend beyond 1,000 Hz. It must be noted that the bell of the stethoscope picks up low frequencies, while the diaphragm picks up the high frequencies. Understanding the frequency characters of the various heart sounds and murmurs heard both in the normal and the abnormal cardiac states will allow one to use the stethoscope appropriately for their detection. The ideal bell chest piece should be shallow with a large internal diameter to pick up low frequencies.

The diaphragm should be thin and stiff. An X-ray film is not stiff enough to be a good diaphragm. Pressing the bell over the chest wall will make the skin taut and make it behave like a diaphragm and may result in bringing out higher frequencies. The optimum tubing of the stethoscope should be made of smooth vinyl or rubber about 10–12 inches or 25 cm in length and the internal diameter should be about 3/16 inches. Most commercially available stethoscopes (The Littman, Harvey, Leatham, Rappaport and Sprague makes) will satisfy these requirements. The metal head pieces should be rotated so that the ear tips face anteriorly toward the external auditory meatus, since the external ear canals are normally oriented slightly backward. Finally, the ear pieces should be comfortably large.

THE METHODICAL WAY OF AUSCULTATION

The methodical way of auscultation needs to incorporate the following elements:

1. *Listening for one thing at a time and one thing at a time only.*
2. *Listening for specific things with predetermined mental filter with the use of cadence (or vocal simulation).*
3. *Application of principles based on sound transmission as related to the site of origin (not related to the traditional areas of auscultation).*
4. *Recognition of location of maximal loudness of sound and/or murmur and not merely the radiation.*
5. *Effect of gradient versus effect of flow on frequency and character of the murmurs.*
6. *Logical application of behavior of timing of sounds based on proper understanding of physiologic alterations.*
7. *Application of the concepts of mechanisms.*
8. *Appropriate use of bedside maneuvers and vasoactive agents.*

Listening for One Thing at a Time and One Thing at a Time Only

This is extremely important and this allows one to focus on all normal and abnormal heart sounds as well as on any murmur that may be heard. One needs to start auscultation by first assessing the S1 and S2. In fact, S2 may be assessed first since it demarcates systole from diastole. When one listens for the S2, one should literally ignore everything else until the S2 has been properly assessed. This means listening for S2 and its components all over the precordium moving from base to the apex, sequentially over all the areas including the second left interspace, the third left interspace, the second right interspace, the lower left sternal border area, the apex, the area between the apex and the left sternal border and if considered necessary over the xiphoid area as well. Similarly, one can focus on S1 and then other sounds such as ejection click, OS, S3 and S4 as well as murmurs sequentially.

Listening for Specific Things with Predetermined Mental Filter

Specific cadence or rhythm is often produced by the various heart sounds and murmurs, which often help in their recognition. These have been mentioned in relation to the various sounds and murmurs that have been discussed previously (Fig 9.1). This method often helps in the recognition of the OS and how widely it is separated from the S2, the S4, the S3, and the presence of A2-P2 and OS, the identification of the ejection murmur and the presence of mitral diastolic murmur. Obviously, these are often specifically looked for depending on the clinical possibilities being considered. For instance, one may specifically listen for an S3 when suspecting a dilated cardiomyopathy or mitral regurgitation. In this instance, one actually applies the specific mental filter as it were with the cadence of S3 in mind, to try and detect its presence or absence. Similarly, one may specifically listen for a mitral diastolic murmur in a patient who already was found to have a loud M1 and OS to detect the presence of mitral stenosis. In this instance, the cadence of the mitral diastolic murmur will apply.

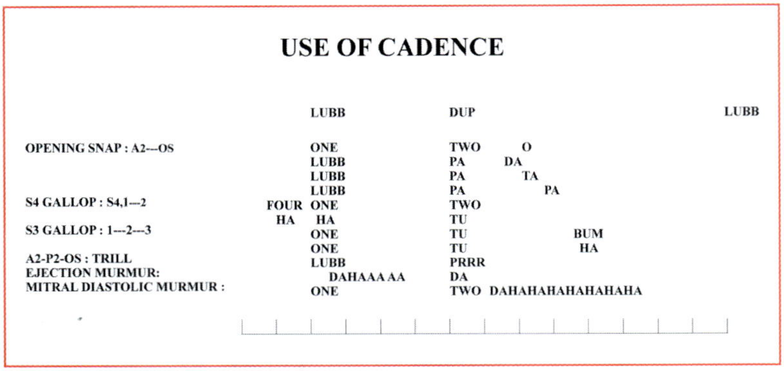

Fig. 9.1: Use of Cadence. The cadence or rhythm produced by the various abnormal heart sounds and murmurs that can be imitated by vocal simulation of syllables are shown. Normal S1 and S2 are represented by syllables LUBB and DUP (shown at the top). The time lines are indicated at the bottom to approximate the length of systole and diastole of an average cardiac cycle. Each of the various abnormal sounds and murmurs is listed in the column on your left. The appropriate syllables are indicated against each of them individually according to their time of occurrence during the cardiac cycle. The cadence for each of the individual abnormal sound or murmur can be simulated vocally by using the syllables in the background rhythm of a cardiac cycle. In the case of the OS, the variations in the S2–OS intervals (short, medium, and late) correspond to three different syllables (PA..DA, PA....TA and PA......PA).

Application of Principles Based on Sound Transmission Related to the Site of Origin

By now it must be clear to everyone who has reviewed the previous sections on auscultation that *the reference to the so-called traditional areas like mitral area referring to the apex, aortic area with reference to the second right interspace and pulmonary area with reference to the second left interspace are not correct terminology and therefore best avoided.* It is better to describe the sounds or murmurs with reference to their locations in terms of the actual interspace (e.g. the second left interspace) on the chest or using chest wall reference terms such as the left lower sternal border, lower sternum, apex area and xiphoid area. It should be recognized that ***the true aortic area*** is actually ***the sash area*** extending from the second right interspace across the left sternal border to the apex and ***the true pulmonary area*** normally is over the second and third left interspace and this may extend into the lower sternum and sometimes to the apex particularly in situations when the right ventricle becomes enlarged and actually form the apex beat as determined by the presence of a lateral retraction. *The sound transmission of A2 and P2 to the chest will be such that they will be, respectively, heard over the true aortic and pulmonary areas depending on the individual patient. This concept allows us to formulate, "The rule of the split S2 at apex".*

The "split S2" at the apex would indicate one of the following:

1. *That it is due to a loud P2 and therefore indicative of the presence of pulmonary hypertension.*
2. *If the P2 is not loud and there is no evidence of pulmonary hypertension, then the right ventricle may be enlarged as in volume overload (e.g. atrial septal defect) forming the apex.*
3. *P2 is normal and audible at apex due to a thin chest (e.g. in children).*
4. *The split S2 effect is being mimicked by a normal single A2 followed by another sound such as an opening snap or S3.*

The rule then can be applied in the specific patient to derive the appropriate conclusions regarding the split S2 at the apex and its significance.

In situations of a split S2 to detect the sequence whether it is A2 followed by the P2 or whether it is P2 followed by the A2, similar conceptual thinking can be applied. The A2 is the component that will remain audible at the normal apex area, which is usually formed by the left ventricle, whereas the P2 will be either absent or become softer and almost inaudible as when one moves over to the apex area. By noting whether the first or the second component that gets softer when one moves ***inching*** from the base to the apex while auscultating, one can develop the skills to decide what the sequence of the two components is in any given patient. This may be useful in situations where the patient is not able to follow instructions about breathing phases.

Recognition of Location of Maximal Loudness of Sound and/or Murmur

The location where a murmur or a sound radiates and therefore is heard does not have any diagnostic value. On the other hand, the location of maximal loudness is often very helpful and gives us clues as to what the sound or the murmur is likely to be. Several examples can be given in this regard. The maximal loudness of an OS is usually between the left sternal border and the apex, whereas the maximal loudness of S3 is usually at the apex.

The regurgitation murmur caused by a VSD is maximally loud at the lower left sternal border, whereas the mitral regurgitation murmur is usually maximally loud over the apex. In acute septal rupture due to myocardial infarction, the murmur may be loudest at the apex. However, it is also equally loud medial to the apex. This is in contrast to acute mitral regurgitation, where the murmur may be loudest at the apex but it will be equally loud lateral to the apex and not medial to the apex. These points relative to the location of maximal loudness obviously have diagnostic significance. When aortic regurgitation murmur is equally loud over the right sternal border as it is over the left sternal border, then aortic root dilatation may be suspected as the cause of the aortic regurgitation. With regard to continuous murmur, the location of maximal loudness correlates best with the chamber that receives the left-to-right shunt. For instance, if the continuous murmur is maximally loud over the second left interspace then the receiving chamber most likely to be the pulmonary artery. If the murmur is loudest at the third left interspace, the right ventricular outflow tract is most likely the receiving chamber.

Effect of Gradient versus Effect of Flow on Frequency and Character of Murmurs

It has been mentioned previously that the frequency of the murmur has a relationship to both the flow and the pressure gradient that is involved in the turbulence. This relationship is such that *the higher the pressure gradient the higher the frequency and the greater the flow the greater the low frequency.* The features of the various murmurs stem from this relationship and this helps in understanding their character. This has been mentioned previously. They are simply listed below:

1. *The harshness of the ejection murmurs.*
2. *Low pitch of the mitral stenosis rumble.*
3. *The blowing character of the early diastolic murmur of aortic regurgitation.*
4. *The high frequency of the pulmonary hypertensive pulmonary regurgitation and the low pitch of the congenital pulmonary regurgitation.*
5. *The harshness and the decrescendo character of acute severe mitral regurgitation secondary to ruptured chordae.*

6. *If a high frequency murmur (e.g. mitral regurgitation) is harsh and has a lot of medium and low frequencies, it will suggest a lot of flow as well as indicate the regurgitation to be probably hemodynamically significant or severe.*

Logical Application of Behavior of Timing of Sounds Based on Proper Understanding of Physiologic Alterations

Physiologic alterations that occur with simple maneuvers such as standing can often be applied during auscultation to help distinguish certain sounds. Thus, one needs to understand the logical reason behind these. Often standing can be used to tell splitting of A2 and P2 from A2 and OS. A2-OS split separates more on standing, whereas A2-P2 tends to narrow. The reason for this is the decreased venous return, which lowers the left atrial pressure, thereby making the OS to occur later. Same maneuver can also be used to tell M1-A1 versus S4-S1. The lower preload on standing leads to prolongation of the isovolumic phase of contraction making the A1 come later, thereby separating it more from M1. The S4, on the other hand, with decreased left atrial pressure may become softer and may tend to come closer to M1.

Application of the Concepts of Mechanisms

Often various maneuvers ranging from simple standing and squatting to the administration of amyl nitrite inhalations are sometimes carried out at the bedside while auscultating for their effects to help distinguish sounds and murmurs in various conditions. It is important to understand the concepts involved in each instance so that the auscultation can be carried out appropriately to achieve the proper conclusion. Some of these are listed below:

1. *S2 components A2 and P2 and how they are affected by the following namely:*
   a. *QRS delay*
   b. *Mechanical ventricular function*
   c. *Impedance, e.g. post-Valsalva effect on the S2 split to distinguish atrial septal defect versus pulmonary hypertension with right ventricular failure*
2. *Effect of long diastole (postextrasystolic pause) on ejection versus regurgitation murmurs.*
3. *Changing S1 intensity in complete A-V block (A-V dissociation).*
4. *Pulmonary ejection click getting softer on expiration.*
5. *Change of murmur intensity with standing and squatting in hypertrophic obstructive cardiomyopathy and mitral valve prolapse with mitral regurgitation.*
6. *Effect of the Valsalva maneuver on the murmur of hypertrophic obstructive cardiomyopathy.*

7. *Amyl nitrite inhalation to distinguish Austin Flint rumble in aortic regurgitation from organic mitral stenosis.*

The Use of Bedside Maneuvers and Vasoactive Agents

Bedside Maneuvers

Simple bedside maneuvers sometimes applied in appropriate situations could be quite useful in sorting out some of the lesions where the distinction is not clearly apparent. Again understanding the physiologic changes induced by the maneuvers is a preliminary step in understanding their likely effects on a given clinical lesion. Under this heading, we discuss the effect of respiration, the application of the Valsalva maneuver, the effect of changes in postures such as standing and squatting and finally the effect of sustained handgrip or isometric exercise.[1-4]

Effect of respiration: The effect of inspiration is of course to increase the venous return by the increased negative intrathoracic pressure. It also expands the pulmonary vasculature, thereby decreasing the pulmonary impedance.[5] All right-sided events that are related to flow through the right heart and right ventricular volume will be expected to increase or intensify on inspiration. In addition to the effect on the timing of the P2 that gets delayed and the slight opposite effect on the timing of the A2, all pulmonary and tricuspid murmurs as well as the right-sided S3, tricuspid inflow rumble and S4 will intensify on inspiration. The inspiratory accentuation of the tricuspid regurgitation murmur goes by the name of Carvallo's sign.[6]

One exception of course is the pulmonary ejection click secondary to congenital pulmonary valvular stenosis.[7] In these patients, the pulmonary artery pressure is usually very low. During inspiration the increased venous return into a hypertrophied and somewhat noncompliant right ventricle, raises the right ventricular end-diastolic pressure during right atrial contraction. This may exceed the diastolic pressure of the pulmonary artery. This effect would cause the doming of the pulmonary valve even before the ventricular contraction starts. Thus with ventricular systole as the column of blood is set into motion, the valve being maximally domed, there is no sudden deceleration against the valve itself, therefore no sound. It must be noted, however, that the pulmonary ejection sound associated with pulmonary hypertension will not be influenced by respiration due to the fact that the pulmonary arterial diastolic pressure is often quite high and also higher than the right ventricular diastolic pressures.

It must also be noted that the respiratory changes in venous return are exaggerated in the sitting and standing position when the venous return is normally low. Thus in order to fully appreciate the effect of respiration it would be important to compare the effects in both the supine and in the erect positions.[8] For instance, the respiratory variations of wide physiologic splitting in young children or adults sometimes may be difficult to distinguish accurately in the supine position. On the other hand, the movements of the two components will be better appreciated in the sitting or standing position. This will help in avoiding the misinterpretation of a wide physiologic split of the S2 as a fixed splitting of the S2, a distinction that is of utmost importance.

Valsalva maneuver: The maneuver involves attempted forceful exhalation against a closed glottis. The effects occur ***in two phases,*** one during the strain phase and the other during the post strain release phase.[8-12] It is usually performed by asking the patient to take a medium breath and hold the breath and forcefully strain as if sitting on the toilet or bear down. One needs to ensure that the patient is in fact straining by placing one's hand on the patient's abdomen to see whether the abdominal muscles become tense. One can also instruct the patient to push the abdominal muscles against the hand. A controlled way of performing the Valsalva maneuver is to have the patient blow through a rubber tube attached to an aneroid manometer to keep the pressure around 40 mm Hg during the period of straining. When performed appropriately, the intrathoracic pressure will become elevated together with elevations of the end-diastolic ventricular pressures. The pulmonary vessels empty into the left atrium, initially raising the arterial pressure slightly. Soon the increased intrathoracic pressure will decrease significantly the venous return. The cardiac output and the systemic arterial pressure will fall with sympathetic stimulation resulting in increased heart rate. Patient is normally asked to strain for about 10 seconds. Usually when performed in the supine position most patients will tolerate the maneuver. However, one should not perform this maneuver in the setting of active ischemic symptoms or acute coronary syndrome.

The effect of ***the strain phase*** is, therefore, to considerably diminish the venous return and filling. Thus, all events and murmurs dependent on flow and filling will diminish. However, in two clinical states, the decrease in the ventricular dimension may become critical enough to aggravate the lesion. One is mitral valve prolapse, where the decreased ventricular size will allow earlier onset of prolapse and mitral regurgitation resulting in the murmur starting earlier and becoming longer. The murmur intensity may not necessarily increase. If there is a whoop, however, it may get louder. The other condition is hypertrophic cardiomyopathy with obstruction. In this condition, the murmur will be expected to increase in intensity because the obstruction tends to become worse due to earlier and easier contact of the anterior mitral leaflet with the hypertrophied septum.[12]

The second part of the effect of the Valsalva maneuver of course is during ***the post-strain release phase.*** During this phase, there is an immediate increase in venous return and flow, which will increase the right-sided volume for the first three to four beats and subsequently also the left ventricular volume. Thus, an immediate return to baseline will be seen on the right-sided events and murmurs, whereas the left-sided events and murmurs will gradually return to the baseline. The post-Valsalva effect on the P2 in distinguishing pulmonary hypertension with right ventricular dysfunction from atrial septal defect was referred to earlier.

The Valsalva maneuver in the assessment of left ventricular function: During the strain phase, with the drop in the output and blood pressure there will be often a marked sympathetic stimulation resulting in a tachycardia. When the strain is released, the increased venous inflow initially into the right side later into the left heart will result in increased cardiac output. The ejection of increased volume into a constricted vascular system will result in significant rise in the arterial pressure, causing an overshoot. The overshoot will be accompanied by reflex bradycardia.

Patients with left ventricular failure and pulmonary congestion do not drop their filling much during the straining and the blood pressure remains flat with very little change in the heart rate. This response is termed ***the square wave response.*** Patients with left ventricular dysfunction who are not in overt failure also often have an abnormal response. They tend to have resting increase in sympathetic tone and fail to exhibit the overshoot in blood pressure as well as the reflex bradycardia. This can be detected at the bedside by taking the resting systolic blood pressure and keeping the cuff inflated about 25 mm Hg above the resting systolic pressure during the strain and for 20–30 seconds after the release. If one detects the Korotkoff sounds coming through, then one can infer there has been an overshoot in blood pressure. Failure to achieve an overshoot of 25 mm Hg has been correlated with resting left ventricular dysfunction with decreased ejection fraction of 40 ± 10%[11,13]

Postural changes

Standing: Assumption of the standing posture from the supine position will have the effect of decreasing the venous return and making the ventricular volume and output to fall together with a drop in the arterial pressure.[14] Events and murmurs dependent on filling and flow will be expected to diminish. Lesions that are critically affected by decrease in dimensions such as mitral regurgitation secondary to the prolapsed mitral leaflets and hypertrophic cardiomyopathy with obstruction will be expected to show the obvious changes, which have been alluded to previously. The prolapse will tend to occur earlier. This will be reflected in clicks moving closer to the S1 and the murmur of mitral regurgitation to start earlier and perhaps become longer. They may also variably change in intensity. The obstruction in the hypertrophic cardiomyopathy will be expected to be either brought on or made worse by this erect posture. This will affect the murmur intensity directly in relation to either the development of the outflow gradient or the accentuation of a resting gradient.

The effect of standing in distinguishing the S2-OS from a split A2-P2 was referred to earlier. This is of course achieved by the decreased venous return resulting in lowering of the left atrial pressure, which makes the OS to occur later.

Squatting: The hemodynamic changes of squatting include an immediate increase in venous return and an increase in the aortic pressure. The latter probably results from the compression of the lower limb arteries, thereby causing some reflex bradycardia. The sum effects of these changes will be to increase the filling volume on both sides together with an increase in the blood pressure.

If a patient is unable to squat, one can mimic the hemodynamic changes by passively bending the knees of the patient toward the abdomen while the patient remains supine.

This maneuver is also quite useful in hypertrophic cardiomyopathy with obstruction, where the gradient will diminish along with the murmur intensity due to the increased left ventricular size and the elevated aortic pressure.[1,15] In mitral valve prolapse, the prolapse will start later. This will result in the click occurring later in systole. The mitral regurgitation murmur will either disappear or become significantly softer.

Exercise: Light walking exercise can be quite useful in bringing out very soft mitral diastolic murmurs in patients with severe mitral stenosis and low cardiac output with secondary pulmonary hypertension. Patient can be instructed to walk back and forth a few times and then asked to lie quickly in the left lateral decubitus position. They must be immediately auscultated before the effect of the exercise wears off. It is also useful in distinguishing wide split S2 in severe pulmonary hypertension and right ventricular dysfunction and/or failure from atrial septal defect. Exercise will further widen the split in right ventricular failure.

Isometric exercise: This can also be applied. This exercise must be done at least for a period of 60–90 seconds to achieve changes in sympathetic tone with increase in heart rate, cardiac output and blood pressure.[16] These effects are best seen in the supine position. As opposed to aerobic exercise such as walking on a treadmill, isometric exercise will result in marked increase in the systemic arterial resistance. The filling pressure will rise in the left ventricle augmenting events related to ventricular filling such as the left-sided filling sounds (S3 and the S4).[17] The elevated left atrial pressure will cause the OS if present to occur earlier. The mitral diastolic murmur of mitral stenosis will become augmented. The effect in hypertrophic obstructive cardiomyopathy will be variable due to the opposing effects of the increased heart rate and the increased blood pressure on the gradient.

The most useful effect will be in bringing out an aortic regurgitation murmur that is not obvious clinically. The effect on mitral regurgitation will be to increase the regurgitation and the intensity of the murmur. Instructing the patient to ***squat and squeeze*** at the same time both of their hands to perform isometric contraction can also be a very useful maneuver in making faint aortic regurgitation murmurs to become easily audible.

Transient arterial occlusion: This technique involves inflating simultaneously two sphygmomanometer cuffs placed one around each arm of the patient to keep the systolic pressure 20–40 mm above that of the resting systolic pressure of the patient for a duration of about 20 seconds. This maneuver does not increase the aortic pressure but increases the aortic impedance.[8,18] The effect will be to augment left-sided regurgitations such as mitral regurgitation, ventricular septal defect (VSD) and aortic regurgitation. This test does not require patient's co-operation and is reported to be better than squatting.

Vasoactive Agents

Vasoactive agents, which have been used in the past to clarify difficult murmurs in cardiac auscultation, include vasopressor agents and amyl nitrite.[19-24] Vasopressors such as phenylephrine require to be administered intravenously by infusion with careful monitoring of blood pressure. Because of this, they are somewhat cumbersome to use and therefore are not used much currently and we have not found the need for their application. Isometric handgrip exercise and/or squeeze and squat maneuver will give reasonable increase in the peripheral arterial resistance and blood pressure to provide equivalent information in its place. Therefore, their application will not be discussed further.

However, amyl nitrite is still an agent that is used from time to time in cardiologic practice in selected instances to clarify certain clinical states. It is reasonably easy to use and quite safe when administered appropriately with patient in the supine position and keeping the patient supine until its effects wear off. For this reason, we will discuss its application here.

Amyl nitrite is a volatile ester of nitrous acid. When administered to the patient it causes a significant decrease in peripheral arterial resistance due to arterial and arteriolar dilatation within a few seconds after inhalation. It is usually dispensed in a cloth-covered ampoule, which can be broken holding it inside gauze with a gloved hand. The patient must be supine and warned to expect to smell some vapors with a sweet almond like fragrance (some compare it to that of dirty socks). Patient should be asked to take two or three whiffs of this by breathing in while the broken ampoule is held close to the patient's nostrils. The administration must be done after baseline auscultation. It is preferable to have someone other than the examiner administer and monitor the systolic blood pressure by the use of a sphygmomanometer cuff and call the level of the blood pressure as the drug takes effect. When properly administered, it will result in a fall in the systemic blood pressure with a reflex tachycardia secondary to the sympathetic stimulation. The hypotensive effect usually wears off in 1–2 minutes. The hemodynamic effects include increase in cardiac output due to increased venous return caused by venoconstriction. This effect, therefore, is different from that of nitroglycerine, which causes venodilatation. The venoconstriction is secondary to the reflex sympathetic stimulation caused by the hypotension. Other effects include increased ventricular contractility and increase in ejection velocity. A small rise in the pulmonary artery pressure may also occur due to increased venous return.[20,25,26] These significant circulatory effects result in modifications of the intensity of the murmur and its duration depending on the nature of the lesion.

The effect of amyl nitrite inhalation on the behavior of the various murmurs encountered in both congenital and acquired lesions can be summarized briefly as follows:

1. Amyl nitrite by increasing forward flow and the velocity of ejection will *increase the intensity of ejection murmurs caused by fixed outflow obstruction* (the right-sided outflow obstruction at the valvular or infundibular level with intact ventricular septum and the left ventricular outflow obstruction).
2. This effect can be used to differentiate the tetralogy of Fallot from pulmonary stenosis with right-to-left shunt at the atrial level.[23,24] In the presence of the tetralogy, the decrease in the systemic pressure will allow more right-to-left shunting through the VSD. This will decrease the forward flow through the pulmonary outflow tract decreasing the murmur intensity. The murmur of pulmonary stenosis with intact ventricular septum, on the other hand, will increase in intensity.[21]
3. Amyl nitrite is classically used to bring out or intensify the long ejection murmur of the hypertrophic cardiomyopathy. Both the drop in the peripheral resistance and the tachycardia with decreased ventricular size will accentuate the outflow obstruction and the murmur.
4. Amyl nitrite will decrease mitral regurgitation by virtue of the increased net forward flow and decreased peripheral resistance.[19]
5. In patients with VSD and normal pulmonary artery pressures, the effect will be similar to that in mitral regurgitation. It will diminish the shunt and the murmur. In VSD with large flow and pulmonary hypertension, there could be a different effect of increasing the flow through the defect due to a disproportionately greater fall in the pulmonary vascular resistance compared to that of the systemic resistance.
6. The response in mitral valve prolapse, however, can be variable. The effect of more complete emptying and increased forward flow may result in critical left ventricular dimension for prolapse to occur earlier in systole due to smaller ventricular size. The late systolic murmur due to mitral regurgitation may disappear and be replaced with an early systolic murmur. Rarely patient may develop pansystolic mitral regurgitation. If only a mid-systolic click is audible, the click will move earlier in systole.

7. Innocent systolic pulmonary outflow murmur will be expected to accentuate due to increased flow.
8. Amyl nitrite classically will diminish aortic regurgitation and its murmur due to decreased peripheral resistance. When the aortic regurgitation is severe, the associated apical low frequency diastolic murmur (Austin Flint murmur) will be either abolished or become softer. This is as a result of the reduction of the severity of aortic regurgitation following amyl nitrite. The effect on the murmur of organic mitral stenosis is, however, to increase its intensity due to the increased cardiac output and mitral flows. This was referred to earlier.
9. The venous hum and the continuous murmur from pulmonary arteriovenous fistulae intensify after amyl nitrite due to excess flow. On the other hand, the murmurs of persistent ductus arteriosus and systemic arteriovenous fistulae shorten and become less loud. When the persistent ductus is associated with pulmonary hypertension, the diastolic component of the continuous murmur would be absent. In these patients, the systolic murmur will also be expected to shorten and become softer.

REFERENCES

1. Cochran PT. Bedside aids to auscultation of the heart. JAMA. 1978;239:54-5.
2. Crawford MH, O'Rourke RA. A systematic approach to the bedside differentiation of cardiac murmurs and abnormal sounds. Curr Probl Cardiol. 1977;1:1-42.
3. Dohan MC, Criscitiello MG. Physiological and pharmacological manipulations of heart sounds and murmurs. Mod Concepts Cardiovasc Dis. 1970;39:121-7.
4. Lembo NJ, Dell'Italia LJ, Crawford MH, O'Rourke RA. Bedside diagnosis of systolic murmurs. New Eng J Med. 1988;318:1572-8.
5. Harrison DC, Goldblatt A, Braunwald E, et al. Studies on cardiac dimensions in intact, unanesthetized man. I. Description of techniques and their validation. II. Effects of respiration. III. Effects of muscular exercise. Circ Res. 1963;13:448-67.
6. Perloff JK. The physiologic mechanisms of cardiac and vascular physical signs. J Am Coll Cardiol. 1983;1:184-98.
7. Hultgren HN, Reeve R, Cohn K, McLeod R. The ejection click of valvular pulmonic stenosis. Circulation. 1969;40:631-40.
8. Grewe K, Crawford MH, O'Rourke RA. Differentiation of cardiac murmurs by dynamic auscultation. Curr Probl Cardiol. 1988;13:669-721.
9. Gorlin R, Knowles JH, Storey CF. The Valsalva maneuver as a test of cardiac function. Pathologic physiology and clinical significance. Am J Med. 1957;22:197.
10. Elisberg EI. Heart rate response to the Valsalva maneuver as a test of circulatory integrity. JAMA. 1963;186:200-205.
11. Little WC, Barr WK, Crawford MH. Altered effect of the Valsalva maneuver on left ventricular volume in patients with cardiomyopathy. Circulation. 1985;71:227-33.
12. Stefadouros MA, Mucha E, Frank MJ. Paradoxic response of the murmur of idiopathic hypertrophic subaortic stenosis to the Valsalva maneuver. Am J Cardiol. 1976;37:89-92.

13. Zema MJ, Caccavano M, Kligfield P. Detection of left ventricular dysfunction in ambulatory subjects with the bedside Valsalva maneuver. Am J Med. 1983;75:241-8.
14. Rapaport E, Wong M, Escobar EE, et al. The effect of upright posture on right ventricular volumes in patients with and without heart failure. Am Heart J. 1966;71:146-52.
15. Nellen M, Gotsman MS, Vogelpoel L, et al. Effects of prompt squatting on the systolic murmur in idiopathic hypertrophic obstructive cardiomyopathy. Br Med J. 1967;3:140-3.
16. McCraw DB, Siegel W, Stonecipher HK, et al. Response of heart murmur intensity to isometric (handgrip) exercise. Br Heart J. 1972;34:605-10.
17. Cohn PF, Thompson P, Strauss W, et al. Diastolic heart sounds during static (handgrip) exercise in patients with chest pain. Circulation. 1973;47:1217-21.
18. Lembo NJ, Dell'Italia LJ, Crawford MH, et al. Diagnosis of left-sided regurgitant murmurs by transient arterial occlusion: a new maneuver using blood pressure cuffs. Ann Intern Med. 1986;105:368-70.
19. Barlow J, Shillingford J. The use of amyl nitrite in differentiating mitral and aortic systolic murmurs. Br Heart J. 1958;20:162-6.
20. Beck W, Schrire V, Vogelpoel L, et al. Hemodynamic effects of amyl nitrite and phenylephrine on the normal human circulation and their relation to changes in cardiac murmurs. Am J Cardiol. 1961;8:341-9.
21. de Leon AC Jr, Harvey WP. Pharmacologic agents and auscultation. Mod Concepts Cardiovasc Dis. 1975;44:23-28.
22. Ronan JA Jr. Effect of vasoactive drugs and maneuvers on heart murmurs. Am Heart Assoc Monogr. 1975;46:183-6.
23. Schrire V, Vogelpoel L, Beck W, et al. The effects of amyl nitrite and phenylephrine on the intracardiac murmurs of small ventricular septal defects. Am Heart J. 1961;62:225-36.
24. Vogelpoel L, Schrire V, Nellen M, et al. The use of amyl nitrite in the differentiation of Fallot's tetralogy and pulmonary stenosis with intact ventricular septum. Am Heart J. 1959;57:803-19.
25. de Leon AC, Jr, Perloff JK. The pulmonary hemodynamic effects of amyl nitrite in normal man. Am Heart J. 1966;72:337-44.
26. Perloff JK, Calvin J, Deleon AC, et al. Systemic hemodynamic effects of amyl nitrite in normal man. Am Heart J. 1963;66:460-9.

Chapter 10 Pathophysiologic Basis of Symptoms and Signs in Cardiac Disease

Snapshot

INTRODUCTION

In this chapter, the pathophysiologic basis of symptoms and signs will be reviewed in the major categories of cardiac lesions seen mainly in the adult patients, including both regurgitant and stenotic valvular lesions, cardiomyopathies both dilated and hypertrophic types, hypertensive heart disease, ischemic heart disease and pericardial lesions with diastolic restriction. Only congenital lesion that will be referred to is atrial septal defect, since more often than not it causes problems only in the adult life.

PATHOPHYSIOLOGY OF MITRAL REGURGITATION

Chronic Mitral Regurgitation

Mitral regurgitation is ***a volume overload state for the left ventricle,*** since during diastole the ventricle receives not only the normal pulmonary venous return but also the extra volume of blood, which goes into the left atrium during systole. *The left ventricle thus has two outlets for systolic emptying in mitral regurgitation, namely the aorta and the left atrium.* The volume overload would result in left ventricular dilatation and enlargement. The left ventricular dilatation is accompanied initially by a better compliance of the left ventricle, which helps to maintain relatively normal left ventricular diastolic pressure despite the large volume of blood entering the left ventricle during diastole. *The left atrium also becomes enlarged when the regurgitation is significant. The left atrial enlargement is accompanied by increased compliance of the left atrium, which helps to maintain a normal left atrial pressure.*

The two-outlet system allows a supernormal emptying and therefore supernormal ejection fraction when the ventricular function is normal and preserved. The ejection fraction can still be maintained at near normal levels even when some left ventricular dysfunction develops because of the systolic advantage that the left ventricle has. The systolic tension is therefore maintained at normal levels.[1-4]

The increased diastolic tension caused by increased dimension (radius) will act as a stimulus to hypertrophy. The hypertrophy is often eccentric rather than concentric.[5] This will decrease the diastolic compliance of the left ventricle, leading to a rise in the diastolic left ventricular filling pressure. The raised diastolic pressure in the left ventricle may impede good sub-endocardial perfusion, since the majority of coronary flow occurs in diastole. The decreased sub-endocardial perfusion may eventually lead to sub-endocardial fibrosis in late stages, which may further depress the compliance and begin to raise the ***"pre a wave pressure"***. Since the latter forms the baseline filling pressure over which the ***a*** and ***v waves*** build up occur in the atrium, the raised ***pre a wave*** pressure will further raise the ***v wave*** pressure height in the left atrium. The upper normal left ventricular diastolic pressure for the end of diastole (post ***a wave***) is usually between 12 and 15 mm Hg, whereas the upper normal left ventricular ***pre a wave*** pressure is between 5 and 8 mm Hg. The normal ***v wave*** in the left atrium may be between 12 and 18 mm Hg. In chronic mitral regurgitation even when the regurgitation is severe, the left atrial ***v wave*** height may only be mild to moderately elevated (20–35 mm Hg). This would mean a persistent pressure difference between the left ventricle and the left atrium throughout systole, making the regurgitant flow to last until the very end of systole and well into the isovolumic relaxation phase. The murmur, therefore, usually lasts for the whole of systole (thus termed pan-systolic) and thus all the way to the S2 and slightly even beyond the S2. In addition, the gradient remains relatively large and constant from the beginning of systole to its end giving rise to a plateau of high-frequency systolic murmur.

The elevated left atrial pressure will cause some secondary pulmonary hypertension. This together with the decreased left ventricular compliance and diastolic dysfunction will eventually lead to systolic dysfunction, causing reduced stroke volume and ejection fraction (Fig. 10.1).[1-4]

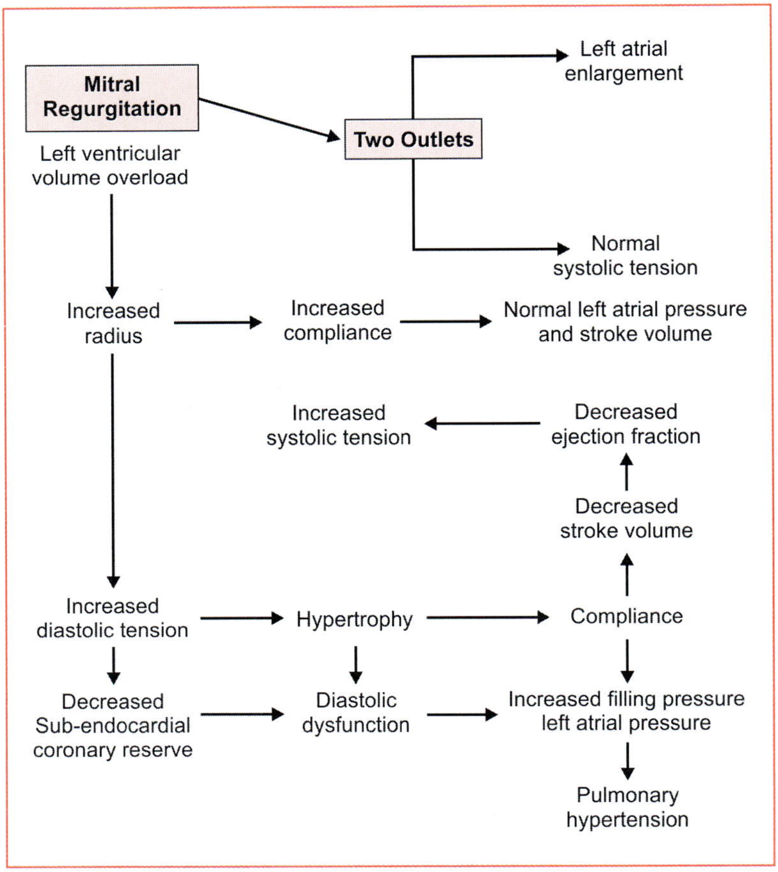

Fig. 10.1.

Acute Mitral Regurgitation

If the mitral regurgitation is severe and acute in onset as with ruptured chordae, then there may *not be enough time to develop compensatory dilatation of either the left atrium or the left ventricle. The large volume of regurgitant blood entering a relatively stiff and non-dilated left atrium will result in steep rise in the v wave pressure in the left atrium (sometimes as high as 50–70 mm Hg).* The entry of large volume of blood during diastole into a non-dilated left ventricle will tend to raise the diastolic filling pressure in the left ventricle. The raised ***pre a wave*** pressure may further add to the ***v wave*** height. *The high v wave build up in the left atrium during systole would mean a decreased and rapidly falling pressure difference between the left ventricle and the left atrium toward the later part of systole. This will, in turn, limit the regurgitant flow during later part of systole making the regurgitant flow and the murmur decrescendo. In addition, the excess flow would cause more low and medium frequencies making the murmur sound harsher (Fig. 10.2).*[6–8]

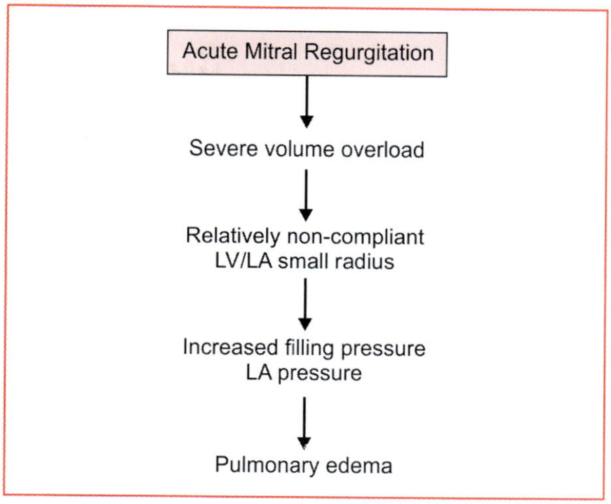

Fig. 10.2.

Clinical Symptoms and Signs in Mitral Regurgitation

The pathophysiologic changes as related to the clinical symptoms and signs in mitral regurgitation together with clinical indicators of the severity of mitral regurgitation are given in Table 10.1.

Even significant degrees of mitral regurgitation when chronic can be tolerated for many years since the left atrial pressure is kept at near normal levels and the stoke volume and the cardiac output maintained. Thus, there is often a long latent period when the patient remains asymptomatic. The left atrial enlargement may eventually lead to the development of atrial arrhythmias especially atrial fibrillation. This may cause symptoms of palpitation. When the left atrial pressure begins to rise, patients may develop symptoms of dyspnea on exertion. When the left atrial pressure is significantly elevated, symptoms of pulmonary congestion such as orthopnea and/or nocturnal dyspnea may also develop. When the mitral regurgitation is severe and acute or abrupt in onset, significant elevations in the left atrial pressure could occur, leading to dramatic symptoms of pulmonary congestion including pulmonary edema.

The enlarged left ventricle with supernormal ejection fraction in the early stages will lead to a hyperdynamic displaced large area left ventricular apical impulse. The systolic advantage that the left ventricle has on account of the two outlets for systole often helps to maintain near normal ejection fraction for a long time and thus the apex beat is unlikely to be sustained. The increased flow across the mitral valve in diastole secondary to the normal pulmonary venous returns together with the regurgitant flow would give rise to an S3 or a mid-diastolic rumble at the apex especially when the mitral regurgitation is severe.

Table 10.1: Chronic Mitral Regurgitation.

Pathophysiological Changes	*Clinical Symptoms/Signs*
• Two outlets • Systolic advantage • Increased LV and LA Compliance	• Long asymptomatic period
• Increased LA size	• Atrial fibrillation • Palpitation
• Increased LA pressure	• Dyspnea • Pulmonary congestion
• Reduced ejection fraction (late sign) • Pulmonary hypertension	• Low output symptoms
• LV volume overload	• Hyperdynamic apex
• Increased radius	• Displaced/Large area apex
• Retrograde flow from high pressure LV into low pressure LA	• Systolic murmur predominantly high frequency
• Incresed flow across mitral valve in diastole due to (normal return + regurgitant flow)	• S3 • Mid diastolic rumble
Signs of Severity	
• Low normal pulse volume • LV enlargement • Wide split S2 due to an early A2 • Harsh low/medium frequencies in the regurgitation murmur indicating a lot of flow • S3 rumble (Inflow rumble) • Signs of pulmonary hypertension	

(LV: Left ventricular; LA: Left atrial)

Reduced ejection fraction and significant pulmonary hypertension are often late signs if present and then may be associated with low output symptoms of fatigue and lassitude.

If mitral regurgitation is detected, the presence of some or all of the following signs (Table 10.1) would indicate that the mitral regurgitation is in fact severe: low normal pulse volume, large area displaced hyperdynamic left ventricular apex beat, wide split S2 due to the early occurrence of the aortic component of S2, harshness of the regurgitant murmur because of excessive flow adding some low and medium frequencies to the usual high frequencies of the regurgitant murmur, S3 and/or inflow mid-diastolic rumble at the apex, signs of pulmonary hypertension such as elevated jugular venous pressure with or without abnormal contour, sustained right ventricular impulse palpable in the sub-xiphoid area and loud or palpable pulmonary component of the S2.

PATHOPHYSIOLOGY OF AORTIC REGURGITATION

Chronic Aortic Regurgitation

If the aortic valve is not competent for any reason, then there will be backward flow of blood from the aorta to the left ventricle in diastole, which will start at the time of A2. *This backward flow will occur under relatively high pressure gradient,* since the aortic diastolic pressure is significantly high soon after the closure of the aortic valve whereas the left ventricular pressure would have fallen close to zero at the onset of diastole. The high-pressure gradient will cause turbulence that will result in *predominantly a high frequency blowing type murmur (Fig. 8.5).* Since the diastolic pressure gradient is high at the onset of diastole and continues to fall gradually during diastole reaching the minimal level at the end of diastole, the murmur has also a decrescendo character.

Aortic regurgitation is also a volume overload lesion for the left ventricle since the filling of the left ventricle during diastole will be augmented due to both the regurgitant volume of blood from the aorta and the normal pulmonary venous return through the mitral inflow (Fig. 10.3). Therefore, the left ventricle will enlarge due to the volume overload effect. The Starling effect of increased stretch caused by the dilatation and the volume overload will not only increase the contractility but also augment the stroke volume. Unlike mitral regurgitation, the left ventricle has only one outlet to eject blood, i.e. eject through aorta only. Thus, it does not have a systolic advantage. The ejection fraction thus does not become supernormal. The increased stroke volume increases the systolic pressure. Peripheral tissue perfusion is maintained by compensatory vasodilatation. This would contribute to the decrease in the arterial diastolic pressure.

The extent of rise in the filling pressure of the left ventricle will depend both on the severity of the regurgitation as well as on the compliance or distensibility of the left ventricle. In ***chronic aortic regurgitation,*** the left ventricle ***initially*** undergoes ***dilatation*** and its compliance is generally preserved. This will help to keep the rise in the diastolic left ventricular pressure to a minimal degree.[1,4,9] On the other hand, the increased dimension of the left ventricle due to dilatation will increase the ventricular wall tension. This will be understandable since the wall tension is directly proportional to the radius by the ***Laplace formula*** (*see* Appendix***). The increased wall tension*** will ***increase the myocardial oxygen demand***. This is one of the reasons that patients with aortic regurgitation may experience symptoms of exertional angina. The increase in the left ventricular wall tension is also a ***stimulus for secondary myocardial hypertrophy.*** In long-standing aortic regurgitation of more than moderate degree therefore, the left ventricle will undergo secondary hypertrophy. Activation of the renin–angiotensin system has been shown to be involved in this process.[10] The hypertrophy is eccentric and is

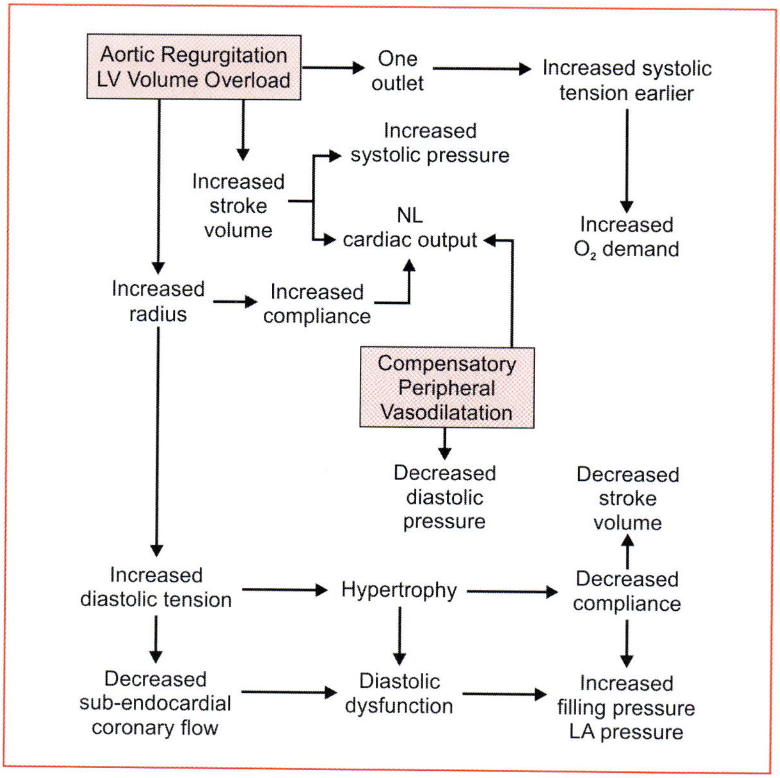

Fig. 10.3.

associated with replication of the sarcomeres in series together with the elongation of the myofibers. The ratio of wall thickness to the radius of the cavity is maintained.[11] This is unlike the concentric hypertrophy that occurs in pressure overload states, where the sarcomeres increase in parallel and the ratio of wall thickness to the radius of the cavity is increased.[5] Thus, in chronic severe aortic regurgitation, the left ventricle is not only dilated and enlarged but also significantly hypertrophied. The markedly hypertrophied and enlarged heart in aortic regurgitation is sometimes massive (***cor bovinum***). The increased wall thickness will help to reduce the wall tension slightly. The hypertrophy will, however, tend to make the left ventricle more stiff and its ***compliance will be diminished.*** This will result in further elevation of the left ventricular diastolic pressure. The increased left ventricular diastolic pressure will tend to interfere with sub-endocardial coronary perfusion. The increased myocardial oxygen demand together with ***decreased sub-endocardial perfusion*** will often result in some myocardial necrosis and replacement ***fibrosis***. This will further depress the compliance of the left ventricle and cause ***additional rise in the left ventricular diastolic pressure***. This will further adversely affect the systolic function.[4,9,12–16]

Since the mitral valve is open in diastole, any elevation of the diastolic pressure before the ***a wave*** will lead to ***increased left atrial pressure.*** The elevated left atrial pressure will be transmitted to the pulmonary capillary bed and will cause symptoms of ***dyspnea.*** When the elevation of the left ventricular diastolic pressure is severe and associated with decreased left ventricular systolic function, the resulting high left atrial pressure will lead to aggravation of symptoms of dyspnea as well as cause orthopnea and paroxysmal nocturnal dyspnea (Fig. 10.3).

Acute Severe Aortic Regurgitation

When the aortic regurgitation is ***severe and acute*** in onset, the left ventricle will ***not have enough time to undergo compensatory dilatation (Fig. 10.4). The severe*** regurgitation into the left ventricle is accommodated only with a significant elevation of the ***left ventricular diastolic pressure.*** The latter can rise to levels not only higher than the prevailing left atrial pressure in diastole but also ***typically reach levels close to the aortic diastolic pressure.*** In fact, often by the end of diastole, the left ventricular diastolic pressure may become equal to the aortic diastolic pressure. The large regurgitant volume of blood from the incompetent aortic valve together with the mitral inflow during the rapid filling phase of diastole often leads to abrupt and large rise in the left ventricular diastolic pressure. The latter will have a significant deceleration effect both on the regurgitant column and on the mitral inflow

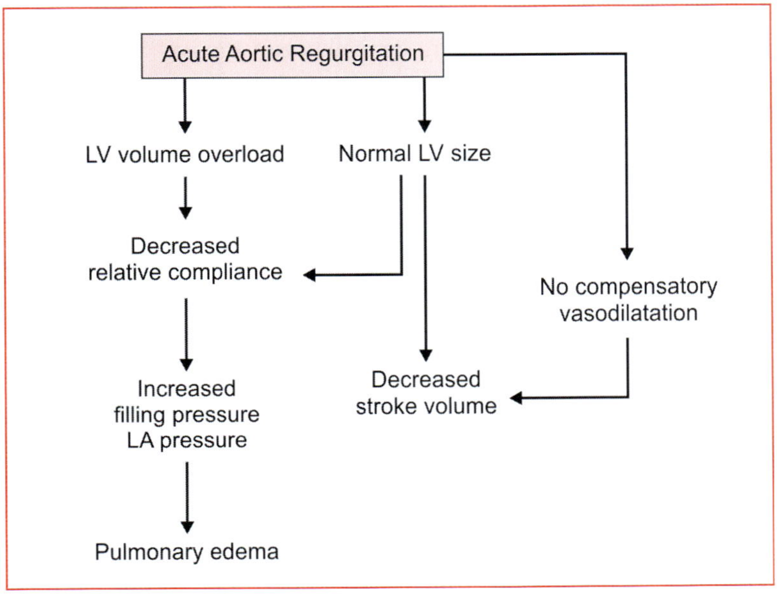

Fig. 10.4.

column of blood. This may result in the production of an S3. In addition, the rapidly rising left ventricular diastolic pressure when it exceeds the left atrial pressure in mid-diastole may ***close the mitral valve prematurely (Fig. 8.6).*** The premature closure of the mitral valve can be seen quite easily in M-mode recordings of the echocardiograms. The premature mitral closure will contribute to the ***S1 becoming soft or even absent.***

The large volume of regurgitant aortic diastolic flow will give rise to predominantly low and medium frequency aortic regurgitation murmur making it harsher in quality. In addition, the rapidly rising left ventricular diastolic pressure will limit the regurgitant flow by diminishing the pressure difference between the aorta and the left ventricle. This will make the murmur somewhat shorter.[17–19]

Clinical Symptoms and Signs in Aortic Regurgitation

The left ventricular enlargement in significant aortic regurgitation will tend to cause a displaced wide area left ventricular apex beat, which will be hyperdynamic. It may also become sustained if the duration of high systolic wall tension is increased. This is likely to happen since the left ventricle has no special systolic advantage unlike mitral regurgitation (Table 10.2). Many of the peripheral signs of aortic regurgitation stem from the large stroke volume, increased ejection velocity and momentum together with decreased peripheral resistance, and widened pulse pressure with low diastolic pressure secondary to retrograde flow into the left ventricle and peripheral vasodilatation (*see* Chapter 2 on Arterial Pulse).[20]

The high diastolic pressure gradient between the left ventricle and the aorta will make the murmur pre-dominantly high frequency and blowing in character. It is also decrescendo since the gradient continues to fall as diastole proceeds. The regurgitant jet from the aorta may prevent full opening of the anterior mitral leaflet when it is severe, causing a state of functional mitral stenosis. This may cause turbulence in the mitral inflow in turn giving rise to a mid-diastolic low-frequency murmur, the ***Austin Flint rumble.*** The presence of this murmur will also indicate that the degree of aortic regurgitation is severe or significant.[21,22] Increased left ventricular diastolic pressure for various reasons mentioned previously will cause elevation of the left atrial pressure and therefore the pulmonary capillary wedge pressures, thereby contributing to the symptoms of dyspnea, paroxysmal nocturnal dyspnea, and orthopnea. The increased myocardial O_2 demand due to increased left ventricular wall tension together with decreased coronary perfusion pressure secondary to decreased aortic diastolic pressure and increased left ventricular intracavitary diastolic pressure will contribute to the symptoms of angina.

Table 10.2: Chronic Aortic Regurgitation.

Pathophysiological Changes	*Clinical Symptoms/Signs*
• LV volume overload • Increased radius • Increased duration of systolic tension	• Hyperdynamic LV apex • Displaced large area apex • Sustained apex
• Increased systolic pressure • Lower diastolic pressure • Peripheral vasodilatation	• Large amplitude carotid pulse • Normal upstroke • Wide pulse pressure • Peripheral signs of aortic regurgitation
• Retrograde flow through aortic valve with a high pressure gradient	• Murmur predominantly high frequency • Decrescendo diastolic
• Regurgitant jet preventing mitral valve from opening freely	• Austin Flint rumble (Relative mitral stenosis)
• Increased filling pressure • Increased LA pressure	• Dyspnea • Paroxysmal nocturnal dyspnea/ orthopnea
• Increased O_2 demand • Decreased subendocardial perfusion	• Angina

(LA: Left atrial; LV: Left ventricular)

PATHOPHYSIOLOGY OF MITRAL STENOSIS

Mitral Stenosis is a left ventricular inflow obstructive lesion. The consequences of mitral inflow obstruction are two-fold:

Under filling of the left ventricle that will cause low stroke volume if the obstruction is severe and low left ventricular systolic tension.

Increased left atrial pressure and left atrial stasis and hence left atrial enlargement (Fig. 10.5).

When there is any significant obstruction to flow at the mitral valve, the left atrial pressure will be elevated due to the obstruction and the flow through the valve in diastole will occur under a higher ***v wave*** pressure gradient. The more severe the obstruction or the stenosis the more persistent will be the elevation in the left atrial pressure. The pressure gradient between the left atrium and the left ventricle will tend to persist throughout diastole. The diastolic flow occurring under a higher and a persistent pressure gradient will contribute to a turbulent flow, which may last throughout diastole. The normal left atrial ***v wave*** pressure is usually about 12–15 mm Hg. When there is significant mitral stenosis, the ***v wave*** pressure may be elevated up to 25–30 mm Hg (Fig. 8.1). *However, the pressure gradient noted even with severe mitral stenosis is still fairly low in terms of the absolute mmHg elevation. On the other hand, the volume of flow through the mitral valve is always significant, since the entire stroke volume of the heart will have to go through*

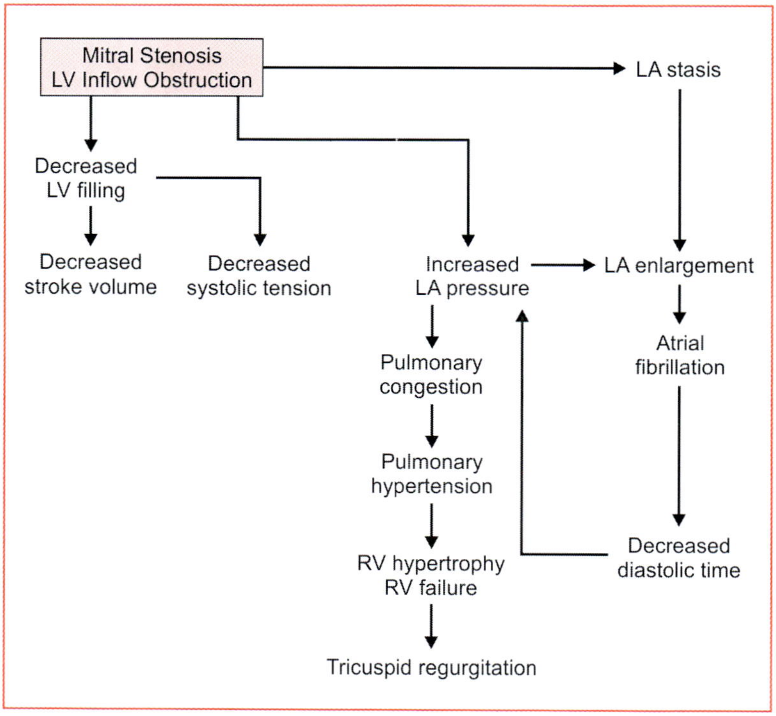

Fig 10.5.

the mitral valve in diastole. Thus, a large volume going through the mitral valve under relatively low levels of pressure will be expected to give rise to turbulence that will produce pre-dominantly low-frequency murmur, the characteristic diastolic rumble.

The elevated left atrial pressure and left atrial stasis will lead to left atrial enlargement, which over a period of time would contribute to the development of atrial fibrillation. The rapid ventricular response during atrial fibrillation and resulting tachycardia will shorten the diastolic filling period. By impeding the left atrial emptying, this will further tend to increase the left atrial pressure.

The elevated left atrial pressure will get transmitted to the pulmonary capillary bed, causing symptoms of pulmonary congestion. Elevation of pulmonary venous pressure eventually will lead to secondary rise in the pulmonary arterial pressure. Persistent and significant elevation of the pulmonary arterial pressure would lead to right ventricular hypertrophy. When the pulmonary hypertension is significant and long-standing, the right ventricle, which remains compensated initially, will eventually fail with right ventricular dilatation. This will eventually lead to the development of significant tricuspid regurgitation.[2,23-26]

Clinical Symptoms and Signs in Mitral Stenosis

The elevated left atrial pressure transmitted to the pulmonary capillary bed will cause symptoms of dyspnea, paroxysmal nocturnal dyspnea and even orthopnea (Table 10.3). The latter may be atypical, for these patients will have a raised left atrial pressure most of the time when the mitral obstruction is significant. Therefore, they may never feel comfortable enough to go to sleep once they are woken up from sleep because of dyspnea and furthermore they may wake up with dyspneic sensation more than once in a night. These features are not seen in classical paroxysmal nocturnal dyspnea due to left ventricular failure where patients usually are able to fall asleep again after they have been up on their feet or up for a while in a recumbent position with their feet dangling. Furthermore, the classical paroxysmal nocturnal dyspnea does not occur more than once in a night.

When atrial fibrillation supervenes due to the various factors mentioned, risk of systemic embolism becomes high. Symptoms will pertain then to the embolic sites or organs. In addition, patients may complain of palpitation as

Table 10.3: Mitral Stenosis.

Pathophysiological Changes	*Clinical Symptoms/Signs*
• Raised LA presuure	• Dyspnea • Orthopnea • Paroxysmal noctumal dyspnea
• LA stasis • LA enlargement	• Atrial fibrillation • Palpitation • Systemic embolism
• Pulmonary hypertension	• Low output symptoms
• RV failure	• Peripheral congestion/edema
• Rapid heart rate • Shortening of diastole (e.g. atrial fibrillation) • Further rise in LA pressure	• Poorly tolerated • Pulmonary congestion
• Volume expansion • Further rise in LA pressure (e.g. pregnancy)	• Poorly tolerated • Pulmonary congestion
• Underfilled LV	• Normal apex • Carotid pulse • Low normal volume
• Mitral closure at higher point of the LV pressure, due to higher LA pressure	• Loud SI "Closing snap"
• Entire LV stroke volume flowing through stenotic valve in diastole at low pressures	• Diastolic murmur • Low frequency rumble
• The higher the LA pressure, (i.e. the more severe the stenosis), the earlier is the mitral valve opening	• S2–OS interval and severity

(LA: Left atrial; LV: Left ventricular; OS: Opening snap; RV: Right ventricular).

well as record an increase in their level of symptoms and decrease in exertional tolerance due to further rise in the left atrial pressure caused by shortened diastolic filling time related to the rapid heart rate. Sometimes patient could develop acute pulmonary edema with sudden onset of rapid atrial fibrillation.

The apex beat is usually normal since the left ventricle is in fact normal except for under filling. The first heart sound may be loud and may become palpable. The loud M1 in mitral stenosis is due to the fact that the mitral closure point occurs at a higher left ventricular pressure due to the raised left atrial pressure. The loud S1 may become palpable. The opening snap (OS) of the mitral valve tends to occur earlier in diastole when the mitral stenosis is severe due to higher left atrial pressure. The diastolic murmur of mitral stenosis is pre-dominantly low frequency due to the fact that the entire left ventricular output goes through the mitral valve in diastole and at relatively low levels of pressure gradients.

PATHOPHYSIOLOGY OF AORTIC STENOSIS

Aortic Stenosis is a lesion that causes left ventricular outflow tract obstruction. This causes the pressure in the left ventricle to rise to overcome the obstruction. The aortic pressure even in the most severe degree of obstruction (>75 mm Hg pressure gradient across the aortic valve) may be maintained close to normal (the systolic pressure of about 100–120 mm Hg). Depending on the severity, the left ventricular systolic pressure can therefore be as high as 200–250 mm Hg. This of course will place a systolic pressure load on the left ventricle. It will raise the systolic tension, thereby increasing the oxygen demand of the myocardium. In addition, the left ventricular pressure takes a longer time to fall to the level of the aortic diastolic pressure. Therefore, the stroke volume is ejected over a longer period of time (prolonged ejection time). The momentum with which the pressure pulse is delivered to the arterial system is slow because of the obstruction. The prolonged slow ejection is felt in the carotid pulse, which has a slow and sustained rise. The left ventricle will be unable to increase the cardiac output due to the fixed nature of the obstruction. With exertion the cardiac output will not sufficiently rise and the peripheral vasodilatation caused by the muscular exertion may actually cause the aortic and the arterial pressure to fall. The increased systolic tension will tend to be a good stimulus to left ventricular hypertrophy. The increased wall thickness is an attempt at normalizing the left ventricular wall tension, since the latter is inversely related to the wall thickness (by Lame's modification of Laplace relationship). But the hypertrophy is often not enough to reduce or normalize the wall tension completely. The hypertrophied left ventricle is stiffer and therefore will offer more resistance to ventricular filling. The decreased left ventricular compliance leads to increased left ventricular diastolic or filling pressures. The increased

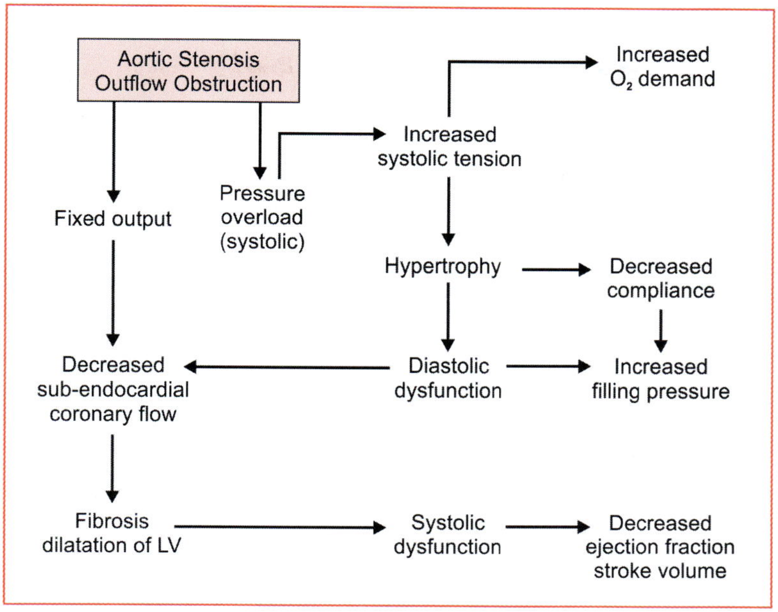

Fig. 10.6.

intraventricular diastolic pressures will offer more resistance to the sub-endocardial capillary flow. Over a period of time, unrelieved severe obstruction can lead to chronic sub-endocardial ischemia that can in turn lead to myocardial necrosis and replacement fibrosis. Eventually the left ventricle may also begin to dilate, and when decompensation sets in, left ventricular systolic function will also deteriorate with reduced ejection fraction (Fig. 10.6).[1,2,5,10,16,27]

Clinical Symptoms and Signs in Aortic Stenosis

In normals, most of the stroke volume is ejected during the first third of systole, causing a rapid rise in the aortic pressure giving rise to a rapid upstroke. In aortic stenosis, this rapid ejection cannot occur. In fact, it takes all of systole to eject the same volume. The decreased mass or volume ejected per unit time leads to considerable decrease in ejection momentum despite increased velocity of ejection. In addition, the increased velocity of flow caused by the significant pressure gradient between the left ventricle and the aorta caused by the stenosis produces a Venturi effect on the lateral walls of the aorta. This has the effect of significantly reducing the net pressure rise in the aorta. *Thus, the rate of rise of the arterial pressure pulse is slow in aortic stenosis. The net effects on the arterial pulse in valvular aortic stenosis are diminished amplitude (small), slow ascending limb (parvus) and a late and poorly defined peak (tardus).* When the stenosis is very severe and accompanied by failing ventricle, the upstroke and the pulse may be poorly felt if felt at all *(pulsus tardus et parvus, meaning late, slow and small).*

Table 10.4: Aortic Stenosis.

Pathophysiological Changes	*Clinical Symptoms/Signs*
• Obstruction at the valve	• Slow, rising carotid pulse
• Increased systolic tension + slow fall in tension due to prolonged ejection	• Sustained LV apex
• Decreased LV compliance	• S4 and atrial kick
• Increased O_2 demand • Decreased subendocardial flow	• Angina
• Fixed output	• Syncope/presyncope on exertion
• Increased LV filling pressure	• Dyspnea • Paroxysmal nocturnal dyspnea/orthopnea
• Dilatation	• Displaced, large area LV apex
• Decreased stroke volume	• Low voloume pulse • Low output symptoms

(LV: Left ventricular).

Increased left ventricular systolic wall tension may cause the left ventricular apex beat to become sustained. Decreased left ventricular compliance may lead to the production of an atrial kick and/or a fourth heart sound (S4).

Increased myocardial oxygen demand caused by the increased left ventricular systolic wall tension and the decreased sub-endocardial capillary flow aggravated by the raised left ventricular diastolic pressures would contribute to the symptoms of angina. Because of the fixed cardiac output, exertional hypotension and syncope and presyncope may also occur. The increased left ventricular filling pressures, which can get transmitted to the pulmonary capillary bed, will give rise to symptoms of dyspnea, paroxysmal nocturnal dyspnea and orthopnea as well as pulmonary congestion.

In recent studies, the degree of diastolic dysfunction correlated best with symptoms of dyspnea. Diastolic function is adversely affected by the pathologic left ventricular hypertrophy. It affects not only the early active relaxation which is related to calcium reuptake by the sarcoplasmic reticulum but also the later phases of diastole where the altered stiffness offers greater resistance to filling. Patients with syncope were found to have small left ventricular mass and volumes with low stroke volume and cardiac output at rest.[28,29]

Eventually when the left ventricle becomes dilated and begins to fail, the dilated enlarged left ventricle can give rise to a large area apex beat. The associated low cardiac output symptoms may be reflected in a very low amplitude arterial pulse (Table 10.4).

PATHOPHYSIOLOGY OF MYOCARDIAL ISCHEMIA/INFARCTION

While myocardial ischemia or infarction could occur in the absence of coronary artery disease and may be caused by other factors such as vasospasm (e.g. patients with vasospastic or Prinzmetal's angina) and coronary emboli (e.g. systemic embolism in patients with atrial fibrillation and mitral stenosis), still its most common cause is atherosclerotic disease of the coronaries. When an atheromatous plaque in a coronary artery develops a crack or a rupture, it would result in the formation of an occlusive thrombus, leading in turn to acute ischemic injury of the myocardium supplied by that artery. When the ischemia is of a sufficiently long duration (usually >20 minutes), then a myocardial infarction could result.

Both contractility and relaxation will be impaired in the ischemic or infarcted myocardial segments. In addition, the affected myocardium will become less compliant and relatively stiffer offering resistance to filling in diastole. When the compliance of the left ventricle is significantly reduced, then the normal left ventricular filling in diastole will be accompanied by a significant rise in the diastolic filling pressures. The increased filling pressures will have a beneficial effect on the non-ischemic or non-infarcted segments inducing them to be stretched more, thereby increasing their contractility. This will have a beneficial effect in maintaining a normal stroke volume. However, the increased filling pressures will also have a detrimental effect on the sub-endocardial capillary flow. It may aggravate or cause sub-endocardial ischemia. This, in turn, can further decrease the ventricular compliance and further raise the diastolic filling pressures.

If the ischemia or infarction involves a large area of the left ventricular myocardium, then the decreased contractility of the ischemic segments will be expected to be associated with a decreased ejection fraction, increased end systolic volume and decreased stroke volume. The greater the increase in the end systolic volume the poorer becomes the clinical outcome. Clinical symptoms of heart failure may develop when > 25% of the myocardium is involved and cardiogenic shock may result if > 40% of the myocardium is infarcted. The latter of course carries with it a high mortality rate.

The infarcted area particularly when large can undergo excessive thinning before formation of a firm scar. This process when it occurs without additional myocardial necrosis is termed ***infarct expansion.*** Pathologically, this involves myocyte and tissue loss with disruption of normal myocardial cells in the infarct zone.

The ischemic or infarcted segments could be dyskinetic and therefore bulge out during systole. This will tend to increase the left ventricular dimension. The resultant increase in the radius will raise the left ventricular wall tension by the Laplace relationship. The increased wall tension could become a stimulus for hypertrophy of the healthy segments of the myocardium. Hypertrophy will eventually lead to further decrease in the left ventricular compliance.

The non-infarcted myocardium could also undergo dilatation. This is a consequence of the degree of elevation of the filling pressures and the underlying systolic and diastolic left ventricular wall tension. In addition to the loading conditions, it is also dependent on the size of the infarct and the patency of the infarct-related artery.

These changes in both the infarcted and the non-infarcted myocardium, which involve varying degrees of hypertrophy and dilatation resulting in changes in the shape and size of the ventricle, are termed ***ventricular remodeling.*** The early and sustained activation of the various neurohormones including the renin-angiotensin and the aldosterone pathway has been shown to be intimately involved in the remodeling that the myocardium undergoes following a myocardial infarction. The blockade of this pathway with the angiotensin converting enzyme inhibitors has been shown to prevent the adverse myocardial remodeling thereby improving the clinical outcome.

The complications that can ensue significant myocardial ischemia/infarction, of course, include ventricular arrhythmias, ventricular rupture, papillary muscle dysfunction and mitral regurgitation. The inhomogeneous repolarization that occurs in the ischemic myocardium and the presence of high sympathetic stimulation accompanying acute ischemia or infarction set the conditions favoring the production of the ventricular arrhythmias. When the myocardium underlying a group of papillary muscle is ischemic or infarcted, then the mitral leaflets would tend to become incompetent. The resulting papillary muscle dysfunction will cause varying degrees of mitral regurgitation (Fig. 10.7).[30–46]

Clinical Symptoms and Signs in Myocardial Ischemia/Infarction

The decreased left ventricular compliance caused by various factors discussed above would favor the production of a fourth heart sound (S4) as long as the left atrium is healthy and the sinus rhythm is preserved. The increased filling pressures in the left ventricle by transmission will raise the pulmonary capillary pressures, thereby causing pulmonary congestion and symptoms of dyspnea. Anginal symptoms will be expected on account of the various factors that increase the myocardial oxygen demand in the face of decreased supply caused by coronary occlusion. When the ejection fraction is decreased and significant left ventricular dysfunction is present, then the increased duration of the raised left ventricular systolic wall tension will make the left ventricular apical impulse to become sustained. When the papillary muscle dysfunction supervenes, one could also hear a mitral regurgitation murmur (Table 10.5). When significant left ventricular dysfunction and failure develop together with elevated left atrial pressure, an S3 may alsobe heard.

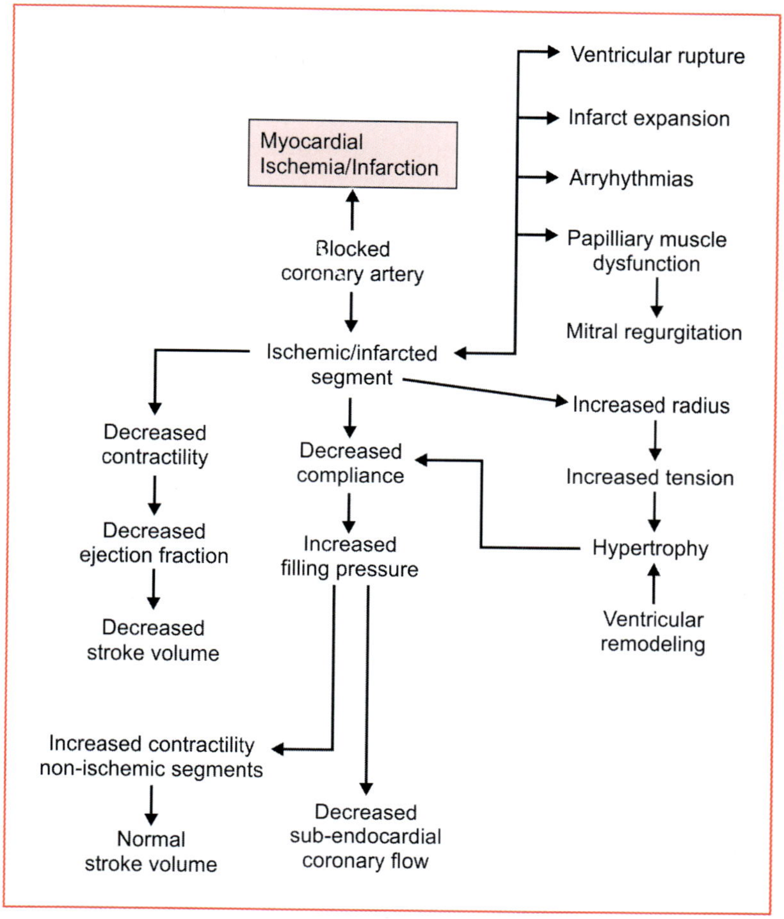

Fig. 10.7.

Table 10.5: Myocardial Ischemia/Infarction.

Pathophysiological Changes	*Clinical Symptoms/Signs*
• Decreased LV compliance	• S4
• Increased LV filling pressure	• Dyspnea • Pulmonary congestion
• Decreased supply • Decreased sub-endocardial flow • Increased tension • Increased O_2 demand	• Angina
• Reduced ejection fraction • Increased duration of systolic tension	• Sustained LV apex
• Papilliary muscle dysfunction	• Mitral regurgitation murmur

(LV: Left ventricular).

PATHOPHYSIOLOGY OF HYPERTENSIVE HEART DISEASE

Significant and long-standing hypertension whether secondary or primary can lead to cardiac pathologic changes and give rise to signs and symptoms. The sequence of these changes pertaining to the heart will be reviewed without attempting to review all of the vascular changes that lead to eventual target organ damage in other parts of the body including the brain and the kidney.

Hypertension, the essential or the primary type, is a fairly common disorder. The disorder is characterized by a reduction in the caliber as well as in the number of small arterioles resulting in increased peripheral vascular resistance. While hypertension by itself can produce significant cardiac changes leading to symptoms and signs, it is also a significant risk factor for the development of atherosclerosis. Therefore, it can aggravate symptoms and signs of ischemic heart disease. The endothelial relaxation factor, nitric oxide is not produced adequately due to the endothelial dysfunction that accompanies hypertension. This will cause poor coronary vasodilatation reserve. In addition, the increased systolic pressure will raise the systolic left ventricular wall tension, thereby increasing the myocardial oxygen demand. The increased wall tension is also a stimulus for left ventricular hypertrophy. The hypertrophied left ventricle is less compliant, thereby raising the left ventricular filling pressures. The latter will compromise the sub-endocardial capillary flow. This will over a period of time contribute to the development of fibrosis particularly in the sub-endocardium. As a result of this, the filling pressures will further rise. The elevated filling pressures could cause the symptoms of pulmonary congestion due to the transmission of pressures to the left atrium and the pulmonary capillary bed. At this stage, the systolic function may be still well preserved with good ejection fraction. In fact, hypertension is an important condition, which is often associated with symptoms of congestive failure in the presence of preserved systolic left ventricular function. Eventually in long-standing cases with significant untreated hypertension, the left ventricle will begin to dilate and enlarge and result in systolic dysfunction.

The interaction of the arterial system with the left ventricular function also needs some clarification. This interaction is a direct result of the properties of the peripheral arteries pertaining to their effects on the arterial wave reflection and pulse wave transmission (*see* Chapter 2 on Arterial Pulse). The properties of the proximal arterial system in healthy young individuals are such that the pulse pressure generated by ventricular ejection is not very high. Also, the component of wave reflection returns to the central aorta in diastole raising the diastolic coronary perfusion pressure without causing any increase in the systolic load on the ventricle. However, with aging both the aorta and the arterial system in general become stiffened. The stiffening of the aorta itself contributes to the increased pulse pressure generated by the ventricular ejection. In addition, the stiffened arteries lead to increased pulse wave velocity. This will result in early return of the reflected pressure wave from the periphery to the heart. As long as the left ventricle is compensated, this will add to the late systolic pressure rise and increase the pressure load on the left ventricle without compromising the aortic forward flow. In fact, early wave reflection is an important contributor for the development of systolic hypertension in the elderly.

When the left ventricle is dilated and its function compromised, it will be unable to accommodate for the early pressure wave reflection. This will negatively impact on the forward aortic flow out of the left ventricle with early deceleration of the flow eventually resulting in decreased ejection time and diminished stroke output. While these peripheral arterial effects could play a role in any patient with compromised left ventricular function, it is particularly relevant in the elderly hypertensive patient developing failure. Recognition of this factor is important in view of its therapeutic implications. Reduction of wave reflection with the use of appropriate vasodilatory agents becomes an important therapeutic goal in the treatment of hypertension.

Often, the raised left atrial pressures will lead to left atrial enlargement and can cause the development of atrial arrhythmias particularly atrial fibrillation that can aggravate or precipitate heart failure symptoms (Fig. 10.8). When ischemic heart disease is coexistent, papillary muscle dysfunction and mitral regurgitation can also supervene.

Clinical Symptoms and Signs in Hypertensive Heart Disease

Hypertension may remain silent for a long time and may go undetected because of lack of specific symptoms associated with it. Therefore, it is called the silent killer. However, it may be detected in patients being evaluated for symptoms of atypical chest pain, angina, dyspnea or palpitation. The increased myocardial oxygen demand, the increased left ventricular diastolic filling pressure as well as the elevated left atrial pressure could be contributing to these symptoms. The strong left atrial contraction evoked by the hypertrophied and less compliant left ventricle in those patients with healthy left atria may give rise to a fourth heart sound and/or a palpable atrial kick in the apex beat. The apical impulse may be sustained only when the systolic pressure is very high or when the left ventricular ejection fraction is decreased. The second heart sound is usually narrowly split and may occasionally show reverse splitting with delayed A2. The latter may occur when severe hypertension is accompanied by ischemia as well. The hypertrophy of the left ventricle may be associated with the voltage criteria of left ventricular hypertrophy on the electrocardiogram (ECG). The sub-endocardial ischemia and the development of fibrosis in the late stages would explain the repolarization (ST-T waves) changes on the ECG (left ventricular hypertrophy strain pattern) (Table 10.6).[14,16,47–52]

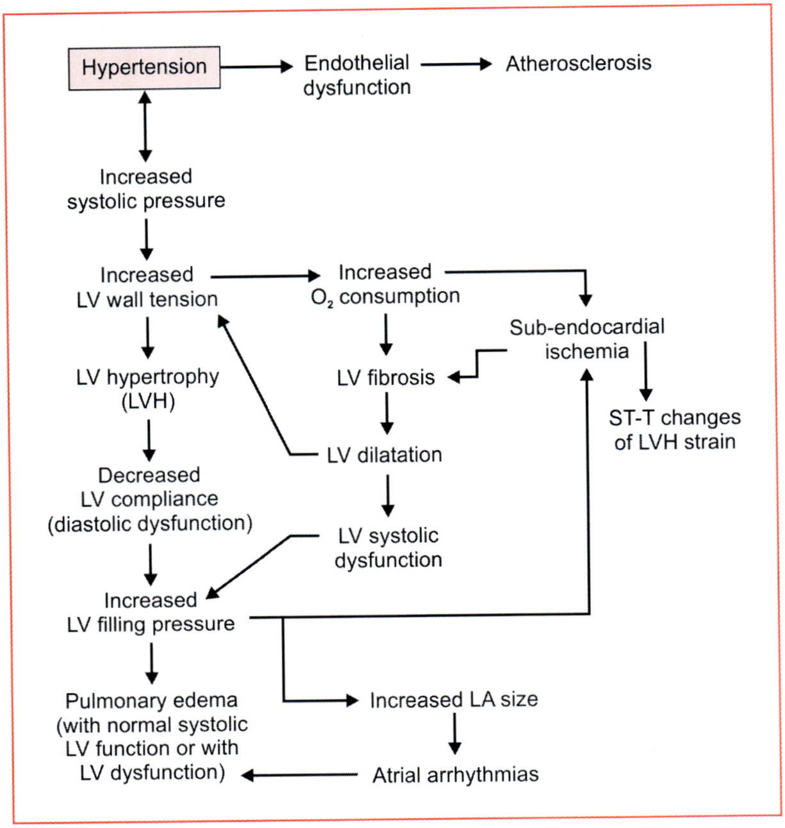

Fig. 10.8.

Table 10.6: Hypertension.

Pathophysiological Changes	*Clinical Symptoms/Signs*
	• Assymptomatic for long time
• Increased systolic LV wall tension	• Atypical chest pain
• Increased O_2 demand	• Angina
• Increased LV filling pressure	• Dyspnea
• Decreased sub-endocardial flow	• Palpitation
• Increased left atrial pressure	
• Decreased LV compliance	• S4/Atrial kick
• Severe hypertension or Decreased LV systolic function	• Sustained LV apex
• Sub-endocardial ischemia ± fibrosis	• ECG—Repolarization, abnormalities LVH strain pattern

(LV: Left ventricular; ECG: Electrocardiogram; LVH: Left ventricular hypertrophy).

Heart Failure with Preserved Ejection Fraction

Some of the elderly patients presenting with symptoms and signs of heart failure with pulmonary and/or systemic congestion may have relatively well preserved systolic function as measured by ejection fraction. Many of these patients often in fact have also hypertension. Currently, these patients comprise the most common form of heart failure in the population.[53] Many of them do have significant diastolic dysfunction and elevated ventricular diastolic pressures due to impaired active relaxation as well as increased wall stiffness and decreased compliance. However, the pathophysiology in this entity is probably more complicated.[54-57] In fact, systolic dysfunction as measured by tissue Doppler strain imaging has been found to be also common when the ejection fraction is in the lower range (between 45% and 54%, normal being 60%) and present in half of the patients when the ejection fraction is normal. Other abnormalities detected include neuroendocrine, autonomic and vascular dysfunction.[55,58] Besides aging, several other comorbidities are also found in these patients including hypertension, obesity, atrial fibrillation and anemia.[59]

PATHOPHYSIOLOGY OF DILATED CARDIOMYOPATHY

Dilated cardiomyopathy refers to intrinsic myocardial disease. The etiology is often idiopathic, while in others it may be related to definable etiologic factors such as ethanol-related myocardial damage or a definite viral myocarditis. Whatever may be the etiology, the hallmark of the disorder is a dilated poorly contracting left ventricle and the process might involve equally the right ventricle. The increased radius caused by the dilatation would increase the oxygen demand by raising the left ventricular wall tension both during systole and diastole. The diastolic dysfunction would contribute to decreased left ventricular compliance. Other factors, which may be involved in the decrease of the ventricular compliance, include myocardial fibrosis in long-standing cases. The decreased compliance will lead to increased filling pressures in the ventricle. This would account for both systemic and pulmonary congestion. In addition, it will contribute to decreased sub-endocardial capillary flow. That will further cause abnormal rise in the filling pressures (Fig. 10.9).

Clinical Symptoms and Signs in Dilated Cardiomyopathy

The increased radius will cause a large area displaced left ventricular apical impulse. If the contractility is significantly reduced, then the accompanying decreased ejection fraction will give rise to a sustained apical impulse. The increased left and right ventricular filling pressures will lead to pulmonary and systemic congestion causing symptoms of dyspnea and peripheral edema. When the ejection fraction is significantly reduced, the stroke volume may be low and give rise to low-amplitude, low-volume pulse. Severe decrease in ejection fraction and stroke volume may actually lead to a very poorly felt apical impulse (Table 10.7).[60,61]

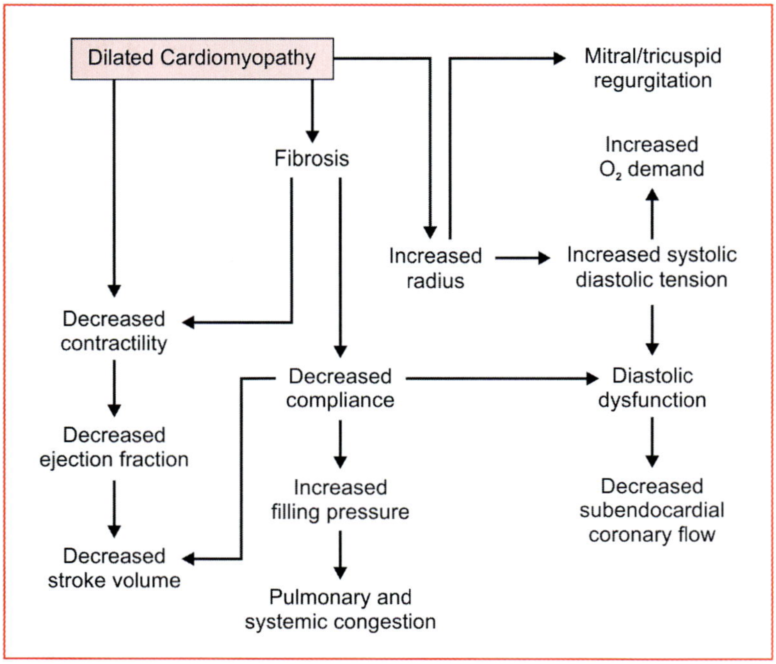

Fig. 10.9.

Table 10.7: Dilated Cardiomyopathy.

Pathophysiological Changes	*Clinical Symptoms/Signs*
• Increased radius	• Displaced large-area LV apex
• Increased duration of systolic tension • Reduced ejection fraction	• Sustained LV apex
• Increased LV/RV filling pressures	• Dyspnea/edema
• Decreased stroke volume	• Low-volume (amplitude) pulse • Low-output symptoms
• Severe reduction in ejection fraction	• Poorly felt apex beat

(LV: Left ventricular; RV: Right ventricular).

PATHOPHYSIOLOGY OF HYPERTROPHIC OBSTRUCTIVE CARDIOMYOPATHY

Hypertrophic cardiomyopathy is characterized by idiopathic hypertrophy of the ventricular myocardium especially of the left ventricle, often with an asymmetric involvement of the septum. The myocardium exhibits considerable disarray of the myocardial fibers. The intraventricular cavity is usually small. The left ventricle is often hypercontractile. The rapid ejection with increased ejection fraction will allow normal systolic tension to be maintained when there is no obstruction. The rapid and forceful ejection may, however, create a Venturi effect on the anterior mitral leaflet. The anterior mitral leaflet then may be pulled forward from its closed position during systole. The systolic anterior motion of the anterior leaflet may bring the leaflet into contact with the interventricular septum, thereby causing obstruction to the left ventricular outflow during the middle of systole. This anterior motion of the anterior mitral leaflet will make the mitral valve incompetent and allow mitral regurgitation to develop when obstruction to the left ventricular outflow tract is produced. In this condition, the obstruction to the left ventricular outflow is often dynamic. It may be exaggerated or increased under conditions of increased inotropic stimulation as may occur with sympathetic stimulation. It also can be increased by maneuvers that decrease the ventricular dimension, which will make the mitral leaflet and septal contact to occur earlier in systole. If the septal hypertrophy is excessive and the intraventricular cavity is small, then obstruction could occur even at rest. When there is significant obstruction during systole, then the left ventricular systolic wall tension will be increased. Increased left ventricular wall tension will increase myocardial oxygen demand.

The hypertrophy of the myocardium as well as the small left ventricular size will decrease the left ventricular compliance. This will increase the filling pressures in the left ventricle. The increased filling pressures will also impede sub-endocardial coronary capillary flow. The latter will contribute to the development of some myocardial fibrosis in the sub-endocardium. In long-standing cases, the left ventricular function could deteriorate with development of myocardial fibrosis and the ejection fraction could actually fall. The decreased left ventricular systolic function, a late phenomenon could further raise the diastolic filling pressures in the ventricle (Fig. 10.10).[62–66]

Clinical Symptoms and Signs in Hypertrophic Obstructive Cardiomyopathy

The hypercontractile left ventricle with rapid ejection will give rise to a sharp and rapid rate of rise of the arterial pulse. In the presence of significant outflow obstruction, the pulse will either have normal or low amplitude. The increased left ventricular wall tension during systole accompanying significant obstruction will be associated with a sustained duration of the apical impulse. Decreased left ventricular compliance will evoke a strong atrial contraction and may result in the production of a fourth heart sound (S4). It may also cause an atrial kick to be felt at the apex. The dynamic nature of the obstruction between the anterior mitral leaflet and the interventricular septum will explain the varying loudness of the ejection murmur depending on the degree of the obstruction. This can be brought out by change in the venous return and the resultant change in the left ventricular dimension caused by change in posture from a supine to the erect position. The murmur will be louder and longer on standing than when supine since the left ventricular size will be smaller in the standing position than when

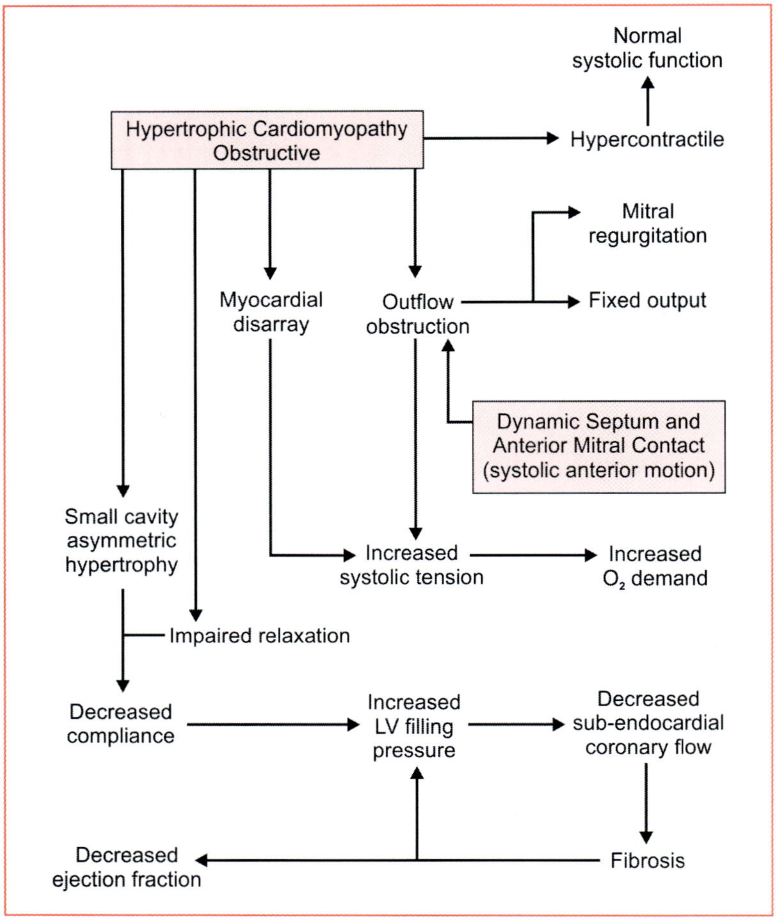

Fig. 10.10.

supine making the septal and mitral leaflet contact to occur earlier. In addition, the increase in the sympathetic tone caused by the assumption of the upright posture will help increase the contractility of the left ventricle. This will further increase the force of ejection. This will generate a greater Venturi effect on the mitral leaflet pulling the anterior leaflet forward more forcefully. The aortic pressure is the distending pressure that will oppose the systolic anterior motion of the anterior mitral leaflet. Standing may actually cause a slight fall in the systemic arterial pressure, thereby decreasing this opposing force. For all these reasons, the ejection murmur tends to be longer and louder on standing than when supine.

The increased left ventricular diastolic filling pressures being transmitted to the pulmonary capillary bed will produce symptoms of pulmonary congestion. Depending on the severity of the elevation of the left atrial and the pulmonary venous pressures, these symptoms can consist of dyspnea, paroxysmal nocturnal dyspnea and/or orthopnea. When the left atrial pressure is significantly increased and the left ventricular compliance markedly diminished, then abrupt deceleration of the early rapid diastolic inflow into the left ventricle could occur causing the production of an S3.

The increased myocardial oxygen demand and the decreased sub-endocardial capillary flow could contribute to symptoms of angina.

When the obstruction to outflow is severe, then the cardiac output becomes fixed and will not significantly increase on exertion. In fact, exercise induced peripheral vasodilatation may actually drop the systemic arterial pressure further and may cause the obstruction to get worse due to the decreased (distending) aortic root pressure (i.e. the opposing force of the systolic anterior motion of the anterior mitral leaflet). This may manifest as symptoms of exertional presyncope or syncope. The mitral regurgitation that accompanies the systolic anterior motion of the anterior mitral leaflet during systole may vary in severity depending on the degree of obstruction. The long-standing effects of mitral regurgitation and the elevated left atrial pressure could result in the development of atrial arrhythmias especially atrial fibrillation. These may manifest as symptoms of palpitation. The underlying myocardial disease and the pathologic changes of myocardial disarray and fibrosis could also set conditions suitable for the development of ventricular arrhythmias (Table 10.8).

Table 10.8: Hypertrophic Obstructive Cardiomyopathy.

Pathophysiological Changes	*Clinical Symptoms/Signs*
• Hypercontractile left ventricle	• Sharp upstroke carotid
• Outflow obstruction	• Normal or low amplitude pulse
• Increased systolic tension with slow fall in tension	• Sustained LV apex
• Decreased LV compliance	• Atrial kick • S4
• Dynamic nature of obstruction anterior leaflet MV and septum	• Ejection murmur varying loudness
• (LV size; systemic resistance—aortic pressure; contractility)	• Murmur louder on standing • Murmur softer on squatting
• Increased LV filling pressure • LA pressure	• Dyspnea • Paroxysmal nocturnal dyspnea/orthopnea
• Increased O_2 demand • Decreased sub-endocardial flow	• Angina
• Increased LA pressure • Decreased compliance	• S3
• Fixed output	• Exertional syncope/presyncope
• Mitral regurgitation	• Atrial fibrillation • Palpitation
• Myocardial disease	• Ventricular arrhythmias

(LV: Left ventricular; LA: Left atrial; MV: Mitral value).

PATHOPHYSIOLOGY OF ATRIAL SEPTAL DEFECT

Atrial septal defect represents the lesion that allows left-to-right shunt at the atrial level. The right ventricular wall is normally thinner compared to the left ventricle. The pulmonary arterial resistance is significantly lower than the systemic vascular resistance. Therefore, the right ventricle is more compliant than the left ventricle. Due to these reasons, the right side offers less resistance to flow than the left side. So the left-to-right shunt is a natural consequence in the presence of a defect in the atrial septum. The right atrium and the right ventricle will therefore receive the usual normal systemic venous return as well as this extra volume of blood received through the atrial septal defect. This leads to a volume overload state of the right ventricle. The large right ventricular stroke volume and the increased pulmonary flow is maintained for a long period of time (i.e. for many years) with normal or even low pulmonary arterial pressures. In some patients, the large flow could be associated with slight or moderate increase in the pulmonary arterial pressures mainly related to the flow. The increased size of the dilated right ventricle will cause increased right ventricular wall tension by Laplace relationship. The increased wall tension being a stimulus for hypertrophy will result in right ventricular hypertrophy. The dilatation of the right ventricle may cause increased tension in the moderator band through which the right bundle normally reaches the free wall of the right ventricle. This may contribute to the right bundle branch block pattern that is commonly seen in patients with atrial septal defect. The long standing shunt and the secondary right ventricular hypertrophy could lead to decreased right ventricular compliance, thereby raising the right ventricular filling pressures and therefore the right atrial pressures. The large pulmonary flow also means increased pulmonary venous inflow into the left atrium contributing also to some left atrial enlargement. With increasing age the left ventricular compliance gets decreased further. This will allow more preferential flow to the right side increasing the magnitude of the left-to-right shunt. The dilated atria would lead to the development of atrial arrhythmias and in particular atrial fibrillation. Since right ventricular dilatation automatically stretches the tricuspid valve ring, tricuspid regurgitation usually ensues. This gets aggravated by the onset of atrial fibrillation. The onset of atrial fibrillation usually heralds the symptoms and signs of peripheral congestion. The tendency for the development of atrial fibrillation and symptoms of heart failure is particularly increased after the fourth decade of life.

The rise in pulmonary vascular resistance caused by pulmonary vascular disease secondary to long-standing increase in the pulmonary flow is usually a very late phenomenon and is seen only in adults and in a small percentage of patients. If the pulmonary hypertension is significant, then it can further cause right ventricular hypertrophy and secondarily increase its filling pressures. The increased resistance in the pulmonary vascular bed together with increased right ventricular and right atrial filling pressures could then reverse

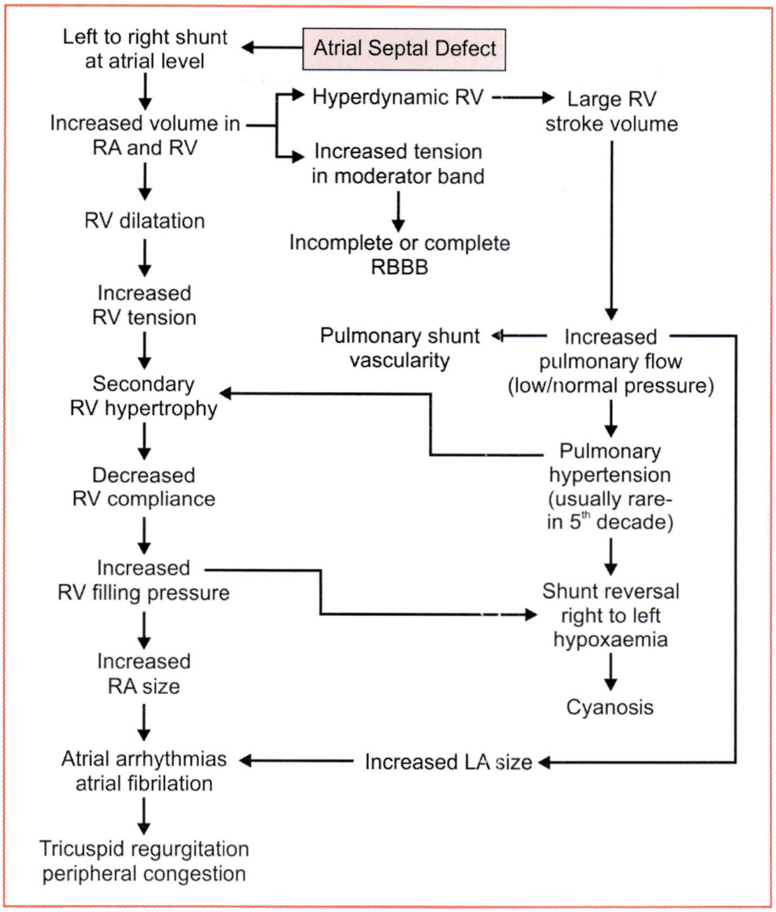

Fig. 10.11.

the shunt and begin to produce cyanosis secondary to hypoxemia. This type of Eisenmenger's syndrome with atrial septal defect secundum is usually rare (Fig. 10.11).[67-71]

Clinical Symptoms and Signs in Atrial Septal Defect

Atrial septal defect may not cause any significant symptoms and may be picked up by the presence of an ejection systolic murmur heard over the second left interspace caused by the increased pulmonary flow and/or a fixed splitting of the second heart sound (S2). The increased venous return on inspiration is accompanied by decreased left-to-right shunt flow. The opposite occurs with expiration, thereby keeping the pulmonary flow from varying very little with respiration. This allows the A2 and P2 separation to remain constant and unchanging with respiration. While this explanation may be simple, there could be other factors involved. The murmur may sometimes be scratchy and harsh and sometimes may be absent.

Table 10.9: Atrial Septal Defect.

Pathophysiological Changes	*Clinical Symptoms/Signs*
	• May be asymptomatic
• Not clearly explainable	• Vague symptoms, fatigue, palpitation, dyspnea
• Onset of atrial fibrillation	• Peripheral congestion
• RV volume overload	• Apex fromed by right ventricle with lateral retraction
• Increased venous return on inspiration • with decrease in left to right shunt and opposite changes on expiration	• Fixed split S2
• Increased pulmonary flow secondary to left to right shunt	• Ejection murmur II and III LICS • Tricuspid inflow rumble

(LICS: Left intercostal space).

Patients with atrial septal defect may also have vague symptoms of fatigue, palpitation and shortness of breath, all of which may not be clearly explainable. The symptoms of peripheral congestion with the onset of atrial fibrillation are usually noteworthy. The left ventricle is usually under filled and displaced posteriorly by the enlarged right ventricle. The enlarged right ventricle may in fact form the apical impulse and may be characterized by the presence of lateral retraction. A short mid-diastolic inflow murmur may accompany the increased flow into the right side across the tricuspid valve, which may be audible over the lower sternal or xiphoid area. The murmur may increase in intensity on inspiration indicating its tricuspid origin. The presence of such a flow murmur is usually indicative of a significant left to right shunt (Table 10.9).[72–74]

PATHOPHYSIOLOGY OF DIASTOLIC DYSFUNCTION

Several factors can affect the compliance of the left ventricle, thereby affecting the filling characteristics as well as its diastolic filling pressures. These include the completeness of ventricular relaxation, the chamber size, the thickness of the wall, the composition of the wall (inflammation, infiltrate, ischemia or infarction, scars etc.), the pericardium and the right ventricular volume and pressure.

The diastolic filling consists of three consecutive phases namely:

1. ***The early rapid filling phase***, which is an active phase beginning with ventricular relaxation
2. ***The slow filling phase***
3. ***The atrial contraction phase*** during end-diastole

The degree of decrease in diastolic compliance may vary. In the early stages, it may restrict only end-diastolic filling. It may evoke a strong atrial

Table 10.10: Diastolic Dysfunction.

1.	Decreased ventricular compliance in end-diastole only	
2.	Progressive stages of decreased compliance affecting the slow filling phase of diastole, leading to eventual increase in mean atrial pressure	
		Etiology
	• Intraluminal	• (Systolic failure)
	• Endocardial	
	• Myocardial	
	• Pericardial	• Pericardial effusion
		• Constriction
3.	Filling restriction also involving the rapid filling phase of diastole (Cardiac tamponade) (Rarely severe heart failure)	

contraction to help achieve better filling and stretch of the ventricular myocardium. At this stage, only the end-diastolic ventricular pressure will be increased and only the ***a wave*** pressure will be increased in the atrium. This will not significantly affect the mean atrial pressure due to the short duration of the ***a wave***. When the degree of diastolic dysfunction is more advanced, it may begin to encroach on the slow filling phase of diastole as well. At this stage, the ***pre a wave*** pressure will also be increased, thereby increasing the mean atrial filling pressure. The etiology of this type of diastolic restriction may be intraluminal as in systolic heart failure, where the ventricle empties poorly due to decreased ejection fraction and therefore gets overfilled quite early in diastole. It may be due to endocardial pathology as in idiopathic endomyocardial fibrosis or fibroelastosis due to myocardial pathology of various etiologies or due to pericardial causes including significant pericardial effusion and/or constrictive pericarditis. In all these situations, the filling in the rapid filling phase is not impaired, but restriction affects the slow filling phase to end of diastole. The third type of restriction is when it involves all of diastole, beginning with the early rapid filling phase. This type of total diastolic restriction is characteristic of cardiac tamponade. The latter is usually due to collection of fluid or blood in the pericardial space, which is under high pressure thereby compressing the ventricle from the very onset of diastole. This type of restriction is rare in systolic heart failure except in some very rare instances of severe degree of heart failure (Fig. 10.12 and Table 10.10).

PATHOPHYSIOLOGY OF CONSTRICTIVE PERICARDITIS

As a result of recurrent episodes of pericarditis or chronic pericarditis and specially those associated with certain specific pathogens such as tuberculous pericarditis, the pericardium may mount excessive reaction and may eventually thicken, become fibrosed and even calcified. In the initial stages, there may be pericardial effusion, but this eventually disappears and the thickened pericardium will become adherent to the underlying epicardium.

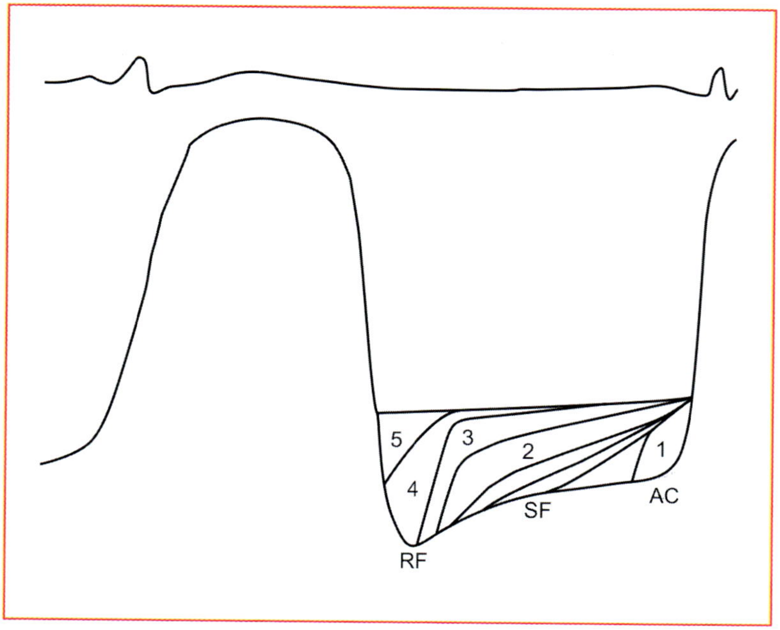

Fig. 10.12: The varying severity of restriction to diastolic ventricular filling is shown with lines to indicate the ventricular diastolic pressure elevations and their timing in diastole. In mild form, the pressure increase is during atrial contraction (AC) at end diastole (line 1). As restriction gets worse the ***pre a wave*** pressure starts to rise gradually and earlier and earlier in diastole. This progression is shown as four successive lines (lines 2). When severe, it may be total during mid- and late-diastole restricting flow into the right ventricle (RV) beginning with the slow filling phase (SF). There will be very rapid inflow only during early diastole or the rapid filling phase (RF) followed by a rapid rise in pressure with no further flow producing the classic dip and plateau or the square root pattern (line 3). This is typical for chronic constrictive pericarditis. If the restriction is severe and involves also the RF phase, the pressures rise quickly in the RV in early diastole limiting inflow altogether. This can occur in severe pericardial effusion leading to cardiac tamponade where the high intrapericardial pressure will limit ventricular expansion altogether. Line 4 depicts pre tamponade and line 5 is full tamponade with no diastolic inflow possible. Such severe elevations in diastolic pressures may rarely also occur in severe cardiomyopathy, cardiac failure and in some patients with severe right ventricular infarctions.

Similar reaction can also follow traumatic, post-surgical or radiation-induced pericarditis. Often, however, the etiology may be difficult to pinpoint and may be truly idiopathic. Occasionally, patients may present during the transitional phase with both effusion and signs of constriction. The signs of constriction may actually become evident when the patient's hemodynamics fail to show improvement even after the effusion is drained. These patients may be termed to have ***effusive-constrictive pericarditis.***

In ***constrictive pericarditis***, the pericardium is very stiff and fibrotic and may even be calcified. The visceral pericardium is thickened (sometimes up to 1 cm thick) and adherent to the underlying myocardium. The

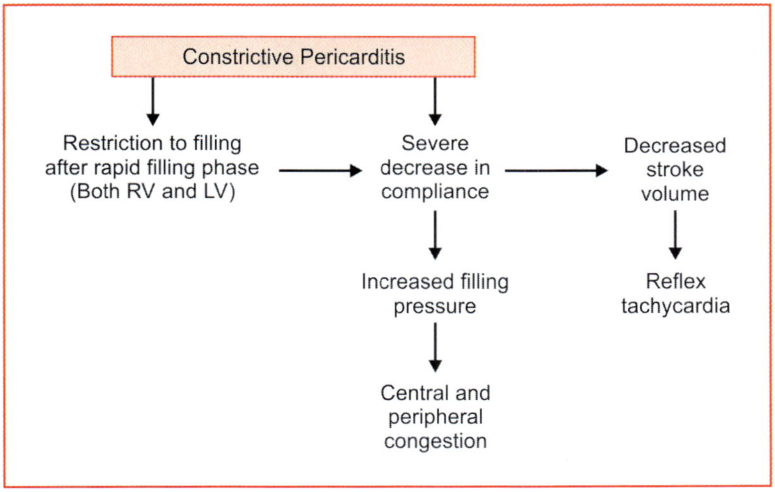

Fig. 10.13.

thickened and fibrotic pericardium acts as a steel armor around the ventricles preventing its full expansion. The ventricles could expand in early diastole but as soon as its size reaches the limits set by the thickened pericardium, the expansion is suddenly restricted and the filling comes to an abrupt end. No further expansion being possible, there is hardly any further filling during the later phases of diastole. The ventricular pressure that dips to zero at the onset of diastole suddenly rises to a peak and flattens out and stays elevated during the remainder of diastole giving rise to the characteristic ***"dip-plateau" square root sign*** of the filling pressures in the ventricles. Since the pericardium restricts both the right ventricle and the left ventricle alike, the filling pressures rise on both sides to similar levels. The increased diastolic ventricular pressures raise the mean pressures in both the atria. The raised right atrial pressure lead to the formation of systemic congestion and the raised left atrial pressure would cause pulmonary congestion. The severe diastolic filling restriction would cause decreased stroke output. This will be felt as low-amplitude arterial pulse. The cardiac output may be maintained by a reflex increase in the heart rate (Fig. 10.13).

Clinical Symptoms and Signs in Constrictive Pericarditis

The jugular venous pressure is not only elevated due to the raised right atrial pressures, it shows the altered contour with a dominant ***y descent***. This is because the ***v wave*** pressure head is raised with sudden restriction to filling at the end of the early rapid filling phase. This abrupt deceleration to the rapid inflow into the ventricles sets also the stage for the production of an early S3, the pericardial knock. The elevation of the atrial pressures will result in central congestion and dyspnea as well as peripheral congestion leading to edema and ascites.

Table 10.11: Constrictive Pericarditis.

Pathophysiological Changes	*Clinical Symptoms/Signs*
• Increased RV diastolic pressure • Restriction after rapid filling	• Elevated JVP • Dominant *y descent*
• Sudden deceleration of early diastolic inflow	• S3 (early) • "Pericardial knock"
• Central and peripheral congestion	• Dyspnea • Acsites • Edema
• Severe decrease in compliance • Inspiratory increase in RV filling pressure	• Kussmaul's sign
• Inspiratory increase in RV filling pressure • Septal shift • Decreased LV filling pressure	• Pulsus paradoxus
• Decreased stroke volume	• Low output symptoms

(LV: Left ventricular; JVP: Jugular venous pulse).

The venous pressure will rise on inspiration with the increased venous return since the right ventricular compliance is significantly decreased due to the pericardial restriction. This is the basis of ***Kussmaul's*** sign. In some patients with constrictive pericarditis, one may also have a pulsus paradoxus. This may happen for the reason that the inspiratory increase in the right ventricular filling pressure may produce some septal shift causing decreased left ventricular filling and pressure and therefore the stroke output on inspiration may fall and the opposite changes will occur on expiration and improve the left ventricular filling, thereby increasing the stroke output. These changes may be reflected on the arterial pressure with the pressure falling on inspiration and rising on expiration significantly. When the filling is considerably impaired then the decreased output will cause the arterial pulse to have low amplitude and this may be associated with low output symptoms of lassitude, fatigue and weakness as well (Table 10.11).

PATHOPHYSIOLOGY OF CARDIAC TAMPONADE

When pericarditis occurs, the inflamed surfaces of both the pericardium and the epicardium moving against each other as a result of heart movement with each cardiac beat cause friction because of the roughened surfaces. This results in an audible pericardial friction rub. The friction rub may disappear as a result of the inflammation settling down and the surfaces becoming smooth again. This is a good sign. But the friction rub may also disappear as a result of fluid accumulation between the two surfaces, which acts as a buffer and eliminates the friction and the friction rub.

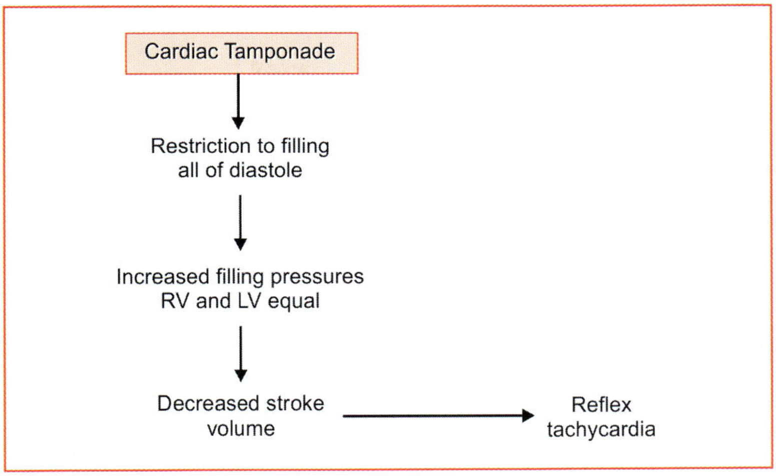

Fig. 10.14.

Table 10.12: Cardiac Tamponade.

Pathophysiological Changes	*Clinical Symptoms/Signs*
• Increased filling pressures	• Elevated JVP • Dyspnea
• Restriction all of diastole including early rapid filling phase	• Absent y descent • x′ descent only
• Severe decrease in stroke volume	• Hypotension • Low pulse pressure • Low output symptoms
• Sympathetic stimulation	• Tachycardia

(JVP: Jugular venous pulse).

If the fluid accumulation of whatever cause (i.e. viral pericarditis, malignancy, systemic lupus and uremia) is slow, the pericardium may adapt and dilate slowly allowing the intrapericardial pressure to stay low. Therefore, a large effusion may be well tolerated by the patient if accumulated over a period of time. Although the intrapericardial pressure may remain low with large effusion, the volume pressure relationship of the pericardium is such that when it has reached its limits of compliance, further accumulation of even a small amount of fluid could suddenly raise the intrapericardial pressure quite dramatically leading to cardiac tamponade. This change could occur within a short period of time.

When there is acute accumulation of pericardial fluid as seen in bleeding into the pericardial space secondary to trauma, ruptured myocardium post-myocardial infarction or following aortic root dissection (type I), the pericardium will be unable to adapt to the sudden accumulation of volume and the intrapericardial pressure will rise acutely and cause cardiac tamponade.

In ***cardiac tamponade***, the restriction involves all of diastole. The filling pressures are increased and equal in both the right and the left ventricles. The ventricles receive blood flow with great difficulty. All the four chambers are boxed in a tight space with high fluid pressure in the pericardial space. The blood can enter the heart only when it leaves the heart namely during systole. The blood that enters the atria during systole is with great difficulty transferred to the ventricles during diastole. The filling becomes inadequate invariably with low stroke output, which will result in reflex tachycardia (Fig. 10.14).

Clinical Symptoms and Signs in Cardiac Tamponade

The increased filling pressures contribute to symptoms of dyspnea and cause the venous pressure to be elevated. The jugular contour ***will show no y descent*** despite high venous pressure, since the restriction involves all of diastole. The contour may show only an ***x′ descent***. That too may be difficult to discern but can best be recorded by Doppler flow over the jugular. The marked decrease in stroke volume will cause hypotension and low systolic and low pulse pressure in addition to causing low output symptoms. The reflex sympathetic stimulation will be reflected in the presence of tachycardia (Table 10.12).[75–81] In addition, in the majority of patients, there will be a significant ***pulsus paradoxus*** (with an inspiratory drop in blood pressure of >15 mm Hg). The increased inspiratory venous return to the right ventricle and the associated right ventricular expansion may shift the interventricular septum as in the case of the constrictive pericarditis. In this situation, the pericardial fluid is squeezed and shifted also to the left side restricting expansion of the left ventricle during diastole. The effects of fluid shift may be seen as collapse or compression of relatively thin and low pressure chambers like the right atrium or the right ventricle during diastole on a two-dimensional echocardiogram.[82,83]

In some patients with large pericardial effusions, the marked increase in cardiac size at times may cause some compression and atelectasis of the adjacent lung, resulting in a small well-defined area of bronchial breathing just below the tip of the left scapula. The same area may also be dull to percussion and show egophony (Ewart's sign). This sign sometimes seen in patients with large pericardial effusions, may also be noted in patients with marked cardiomegaly of other causes. Since bronchial breathing and dullness may be present as a result of other pulmonary causes, this sign is not very specific.

APPENDIX

Laplace's Law

This law defines the relationship between the wall tension (***T***) and the pressure (***P***) and the radius (***r***) for a thin walled cylindrical shell (Fig.10.15). The

Laplace's law

for a thin walled cylindrical shell.

Tension = P (pressure) x r (radius)

Lamé's equation

If the wall has a thickness, then the circumferential wall stress is given by

$$\text{Tension} \propto \frac{\text{P (pressure) x r (radius)}}{\text{2h (wall thickness)}}$$

Fig. 10.15.

Table 10.13: Factors Determining Myocardial O_2 Consumption.

• Heart rate	• Systolic pressure, LV volume
• Wall tension (Laplace's Law)	• Contractility (Inontropic state)

(LV: Left ventricular).

tension is directly related to the pressure and the radius. If the wall has a thickness, then the circumferential wall stress is given by ***Lame's equation*** where the wall tension (***T***) is related to the pressure (***P***) and the radius (***r***) and inversely related to the wall thickness (***h***) (Fig. 10.15). In other words, hypertrophy of the wall is a compensatory mechanism, which tends to bring back the wall tension to near normal levels. Dilatation or enlargement, on the other hand, significantly increases the wall tension. This relationship needs to be kept in mind for it operates in many disorders both physiologic and pathologic. One of the important determinants of myocardial oxygen consumption is the wall tension developed in the left ventricle. The other factors include heart rate and contractility or inotropic state (Table 10.13).

Symptoms of High Left Atrial Pressure

High left atrial pressure, however, produced will lead to elevated pulmonary venous and capillary bed pressure. This in turn will cause symptoms of dyspnea. When the pressure is significantly elevated, it can produce symptoms of ***orthopnea***, which is dyspnea on assuming supine position relieved by raising the head or sitting up, as well as ***paroxysmal nocturnal dyspnea***. The latter requires the sleep mechanism and it usually occurs at night. The patient will give history of waking up short of breath from sleep after having gone to sleep a few hours prior to the episode. Sitting up and dangling the feet or getting up and standing for a while relieve the dyspnea. The extravascular fluid shifts gradually into the vascular compartment during sleep. This expands the blood volume and raises the left atrial pressure. In the normal subjects, the left ventricle accommodates the extra volume by increasing the output and the consequent increase in renal blood flow increases the urine output. However, when the left atrial pressure is somewhat elevated already, this shift from the extravascular to the intravascular compartment is not tolerated and results in symptoms of pulmonary congestion. The classical paroxysmal nocturnal dyspnea occurs in patients with decompensated left ventricles. In mitral stenosis, where the left ventricle is under filled and normal, one may get the history of paroxysmal nocturnal dyspnea. However, it is often atypical. The patient never gets comfortable completely after being up or tends to wake up more than once in the night since the left atrial pressure is significantly elevated due to the mitral obstruction. Occasionally, the patient with elevated left atrial pressure may complain of a nocturnal cough instead of dyspnea.

Clinical Signs of High left Atrial Pressure

In the absence of mitral stenosis, high left atrial pressure secondary to heart failure will often be associated with the presence of a pathological S3.

The pulmonary congestion may result in basal rales or crepitations (crackles) when the lungs are auscultated. These crepitations result from the congestion of the smaller airways with swelling, resulting in the closure of the airways during expiration as the lungs collapse. With expansion of the lungs on inspiration, the closed airways snap open, causing these snapping sounds. These crackles heard when the patient is supine may sometimes clear up on patients assuming erect posture due to a decrease in the venous return, resulting in lowered left atrial pressure. When the pulmonary congestion is significant, it would require active therapy for improvement. When untreated or ineffectively treated, it may end in a vicious cycle of hypoxemia, worsening left ventricular function, further rise in left atrial pressure and worse pulmonary congestion. Acute pulmonary edema may follow with marked shortness of breath associated with labored breathing with the use of the accessory muscles. Cyanosis may occur and the patient may start coughing up pink froth. Due to pulmonary venous congestion, the fluid is blood tinged making it pink. The surfactant in the lung causes the fluid to bubble hence the froth. Hypoxemia and low cardiac output will be associated with sinus tachycardia. Untreated this may deteriorate. There could be gradual slowing of the heart rate with the patient losing consciousness, resulting in hypoxemic cardiorespiratory arrest.

The pulmonary signs of crackles, however, are not specific for high left atrial pressure and more often present in other causes of pulmonary disease including pneumonia, chronic obstructive pulmonary disease and pulmonary fibrosis. Furthermore, pulmonary edema can also occur in the absence of elevated left trial pressure.

Symptoms of Pulmonary Hypertension

When pulmonary hypertension is severe, the vascular changes that develop in the pulmonary arterial bed not only raise the pulmonary vascular resistance but also act as severe obstructive lesion peripherally reducing flow and output. This gets further aggravated when the right ventricle gets decompensated. The main symptoms of pulmonary hypertension are therefore one of low output. The output may become relatively fixed and fail to increase with exertion and may actually paradoxically fall causing symptoms of presyncope and/or syncope with exertion. The oxygen saturation may also fall with exertion. The hypoxemia may also predispose to the development of arrhythmias. Often patients may also complain of vague atypical chest pain. The cause of this is not easily explainable (Table 10.14).

Signs of Pulmonary Hypertension

Pulmonary hypertension would make the pulmonary component of the second heart sound (P2) to become more sharp and loud. The P2 may become palpable in the second left interspace where it is often best heard. A palpable S2 (when confirmed to be due to the loud P2 by auscultation) in the second left interspace usually is a good sign of pulmonary hypertension and the pulmonary systolic pressure may be 75 mmHg or higher when this sign is present. The S2 split is usually narrow when the right ventricle is still compensated since the effect of the higher pulmonary impedance will be to bring the P2 earlier making the split narrower. When the right ventricle is decompensated, however, the S2 split may become wide due to a delayed P2 component as a result of poor and delayed right ventricular relaxation. The split may not vary well with respiration when this happens, it may be confused with a fixed splitting of S2. However, following exercise or in the post-Valsalva strain phase, the S2 split can be shown to vary making this a useful maneuver during auscultation.

The increased right ventricular pressure and the consequent increase in its wall tension may give rise to a sustained right ventricular impulse on sub-xiphoid palpation. One may also feel along with it an atrial kick due to a strong right atrial contraction. This is usually present only in the early compensated state of significant pulmonary hypertension.

The decreased right ventricular compliance due to diastolic dysfunction and right ventricular hypertrophy will lead to increased right ventricular

Table 10.14: Clinical Features of Left atrial and Pulmonary Hypertension.
Symptoms of High Left Atrial Pressure
• Dyspnea • Orthopnea • Paroxysmal nocturnal dyspnea • Palpitation if in atrial fibrillation
Symptoms of Pulmonary Hypertension
• Low output symptoms • Exertional presyncope/syncope (due to fixed output) • Chest pain
Signs of Pulmonary Hypertension
• Loud P2 (may be palpable in II LICS) • Narrow split S2 • Wide split S2 if RV failure • Sustained subxiphoid impulse • Elevated JVP • JVP Contours x′ > y (RV compensated) x′ = y (RV diastolic dysfunction with raised RV filling pressure) x′ < y (early RV systolic failure) y descent with large v wave (tricuspid regurgitation with RV dilatation)

(JVP: Jugular venous pulse; LICS: Left intercostal space: RV: Right ventricular).

diastolic pressure. This is reflected in the right atrial and the jugular venous pressures. Thus, pulmonary hypertension will often lead to elevated jugular venous pressure and abnormal jugular venous pulse contour. This has been discussed in detail in the Chapter 4 on Jugular Venous Pulsations. Here, it suffices to summarize the sequence of jugular contour changes in pulmonary hypertension. In the presence of pulmonary hypertension, the JVP contour of $x' > y$ indicates compensated right ventricular function, $x' = y$ indicates right ventricular diastolic dysfunction with raised filling pressures, $x' < y$ indicates early right ventricular systolic failure, ***y descent*** with large ***v wave*** denotes tricuspid regurgitation and right ventricular dilatation (Table 10.14).

Signs of Wide Pulse Pressure with Decreased Peripheral Resistance

These are listed in the Table 10.15.

Splitting of the Second Heart Sound

The respiratory variations in the timing of both the A2 and the P2 components of the S2 and their effects on the splitting of the S2 are shown in Figure 10.16.

Table 10.15: Signs of Wide Pulse Pressure with Decreased Peripheral Resistance.

- Corrigan Pulse (visible carotid pulse)
- Quincke's Sign (increased capillary pulsation)
- Pistol shot sounds
- Duroziez's Bruit (systolic and diastolic bruit over femorals, brought out by compression)
- Collapsing pulse
- de Musset's sign (rocking head movement)
- Positive Hill's sign (Blood pressure in the leg higher than in the arm > 15 mm Hg)

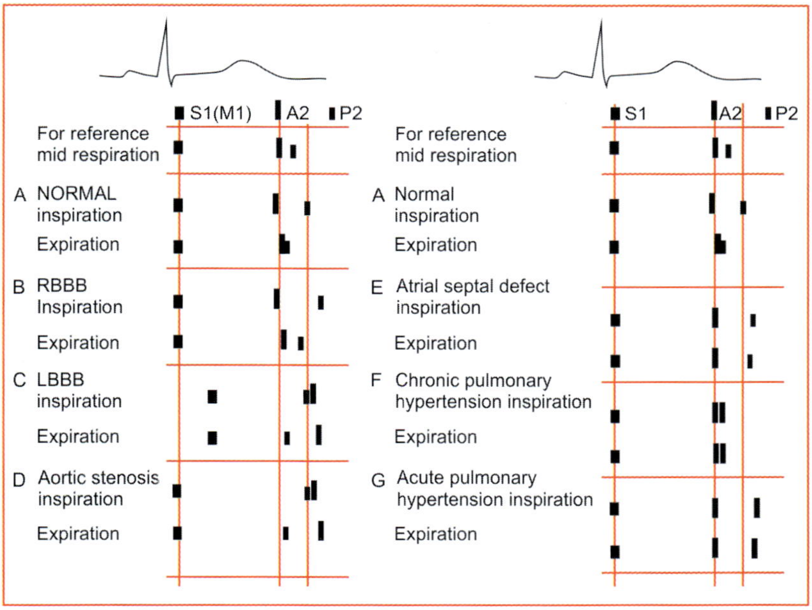

Fig. 10.16.

In the ***normals,*** the sequence of the components is A2 followed by P2, since the left ventricle is a more powerful chamber. Its contraction and relaxation are much faster than that of the right ventricle. On inspiration, there is decreased intrathoracic pressure with increased venous return to the right side. The lungs expand and the pulmonary impedance falls. Thus, the increased right ventricular volume and the decreased pulmonary impedance make the P2 come later on inspiration. The expansion of the lungs on inspiration diminishes the pulmonary venous return to the left heart. This may make the A2 come slightly earlier on inspiration. The effect of these changes on inspiration is to make both the A2 and the P2 to move away from each other resulting in a split. The reverse changes occur on expiration. The A2 comes later and the P2 comes earlier. The components come together with the splitting narrowing.

Right Bundle Branch Block

In right bundle branch block, the right ventricular electrical depolarization is delayed; therefore, the right ventricular mechanical events are also delayed by the same amount. Otherwise, the variations are the same as in the "***Normal***". The right ventricular delay causes a wider splitting of S2 due to delayed P2 on inspiration. The P2 does not come close to A2 during expiration. Thus, the split remains on expiration (***audible expiratory splitting***), although there is significant movement in A2–P2 intervals with respiration.

Left Bundle Branch Block

In left bundle branch block, the left ventricular depolarization and mechanical events are delayed. Therefore, both the mitral component of the S1 (M1) and the A2 are delayed. This delay causes the A2 to occur after P2, resulting in an abnormal sequence. This leads to a reversal of the splitting on inspiration called "***the paradoxical splitting***". The P2 moves as in the "normal", but due to the delay in A2, the two components come together during inspiration and move away from each other during expiration.

Aortic Stenosis

In aortic stenosis, a paradoxical splitting of the S2 can occur as a result of delayed A2 (closure of aortic valve). This is not because of an electromechanical delay as in LBBB, but rather due to increased ejection time as a result of the stenotic valve causing outflow obstruction. Unlike the case in LBBB, the M1 in this case is not delayed. Ischaemia can also cause similar change.

Atrial Septal Defect

In atrial septal defect, there is a left-to-right shunt across the atrial septum. The respiratory variations in the venous return and the consequent right-sided filling are compensated by the variations in the shunt with the result that the right ventricle receives more or less the same amount of blood on both inspiration and expiration. In addition, the overfilled pulmonary arterial bed from the left-to-right shunt does not allow any significant changes in the pulmonary impedance on inspiration. The left-sided filling also remains relatively the same for similar reasons. This results in a relatively ***fixed splitting of A2 and P2***.

Chronic Pulmonary Hypertension

In chronic pulmonary hypertension, the P2 becomes louder due to significant increase in the pulmonary arterial pressure and the high pulmonary arterial resistance. The high pulmonary impedance does not drop much with inspiration. This will result in a P2 that occurs somewhat early and does not change much with respiration. This will result in a narrow split of the S2 or a single S2.

Acute Pulmonary Hypertension

In acute pulmonary hypertension as seen in large acute pulmonary embolism, the P2 is not only loud and in fact may be delayed resulting in a wide split S2. It may remain wide until full compensatory mechanisms come into play. The wide split may become normal eventually unless recurrent embolism leads to the development of chronic pulmonary hypertension.

REFERENCES

1. Bonow RO, Carabello B, de Leon AC, et al. ACC/AHA guidelines for the management of patients with valvular heart disease. A report of the American College of Cardiology/American Heart Association. Task Force on Practice Guidelines (Committee on Management of Patients with Valvular Heart Disease). J Am Coll Cardiol. 1998;32:1486-588.
2. Carabello BA, Crawford FA Jr. Valvular heart disease. N Engl J Med. 1997;337 (1):32-41.
3. Carabello BA. The pathophysiology of mitral regurgitation. J Heart Valve Dis. 2000;9(5):600-608.
4. Carabello BA. Progress in mitral and aortic regurgitation. Prog Cardiovasc Dis. 2001;43(6):457-75.
5. Carabello BA. Concentric versus eccentric remodeling. J Card Fail. 2002;8(6 Suppl):S258-63.
6. DePace NL, Nestico PF, Morganroth J. Acute severe mitral regurgitation. Pathophysiology, clinical recognition, and management. Am J Med. 1985;78 (2):293-306.
7. Roberts WC, Braunwald E, Morrow AG. Acute severe mitral regurgitation secondary to ruptured chordae tendineae: clinical, hemodynamic, and pathologic considerations. Circulation. 1966;33(1):58-70.
8. Ronan JA, Jr., Steelman RB, DeLeon AC Jr, et al. The clinical diagnosis of acute severe mitral insufficiency. Am J Cardiol. 1971;27 (3):284-90.
9. Bonow RO. Chronic aortic regurgitation, 3rd edition. In Valvular Heart Disease. Alpert JS, Dalen JE, Rahimtoola SH (Eds). Philadelphia: Lippincott Williams & Wilkins; 2000.
10. Fielitz J, Hein S, Mitrovic V, et al. Activation of the cardiac renin-angiotensin system and increased myocardial collagen expression in human aortic valve disease. J Am Coll Cardiol. 2001;37(5):1443-9.
11. Gaasch WH, Carroll JD, Levine HJ, et al. Chronic aortic regurgitation: prognostic value of left ventricular end-systolic dimension and end-diastolic radius/thickness ratio. J Am Coll Cardiol. 1983;1(3):775-82.
12. Borer JS, Truter S, Herrold EM, et al. Myocardial fibrosis in chronic aortic regurgitation: molecular and cellular responses to volume overload. Circulation. 2002;105(15):1837-42.
13. Otto CM. Aortic Regurgitation, 2nd edition. Otto CM (Ed). Philadelphia: WB Saunders; 2004.

14. Vatner SF, Shannon R, Hittinger L. Reduced sub-endocardial coronary reserve. A potential mechanism for impaired diastolic function in the hypertrophied and failing heart. Circulation. 1990;81(2 Suppl):III8-14.
15. Hittinger L, Mirsky I, Shen YT, et al. Hemodynamic mechanisms responsible for reduced sub-endocardial coronary reserve in dogs with severe left ventricular hypertrophy. Circulation. 1995;92(4):978-86.
16. Vatner SF, Hittinger L. Coronary vascular mechanisms involved in decompensation from hypertrophy to heart failure. J Am Coll Cardiol. 1993;22(4 Suppl A):34A-40A.
17. Reddy PS, Leon DF, Krishnaswami V, et al. Syndrome of acute aortic regurgitation. American Heart Association Monograph 1975;46:166-74.
18. Wigle ED, Labrosse CJ. Sudden, severe aortic insufficiency. Circulation. 1965;32 (5):708-20.
19. Meadows WR, Vanpraagh S, Indreika M, et al. Premature mitral valve closure: a hemodynamic explanation for absence of the first sound in aortic insufficiency. Circulation. 1963;28:251-8.
20. Sapira JD. Quincke, de Musset, Duroziez, and Hill: some aortic regurgitations. South Med J. 1981;74(4):459-67.
21. Reddy PS, Curtiss EI, Salerni R, et al. Sound pressure correlates of the Austin Flint murmur. An intracardiac sound study. Circulation. 1976;53(2):210-7.
22. Constant J. Bedside Cardiology, 2nd edition. Boston: Little, Brown and Company; 1976.
23. Wood.P. An appreciation of mitral stenosis I Clinical features. BMJ. 1954;1: 1051-113.
24. Wood P. An appreciation of mitral stenosis II Investigations and results. BMJ. 1954;1:1113-24.
25. Rahimtoola SH, Durairaj A, Mehra A, et al. Current evaluation and management of patients with mitral stenosis. Circulation. 2002;106(10):1183-8.
26. Otto CM. Mitral stenosis, 2nd edition. Otto CM (Ed). Philadelphia: WB Saunders; 2004.
27. Gould KL, Carabello BA. Why angina in aortic stenosis with normal coronary arteriograms? Circulation. 2003;107(25):3121-3.
28. Park SJ, Enriquez-Sarano M, Chang SA, et al. Hemodynamic patterns for symptomatic presentations of severe aortic stenosis. JACC Cardiovasc Imaging. 2013;6(2):137-46.
29. Carabello BA. The symptoms of aortic stenosis: a step closer to understanding their cause. JACC Cardiovasc Imaging. 2013;6(2):147-9.
30. Braunwald E, Antman EM, Beasley JW, et al. ACC/AHA guidelines for the management of patients with unstable angina and non-ST-segment elevation myocardial infarction. A report of the American College of Cardiology/ American Heart Association Task Force on Practice Guidelines (Committee on the Management of Patients With Unstable Angina). J Am Coll Cardiol. 2000;36(3):970-1062.
31. Braunwald E, Antman EM, Beasley JW, et al. ACC/AHA guideline update for the management of patients with unstable angina and non-ST-segment elevation myocardial infarction—2002: summary article: a report of the American College of Cardiology/American Heart Association Task Force on Practice Guidelines (Committee on the Management of Patients With Unstable Angina). Circulation. 2002;106(14):1893-900.
32. Corti R, Fuster V, Badimon JJ. Pathogenetic concepts of acute coronary syndromes. J Am Coll Cardiol. 2003;41(4 Suppl S):7S-14S.

33. Forrester JS, Wyatt HL, Da Luz PL, et al. Functional significance of regional ischemic contraction abnormalities. Circulation. 1976;54(1):64-70.
34. Fuster V, Corti R, Fayad ZA, et al. Integration of vascular biology and magnetic resonance imaging in the understanding of atherothrombosis and acute coronary syndromes. J Thromb Haemost. 2003;1(7):1410-21.
35. Pfeffer MA, Braunwald E. Ventricular remodeling after myocardial infarction. Experimental observations and clinical implications. Circulation. 1990;81(4):1161-72.
36. St John Sutton M, Lee D, Rouleau JL, et al. Left ventricular remodeling and ventricular arrhythmias after myocardial infarction. Circulation. 2003;107(20):2577-82.
37. Swan HJ, Forrester JS, Diamond G, et al. Hemodynamic spectrum of myocardial infarction and cardiogenic shock. A conceptual model. Circulation. 1972;45(5):1097-110.
38. Antman EM, Anbe DT, Armstrong PW, et al. ACC/AHA guidelines for the management of patients with ST-elevation myocardial infarction--executive summary. A report of the American College of Cardiology/American Heart Association Task Force on Practice Guidelines (Writing Committee to revise the 1999 guidelines for the management of patients with acute myocardial infarction). J Am Coll Cardiol. 2004;44(3):671-719.
39. Boersma E, Mercado N, Poldermans D, et al. Acute myocardial infarction. Lancet. 2003;361(9360):847-58.
40. Libby P. Current concepts of the pathogenesis of the acute coronary syndromes. Circulation. 2001;104:365-81.
41. Goodman SG, Langer A, Ross AM, et al. Non-Q-wave versus Q-wave myocardial infarction after thrombolytic therapy: angiographic and prognostic insights from the global utilization of streptokinase and tissue plasminogen activator for occluded coronary arteries-I angiographic sub-study. GUSTO-I Angiographic Investigators. Circulation. 1998;97(5):444-50.
42. White HD, Norris RM, Brown MA, et al. Left Ventricular end-systolic volume as a major determinant of survival after recovery from myocardial infarction. Circulation. 1987;76:44-51.
43. Sadanandan S, Buller C, Menon V. The late open artery hypothesis-A decade later. Am Heart J. 2001;142:411-21.
44. Pfeffer MA, Lamas GA, Vaughan DE, et al. Effect of captopril on progressive ventricular dilatation after anterior myocardial infarction. N Engl J Med. 1988;319(2):80-6.
45. Weisman HF, Bush DE, Mannisi JA, et al. Cellular mechanisms of myocardial infarct expansion. Circulation. 1988;78(1):186-201.
46. Pfeffer MA. Left ventricular remodeling after acute myocardial infarction. Ann Rev Med. 1995;46:455-66.
47. Laskey WK, Kussmaul WG. Arterial wave reflection in heart failure. Circulation. 1987;75(4):711-22.
48. London GM, Guerin A. Influence of arterial pulse and reflective waves on systolic blood pressure and cardiac function. J Hypertens Suppl. 1999;17(2):S3-6.
49. Nichols WW, O'Rourke MF. McDonald's blood flow in Arteries, 4th edition. London: Edward Arnold; 1998.
50. O'Rourke MF, Kelly R, Avolio A. The arterial pulse. Philadelphia: Lea & Febiger; 1992.
51. Westerhof N, O'Rourke MF. Haemodynamic basis for the development of left ventricular failure in systolic hypertension and for its logical therapy. J Hypertens. 1995;13(9):943-52.

52. Hein S, Arnon E, Kostin S, et al. Progression from compensated hypertrophy to failure in the pressure-overloaded human heart: structural deterioration and compensatory mechanisms. Circulation. 2003;107(7):984-91.
53. Kitzman DW, Gardin JM, Gottdiener JS, et al. Importance of heart failure with preserved systolic function in patients > or = 65 years of age. CHS Research Group. Cardiovascular Health Study. Am J Cardiol. 2001;87(4):413-9.
54. Kitzman DW, Little WC, Brubaker PH, et al. Pathophysiological characterization of isolated diastolic heart failure in comparison to systolic heart failure. JAMA. 2002;288(17):2144-50.
55. Kitzman DW, Upadhya B. Heart failure with preserved ejection fraction: a heterogenous disorder with multifactorial pathophysiology. J Am Coll Cardiol. [Editorial]. 2014;63(5):457-9.
56. Gottdiener JS, Arnold AM, Aurigemma GP, et al. Predictors of congestive heart failure in the elderly: the Cardiovascular Health Study. J Am Coll Cardiol. 2000;35(6):1628-37.
57. Owan TE, Hodge DO, Herges RM, et al. Trends in prevalence and outcome of heart failure with preserved ejection fraction. N Engl J Med. 2006;355(3):251-9.
58. Kraigher-Krainer E, Shah AM, Gupta DK, et al. Impaired systolic function by strain imaging in heart failure with preserved ejection fraction. J Am Coll Cardiol. [Randomized Controlled Trial]. 2014;63(5):447-56.
59. Ather S, Chan W, Bozkurt B, et al. Impact of non-cardiac comorbidities on morbidity and mortality in a pre-dominantly male population with heart failure and preserved versus reduced ejection fraction. J Am Coll Cardiol. 2012;59(11):998-1005.
60. Deedwania PC. The key to unraveling the mystery of mortality in heart failure: an integrated approach. Circulation. 2003;107(13):1719-21.
61. Braunwald E, Bristow MR. Congestive heart failure: fifty years of progress. Circulation. 2000;102(20 Suppl 4):IV14-23.
62. Braunwald E, Morrow AG, Cornell WP, et al. Idiopathic Hypertrophic sub-aortic stenosis. Clinical, hemodynamic and angiographic manifestations. Am J Med. 1960;29:924.
63. Glancy DL, Shepherd RL, Beiser D, et al. The dynamic nature of left ventricular outflow obstruction in idiopathic hypertrophic sub-aortic stenosis. Ann Intern Med. 1971;75(4):589-93.
64. Murgo JP, Alter BR, Dorethy JF, et al. Dynamics of left ventricular ejection in obstructive and non-obstructive hypertrophic cardiomyopathy. J Clin Invest. 1980;66(6):1369-82.
65. Ross J Jr, Braunwald E, Gault JH, et al. The mechanism of intra-ventricular pressure gradient in idiopathic hypertrophic sub-aortic stenosis. Circulation. 1966;34:558.
66. Sherrid MV, Gunsburg DZ, Moldenhauer S, et al. Systolic anterior motion begins at low left ventricular outflow tract velocity in obstructive hypertrophic cardiomyopathy. J Am Coll Cardiol. 2000;36(4):1344-54.
67. Perloff JK. The Clinical Recognition of Congenital Heart Disease. Philadelphia: WB Saunders; 2001.
68. Campbell M. Natural history of atrial septal defect. Brit Heart J. 1970;32:820-6.
69. Craig RJ, Selzer A. Natural history and prognosis of atrial septal defect. Circulation. 1968 May;37(5):805-15.
70. Therrien J, Dore A, Gersony W, et al. CCS Consensus Conference 2001 update: recommendations for the management of adults with congenital heart disease. Part I. Can J Cardiol. 2001;17(9):940-59.

71. Wood P. The Eisenmenger syndrome or Pulmonary hypertension with reversed central shunt. Br Heart J. 1963;2:701.
72. Aygen MM, Braunwald E. The splitting of the second heart sound in normal subjects and in patients with congenital heart disease. Circulation. 1962;25: 328-45.
73. Perloff JK, Harvey WP. Mechanisms of fixed splitting of the second heart sound. Circulation. 1958;18(5):998-1009.
74. O'Toole JD, Reddy PS, Curtiss EI, et al. The mechanism of splitting of the second heart sound in atrial septal defect. Circulation. 1977;56(6):1047-53.
75. Dornhorst A, Howard P, Leathart GL. Pulsus Paradoxus. Lancet. 1952;1:746-8.
76. Gibson R. Atypical constrictive pericarditis. Brit Heart J. 1959;21:583.
77. Ranganathan N, Sivaciyan V. Jugular venous flow velocity pattern, application to bedside recognition of jugular venous pulse contour and right heart hemodynamics. Am J Noninvas Cardiol. 1993;7:75-88.
78. Reddy PS, Curtiss EI, O'Toole JD, et al. Cardiac tamponade: hemodynamic observations in man. Circulation. 1978;58(2):265-72.
79. Shabetai R, Fowler NO, Guntheroth WG. The hemodynamics of cardiac tamponade and constrictive pericarditis. Am J Cardiol. 1970;26(5):480-9.
80. Wood P. Chronic constrictive pericarditis. Am J Cardiol. 1961;7:48-61.
81. Bilchick KC, Wise RA. Paradoxical physical findings described by Kussmaul: pulsus paradoxus and Kussmaul's sign. Lancet. 2002;359:1940-2.
82. Fowler NO, Gabel M, Buncher CR. Cardiac tamponade: a comparison of right versus left heart compression. J Am Coll Cardiol. 1988;12(1):187-93.
83. Spodick DW. Pericardial diseases, 6th edition. Braunwald E, Zipes D, Libby P (Eds). Philadelphia: WB Saunders; 2001.

Chapter 11

Local and Systemic Manifestation of Cardiovascular Disease

Franklin Saksena

Snapshot

A good deal of information about cardiovascular diseases can be obtained by the thorough inspection of a patient using only the unaided senses. Inspection is a frequently overlooked aspect of cardiovascular physical diagnosis. This section aims to promote the recognition of the local and systemic manifestations of cardiovascular disease under the following headings: General Observations, Congenital Syndromes, Vascular Diseases, Valvular Heart Disease, Endocrine and Metabolic Diseases, Inflammatory Diseases, Pharmacologic Agents, Musculoskeletal Diseases and Tumors. Associated cardiovascular findings are placed in brackets.

GENERAL OBSERVATIONS

The patient's height, weight, degree of alertness, skin, nails, and clothing are initially evaluated.[1]

Height

A tall thin patient with an arm span exceeding the height, ectopia lentis, long thin fingers, hyper extensible joints, high arched palate suggests ***Marfan's syndrome.*** Such patients often have *aortic regurgitation, dissecting aneurysm of the aorta and mitral valve prolapse*[2] (Figs. 11.1A and B).

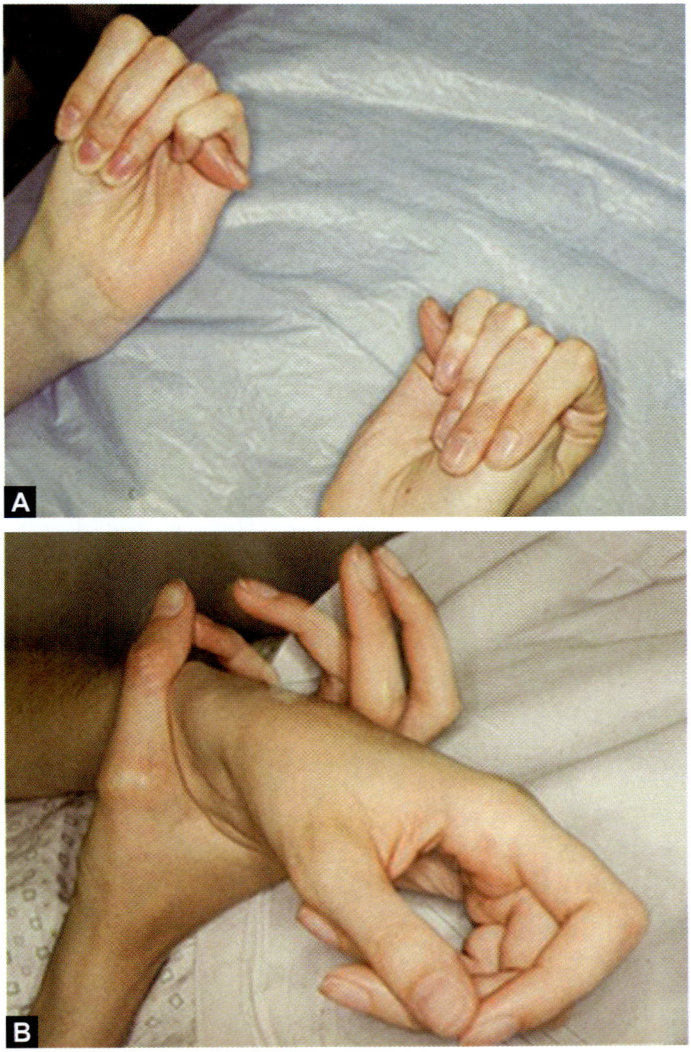

Figs. 11.1A and B: A 27-year-old female with Marfan's syndrome showing arachnodactyly (positive thumb and wrist signs). Her arm span = height = 73 inches. She had aortic insufficiency and a dilated aortic root measuring 6 cm in diameter.

A short female patient usually <5 feet tall with webbing of the neck, widely spaced nipples, short fourth finger are characteristic of Turner's syndrome (coarctation of the aorta).[3]

Weight

Obese patients have a body mass index exceeding 26 kg/m^2. Obesity localized to the abdomen (android or central type) has a higher incidence of hypertension and diabetes.[4]

A large protuberant abdomen may be due to central obesity or ascites. Patients with ascites may have liver disease or less commonly right heart failure.[5]

Weight gain or loss can be visually assessed by noting the changing position of the belt buckle markings, how well the clothing fits or whether a wedding ring is too loose or too tight.[1]

Degree of Alertness

Patients who fall asleep frequently during an interview may have the sleep apnea syndrome. Such patients may or may not be obese and may have coexisting polycythemia, cor pulmonale or systemic hypertension.[6]

Skin

Skin color alterations and edema provide useful clues in the detection of underlying cardiovascular disease. Alterations in skin color may be due to cyanosis, polycythemia, anemia, periodic facial flushing, jaundice or bronzed pigmentation.

Cyanosis is a bluish discoloration of the skin that occurs when there is at least 5 gm% of reduced hemoglobin circulating in the capillaries and venules. Cyanosis may be of central, peripheral or mixed origin.

Central cyanosis is often associated with clubbing and polycythemia. It is visually detected when the arterial saturation is <80% and is best seen under the tongue.[7] Central cyanosis is seen in patients with intracardiac right-to-left shunts (e.g. tetralogy of Fallot and Eisenmenger's syndrome), A-V fistula or intrapulmonary shunts (e.g. chronic obstructive lung disease and pulmonary infarction).

Differential cyanosis may occur in persistent ductus arteriosus with right-to-left shunting of blood. The cyanosis may be more pronounced in the legs and left arm than in the right arm and head. Coexisting coarctation of the aorta will aggravate this differential cyanosis.[8,9] If transposition of the great vessels coexists with a persistent ductus arteriosus with right-to-left shunting, then cyanosis is more prominent in the upper extremities and head than in the lower extremities.[9a]

Peripheral cyanosis is seen in low output states or localized venous obstruction. Thus, it is common in congestive heart failure, Raynaud's disease or vena caval obstruction. It may be detected in the ears, nail beds or the lips. Clubbing and polycythemia are absent.[9]

Patients with ***polycythemia*** have a ruddy complexion and brick red conjunctiva. Polycythemia is of primary or secondary origin. Secondary polycythemia is seen in patients with arterial hypoxemia due to right-to-left intracardiac shunting or due to intrapulmonary shunting (e.g. COPD). There is an increased incidence of myocardial infarction and thromboembolism in patients with primary polcythemia.[10] Secondary polycythemia is rarely a cause of myocardial infarction.[10a]

Anemia is best detected by looking for conjunctival pallor.[11] Nail bed and palmar crease pallor are unreliable signs of anemia.[11] Anemia may account for a pulmonary flow murmur, bruit de diable, venous hum and high output failure. Although the cardiac output is almost always raised when the hemoglobin is <6 gm%,[12] high output failure may occur at higher levels of hemoglobin concentration in the presence of underlying ventricular dysfunction.

Periodic flushing of the skin of the face, neck and chest is seen in patients with carcinoid syndrome. Patients with carcinoid syndrome have a high incidence of tricuspid regurgitation and pulmonic stenosis.[13]

Jaundice may be detected as a yellowish tint of the skin, the sub-glossal mucosa or sclera, and is usually mild in cardiac disease. Jaundice is seen in patients with (a) hepatic congestion due to right heart failure, tricuspid regurgitation, constrictive pericarditis or (b) hemolysis associated with prosthetic valve dysfunction.

Patients with ***hemochromatosis*** have iron and melanin deposits in the skin producing a diffuse slate grey or bronzed appearance especially prominent in the face, neck and distal parts of the extremities. Diabetes and hepatic dysfunction frequently co-exist along with a restrictive or a dilated cardiomyopathy.[14]

Multiple café au lait macules over 1.5 cm in diameter occur in neurofibromatosis. Other skin lesions consist of neurofibromas, axillary or inguinal freckling. These skin lesions are randomly distributed, but appear most commonly over the back and chest. Neurofibromatosis (Von Recklinghausens's disease) is associated with hypertension due to renal artery stenosis or pheochromocytoma.[15] Cardiac neurofibromas may produce outflow obstruction.[16]

Bilateral edema of the legs is seen in heart failure, venous insufficiency, venous thrombosis, lymphedema, hypoalbuminemia or severe anemia.[17] Of the causes of bilateral leg edema, only heart failure is associated with an elevated jugular venous pressure.[17] Unilateral leg edema is usually due to local venous obstruction. Edema of the upper extremity is seen in superior vena cava syndrome, sub-clavian vein thrombosis, thoracic outlet syndrome, or lymphatic obstruction due to breast cancer.[17,18] Edema of the hand may be caused by all the causes mentioned for upper extremity edema as well as local causes such as infection or trauma.[19] The shoulder hand syndrome as a cause of hand edema is rarely seen now.

Nails

The nails are examined for clubbing, sub-ungal hemorrhages, sub-ungal fibromas, and any distinctive color of the nails.

Sub-ungal hemorrhages (splinter hemorrhages) are seen in endocarditis and usually involve the middle portion of the nail. Sub-ungal hemorrhages may also be seen in trauma, vasculitis or systemic embolism.[20,21]

Sub-ungal fibromas (hands, feet) are a feature of tuberous sclerosis.[22]

White nails (Terry's nails) are in my opinion commonly seen in chronic hepatic congestion due to heart failure but may also be seen in liver cirrhosis.[23] ***Blue gray nails*** are seen in hemochromatosis (cardiomyopathy), Wilson's disease (cardiomyopathy), ochronosis (aortic or mitral valvular disease).[24] ***Black nails*** are seen in Cushing's syndrome (hypertension).[24]

Onycholysis (Plummer's nails) is seen in hyperthyroidism, but may also occur in trauma, psoriasis, or syphilis.[25] A ***red lunula*** is associated with heart failure, but is also seen in psoriasis and collagen diseases.[26]

Gait

A ***high steppage*** gait is seen in muscular dystrophy (cardiomyopathy), whereas sensory ataxia and pes cavus are seen in Friedreich's ataxia (cardiomyopathy).

Tabes dorsalis, a manifestation of tertiary syphilis is characterized by sensory ataxia, ***Argyll Robertson pupil*** and optic atrophy (aortic regurgitation).

A ***festinating gait*** with orthostatic hypotension is seen not only in Parkinson's disease but also in the Shy-Drager syndrome.[27]

CONGENITAL SYNDROMES/DISEASES

Inspection of the head and/or hands[8] is often useful in detecting congenital disorders associated with underlying heart disease. In this section, I will mention Down, LEOPARD, Noonan, William, Osler-Weber-Rendu, and Holt-Oram syndromes, as well as tuberous sclerosis and cyanotic heart disease. The importance of clubbing will be discussed under the latter heading.

Down's Syndrome

Down's syndrome occurs 1:1,000 newborns and is characterized by a vacant expression on the face, mental retardation, slanting of the palpebral fissures, Brushfield spots, small ears, macroglossia, a simian crease and a small fifth digit[28] (AV canal, ventricular septal defect, tetralogy of Fallot).[29]

LEOPARD Syndrome

These patients have **L**entigines (1–5 mm size brown macules on back, thorax and neck), **E**CG conduction defects, **O**cular-hypertelorism, **P**ulmonic stenosis (and other CVS abnormalities such as ***hypertrophic cardiomyopathy***), **A**bnormalities of genitalia (hypogonadism), **R**etardation of growth and **D**eafness sensorineural[30] (Figs. 11.2A to C). Patients with the LEOPARD syndrome are predisposed to sudden death if there is coexistent hypertrophic cardiomyopathy.[31]

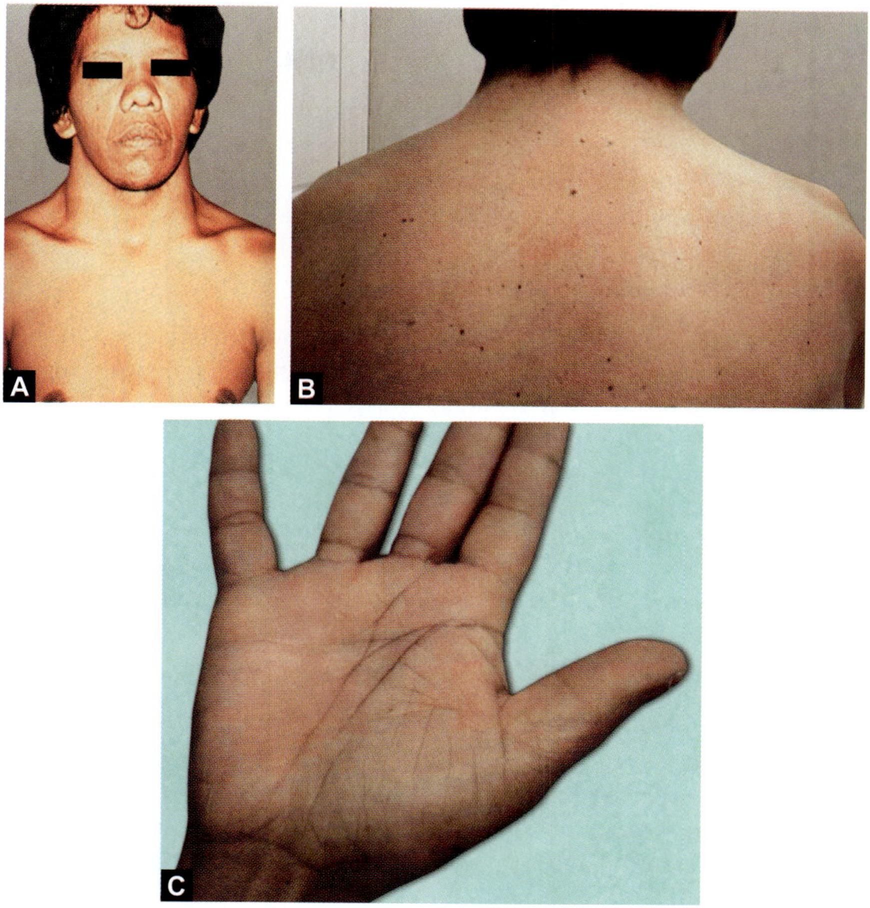

Figs. 11.2A to C: A 35-year-old Mexican male with features of LEOPARD and Noonan's syndromes showing chest wall lentigines, webbing of the neck, hypertelorism (A and B), and a variant of a Simian crease (C). He had mental retardation and pulmonary stenosis.

Noonan's Syndrome

This syndrome consists of hypertelorism, mental retardation, high-arched palate, webbing of neck, a Simian crease and cryptorchidism ***(pulmonic stenosis).***[32,33]

Tuberous Sclerosis

This entity is inherited as an autosomal dominant trait (1:10,000) and diagnosed by detecting angiofibromata of the lower half of the face (adenoma sebaceum). There is often a history of mental retardation, seizure disorder and multiple sub-ungal fibromas. These patients often have a ***rhabdomyoma,*** which may occasionally obstruct the RV or LV outflow tract.[22]

William's Syndrome

These patients have a large forehead, upturned nose, a long philtrum, an enlarged overhanging upper lip, deformed teeth, puffy cheeks and a friendly disposition (i.e. an elfin like appearance). The voice is hoarse and has a metallic tone.[34] Patients have supravalvular aortic stenosis and may occasionally have a pulmonary artery branch stenosis.[35]

Osler-Weber-Rendu Syndrome

This autosomal dominant entity is characterized by capillary angiomata of the tongue and lips[36] (Fig. 11.3). Epistaxis and GI bleeding may also occur (pulmonary A-V fistula).[37]

Holt-Oram Syndrome

An autosomal dominant condition in which patients with a ***secundum atrial septal defect*** have various hand abnormalities such as a long first proximal phalanx (fingerized thumb), or a missing thumb or an extra digit.[38]

Cyanotic Heart Disease

Patients with clubbing, cyanosis and polycythemia often have cyanotic heart disease *(tetralogy of Fallot, tricuspid atresia with right-to-left shunt at atrial level, or the Eisenmenger's syndrome).*

Clubbing is a very important physical finding in the detection of cardiopulmonary disease and needs some discussion as to its detection and usefulness.

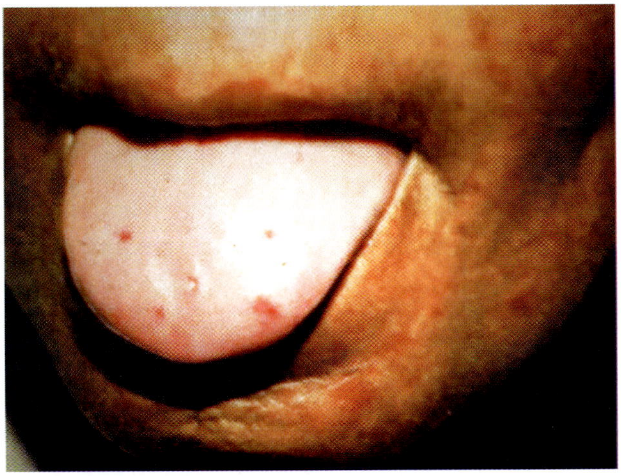

Fig. 11.3: Osler-Weber-Rendu syndrome. This 44-year-old female had capillary angiomata on the tongue and telangiectasia of the cheeks. No history of epistaxis or GI bleeding.

The normal angle that the nail plate makes with the adjacent skin fold is 150–170° degrees[39] (Fig. 11.4A) and the hyponychial angle (nail plate to distal nail angle) is 178–192°,[40] (Fig. 11.4B). In clubbing, the nail bed angle or profile angle exceeds 180° and the hyponychial angle is increased. Normally, there is a window formed between the thumbnails when they are held together and seen in profile. In clubbing, the hyponychial angle is increased and the window between the two pressed together thumbnails is lost ***(Shamroth's clubbing sign).***[41]

A useful sign of early clubbing is to determine if the ratio of the distal phalangeal depth to the interphalangeal joint depth in the index finger exceeds 1.0 (normal ratio using a micrometer is 0.9).[42] This distal/interphalangeal ratio may also be visually assessed at the bedside with a "shadowgram" of the finger in profile.[43]

Sub-cuticular edema and ballotability of the nail itself are often present, but may be a late sign of clubbing.[44] Clubbing needs to be distinguished from

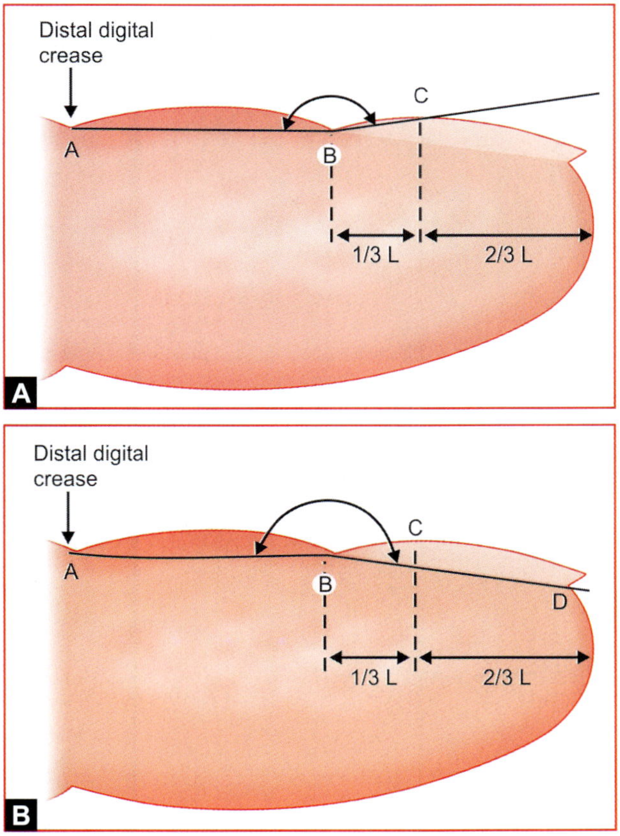

Figs. 11.4A and B: In (A) the profile nail bed angle ABC is depicted (normal = 150–170°) and in (B) the hyponychial nail bed angle is ABD is seen (normal = 178–192°).
Source: Modified from Regan GM, Tagg B, Thomson ML. Subjective assessment and objective measurement of finger clubbing. Lancet. 1967;1:530-2.

nail beaking. In nail beaking the nail is curved, the hyponychial angle is preserved and there is loss of pulp tissue.[45] Nail beaking is not associated with cardiac disease.[46]

Clubbing of the fingers is usually associated with pulmonary disease (80% of cases), with cardiac disease accounting for 10–15% of cases.[47] Cardiovascular associations include ***right-to-left shunts*** (e.g. tetralogy of Fallot and transposition of the great vessels), ***infective endocarditis***[47] (Figs. 11.5A and B) ***myxoma of left atrium***[48] and rarely an infected abdominal aortic graft.[49]

Unilateral finger clubbing is seen in aortic or sub-clavian aneurysm or rarely persistent ductus arteriosus with right-to-left shunting and an absent aortic arch.[50]

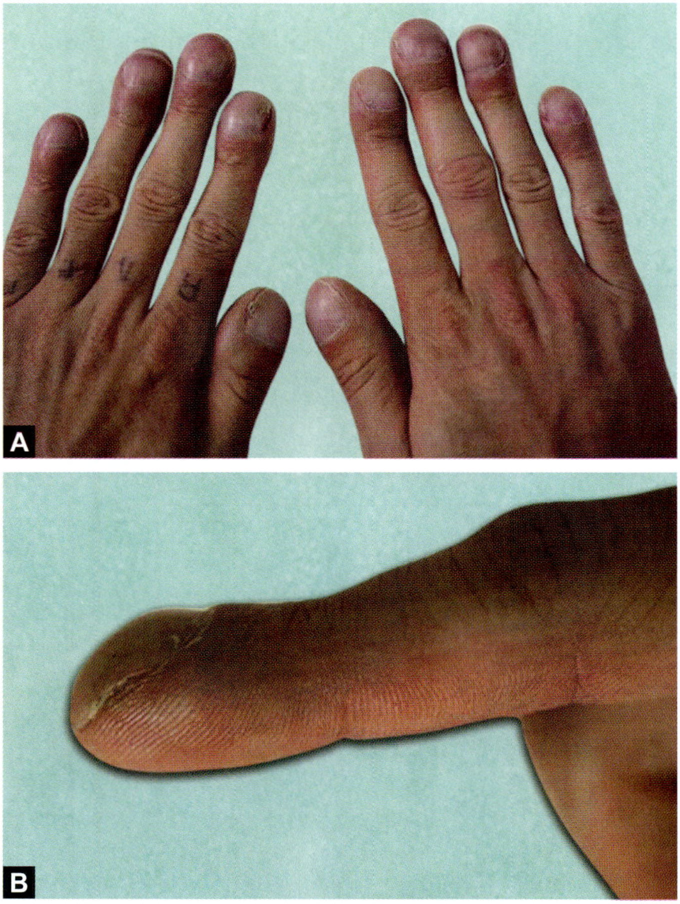

Figs. 11.5A and B: Tetralogy of Fallot: a 23-year-old man with polycythemia (hemoglobin 21 gm%) and advanced clubbing and cyanosis (hyponychial angle = 210°). The hands show sub-cuticular edema and bulbous fingertips. Right ventricular pressure was 135/1. Pulmonary artery pressure 13/5. There was a ventricular septal defect with a pulmonary/systemic blood flow ratio of 0.8.

Differential clubbing, in which clubbing is more prominent in the feet than in the hands, occurs in persistent ductus arteriosus when there is a right-to-left shunt or an infected abdominal aortic graft.[49]

VASCULAR DISEASES

Coronary Artery Disease (CAD)

Coronary artery may be suspected if any of the ***cardiac risk factors*** are present (hypertension, hyperlipidemia, smoking, diabetes, obesity) or in the presence of a diagonal ear crease sign, prior mediastinal radiation, progeria, polycythemia, Tangier's disease, or in a cocaine user.

Hypertension may be detected by a funduscopic examination. ***Hypertensive retinopathy*** is graded by ***the Keith-Wagner-Barker criteria:***[51]

Grade 1: There is generalized narrowing of the arterioles with the A/V ratio falling to one third from the normal value of two thirds.

Grade 2: There is further narrowing of the arterioles with focal areas of spasm.

Grade 3: The arteriolar walls thicken and take on a copper wire appearance. Hemorrhages and exudates appear.

Grade 4: The arterioles thicken further and appear like silver threads. There are pronounced AV nicking, hemorrhages and exudates and papilledema is now seen.

Hyperlipidemia may be suspected if there is arcus cornealis or xanthomas are seen. An arcus cornea is a gray yellow band up to 1.5 mm wide that may surround the rim of the cornea. It occurs with aging, but if seen before the age of 40 in the Caucasian may be a marker of CAD.[52]

Xanthomas are seen in hyperlipidemia as follows.

Hypercholesterolemia

Eyelid xanthomas (xanthelasma) are multiple soft elevated yellow plaques that usually occur near the inner canthi bilaterally. About 50% of patients will have normal lipid levels and the rest have an elevated serum cholesterol (Frederickson type II).[53]

Tendon xanthomas are yellow papular-nodular lesions found on the dorsum of the feet, the tendon Achilles or on the extensor tendons over the metacarpals (type II).[54]

Hypertriglyceridemia

Eruptive xanthoma are discrete yellow papular lesions surrounded by a red base and most commonly are found on the buttocks, back, elbow, and knees (Fig. 11.6). These lesions may be mistaken for acne. The lesions appear in crops and may coalesce to form plaques. Eruptive xanthomas usually appear

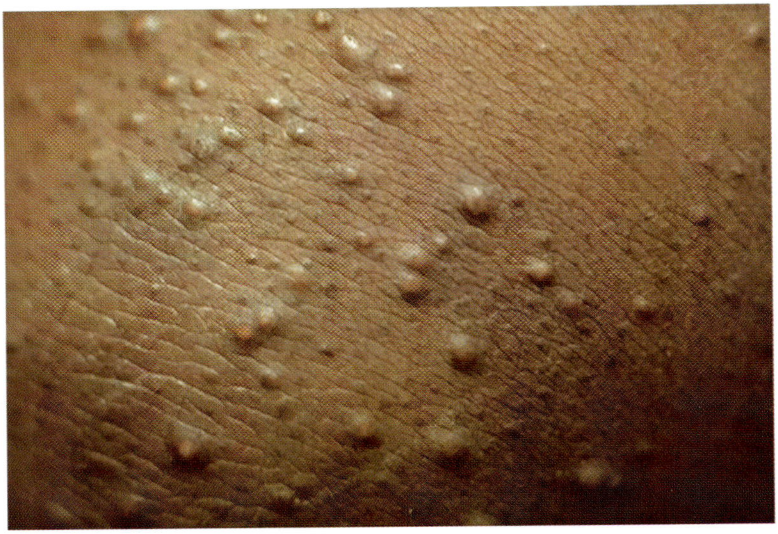

Fig. 11.6: Eruptive xanthoma: the skin lesions were seen over the back and chest and resemble acne. Serum triglyceride level was over 2,000 mg%.

when the plasma triglyceride exceeds 1,000 mg/dL.[55] Lipemia retinalis may be detected when the plasma triglycerides are over 3,000 mg/dL.[56] A milky white serum occurs when the plasma triglycerides are over 600 mg/dL.[57] Eruptive xanthoma may thus be seen in Frederickson types I, III and V.

Dysbetalipoproteinemia (Type III)

These patients have an elevated serum cholesterol and triglyceride levels and exhibit characteristic ***palmar xanthoma.*** Palmar xanthomas consist of yellow infiltrations of the palmar and digital creases of the hand.[58]

Tuberous xanthomas and eruptive xanthomas may also be seen in dysbetalipoproteinemia.[58]

Tuberous xanthomas are flat or elevated yellow nodules surrounded by a red margin seen mainly on the knees or elbows.

Patients who are smokers may exhibit tobacco stained fingers, a tobacco odor to the clothing or their medicine bag along with cigarette burns to their clothing. Excessive and pre-mature wrinkling (especially "crow's feet" around the eyes) is seen in heavy smokers, but can also be seen in non-smokers chronically exposed to sunlight.[59]

Central obesity with a waist measurement exceeding 35 inches in a woman and 40 inches in a man represents another easily recognizable coronary risk factor.[60]

Diabetes may be suspected by detecting vascular changes on funduscopic examination and the presence of small vessel disease in the feet.

The ***diagonal ear crease sign*** is said to be a marker for coronary artery disease, but its utility is controversial.[61] If seen in patients <40 years of age, I believe other coronary artery risk factors should be sought after.

Patients who have received extensive ***radiation therapy*** to the mediastinum may show atrophy of the paravertebral muscles of the back as well as chronic radiation dermatitis. Such patients have a higher incidence of coronary artery stenosis.[62]

Progeria is characterized by pre-mature aging, best seen by examining the face. The skin is thin and translucent and lacks wrinkles. There is also alopecia and dwarfism. These patients usually die before the age of 15 of a myocardial infarction.[63]

Patients with primary polycythemia have a higher incidence of coronary artery disease.[9]

Tangier disease (hypoalphalipoproteinemia) is a very rare condition characterized by a very low HDL (high-density lipoprotein) cholesterol and low total cholesterol blood levels.[64] Cholesterol esters are deposited on the tonsils producing a characteristic orange tiger striped appearance. These patients have pre-mature coronary artery disease[65,66] and peripheral neuropathy.[67]

Cocaine use may be suspected if there is perforation of the nasal septum[68] speckled enamel loss on the buccal surfaces of the teeth[69] skin popping or venous track sites. Cocaine use is associated with ***myocardial ischemia or necrosis, hypertension or endocarditis.***[70]

Pseudoxanthoma elasticum (PXE) is characterized by a network of closely grouped yellow papules (plucked chicken skin appearance). The skin is lax and hangs in folds. Pseudoxanthoma elasticum occurs in the neck, axilla, abdomen, and thighs.[71] There may be associated angioid streaks and retinal hemorrhages. Pseudoxanthoma elasticum is associated with *mitral valve prolapse, hypertension, peripheral vascular disease, and pre-mature coronary artery disease,*[72] the latter being a common cause of early death.[72]

Scars of a median sternotomy, radial artery, or saphenous vein harvesting sites, point to prior coronary artery bypass surgery.

Unilateral Internal Carotid Artery Disease

Internal carotid artery disease may be suspected if the external carotid or unilateral arcus signs are present along with a Hollenhorst plaque seen on fundoscopy. Patients with internal carotid artery stenosis have an increase in blood flow in the ipsilateral external carotid artery, so that its superficial temporal artery branch is more prominent than on the non-obstructed side (Olivarius's external carotid sign).[73] This is a useful sign especially if combined with greater prominence of the ipsilateral brow arterial pulse.[73]

Unilateral arcus is very rare and suggests internal carotid artery stenosis on the non-arcus side,[74] provided that ocular hypotony has been excluded.[75]

A ***Hollenhorst plaque*** is a cholesterol-laden crystal that embolizes to a retinal arteriole usually from an ipsilateral atherosclerotic internal carotid artery or less often from the aorta or cardiac valves.[75] These emboli are pale yellow and refractile.

Temporal Arteritis

This occurs in patients over the age of 50 and is characterized by scalp tenderness in the temporal area followed occasionally by scalp necrosis. The superficial temporal artery is tender, pulseless, and feels ropy. There may be lingual gangrene and jaw claudication. Polymyalgia rheumatica may coexist. Blindness may occur in <5 months after the onset of symptoms.[75a]

Cholesterol Emboli to the Lower Extremities

These emboli originate from an atherosclerotic descending aorta in which plaques may break off from the aorta either spontaneously, following surgical manipulation of the aorta[76] or angiography, or associated with the use of anticoagulants,[77] or fibrinolytic agents.[78] Cholesterol emboli may present as either livedo reticularis, gangrene or the purple toe syndrome. Livedo reticularis is a red pruritic macular eruption resembling the imprint of fine wire mesh on the skin of the legs and especially of the feet. The foot pulses are usually present, but often diminished.[79] The purple toe syndrome is characterized by multiple bluish red toes and palpable arterial pulses.[76,79]

Buerger's Disease (Thromboangiitis Obliterans)

Buerger's disease is a non-atherosclerotic inflammatory obliterative disease characterized by thrombotic occlusion of the small- and median-sized vessels of the lower extremities, and less commonly the upper extremities. Gangrene of one or more digits may occur. Buerger's disease has usually been regarded as occurring mostly in males <40 years of age who are heavy smokers. Recent studies[80] show that Buerger's disease is now more common in the 40–60 age group and that the male/female ratio has dropped from 9/1 to 3/1. Thirty percent of patients have an associated superficial thrombophlebitis.[80]

Raynaud's Phenomenon

Patients with Raynaud's phenomenon have reversible digital artery spasm precipitated by cold or emotional stress. The digits become pallid, then blue, and on rewarming, or relief of the emotional stress become hyperemic. It is most commonly associated with collagen vascular disease (scleroderma or disseminated lupus erythematosus), but may also be associated with Buerger's disease, primary pulmonary hypertension or thoracic outlet syndromes.[81]

Patients with scleroderma and Raynaud's phenomenon may show digital ischemia, fingertip necrosis (rat bite lesions) and even autoamputation.[82]

Superior Vena Caval Syndrome

Obstruction of the superior vena cava may be caused by encroachment of the superior vena cava by an intrathoracic tumor,[83] an aortic aneurysm[84] or thrombosis associated with a transvenous pacemaker.[85] Patients may have a ruddy complexion aggravated by recumbency, bluish red discoloration of the upper chest and neck, edema of the head and neck and upper extremities, neck vein distention, venous stars and collateral veins on the anterior chest wall. The extent and location of these collateral veins depend on how rapidly the obstruction occurs and whether the obstruction of the superior vena occurs above at or below the azygos vein.[83]

Sub-clavian Vein Thrombosis

Sub-clavian vein thrombosis gives rise to a swollen arm, distended veins in the arms and cyanosis. As the arm may be painful to move, eliciting Palmerton's sign (suffusion of face with arms held above the head)[86] is, I believe, impractical.

Inferior Vena Caval Syndrome

Obstruction of the inferior vena cava may be due to a malignancy or an underlying thrombophlebitis or thrombosis.[87] Distended venous collaterals are seen on the lateral aspect of the abdominal wall. There may be bilateral leg edema. Coexistent ascites points to an inferior vena caval obstruction superior to the renal veins.[87]

VALVULAR HEART DISEASE

Only the more advanced forms of valvular heart disease may be visually detected.

Tricuspid Regurgitation

Tricuspid regurgitation may be suspected on observation if there are ear lobe pulsations, a ***prominent v wave*** in the jugular venous pulse, as well as hepatic pulsations.

Mitral Stenosis

Caucasian patients with mitral stenosis may have venous telangiectasia of the cheeks ***(malar flush)*** because of a low output state and an elevated pulmonary vascular resistance[88] (Fig. 11.7).

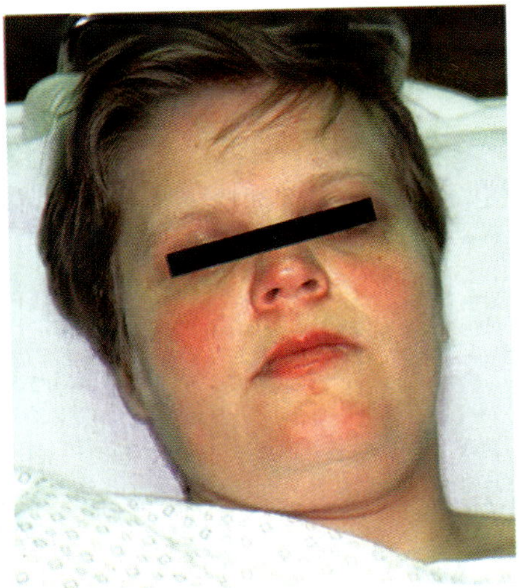

Fig. 11.7: Mitral facies. A 35-year-old Polish female P1 G6 Ab4 showing a malar flush. She had mitral stenosis and mitral regurgitation.

Aortic Regurgitation

A patient may be suspected of having aortic regurgitation if he presents with dyspnea, a head that shakes with each arterial pulsation ***(De Musset's sign)*** and prominent arterial pulsations in the neck.

ENDOCRINE AND METABOLIC DISEASES

A careful examination of the face will detect patients with acromegaly, thyroid disease, Cushing's disease, amyloidosis, gout and ochronosis.

Acromegaly

Acromegaly is detected by looking at the head and the hands. These patients have a lantern jaw, coarsening of the facial features (best determined by comparing old photographs), widely spaced teeth, macroglossia, and spade shaped hands (Figs. 11.8A and B). Acromegaly is associated with hypertension of the low renin type.[89] There is an increased incidence of pre-mature coronary atherosclerosis in acromegaly because of coexistent diabetes and hypertension.

Hyperthyroidism

Patients with hyperthyroidism often are detected by looking at the face. There may be ***lid lag, exophthalmos, ophthalmoplegia*** and ***temporal muscle wasting.*** Other features include palmar erythema, warm moist palms, fine tremor of the outstretched hands, proximal myopathy, pretibial myxedema

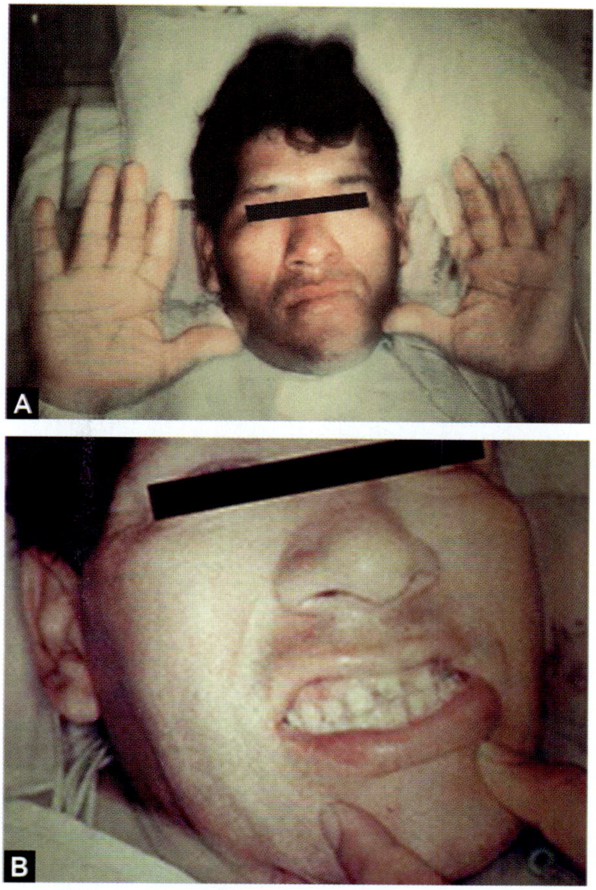

Figs. 11.8A and B: Acromegaly. A 40-year-old man admitted to the hospital with an acute anterior wall myocardial infarction. He had a lantern jaw, coarse facial features, spade like hands and widely spaced teeth.

and an enlarged thyroid (Fig. 11.9). The patient may appear restless and show evidence of weight loss by her loose fitting clothes. Hyperthyroidism may be associated with a ***high output failure, atrial fibrillation or a cardiomyopathy.***[90] Some elderly patients with hyperthyroidism may not have the above eye or skin changes, but present with heart failure or atrial fibrillation ***(apathetic hyperthyroidism).***

Myxedema

Periorbital puffiness, *brittle hair, dry skin, slowing of cerebration, low husky voice macroglossia, and delayed relaxation of heel reflexes* are the main clinical features of myxedema (Fig. 11.10). Thyroid replacement therapy may lead to a striking improvement of the facies. Myxedema is associated with ***pericardial effusion,*** which rarely leads to cardiac tamponade.[91]

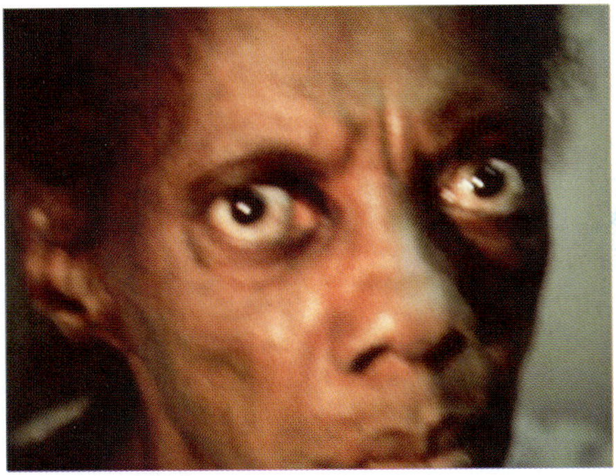

Fig. 11.9: Hyperthyroidism. A 60-year-old female with lid retraction, exophthalmos and facial muscle wasting.

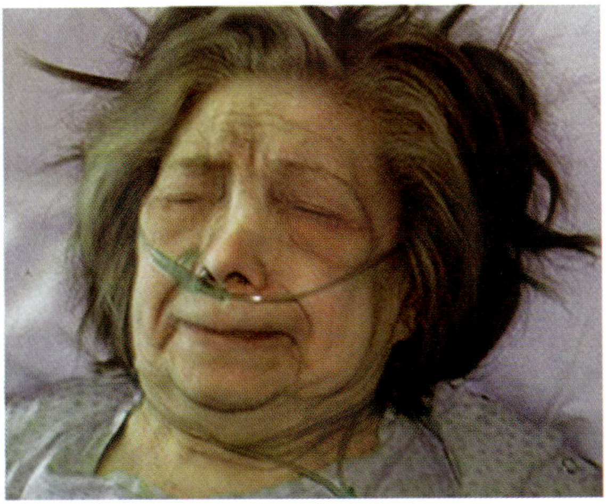

Fig. 11.10: Myxedema. A 80-year-old female admitted in heart failure. She had stopped taking her thyroid medicine a year ago. She has a pasty face, some periorbital puffiness, dry skin and coarse hair. Thyroid stimulating hormone level was 100 lu/mL.

Cushing's Disease

The moon facies, buffalo hump, truncal obesity with thin limbs, and red abdominal striae are the usual features of Cushing's disease. It is associated with ***hypertension*** in 80% of cases.[92]

Amyloidosis

Primary or hereditofamilial amyloidosis may involve the deposition of an amyloid protein consisting of light chain immunoglobulins in the heart, skin

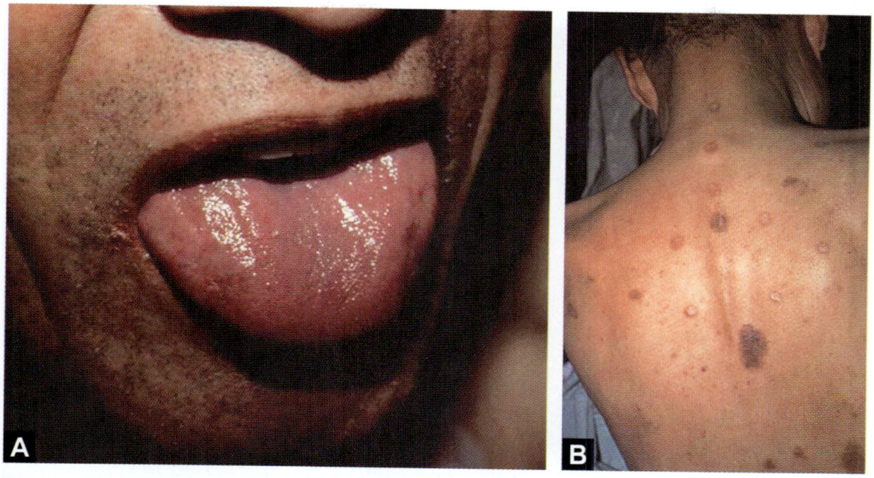

Figs. 11.11A and B: Amyloidosis. A 60-year-old man with large tongue, brown maculopapular lesions on the back. He was admitted in heart failure due to a restrictive cardiomyopathy. Echocardiography showed biventricular hypertrophy and a sparkling appearance to the myocardium. He had biopsy proven amyloidosis.

or tongue.[93] Patients with amyloidosis may have waxy yellow translucent papules and plaques on the eyelids, nasolabial folds, and mouth.[94] Purpura frequently occurs in these areas after minor trauma.[94] The tongue may be diffusely or irregularly enlarged.[94] ***Restrictive cardiomyopathy*** is often seen in amyloidosis[93,94] (Figs. 11.11A and B).

Hemochromatosis

See under skin color, page 442.

Gout

The patient may have gouty tophi (urate deposits) on the ears or the small joints of the hand. Rarely urate deposits may involve the heart valves or the conducting system causing complete heart block.[95] Patients with gout via its association with elevated serum uric acid levels have a higher incidence of ***hypertension***[96] and possibly ***coronary artery disease.***[97]

Alkaptonuria (Ochronosis)

Alkaptonuria is a defect in tyrosine metabolism in which homogentisic acid is deposited in the skin, joints, ear and the mitral and aortic valves. The skin on the ears gradually darkens and the fingernails show a blue-gray discoloration. ***Aortic stenosis*** is the most significant lesion associated with it.[98]

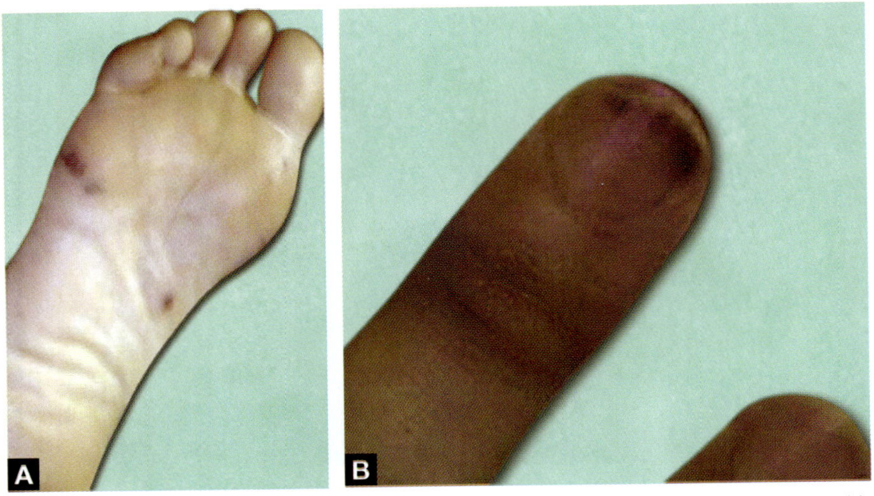

Figs. 11.12A and B: Infective endocarditis. A 50-year-old drug addict admitted with fever and mitral regurgitation. She had sub-ungal hemorrhages and Janeway lesions on the soles of her feet. There was vegetation on the mitral valve.

INFLAMMATORY DISEASES

Inflammation may be caused by chemical or physical agents or infections. Under the heading of inflammatory diseases infective endocarditis, syphilis and sarcoidosis will be discussed.

Infective Endocarditis (IE)

Patients with infective endocarditis may or not have evidence of recreational drug use (e.g. skin popping, venous tracks). Systemic manifestations of infective endocarditis are said to be less frequent now, but are still quite common in the poorer patients who are often late in coming to get medical attention. The fundi may show flame-shaped hemorrhages and ***Roth spots*** (i.e. micro-infarct of the retina). The hand may reveal ***Osler nodes*** (red sub-cutaneous nodules 2 mm in size on the tips of the fingers, thenar or hypothenar areas that disappear after a few days).[99] ***Splinter*** nail bed ***hemorrhages*** may also be seen, but can also occur with local trauma, vasculitis or systemic embolism.[20] ***Janeway lesions*** are painless red macules or nodules seen on the palms or soles of the feet[100] (Figs. 11.12A and B). Clubbing may occur in late cases of I.E.[99] Petechial hemorrhages are seen in the conjunctiva, palate, buccal mucosa and extremities.[17]

Syphilis

Patients with tertiary syphilis may have a saddle-shaped nose, optic atrophy, Argyll Robertson pupil and evidence of ***aortic regurgitation.***

Sarcoidosis

Patients with sarcoidosis may have skin and cardiac involvement. The skin lesions that involve the face may take two forms: red papules around the eyes, nose and mouth that are pruritic and do not ulcerate; purple plaques that produce a bulbous nose, thickened cheeks and thickened ears (lupus pernio).[101] There may also be erythema nodosum (red nodules on the legs).[101] Twenty percent of patients with sarcoidosis have cardiovascular findings at autopsy.[102,103] Clinical manifestations include *congestive heart failure, ventricular tachycardia, complete heart block or cor pulmonale.*[102,103]

DISEASES OF CONNECTIVE TISSUE AND JOINTS

In this section, *inherited disorders* of connective tissue *(Ehlers-Danlos syndrome, osteogenesis imperfecta, Marfan's syndrome, pseudoxanthoma elasticum)* and *immune-mediated diseases* of connective tissue *(systemic lupus erythematosus, scleroderma, polyarteritis nodosa, rheumatic fever, ankylosing spondylitis and Reiter's syndrome)* are discussed.

Ehlers–Danlos Syndrome

Usually the Ehlers-Danlos syndrome is characterized by excessive mobility of joints and a thin stretchable skin. However in type 4 Ehlers-Danlos syndrome, these findings are attenuated and patients have bruises and pigmented scars over the bony prominences. Patients with type 4 Ehlers-Danlos syndrome may have an *aortic aneurysm and rupture as well as mitral valve prolapse.*[103a]

Osteogenesis Imperfecta

Patients with osteogenesis imperfecta have a decrease in bone mass and thus a tendency to have multiple bone fractures on minor trauma. Blue sclera and kyphoscoliosis are seen along with ***aortic and mitral regurgitations***.

Marfan's syndrome: *See* previous section page 440-441.

Pseudoxanthoma elasticum: *See* previous section page 451.

Systemic Lupus Erythematosus

The diagnosis of systemic lupus erythematosus (SLE) may often be made by inspection of the face and the hands. In the Caucasian 10–61% (average 45%) of patients with SLE will have a characteristic malar butterfly skin lesion consisting of a red confluent maculopapular eruption with fine scaling involving the nose and cheeks.[104] However, in Black patients with SLE there is depigmentation in the malar area (Figs. 11.13A and B). The dorsum of the hands may show red plaques or confluent red papules that spare the skin

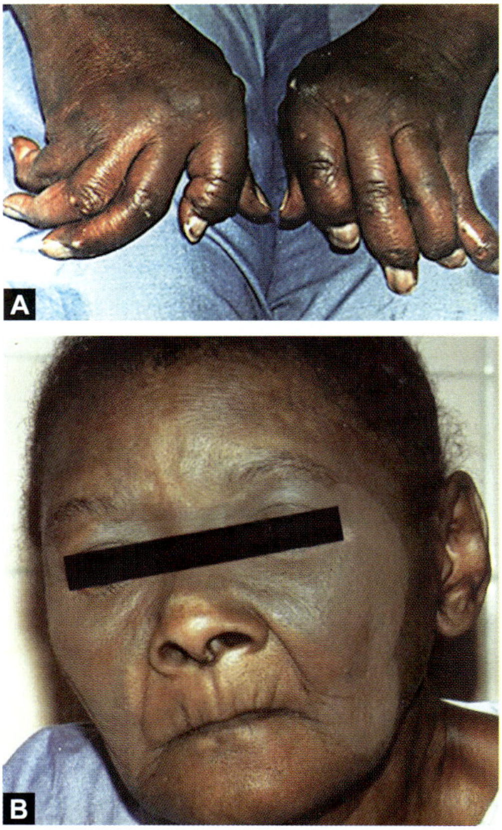

Figs. 11.13A and B: Mixed connective tissue diseases (lupus, rheumatoid arthritis, scleroderma). The patient had a mask facies with puckering of skin around lips, malar depigmentation in Figure B. In Figure A, the patient's hand showed ulnar deviation of the MP joints as well as a taut shiny skin.

creases of the joints.[105] As vasculitis is a feature of SLE, leg ulcers or livedo reticularis may be seen. Raynaud's phenomenon occurs in 27% of cases of SLE.[104]

Systemic lupus erythematosus is associated with clinically evident ***pericarditis*** in 25% of cases, ***hypertension*** in 16%, ***cardiomyopathy*** in 10%, symptomatic ***coronary arteriosclerosis*** in 10%, ***pulmonary hypertension*** in 5% and rarely aortic or mitral regurgitation or complete AV block.[106-108]

Scleroderma

Patients with scleroderma may initially develop Raynaud's phenomenon and then skin changes involving the face and hands. Facial edema occurs followed by the development of smooth, shiny taut skin, resulting in a loss of facial wrinkling, puckering of the skin around the mouth and difficulty in opening the mouth wide.

The dorsum of the hands may also show skin tightening and the development of flexion contractures of the IP joints (claw hand). Focal areas of skin necrosis may be seen on the finger tips ("rat bite" necrosis).[82] Loss of one or more of the distal phalanges may ensue. Telangiectasias are frequently seen in the skin of the face and the limbs.[109] Patients with scleroderma commonly have ***pulmonary hypertension*** and may have symptomatic ***pericarditis*** in 15% of case[110] and depressed left ventricular function in <5% of cases.[111]

Dermatomyositis

Patients with dermatomyositis develop a dusky heliotrope eruption in the periorbital areas and may have facial fold erythema.[112] Violaceous papules are seen over the knuckles (Gottron's papules), which are virtually pathognomonic of dermatomyositis.[113] Raynaud's phenomenon and proximal muscle weakness also occur.

Patients with dermatomyositis may develop ***myocarditis*** leading to congestive heart failure. Pericarditis and heart block rarely occur.[114]

Polyarteritis Nodosa

Polyarteritis nodosa is a necrotizing arteritis involving the small- and medium-sized arteries of the body. Visual findings are somewhat limited as skin lesions are only seen in 15% of cases.[115] There may be sub-cutaneous red nodules following the course of a leg artery, which may ulcerate and become necrotic. Livedo reticularis may be seen over the thighs. There is often ***hypertension*** and ***congestive heart failure*** and although ***coronary arteritis*** occurs in 50% of cases, myocardial infarction is uncommon.[116]

Rheumatic Fever

Rheumatic fever remains quite common in the developing countries. Boyd described rheumatic fever as a disease that licks the joints and bites the heart. The visible manifestations of rheumatic fever are erythema marginatum, sub-cutaneous nodules and Jaccoud's syndrome. Erythema marginatum is a pink circular eruption with a pale center and raised red margins that is usually seen on the trunk, limbs or axillae. It often precedes carditis and joint involvement. Erythema marginatum may occur in 10–25% of cases of rheumatic fever.[117] Sub-cutaneous nodules are uncommon now. They occur around the elbow, the knuckles and spinous processes and usually signify cardiac involvement.[118] Jaccoud's syndrome is a rare rheumatoid arthritis like deformity of the hand following one or more attacks of rheumatic fever.[119] Patients with rheumatic fever may develop a pancarditis in the acute stage consisting of (a) valvulitis (mitral regurgitation or occasionally aortic regurgitation), (b) myocarditis and rarely heart block and (c) pericarditis. Subsequently, mitral stenosis occurs in the established case of rheumatic heart disease.

Ankylosing Spondylitis

Patients with ankylosing spondylitis have limited mobility of the spine (Schober test),[120] which eventually becomes rigid (bamboo spine). The mobility of the sacroiliac joint is reduced and chest expansion limited. ***Aortic regurgitation*** is seen in 3% of cases of long-standing ankylosing spondylitis.[120] Complete heart block is very rarely seen.[120]

Reiter's Syndrome

The diagnosis of Reiter's syndrome (conjunctivitis, arthritis and urethritis) may also be considered in the presence of keratoderma blennorrhagica, the latter occurring in 60% of cases of Reiter's syndrome.[121] Keratoderma blennorrhagica occurs on the soles of the feet or the palms of the hand mostly in Caucasian males. The skin lesions consist of red macules that become hyperkeratotic waxy papules with a central zone of yellow surrounded by a red halo. The papules coalesce to form plaques with subsequent crusting. ***Aortic regurgitation*** may occur in 60% of cases of Reiter's syndrome.[121] Complete heart block occurs rarely.[121]

PHARMACOLOGICAL DRUGS

Nifedipine

The side effects of nifedipine include postural hypotension, pedal edema and gum hyperplasia. Pedal edema may occur with higher doses (over 60 mg/day) in 5–10% of cases.[122] Gum hyperplasia may occur in 38% of patients who have been on nifedipine for 3 months or more.[123] Patients with poor dental hygiene are more liable to have ***gum hyperplasia.*** Dilantin and cyclosporine are other drugs that may give rise to gum hyperplasia.[124]

Angiotensin Converting Enzyme Inhibitors

These drugs produce rapid swelling of the face, tongue and larynx (angioedema) in 0.2% of cases. It is more common in black patients and may be fatal.[125,126]

Anticoagulants (Heparin and Coumadin)

Heparin-induced skin necrosis may be seen in the arms and is attributed to hypersensitivity angiitis.[127] Bleeding into the skin or mucous linings is readily detected if the heparin dose is excessive, or in the rare instance of heparin-induced thrombocytopenia[128] (Fig. 11.14).

Coumadin may also rarely (0.01%) produce extensive purpuric areas of skin in necrosis involving the breasts, thighs and extremities.[129] It is common in middle-aged obese females.[129]

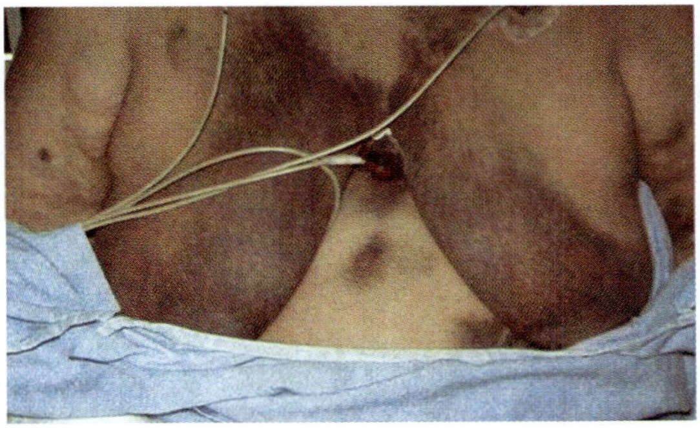

Fig. 11.14: Heparin-induced thrombocytopenia. A 80-year-old female who developed an extensive area of ecchymosis over the anterior chest wall and severe thrombocytopenia. Four days previously she had received DC shock for ventricular tachycardia as well as heparin for an acute myocardial infarction. She had received heparin for a DVT in the past without any ill effects.

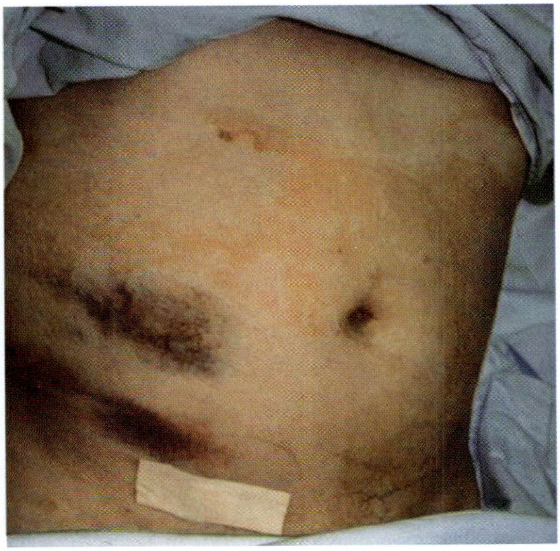

Fig. 11.15: Gray-Turner's sign. A 60-year-old female with retroperitoneal bleeding following the use of heparin. Extensive ecchymoses seen in the right flank.

Anticoagulants may also give rise to retroperitoneal bleeding and can be detected by seeing bruising of the flanks (Gray-Turner's sign) (Fig. 11.15) or around the umbilicus (Cullen's sign)[130] (Fig. 11.16). Swelling of the tongue due to bleeding may also be occasionally seen if a patient is over anticoagulated.

Amiodarone

Patients on long-term high-dose amiodarone, i.e. 600 mg/day for 2 years, may develop a blue-gray dermal melanosis of the face especially of the areas exposed to the sun.[131] It may take several months for the skin discoloration

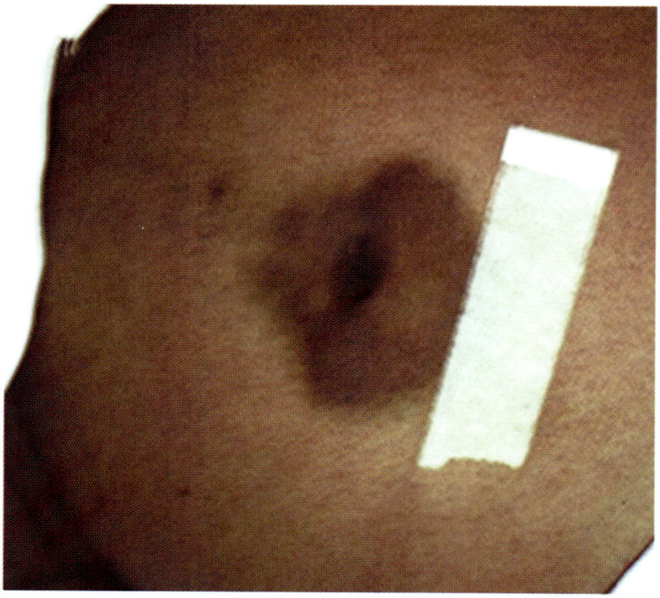

Fig. 11.16: Cullen's sign. This patient came into the hospital with retroperitoneal bleeding due to coumadin overdose. Ecchymosis is seen around the umbilicus. Prothrombin time was 110 seconds.

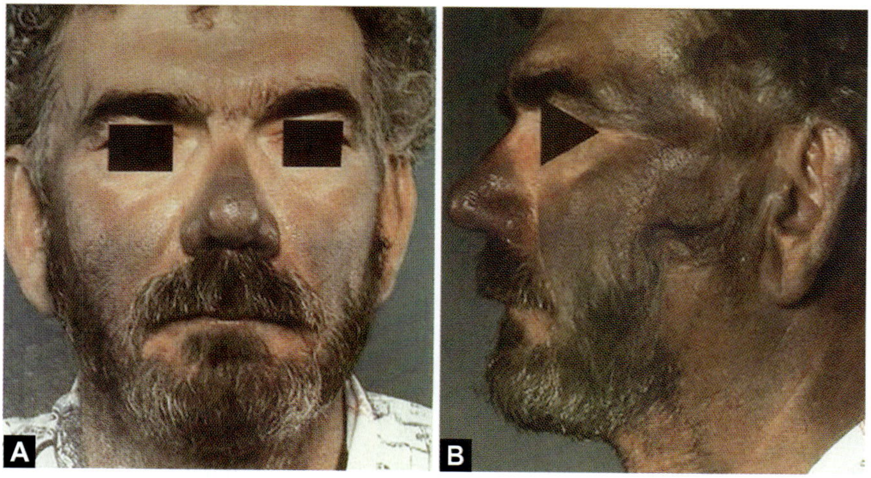

Figs. 11.17A and B: Amiodarone skin toxicity. There is a blue-gray dermal melanosis of the face, which partially improved in 9 months after amiodarone was stopped.
Source: Blackshear JL, Randle HW. Reversibility of blue-gray cutaneous discoloration from amiodarone. Mayo Clin Proc. 1991;66:721-6.

to resolve after stopping the drug, owing to its long half life[132,133] (Figs. 11.17A and B). A lupus like syndrome has also been reported with amiodarone.[134] Hyperthyroidism, hypothyroidism, liver dysfunction and pulmonary fibrosis are other side effects of amiodarone.[131]

Procaine Amide

A lupus like syndrome may occur with the use of procaine amide, but the butterfly rash is rarely seen.[135] Pericarditis may also occasionally be seen.[136]

Hydralazine

This drug may also produce a lupus like syndrome and rarely a pericarditis.[136] A malar butterfly rash is more often seen than in procaine amide induced lupus.[136]

Alpha Methyl Dopa

This drug may produce a lupus like syndrome but without the malar butterfly rash.[135]

Digitalis, Spironolactone, Estrogens

Gynecomastia is seen occasionally with these drugs.

Recreational Drugs

Venous tracks or skin popping sites (Figs. 11.18A and B) are some of the suggestive findings in a drug abuser. Additional findings in a cocaine abuser are described elsewhere[68] including its association with coronary artery disease and hypertension.[70] Venous tracks may be seen in drug users who repeatedly inject heroin intravenously. They are usually found in the forearm or less commonly the neck. Heroin addicts are at risk for infective endocarditis.

Skin popping sites are rounded scars 1–3 cm in diameter, seen on the legs and arms of drug abusers who inject heroin or cocaine sub-cutaneously. Extensive cellulitis and scarring on the thighs occur with deep and repeated sub-cutaneous drug injections (Fig. 11.18C).

MUSCULOSKELETAL DISEASES

Muscular Dystrophies

Myotonic dystrophy is the commonest of the muscular dystrophies. This autosomal dominant disease shows characteristic facial features (a thin narrow face with drooping eyelids, frontal baldness) and muscle weakness of the neck, hands and extremities. The patient has a high steppage gait and difficulty in grasp relaxation (myotonia). Fifty percent of such patients have a cardiomyopathy[137] and occasionally complete heart block.[138]

Duchenne dystrophy is a sex-linked recessive entity seen in boys characterized by proximal muscle weakness, waddling gait and pseudohypertrophy of the calf muscles. Cardiomyopathy or atrial arrhythmias are often present.[138]

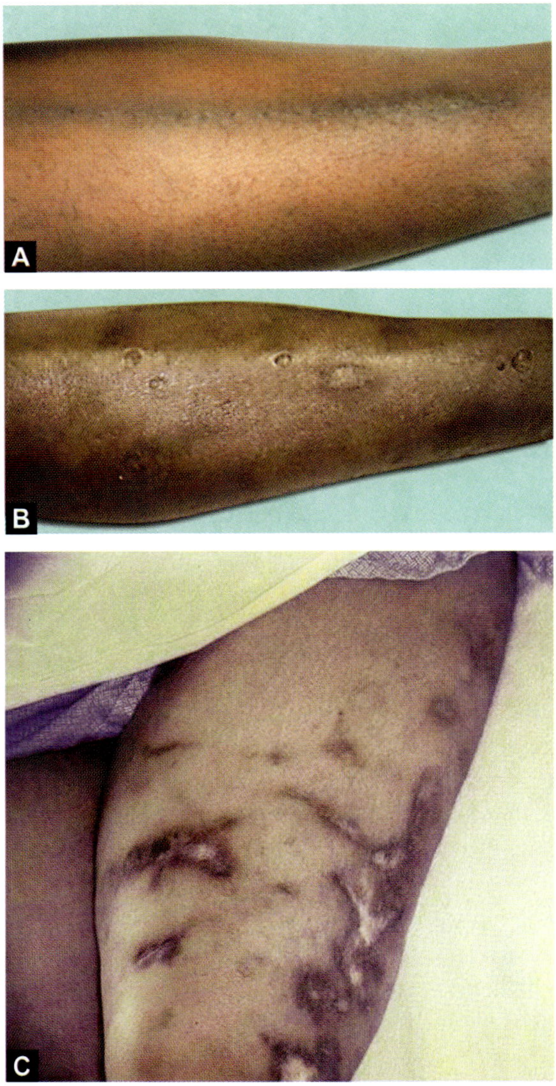

Figs. 11.18A to C: Signs of drug addiction. (A) venous tracks in arm. (B) skin-popping sites in leg. (C) extensive cellulitis and scarring of thigh due to extensive sub-cutaneous injections of heroin.

The ***Kearns–Sayre syndrome*** is characterized by ophthalmoplegia, short stature, retinitis pigmentosa and is associated with complete heart block and cardiomyopathy.[34]

Friedreich's Ataxia

Patients with Friedreich's ataxia are characterized by pes cavus, nystagmus and sensory ataxia. A cardiomyopathy is seen in over 50% of cases.[138]

Osteogenesis Imperfecta

In this autosomal dominant entity, patients have multiple bone fractures, bowing of the long bones, kyphoscoliosis, pectus excavatum and blue sclera (due to loss of scleral collagen). Aortic or mitral regurgitation may be found in patients with osteogenesis imperfecta.[139,140]

Thoracic Cage Deformities

Thoracic cage deformities may provide a clue to the presence of underlying cardiovascular diseases. A patient with ***the straight back syndrome*** (transverse diameter/anteroposterior ratio >3: and loss of normal kyphosis) may have an innocent pulmonary flow murmur, which may be confused with pulmonic stenosis or an atrial septal defect.[141]

A ***shield chest*** is a broad chest with widely spaced nipples and an increased angle between manubrium and the body of the sternum. It is seen in Turner's syndrome (coarctation of aorta)[3] and LEOPARD syndrome (pulmonic stenosis).[30]

Pectus carinatum (pigeon chest) is associated with Marfan's syndrome (aortic regurgitation, dissecting aneurysm).[2]

Pectus excavatum is seen in Marfan's syndrome,[2] Noonan's syndrome (pulmonary stenosis),[32] homocystinuria (coronary artery disease), Ehlers–Danlos syndrome (aortic dissection, spontaneous aortic rupture and mitral valve prolapse)[34] and gargoylism (mitral valve disease, ischemic heart disease, cardiomyopathy)[34] and osteogenesis imperfecta (aortic and mitral regurgitation).[139]

A ***bamboo spine*** is seen in ankylosing spondylitis (aortic regurgitation).[120]

Kyphoscoliosis occurs in Friedreich's ataxia (cardiomyopathy),[138] Gargoylism,[34] neurofibromatosis (hypertension, outflow tract obstruction)[15] and osteogenesis imperfecta.[139]

A ***barrel shaped chest*** (transverse/AP diameter ratio of 1) is an unreliable sign of chronic obstructive lung disease, as it can also be found in the elderly patients without chronic obstructive lung disease.[142]

Paget's Disease of Bone

Patients with Paget's disease may have a progressive increase in hat size (due to a thickening skull), a decline in height (due to kyphoscoliosis) as well as sabre shins.[143] Aortic stenosis[144] and left ventricular systolic dysfunction[145] occur in moderately severe Paget's disease of bone, whereas high output failure occurs in patients with more extensive osseous involvement.[145]

TUMORS

Atrial myxomas may be considered in the differential diagnosis of ***clubbing.***[48] The ***LAMB syndrome*** comprises 7% of all atrial myxomas and consists of

Lentiginous macules of the face or "freckling," **A**trial myxoma, **M**ucocutaneous myxomas of the breast and skin, and **B**lue nevi.[146,147] Rhabdomyomas are seen in tuberous sclerosis in 66% of cases.[22] Neurofibromas of the heart are seen in neurofibromatosis (von Recklinghausen's disease).[16]

SYNOPSIS

Step 1: Detection of the Physical Signs

General Observations

Is the patient excessively tall or short? Body build should be noted. Is the patient alert or somnolent? Are there any abnormalities in the gait? Note the clothing for evidence of weight change or tobacco use.

Head

Are there any facial features to suggest a collagen or endocrine disorder such as butterfly eruption or exophthalmos, respectively? A mask like face may suggest Parkinsonism, scleroderma or myotonia dystrophica, whereas a vacant expression suggests Down's syndrome.

Are the eyes widely spaced apart (hypertelorism)? Do the conjunctiva appear pale or brick red? Are there any xanthelasma, waxy eyelid plaques, or drooping eyelids? Is the sclera discolored (e.g. blue or yellow)? Is there an Argyll Robertson pupil or sub-luxation of the lens? Is there an arcus cornealis (unilateral or bilateral)? Fundi should be checked for hypertension, diabetes, dyslipidemias or embolic changes due to carotid artery disease or infective endocarditis.

Is there unilateral temporal artery prominence to suggest ipsilateral carotid disease or temporal arteritis? Skin findings such as malar flush, angiofibromata, slate gray pigmentation due to amiodarone, lupus pernio, facial edema, or pre-mature aging should be noted.

The mouth should be inspected for dental hygiene or enamel erosions, gum hyperplasia, widely spaced teeth, macroglossia, tongue angiomata or sub-lingual cyanosis. Are there any tonsillar lesions to suggest Tangier disease? Are there any petechiae on the hard palate? Is the nose saddle shaped? Do the ears show evidence of gout, ***alkaptonuria*** or a diagonal crease sign?

Neck

Is there any webbing of the neck? Is the thyroid enlarged? Are there any surgical scars to suggest carotid or thyroid operations? Is there unilateral or bilateral jugular venous distention? Plucked chicken skin appearance of the neck?

Chest

Are there any deformities of the thoracic cage such as kyphoscoliosis, straight back syndrome, pectus excavatum, shield chest, or bamboo spine? Are there any surgical scars (thoracotomy, pacemaker, IV access site, or vascular surgery)? Are the ribs or sternum still intact? Are there any venous collaterals on the chest wall to suggest superior vena cava (SVC) syndrome? Is there gynecomastia?

Upper Extremity

The hand should be examined for:
1. Size and shape: Acromegaly (spade like), Marfan's syndrome (arachnodactyly), rheumatoid arthritis with an ulnar drift, Ehlers-Danlos syndrome with hyper extensible joints, Holt-Oram syndrome with fingerized thumb. Absent digits or deformed digits are also noted. Is there clubbing?
2. Edema: superior vena cava syndrome, thoracic outlet syndrome.
3. Neuromuscular disease: Myotonia dystrophica, fine tremor of hyperthyroidism.
4. Color change: Nicotine staining, cyanosis of nail beds, Raynaud's phenomenon, Osler's nodes, Janeway lesions, tissue necrosis associated with vasculitis.
5. Nail abnormalities: Splinter hemorrhages, Terry nails, red lunula, onycholysis, sub-ungal fibromas.
6. Palmar changes: Palmar erythema, simian crease, and yellow palmar creases.
7. Temperature change: Warm hands (e.g. hyperthyroidism) cold hands (e.g. vasculitis and arterial occlusion).
8. Any xanthomas (elbows, hands): Any surgical scars [brachial artery cut down, radial artery harvesting site for coronary artery bypass graft (CABG)]? Any venous tracks from IV drug abuse?

Abdomen

Is there ascites or central obesity? Is the liver enlarged, tender or pulsating? Are there prominent venous collaterals due to inferior vena cava (IVC) obstruction? Any signs of red abdominal striae of Cushing's disease; flank or periumbilical ecchymoses?

Back

Deformities such as kyphoscoliosis or bamboo spine are noted. The skin lesions of neurofibromatosis or eruptive xanthoma are often seen here. Any radiation dermatitis associated with paravertebral muscle atrophy noted?

Lower Extremities

Skin lesions of erythema marginatum (thighs), erythema nodosum (legs), keratoderma, blennorrhagica, or Janeway lesions (soles of feet) are noted. Are skin-popping sites (legs, thighs) seen?

Is there leg swelling (unilateral or bilateral)? Does the swelling pit or is it firm? Note evidence of pseudohypertrophy of calf muscles and Sabre shins. Xanthomas of the nodular or tendinous type should be noted. Check for evidence of vascular insufficiency and gangrene of toes.

Step 2: Correlation of the Physical Signs with a Cardiovascular Entity

Congenital Heart Disease

Holt-Oram syndrome (atrial septal defect), Down's syndrome (AV communis, ventricular septal defect, persistent ductus arteriosus), Turner's syndrome (coarctation of the aorta), central cyanosis, polycythemia and clubbing point to a right-to-left shunt.

Vascular Disease

Hypertension, hyperlipidemia, smoking, diabetes, and obesity are detectible as coronary artery disease risk factors. Coronary artery disease may also be suspected in the presence of an ear crease sign, evidence of mediastinal radiation, progeria, polycythemia, PXE, Tangier disease, acromegaly, and in a cocaine addict. Sleep apnea, polyarteritis nodosa, Von Recklinghausen's disease, Cushing's syndrome, acromegaly and gout are associated with hypertension.

Arcus cornealis, xanthoma, lipemia retinalis suggest hyperlipidemia. Hyperlipidemia is seen in acromegaly and myxedema. Olivarius's sign, unilateral arcus cornealis and a Hollenhorst plaque occur in internal carotid artery disease.

Marfan's syndrome and Ehlers-Danlos syndrome are associated with aortic aneurysms/rupture. Sleep apnea, sarcoidosis, scleroderma and tricuspid regurgitation are associated with pulmonary hypertension. The Shy-Drager syndrome gives rise to postural hypotension.

Limb ischemia/necrosis may be due to atherosclerosis, cholesterol embolism, Buerger's disease, diabetes, Raynaud's phenomenon, or a collagen disease.

Facial edema, neck vein distention, prominent venous collateral circulation on the chest wall and venous stars are seen in the superior vena caval syndrome, whereas prominent abdominal venous collateral circulation, leg edema and possibly ascites point to the inferior vena caval syndrome.

Patients with the Osler-Weber-Rendu syndrome may have pulmonary AV fistula.

Infective Endocarditis (IE)

The physical signs are Roth spots, retinal hemorrhages, sub-ungal hemorrhages, petechiae involving the conjunctiva or palate, Osler's nodes and Janeway lesions. Valvular heart disease may also be present.

Valvular Heart Disease

Carcinoid syndrome, pulmonary hypertension (tricuspid regurgitation). Carcinoid, LEOPARD and Noonan's syndromes (pulmonic stenosis). Osteogenesis imperfecta, PXE, and Marfan's syndrome, I.E. (mitral regurgitation). Mitral valve prolapse is seen in PXE, Ehlers-Danlos syndrome and Marfan's syndrome. Marfan's, Reiter's, ankylosing spondylitis, tertiary syphilis, I.E. and osteogenesis imperfecta (aortic regurgitation). Ochronosis and Paget's disease of bone (aortic stenosis). LEOPARD syndrome (hypertrophic cardiomyopathy). William's syndrome (supravalvular aortic stenosis).

Heart Failure

Patients with heart failure may have peripheral cyanosis, edema, neck vein distention, leuconychia and mild jaundice (hypertension, coronary artery disease, valvular heart disease, myocarditis, cardiomyopathy or pericardial disease may be the underlying cause). High-output failure is seen in Paget's disease of bone and hyperthyroidism.

Myocardial and Pericardial Disease

Hemochromatosis, muscular dystrophy, Friedreich's ataxia, hyperthyroidism, amyloidosis (cardiomyopathy), rheumatic fever, Reiter's syndrome (myocarditis), scleroderma, dermatomyositis, and sarcoidosis (pericarditis), pericardial effusion and possibly tamponade (myxedema)

Heart Block

Sarcoidosis, gout, rheumatic fever, Reiter's syndrome, SLE and ankylosing spondylitis

Cardiac Tumors

Examples are neurofibromatosis, tuberous sclerosis and LAMB.

ACKNOWLEDGMENT

The author is indebted to the secretarial skills of Mrs. Ruby N. Stubbs-Stamps.

REFERENCES

1. Fitzgerald FT, Tierney Jr. LM: The bedside Sherlock Holmes. West J Med. 1982;137:169-75.
2. Pyeritz RE. The Marfan syndrome. Ann Rev Med. 2000;51:481-510.
3. Rudolph AM, Hoffman JIE, Rudolph CD. In: Appleton & Lange Rudolph's Pediatrics, Stamford, Connecticut, 20th edition; 1996. p. 1782.
4. Pi-Sunyer FX, Becker DM, Bouchard C, et al. Clinical guidelines on the identification evaluation and treatment of overweight and obesity in adults—the evidence report—NIH. Obes Res Suppl. 1998;2: 51S-209S.
5. Ruyon BA. Cardiac ascites. J Clin Gastroenterol. 1988;10:410-12.
6. Fraser RS, Colman N, Muller NL, et al. Obesity hypoventilation syndrome. In: Fraser & Pare's Diagnosis of Diseases of the Chest, 4th edition. Philadelphia: WB Saunders Co; 1999. p. 3053.
7. Lin YT, Yeh L, Oka Y. Pathophysiology of general cyanosis. NY State J Med. 1977;77:1393-6.
8. Silverman ME, Hurst JW. The hand and the heart. Am J Cardiol. 1968;22:718-28.
9. Blount Jr SG. Cyanosis: pathophysiology and differential diagnosis. In: CK Friedberg(Ed). Pathophysiology and Differential Diagnosis in Cardiovascular Disease. New York: Grune & Stratton; 1971. pp. 89-99.

9a. Aziz K, Sanyal SS, Goldblatt E. Reversed differential cyanosis. Br Heart J. 1968;30:288-90.

10. Saif MW, Khan U, Greenberg BR. Cardiovascular manifestations of myeloproliferative disorders: a review of the literature. Hosp Phys. 1999;35:43-54.

10a. Grant P, Patel P, Singh S. Acute myocardial infarction secondary to polycythemia in a case of cyanotic congenital heart disease. Int J Cardiol. 1985;9:108-10.

11. Nardone DA, Roth KM, Mazur DJ, et al. Usefulness of physical examination in detecting the presence or absence of anemia. Arch Intern Med. 1990;150:201-4.
12. Wade OL, Bishop JM. Cardiac Output and Regional Blood Flow. Oxford: Blackwell; 1962. p. 187.
13. Strickman NE, Rossi PA, Massumkhani GA, et al. Carcinoid heart disease: a clinical pathologic and therapeutic update. Curr Probl Cardiol. 1982;6:4-42.
14. Porter J, Cary N, Schofield P. Hemochromatosis presenting as congestive cardiac failure. Br Heart J. 1995;73:73-5.
15. Karnes PS. Neurofibromatosis: a common neurocutaneous disorder. Mayo Clin Proc. 1998;73:1071-6.
16. Alaeddini J, Frater RW, Shirani J. Cardiac involvement in neurofibromatosis. Tex Heart Inst J. 2000;27:218-19.
17. Friedberg CK. Edema and pulmonary edema. In: Friedberg CK, Grune, Stratton (Eds). Pathophysiology and Differential Diagnosis in Cardiovascular Disease. New York; 1971. pp. 40-71.
18. Berry TJ. The Hand as a Mirror of Systemic Disease. Philadelphia: FA Davis; 1963. pp. 193-204.
19. Byrne JJ. The Hand: Its Anatomy and Diseases, Vol. 76. Springfield: CC Thomas; 1959. pp. 194-5.
20. Daniel CR, Sams WM, Scher RK. Nails in systemic disease. In: Scher RK, Daniel CR (Eds). Nails: Therapy, Surgery, and Diagnosis. Philadelphia: WB Saunders Company; 1990. pp. 167-91.

21. Doughty RN, Haydock DA, Wattie J, et al. Systemic embolism from a large ascending aortic aneurysm. Circulation. 1998;97:1421-2.
22. Weiner DM, Ewalt DH, Roach ES, et al. Tuberous sclerosis complex: a comprehensive review. J Am Coll Surg. 1998;187:548-61.
23. Holzberg M, Walker HK. Terry's nails: Revised definition and new correlations. Lancet. 1984;1:896-9.
24. Fitzpatrick TB, Johnson RA, Wolff K. Blue-gray nails. In: Color atlas and synopsis of clinical dermatology, 3rd edition. New York: McGraw Hill; 1997. pp. 498-9.
25. Friedberg IM, Vogel LN. Thyrotoxicosis—onycholysis. In: Werner & Ingbar's The Thyroid, 6th edition. Philadelphia: JB Lippincott; 1986. p. 732.
26. Terry RC. Red half moons in cardiac failure. Lancet. 1954;11:842-4.
27. Cuetter AC, Pearl W, Ferrans VJ. Neurological conditions affecting the cardiovascular system. Curr Probl Cardiol. 1990;15:475-568.
28. Rudolph AM, Hoffman JIE, Rudolph CD. Down syndrome. In: Appleton & Lange, Stamford, Connecticut, Rudolph's Pediatrics, 20th edition. 1996. p. 298.
29. Tandon R, Edward JE. Cardiac malformation associated with Down syndrome. Circulation. 1973;47:1349-55.
30. Gorlin RJ, Anderson RC, Blaw M. Multiple Lentigines syndrome. Am J Dis Children. 1969;117:652-62.
31. Woywodt A, Welzel J, Haase H, et al. Cardiomyopathic Lentiginosis/LEOPARD syndrome presenting as sudden cardiac arrest. Chest. 1998;113:1415-7.
32. Grumbach MM, Conte FA. Noonan's syndrome. In: William's Textbook of Endocrinology, 9th edition. Philadelphia: WB Saunders; 1998. p. 1355.
33. Burch M, Sharland M, Shinebourne E, at al. Cardiologic abnormalities in Noonan syndrome. Phenotypic diagnosis and echocardiographic assessment of 118 patients. J Am Coll Cardiol. 1993;22:1189-92.
34. Sternberg MA, Neufeld HN. Physical diagnosis in syndromes with cardiovascular disease. In: CK Friedberg (Ed). Physical Diagnosis in CVS Disease., New York: Grune & Stratton; 1969. pp. 16-40.
35. Zalzstein E, Moes CAF, Musew NN, et al. Spectrum of cardiovascular anomalies in Williams-Beuren syndrome. Pediatr Cardiol. 1991;12:219-23.
36. Peery WH. Clinical spectrum of hereditary hemorrhagic telangiectasia (Osler-Weber-Rendu disease). Am J Med. 1987;82:989-97.
37. Swanson KL, Prakash UBS, Stanson AW. Pulmonary arteriovenous fistulas: Mayo Clinic experience. Mayo Clin Proc. 1999;74:671-80.
38. Basson CT, Solomon SD, Weissman B, et al. The clinical and genetic spectrum of the Holt-Oram syndrome (heart-hand syndrome). N Eng J Med. 1994;330: 885-91.
39. Lovibond JL. The diagnosis of clubbed fingers. Lancet. 1938;1:363-4.
40. Regan GM, Tagg B, Thomson ML. Subjective assessment and objective measurement of finger clubbing. Lancet. 1967;1:530-2.
41. Shamroth L. Personal experience. S Afr Med J. 1976;50:297-300.
42. Waring WW, Wilkinson RW, Wiebe RA, et al. Quantitation of digital clubbing in children. Measurements of casts of the index finger. Am Rev Resp Dis. 1971; 104:166-74.
43. Bentley D, Moore A, Schwachman H. Finger clubbing: a quantitative survey by analysis of the shadograph. Lancet. 1976;2:164-7.
44. Lovell RRH. Observation on the structure of clubbed fingers. Clin Sci. 1950; 9:299-317.
45. Carroll Jr DG. Curvature of the nails, clubbing of the fingers and hypertrophic pulmonary osteoarthropathy. Trans Am Clin Clim Assoc. 1971;83:198-208.

46. Schneiderman H. Digital clubbing due to idiopathic pulmonary fibrosis. Consultant. 1996;36:1249-56.
47. Coury C. Hippocratic fingers and hypertrophic osteoarthropathy. A study of 350 cases. Brit J Dis Chest. 1960;54:202-9.
48. Goodwin JR. Diagnosis of left atrial myxoma. Lancet. 1963;1:464-7.
49. Hansen-Flaschen J, Nordberg J. Clubbing and hypertrophic osteoarthropathy. Clin Chest Med. 1987;8:287-98.
50. Dorney ER. Unilateral clubbing of the fingers due to absence of the aortic arch. Am J Med. 1955;18:150-4.
51. Kanski JJ. Clinical Ophthalmology, 4th edition. Oxford: Butterworth; 1999. pp.495-7.
52. Barchiesi BJ, Eckel RH, Ellis PP. The cornea and disorders of lipid metabolism. Surv Ophthalmol. 1991;36:1-22.
53. Allander E, Bjornsson OJ, Kolbeinsson A, et al. Incidence of xanthelasma in the general population. Int J Epidermiol. 1972;1:211.
54. Parker F. Xanthomas and hyperlipidemia. J Am Acad Dermatol. 1985;13:1-30.
55. Borrie P, Slack J. A clinical syndrome characteristic of primary Type IV-V hyperlipoproteinemia. Brit J Dermatol. 1974;90:245-53.
56. Polano MK. Xanthomatoses. In: Fitzpatrick TB, Eisen OZ, Wolff K, et al. (Eds) Dermatology in Medicine, 4th edition. New York: McGraw-Hill, Inc; 1993. p. 1910.
57. Glueck CJ. Triglyceride analysis in hyperlipidemia. In: Rifkind BM, Levy RI, (Eds). Diagnosis & Therapy. New York: Grune & Stratton,; 1977. p. 22.
58. Brewer MB, Zech LA, Gregg RE, et al. Type III hyperlipoproteinemia: diagnosis, molecular defects, pathology and treatment. Ann Int Med. 1983:98:623-40.
59. Daniell MW. Smoker's wrinkles: a study in the epidemiology of crow's feet. Ann Intern Med. 1971;75:873-80.
60. Pouliot MC, Després JP, Lemieux S, et al. Waist circumference and abdominal sagittal diameter: best simple anthropometric indexes of abdominal visceral adipose tissue accumulation and related cardiovascular risk in men and women. Am J Cardiol. 1994;73:460-8.
61. Eber B, Delgado P. More on the diagonal earlobe crease as a marker of coronary artery disease; Belin TR earlobes, obesity and bias in observational studies (letters). Am J Card. 1993;72:861.
62. Stewart JR, Fajardo LF, Gillette SM, et al. Radiation injury to the heart. Special feature—late effects. Consensus conference. Int J Radiat Oncol Biol Phys. 1995;31:1205-11.
63. George WM. Cutaneous findings related to cardiovascular disorders. Int J Derm. 1998;37:161-72.
64. Frederickson DS, Altrocchi PH. Tangier disease. In: Aronson SM, Volk BW (Eds). Cerebral Sphingolipidoses. New York: Academic Press; 1962. pp. 343-57.
65. Mahley RW, Weisgraber KH, Farese RV Jr. Disorders of lipid metabolism. In: William's Textbook of Endocrinology 9th edition. Philadelphia: WB Saunders Co; 1998. p. 1134.
66. Komuro R, Yamashita S, Sumitsuji S, et al. Tangier disease with continuous massive and longitudinal diffuse calcification in the coronary arteries. Circulation. 2000;101:2446-8.
67. Pietrini V, Ruzzuto N, Vergani C. Neuropathy in Tangier disease: A clinicopathologic study and a review of the literature. Acta Neurol Scand. 1985;72:495-505.
68. Warner EA. Cocaine abuse. Ann Intern Med. 1993;119:226-35.

69. Krutchkoff DJ, Eisenberg E, O'Brien JE, et al (letter). Cocaine-induced dental erosions. N Engl J Med. 1990;322:408.
70. Pitts WR, Lange RA, Cigarroa JE, et al. Cocaine-induced myocardial ischemia and infarction: pathophysiology, recognition and management. Prog Cardiovasc Dis. 1997;40:65-76.
71. Franks Jr. AG: Cutaneous aspects of cardiopulmonary disease. In: Fitzpatrick TB, Eisen AZ, Wolff K, Austen KF (Eds). Dermatology in General Medicine, 3rd edition. New York: McGraw Hill Book Co; 1997. p. 1981.
72. Lebwohl M, Halperin J, Phelps RG. Brief report: occult pseudoxanthoma elasticum in patients with premature cardiovascular disease. New Eng J Med. 1993;329:1237-9.
73. Fischer CM. Facial pulses in internal carotid artery occlusion. Neurology. 1970;20:476-8.
74. Smith JL, Susac JO. Unilateral arcus senilis: sign of occlusive disease of the carotid artery. JAMA. 1973;226:676.
75. Sapira JD. An internist looks at the fundus oculi: Disease A month. 1984;30:1-64.
75a. Hellmann DB. Temporal arteritis: a cough, toothache and tongue infarction. JAMA. 2002;287:2996-3000.
76. Blackshear JL, Jahanger A, Owenburg WA, et al. Digital embolization from plaque-related thrombus in the thoracic aorta: Identification with transesophageal echocardiography and resolution with Warfarin therapy. Mayo Clin Proc. 1993;68:268-72.
77. Feder W, Auerbach RM. "Purple Toes": an uncommon sequela of oral Coumadin therapy. Ann Int Med. 1961;55:911-7.
78. Pettelot G, Bracco J, Barrillon D, et al. Cholesterol embolization. Unrecognized complication of thrombolysis. Circulation. 1998;97:1522.
79. Falanga V, Fine MJ, Kapor WN. The cutaneous manifestations of cholesterol crystal embolization. Arch Dermat. 1986;122:1194-8.
80. Olin JW, Young JR, Graor RA, et al. The changing clinical spectrum of thromboangiitis obliterans (Buerger's disease). Circulation. 1990;82(Suppl IV):IV-3-IV-8.
81. Spittell JA Jr. The vasospastic disorders. Curr Probl Cardiol. 1984;8:5-27.
82. Fitzpatrick TB, Johnson RA, Wolff K. Vasculitis. In: Color atlas and synopsis of clinical dermatology, 4th edition. New York: McGraw Hill; 2001. pp. 373-7.
83. Ricca J. Obstruction of the superior vena caval system: an extensive review. NY State J Med. 1959;59:4171-7.
84. Parish JM, Marschlke RF, Dines DE, et al. Etiologic considerations in superior vena cava syndrome. Mayo Clin Proc. 1981;56:407-13.
85. Blackburn T, Dunn M. Pacemaker-induced superior vena cava syndrome: consideration of management. Am Heart J. 1988;116:893-6.
86. Wallace C, Siminoski K. The Pemberton sign. Ann Intern Med. 1996;125:568-9.
87. Berlin L, Waldman I, Fong JK. Occlusion of the inferior vena cava. A major roentgenographic abnormality with minor clinical manifestations. JAMA. 1965;194:136-8.
88. Wood P. An appreciation of mitral stenosis. Br Med J. 1954;1:1051 & 1113.
89. Thorner MO, Vance ML. Acromegaly. In: William's textbook of Endocrinology, 9th edition. Philadelphia: Saunders; 1998. pp. 298-9.
90. McKenzie JM, Zakarija M. Hyperthyroidism. In: LJ De Groot (Ed). Endocrinology, 3rd edition. Philadelphia: WB Saunders; 1995. pp. 676-712.
91. Manolis AS, Varriale P, Ostrowski RM. Hypothyroid cardiac tamponade. Arch Intern Med. 1987;147:1167-9.

92. David DS, Grieco MH, Cushman P. Adrenal glucocorticoids after 20 years. A review of their clinically relevant consequences. J Chron Dis. 1970;22:637-711.
93. Gertz MA, Lacy MQ, Dispensieri A. Amyloidosis: recognition, confirmation, prognosis and therapy. Mayo Clin Proc. 1999;74:490-4.
94. Braverman IM. Amyloidosis. In: Skin Signs of Systemic Disease, 3rd edition. Philadelphia: WB Saunders; 1998 pp. 190-7.
95. Pund EE, Hawley RL, McGee HJ, et al. "Gouty Heart." New Eng J Med. 1960;263:835-8.
96. Messerli FH, Frohlich ED, Dreslinski GL, et al. Serum uric acid in essential hypertension. Ann Intern Med. 1980;93:817-21.
97. Maxwell AJ, Bruinsma KA. Uric acid is closely linked to vascular nitric oxide activity. Evidence for mechanism of association with cardiovascular disease. J Am Coll Cardiol. 2001;38:1850-8.
98. Kenny D, Ptacin M, Bamrah VS, et al. Cardiovascular ochronosis: a case report and review of the medical literature. Cardiology. 1990;77:477-83.
99. Scheld WM, Sande MA. Endocarditis and intravascular infections. In: Mandell GL, Bennett JE, Dolin R (Eds). Principles & Practice of Infectious Diseases, 4th edition; part 2. New York: Churchill Livingstone; 1995. p. 748.
100. Proudfit WL. Skin signs of infective endocarditis. Am Heart J. 1983;106:1451-3.
101. James DG, et al. A worldwide review of sarcoidosis. Ann NY Acad Sci. 1976;278:321-34.
102. Matsui Y, Iwai K, Tachibana T, et al. Clinical pathological study of fatal myocardial sarcoidosis. Ann NY Acad Sci. 1976;278:455-69.
103. Roberts WC, McAllister HA, Ferrans VJ. Sarcoidosis of heart. Am J Med. 1977;63:86-108.
103a. Pepin M, Schwarze U, Superti-Furga A, et al. Clinical and genetic features of Ehlers-Danlos syndrome type IV, the vascular type. New Engl J Med. 2000; 342:673-80.
104. Ed. Wallace DJ, Hahn BH. Dubois' Lupus Erythematosus, 6th edition. Philadelphia: Lippincott, William & Wilkins; 2001. p. 622.
105. Fitzpatrick TB, Johnson RA, Wolff K, et al: DLE. Color Atlas and Synopsis of Clinical Dermatology, 4th edition. NY: McGraw Hill; 2001. pp. 361-7.
106. Moder KE, Miller TD, Tazelaar HD. Cardiac involvement in systemic lupus erythematosus. Mayo Clin Proc. 1999;74:275-84.
107. Doherty NE, Siegel RJ. Cardiovascular manifestations of systemic lupus erythematosus. Am Heart J. 1985;110:1257-65.
108. Roberts WC, High ST. The heart in systemic lupus erythematosus. Curr Probl Cardiol. 1999;24:1-56.
109. Braverman IM. Scleroderma. In: Skins Signs of Systemic Disease, 3rd edition. Philadelphia: WB Saunders; 1998. pp. 235-41.
110. Follansbee WP. The cardiovascular manifestation of systemic sclerosis (scleroderma). Curr Probl Cardiol. 1986;11:245-98.
111. Anuari A, Graninger W, Schneider B, et al. Cardiac involvement in systemic sclerosis. Arthritis Rheum. 1992;35:1356-61.
112. Katayama I, Sawada Y, Nishioka K. Facial fold erythema—dermatomyositis: seborrheic pattern of dermatomyositis. Brit J Derm. 1999;140:978-9.
113. Plotz PH, Moderator. Current concepts in the idiopathic inflammatory myopathies: polymyositis, dermatomyositis and related disorders. Ann Intern Med. 1989;111:143-57.
114. Braunwald E. Dermatomyositis in Heart disease, 5th edition. Philadelphia: WB Saunders; 1997. pp. 1779-80.

115. Fitzpatrick TB, Johnson RA, Wolff K, et al. Polyarteritis Nodosa. In: Color Atlas and synopsis of clinical dermatology. 3rd edition. New York: McGraw-Hill; 1997. pp. 372-5.
116. Schrader ML, Hockman JS, Bulkley BH. The heart in polyarteritis nodosa: A clinico-pathologic study. Am Heart J. 1985;109:1353-9.
117. Sahn EE, Maize JC, Silver RM. Erythema Marginatum: An unusual histopathological manifestation. J Am Acad Dermatol. 1989;21:145-7.
118. Scott JT. Rheumatic fever. In: Copeman's textbook of the rheumatic diseases, Churchill Livingstone, Edinburgh, London & New York, 5th edition; 1978. pp. 781-2.
119. Bywaters EGL. Relationship between heart and joint disease including 'rheumatoid heart disease' and chronic post-rheumatic arthritis (type Jaccoud). Brit Heart J. 1950;12:101-31.
120. Scott JT. Ankylosing spondylitis. In: Copeman's textbook of the rheumatic diseases, 5th edition. London & New York: Churchill Livingstone, Edinburgh; , 1978. pp. 513-6.
121. Weinberger HS, Ropes MW, Kulka JP, et al. Reiters syndrome; clinical and pathological considerations. A long term study of 16 cases. Medicine (Baltimore). 1962;41:35-91.
122. Freher M, Challapalli S, Pinto JV, et al. Current status of calcium channel blockers in patients with cardiovascular disease. Curr Probl Cardiol. 1999;25:229-340.
123. Steele RM, Schuna AA, Schreiler RT. Calcium antagonist-induced gingival hyperplasia. Ann Intern Med. 1994; 120:663-4.
124. Meraw SJ, Sheridan PJ. Medically induced gingival hyperplasia. Mayo Clinic Proc. 1998;73:1196-9.
125. Opie LH, Gersh BJ. Drugs for the heart. Philadelphia: WB Saunders; 2001. p. 118.
126. Lapostolle F, Borron SW, Bekka R, et al. Lingual angioedema after perindopril use. Am J Cardiol. 1998;81:523.
127. Hirsh J, Dalen JE, Deykin D, et al. Heparin: Mechanism of action, pharmacokinetics, dosing considerations monitoring, efficacy and safety. Chest. 1992;102 (suppl) 337S-51S.
128. Warkentin TE. Heparin induced thrombocytopenia, Part 1. The diagnostic clues. J Crit Illness. 2002;17:172-8.
129. Pineo GF, Hull RD. Adverse effects of coumadin anticoagulants. Drug Safety. 1993;9:263-71.
130. Silen W. Cope's Early Diagnosis of the Acute Abdomen, 16th edition. Oxford: Oxford University Press; 1983. p. 119.
131. Harris L, McKenna WJ, Rowland E, et al. Side effects of long-term Amiodarone therapy. Circulation. 1983;67:45-51.
132. Blackshear JL, Randle HW. Reversibility of blue-gray cutaneous discoloration from amiodarone. Mayo Clin Proc. 1991;66:721-6.
133. Sra J, Bremner S. Amiodarone skin toxicity. Images in cardiovascular medicine. Circulation. 1998;97:1105.
134. Sheikhzadeh A, Schafer V, Schnabel A. Drug induced lupus erythematosus by amiodarone. Arch Intern Med. 2002;162:834-6.
135. Solinger AM. Drug related lupus. Clinical and etiological considerations. Rheum Dis Clin N Am. 1988;14:187-202.
136. Wallace DJ, Hahn BH. Drug induced lupus. In: Dubuois' Lupus Erythematosus, 6th edition. Philadelphia: Lippincott, Williams & Wilkins; 2001. pp. 891-6.

137. Victor M, Ropper AH. Adams & Victor's Principles of Neurology, 7th edition. New York: McGraw Hill; 2001. p. 1145.
138. Perloff JK. The heart in neuromuscular disease. Curr Probl Cardiol. 1986;11: 511-57.
139. White NJ, Winearls CG, Smith R. Cardiovascular abnormalities in osteogenesis imperfecta. Am Heart J. 1983;106:1416-20.
140. Wong RS, Follis FM. Shively BK, et al. Osteogenesis imperfecta and cardiovascular diseases. Ann Thorac Surg. 1995;60:1439-43.
141. Datey KK, Deshmukh MM, Engineer SD, et al. Straight Back Syndrome. Brit Heart J. 1964;26:614-9.
142. Pierce JA, Ebert RV. The barrel deformity of the chest, the senile lung and obstructive pulmonary emphysema. Am J Med. 1958;25:13-22.
143. Bailey H. Demonstration of Physical Signs in Clinical Surgery, 13th edition. Bristol: John Wright & Sons Ltd; 1960. p. 802.
144. Hultgren HN. Osteitis deformans (Paget's disease) and calcific disease of the heart valves. Am J Cardiol. 1998;81:1461-4.
145. Arnalich F, Plaza JA, Sabrino J, et al. Cardiac size and function in Paget's disease of bone. Internat J Cardiol. 1984;5:491-505.
146. Rhodes AR, Silverman RA, Harrist TJ, et al. Mucocutaneous lentigines, cardiomucocutaneous myxomas, and multiple blue nevi: The Lamb syndrome. J Am Acad Dermatol. 1984;10:72-82.
147. Vidaillet Jr HJ, Seward JB, Fyke FE, et al. "Syndrome Myxoma": a sub-set of patients with cardiac myxoma associated with pigmented skin lesions and peripheral and endocrine neoplasms. Brit Heart J. 1987;57:247-55.

Chapter

12 12-Lead Electrocardiogram Interpretation

Snapshot

- Section I Basic Principles and the Electrocardiogram (ECG) of the Normal Patients
- Section II: Axis Deviations and Intra-Ventricular Conduction Defects
- Section III: Chamber Enlargement, Hypertrophy, Overloads
- Section IV: Myocardial Infarction
- Section V: Ventricular Pre-Excitation/Pericarditis:
- Section VI: Abnormalities of ST-T Waves/QT Intervals/ST Segment Deviations/T Waves
- Appendix

SECTION I BASIC PRINCIPLES AND THE ELECTROCARDIOGRAM (ECG) OF THE NORMAL PATIENTS

Electrocardiography is one of the earliest non-invasive techniques that was introduced in the field of cardiac assessment and still remains an important tool in cardiac physical diagnosis. In fact, it is considered an integral part of cardiac examination since it can be quickly and easily performed during a visit to any physician's office as long as one has access to an electrocardiographic machine. It is an indispensable tool in the evaluation of acute chest pain syndromes and arrhythmias. Although recordings of electrical activity of the heart were first made by use of a capillary electrometer in 1887,[1] modern electrocardiography can be considered to have taken roots in the pioneering work of Einthoven[2] and later advanced into clinical realm by the work of Wilson and others.[3-12] Several textbooks have also been published with regard to teaching electrocardiographic interpretation.[13-21] The impediment to clear and easier understanding inherent in the pattern recognition method of teaching ECG interpretation was overcome by the spatial vector approach advanced by Grant.[10] In this chapter, we will provide the basics of the 12 lead ECG interpretations and in the subsequent chapter we will discuss the integration of ECG into clinical cardiac diagnosis.

Anatomic Considerations of the Conduction System of the Heart

Basic to the understanding of the electrocardiogram in the normal humans is the anatomic considerations of the human heart and its specialized conduction system.[22,23] The normal human heart is an intrathoracic organ located in the mediastinum partially overlapped by the lung. The right atrium and the right ventricle are mostly anterior lying directly behind the sternum. The left atrium is the most posterior chamber in the heart. The right ventricle is somewhat crescent-shaped and has a thin outer layer of muscle. It has marked trabeculations in its walls toward its apex anteriorly and inferiorly. Often a muscle bundle called the ***moderator band*** is seen to cross from the lower inter-ventricular septum to the base of the anterior papillary muscle. The left ventricle is more like an ellipsoidal (or conical) chamber formed by thicker muscle and a large portion of its muscle mass extends antero-laterally as well as infero-laterally and the basal most portion of the inferior wall is also posterior.

The Sinoatrial (SA) Node and the Atrioventricular (AV) Node

The cardiac conduction system with the component parts is shown in the diagram (Fig. 12.1). It is well known that the electrical activation of the normal heart originates in the SA node, which is located in the upper part of the right atrium near the entrance of the superior vena cava. The SA node is an epicardial structure and therefore is closer to the pericardium. It can therefore be easily involved in pericardial diseases. The electrical activation arising from the SA node not only spreads through the atrial myocardial cells activating them, it is also transmitted through specialized pathways called the internodal tracts, to the subsidiary electrical center called the AV node. Three discrete internodal tracts have been recognized in histological studies of the human atrium. These are termed the anterior, middle and the posterior internodal tracts. In addition, a branch of the anterior internodal tract called the Bachmann's bundle provides for transmission across the atrial septum to the left atrium. In the normal hearts, the AV node is located in the basal part of the right side of the interatrial septum, in proximity to and anterior to the coronary sinus opening in the right atrium, which drains the venous blood from the coronary veins. The AV node is connected proximally at its upper part to the internodal tract and the atrium through the cells of the conduction system in the atrionodal (AN) region and distally through the Nodal-His (NH) region to the Bundle of His.

His Bundle, Bundle Branches, Divisions of the Left Bundle and the Purkinje System

The H penetrates the middle of the central fibrous body that forms the skeleton to which the two AV valves are attached along with the aortic valve. The

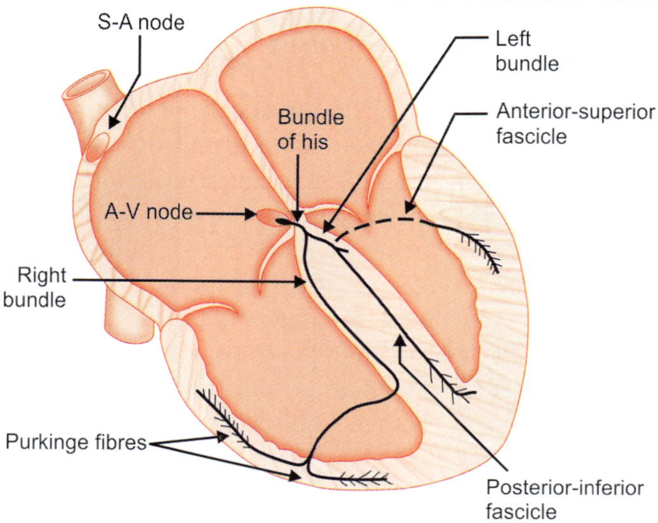

Fig. 12.1: The diagram showing the cardiac conduction system. Sinoatrial node (SA node) is in the epicardium of the top of the right atrium close to the superior vena cava. Atrioventricular node (AV node) is in the lower part of the right atrium near the atrial septum in front of the orifice of the coronary sinus into which the cardiac veins drain. The Bundle of His runs through the central fibrous body that provides attachment to the aortic, mitral and the tricuspid valves. His bundle divides at the top of the inter-ventricular septum into the right and the left bundle branches. The right bundle runs underneath the endocardium of the inter-ventricular septum on the right side, crosses the right ventricular cavity though the moderator band and divides into Purkinje fibers under the right ventricular endocardium. The left bundle divides into two thick fascicles with radiating fibers; one is the anterior superior fascicle that provides Purkinje network of connections to the upper part of the anterior septum, and adjacent anterior wall and the lateral wall of the left ventricle. The second set of fibers that run inferiorly and posterior is termed the infero-posterior fascicle.

pulmonary valve is well separated from this, situated at a higher level at the base of the root of the pulmonary artery trunk. Immediately below the pulmonary valve is the outflow tract of the right ventricle formed by the crista supraventricularis muscle. The H in normal hearts usually runs along the inferior edge of the membranous septum to the apex of the muscular inter-ventricular septum. It bifurcates at the top of the inter-ventricular septum (at the level of the junction of the right coronary and the posterior non-coronary cusps of the aortic valve) into two main bundles called the right bundle branch and the left bundle branch. The right bundle is a long thin fascicle and runs under the endocardium of the right side of the inter-ventricular septum. At the bottom of the right ventricle, it is seen to course through the moderator band. Once it reaches the base of the anterior papillary muscle of the right ventricle it arborizes into fine branches called the Purkinje fibers through which the electrical activation can spread to all of the right ventricular myocardium. Unlike the right bundle, the left bundle is a thick fascicle.

It often divides early at the top and on the left side of the inter-ventricular septum, into two main radiating fascicles or divisions. Sometimes, a third branch called "septal branch" has also been described that might actually be involved in the initial electrical activation of the left side of the septum. One of the two main fascicles is normally oriented anteriorly and superiorly (the anterior division or fascicle) and the other one is oriented posteriorly and also inferiorly (the inferior division). The two divisions can be traced further down and seen to arborize into fine branches (Purkinje fibers) conducting and spreading the electrical activity directly to the myocardium. The antero-superior division arborizes into the anterior septum and the free antero-lateral walls and the infero-posterior division into the posterior septum and the infero-lateral walls. Purkinje fibers essentially provide the final sub-endocardial and intra-myocardial network in both the right and the left ventricles.

The Arterial Supply of the Conduction System

The arterial supply of the SA node in two-thirds of normal subjects arises from the right coronary artery (RCA). The SA nodal branch of the RCA is often the first and the cephalad-oriented branch of the RCA.[24] When the left coronary artery provides the arterial supply as in one-third of normal subjects, it usually arises from the left atrial branch of the left circumflex (LCx) that often runs along the AV groove on the left side. The AV node often is supplied in the majority by a branch of the RCA as it courses through the AV groove on the right side and makes a "U" bend posteriorly. The AV node artery arises often from the tip of this U bend. The right bundle and the anterior fascicle of the left bundle derive their arterial supply from the septal branches of the left anterior descending (LAD) coronary artery. The infero-posterior division of the left bundle gets its arterial supply from the posterior inter-ventricular branch, which can arise either from the RCA or the LCx depending on which of these two arteries is dominant in the individual subject. The RCA tends to be dominant in two-thirds of normal subjects and the LCx in the remaining one-third.[25]

The Function of the Conduction System

The above anatomic considerations are important not only in relation to some of the features of the normal electrocardiograms as well as in understanding the effects of conduction system involvement on the electrocardiograms in abnormal states. The pacemaker cells in the SA node produce the onset of the normal electrical activation of the heart resulting in what is normally termed the sinus rhythm. The wave of excitation spreads to the atria and causes the atrial depolarization that results in the P wave on the surface ECG. The cells in the specialized internodal tracts in the atria conduct the electrical activation down to the AV node. The normal AV node essentially acts to slow down the impulse transmission to the ventricles. The conduction down the normal His-Purkinje system is usually rapid and allows an orderly transmission of the electrical impulse to the working myocardial cells of the ventricles and results in the ventricular depolarization, which causes the QRS complex on the surface ECG.

The PR interval is the time from the onset of the P wave that represents the atrial depolarization to the onset of the QRS complex that represents the ventricular depolarization. It usually varies in the normal hearts from about 0.12 second [120 milliseconds (ms)] the minimum to 0.20 second (200 ms) the maximum. The onset of the P wave only tells us when the atrium begins to depolarize. The SA node pacemaker cells actually fire several ms before the impulse arrives in the atrium and activates the same. This SA conduction time is not usually measurable during normal sinus rhythm. It is usually about 40-60 ms (*see* Appendix).

One can measure the intra-atrial conduction time for the impulse to reach from the top of the atrium to the bottom of the atrium by recording through two electrode tipped catheters placed inside the atrium transvenously from a femoral venous site in such a way that one catheter tip is positioned in the high right atrium and another in the low atrium across the tricuspid valve that also will help to pick up the His bundle potential (H) (Figs. 12.2A and B). One can see that the atrial depolarization marked A in the intracardiac recordings corresponds to the P wave on the surface ECG lead. It will also be seen that the atrial depolarization in the high right atrium begins before the atrial depolarization in the lower atrial recording with the H potential. The interval from the onset of the atrial depolarization (A) in the lower intracardiac recording to the onset of the H potential, marked AH interval represents the conduction time taken for the normal impulse to travel from the low atrium essentially through the AV node and activate the Bundle of His. In the normal subjects, this varies between 80 and 120 ms (maximum). However, the time interval from the onset of the H activation to the onset of the ventricular depolarization that corresponds to the QRS complex on the surface ECG, marked HV interval is only about 45 ms indicating that His-Purkinje conduction is quite rapid. Even when the PR interval is at the normal maximum of about 0.20 second (200 ms), the major portion of that delay is in the AV node being about two-thirds of that time. Thus it is important to understand the normal AV node function. It essentially acts to slow down the impulse transmission to the ventricles. The delay allows for the needed time for effective blood transfer from the atria to the ventricles, before the ventricles contract. In addition, this offers a protective mechanism so that the ventricular rate is not excessive in situations of abnormal tachycardias arising or involving the atria. For example, when an arrhythmia such as atrial flutter develops, the atrial rate is about 300/min although it is regular. If all the atrial impulses were to be conducted to the ventricles, it would result in a ventricular rate of

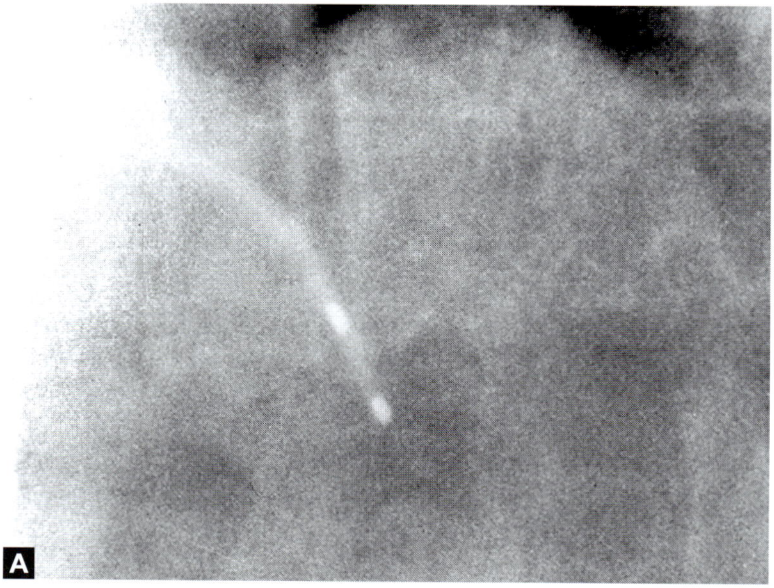

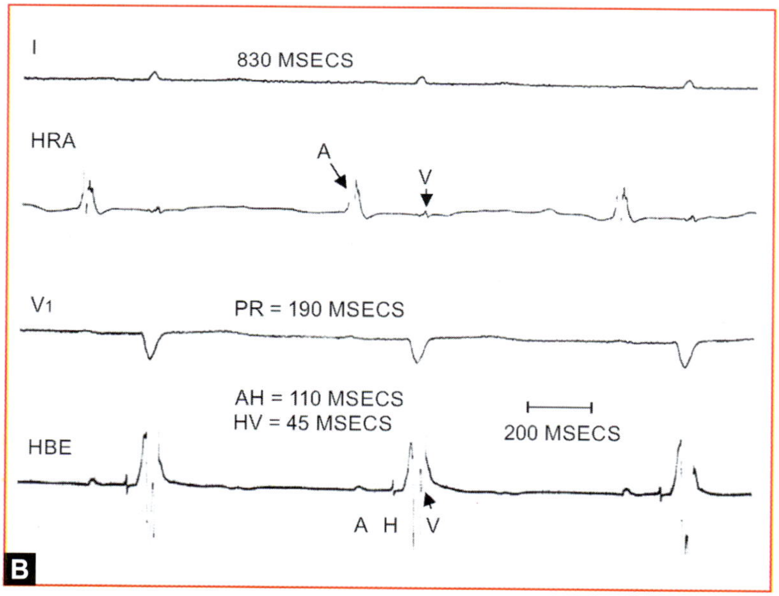

Figs. 12.2A and B: (A) Electrode catheter with two electrodes at the tip in the lower part of the right atrium across the tricuspid valve to record intracardiac recording of bundle of His activation. (B) Shows two intracardiac recordings, one from the high right atrium (HRA) and the other from the region of the Bundle of His (HBE) in the lower part of the right atrium. Lead I and lead V1 are surface reference electrocardiogram (ECG). Atrial activation (A) and ventricular activation (V) correspond to P and QRS on surface ECG. H is HBE potential. "A" in HRA precedes "A" in HBE. The time difference represents intra-atrial conduction time. AH interval represents conduction time through the AV node. HV interval represents conduction time through the His-Purkinje system.

300, which would cause low cardiac output and shock and would result in death within a short period of time. However, the normal AV node will not allow 1:1 conduction at that rate. It will automatically go to a 2:1 AV conduction resulting in an acceptable rate of 150/min, which may cause symptoms but not necessarily end in dire consequences in a short period.

Another important feature of the electrical transmission in the heart is when one cell is activated, the spread of excitation wave will continue in a domino fashion and result in the activation of all cells in the heart unless there is a physiologic or pathologic block in the conduction system.

Basic Principles of ECG

The heart is made of a syncytial network of several millions of striated muscle cells interconnected at the individual cell level to each other at their ends through the ***intercalated discs***. Each individual myocardial cell (cardiomyocyte) contains the actin and the myosin filaments, which provide the contractile mechanisms when electrically activated. The intercalated discs are membrane-like in structure and offer least resistance for electrical conduction. When a cardiac cell is impaled by a microelectrode to record the electrical potential across the cell membrane during the resting state, the inside of the cells is found to be negative relative to the outside by about -90 millivolts (mv). This potential difference is due to the semipermeability of the cell membrane. The cell is said to be in a polarized state at rest with the outside of the cell being rich in the anions (Na^+ and Ca^{2+} ions) and more positive while the inside of the cell is rich in the cations (Cl^- ions) and therefore more negative. This weak electric dipole that exists between the inside and the outside of the cell at rest however has no significant electrical field around it. The movement of the various ions across the membrane is controlled by specific ion channels. These have been more clearly identified and characterized in the last several years. The genes encoding them have been also cloned and sequenced. These ion channels have two properties. One is the selective permeability to the ions. This is the basis of classification of the channels into Na^+, K^+ and Ca^{2+} channels. The other property is the gating mechanism by which the channel opens and closes. These can be voltage-dependent, ligand-dependent (e.g. acetylcholine and ADP-activated K^+ channels) and mechanosensitive gating (activated by mechanical stress).[26]

Action Potential

When the cardiomyocyte is stimulated by a weak electric current or activated by the normal spread of excitation resulting from the discharge of the normal pacemaker cells in the SA node, an action potential develops, which can be shown to have four phases (Fig. 12.3).

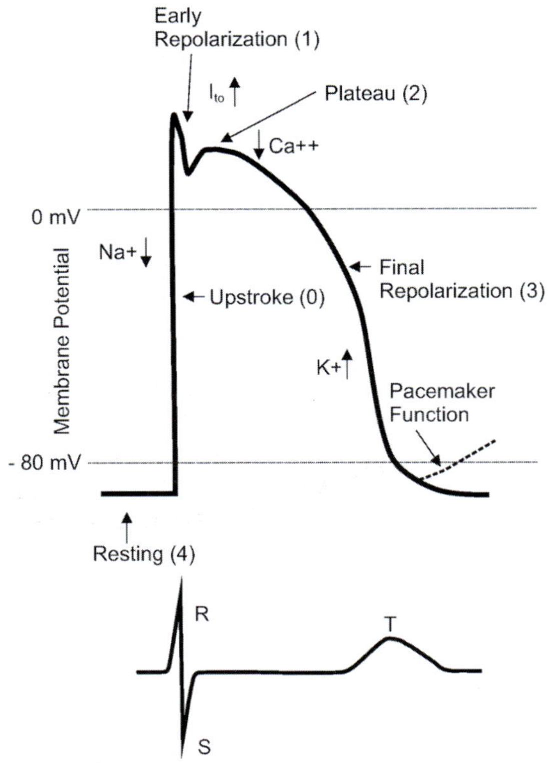

Fig. 12.3: Transmembrane action potential with its four phases resulting from electrical activation of a cardiomyocyte recorded with a micro tip electrode placed across the cell membrane. Surface electrocardiogram shown for reference at the bottom. Ventricular depolarization of the whole heart corresponds to the upstroke (phase 0). The ST segment and the T wave correspond to the repolarization phases 1–3. Phase 4 is the resting phase in electrical diastole. The transmembrane potential during this phase is about –90 mV and remains relatively flat in all working myocardial cells until the cell is activated. However all pacemaker cells of the conduction system show the potential during this phase 4 to rise gradually until it reaches the threshold level for excitation. The slope of this rise is the steepest in the sinoatrial node that is the normal dominant pacemaker.

The Phase 0 is ***the phase of rapid depolarization***. It corresponds to the upstroke of the action potential. The membrane potential becomes more positive. It is usually associated with rapid entry of sodium ions (Na^+) into the cells. This phase corresponds to the QRS complex produced by the depolarization of the ventricles in the whole heart as recorded on the surface ECG.

The Phase 1 is a phase of rapid repolarization.

The Phase 2 is ***the plateau phase***. This is the longest phase and marks the phase of calcium entry into the cells.

The Phase 3 is ***the phase of rapid repolarization,*** which restores the membrane potential back to its resting value. These three phases together correspond to the ST-T waves of the whole heart, which represent the ventricular repolarization. The total duration of the action potential corresponds to the QT interval representing the interval from the onset of the QRS complex to the end of the T wave.

The Phase 4 is ***the electrical diastolic phase***. This phase is usually a quiescent phase in the working myocardial cells, the membrane voltage remaining constant at the resting level until the next wave of excitation arrives.

However, in all of the pacemaker cells in the conduction system, the Phase 4 is characterized by gradual decrease in the potential toward less negative values. When it reaches a threshold level that is usually about -60 mv, the cell will automatically undergo depolarization. The slope of this spontaneous diastolic depolarization is steeper as one moves up the conduction system. It is the steepest in the cells of the SA node making them the most favored natural pacemaker of the heart. The slope in the SA node is such that the normal discharge rate of the SA node is at least above 60 beats/min. In the normal state, the middle portion of the AV node (the N-region) does not have any pacemaker cells. However, the AN region and the NH regions do. Thus when the cardiac rhythm arises from the AV junction, it is best described as junctional as opposed to the old term Nodal Rhythm. The other location of the junctional rhythm is actually the H. Its Phase 4 slope is such that its normal rate of discharge is between 40 and 60/min. However, as one goes down further into the His-Purkinje system, the rate becomes much slower, into the lower 30s or less.

The Electric Dipole Concept in Electrocardiography

An electric dipole is considered when two equal and opposite charges (+q and –q) are separated by a very small distance (d). The strength or the magnitude of the dipole (the dipole moment) is the product of the current and the distance (qd) (Fig. 12.4). The strength alone does not define it clearly. The direction in space also needs to be considered that lines up along the negative to the positive since the dipole moment is a vector. It is an electrical force like any other force. Thus it is a vector with both magnitude and direction. It may be good to recall here that electric current results from flow of electrons that are negatively charged particles. Since opposite charges attract, the negative charges are attracted toward the positive. The electric current flows from the negative to the positive. However, by convention, the current is often depicted in the electric circuit diagrams as flowing from the positive to the negative. This is mainly to avoid a negative sign in front of the numbers in calculating the strength of the current (usually expressed in amperes or as amperage), the pressure pushing the current (usually measured in volts or as voltage) and the resistance in the lines of the circuit (usually expressed in ohms).

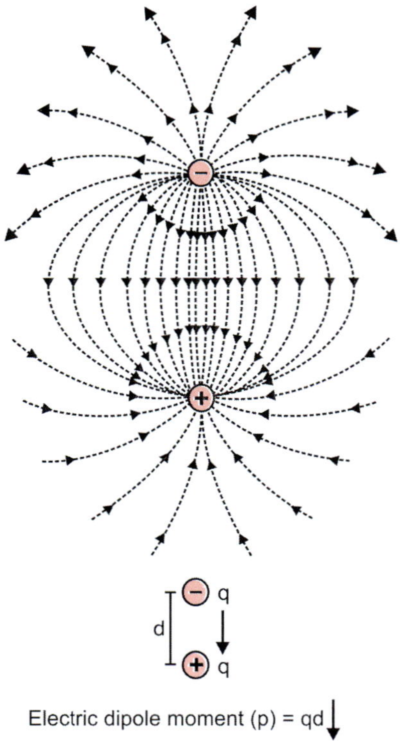

Fig. 12.4: Diagrammatic representation of an electric dipole when two equal and opposite charges (+q and –q) are separated by a very small distance (d). The magnitude of the dipole is the dipole moment.

When cardiac cells are activated by a propagating wave of excitation spreading through the conduction system from the SA node pacemaker cell initiated electrical discharge, a potential difference develops between the activated (the depolarized cells) that becomes more negative on the outside and the non-activated (non-depolarized) cells that are more positive on the outside. This results in the development of electric dipoles between adjacent cells with the negative end in the depolarized cells and the positive end in the non-depolarized cells. As activation progresses and as more and more cells become depolarized, *the electric dipole orientation lines up along the direction of the spread of the wave of excitation* (Fig. 12.5). Since there are several millions of cells in the heart, this sequential activation will end up producing multiple electric dipoles at the various instants each with its own magnitude and direction, each being a vector. The resultant of all these vectors at any given instant can be conceived of as a major single electric dipole with its own magnitude and direction. The latter therefore can have an electrical field around it and also be conducted to the surface since the torso of the human

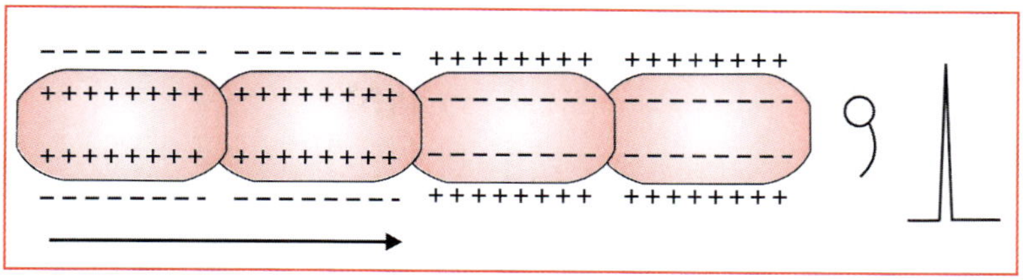

Fig. 12.5: Shows a propagating wave of excitation of adjacent myocardial cells. The arrow shows electric dipole orientation to be along the direction of the spread of the wave of excitation.

body acts essentially as a volume conductor of this electric current. This is understandable since the extracellular spaces of the tissues in the body consist essentially of salt and water.

Electrocardiogram machine is designed to pick up the surface potentials through the electrodes placed on the body surface called the "Leads". An ECG lead is usually made up of two sets of electrodes placed on two specific sites of the human body. One is usually called the positive electrode and another negative electrode as is the case in all bipolar leads, which essentially give the potential difference between the two sites. In case of the unipolar leads, the exploring electrode is placed at the designated sites and can be labeled as positive and it usually will register the actual potential at the site of placement since the negative electrode of this lead is usually a central reference terminal that registers only zero potential.

The ECG machine is set up in such a way that it not only shows the voltage recorded by any specific electrode but also shows whether the current is flowing toward the direction or away from the specific electrode. To state this more precisely, when the direction of the activation spread is oriented toward the site of the positive electrode of a lead, the galvanometer needle in the ECG machine moves up and causes an upward or positive wave whereas when it is oriented away or opposite to that of the site of the positive electrode, it causes a downward or negative wave. When the orientation of the activation (the electric dipole) is at right angles to the positive electrode site of the ECG lead, then it will cause no net positive or negative deflection. It is therefore isoelectric like the baseline or have an equal area of positive and negative deflection on the recorded tracing (Fig. 12.6). The amplitude or the height of the wave represents the voltage and the width of the wave from the beginning to the end represents the time in duration. In other words, the angle of orientation of the lead axis in relation to the orientation of the resultant electric dipole vector at any given instant (that usually lines up along the spread of the wave of activation as mentioned earlier) will determine what is registered on the ECG, as a positive wave, negative wave or otherwise.

During repolarization also, similar electric dipoles develop as a result of the potential differences between the less repolarized cells, which are more

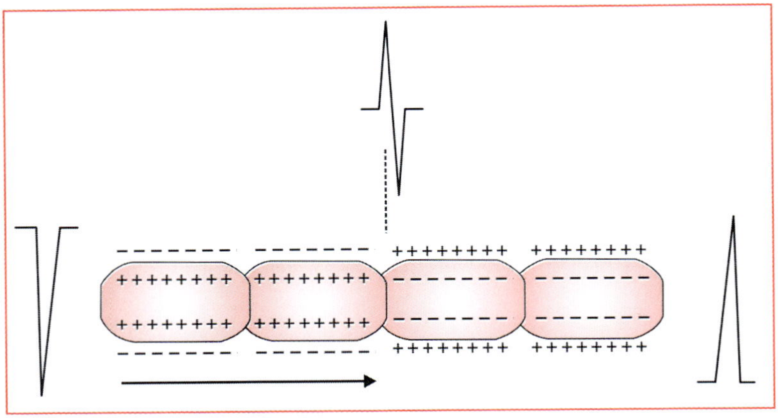

Fig. 12.6: Shows the direction of the activation spread in relation to the site of the positive electrode of an ECG machine. If the orientation of the positive electrode of the lead is toward the direction of activation spread, it will register an upward deflection. If the orientation of the positive electrode is opposite to the direction of the spread of excitation, it will register a downward (negative) deflection. If it is at right angles, it will register an equally positive and negative deflection.

negative on the outside, and the more repolarized cells, which are more positive on the outside. The orientation will be the opposite of the depolarization when studied in isolated strips of cardiac muscle fiber. The situation is somewhat different, as we shall see later with reference to the direction of the QRS complex, which represents the ventricular activation, versus the ST-T waves, which represent the ventricular repolarization in the intact normal heart.

The conduction of the electrical field produced in the heart to the surface and its effects on the ECG recorded by the electrodes on the body surface is also influenced by other factors such as the character of the intervening tissues and the physical distance of the recording site of the electrode. Thus emphysematous lungs surrounding the heart act as poor conductors of cardiac electric dipole vector oriented along the X-axis, although up and down vectors of the heart oriented vertically are unaltered. Pericardial effusion and marked obesity also tend to diminish the voltages of recorded ECG, with leads on the surface of the body.

The concept that the ECG as recorded on the surface of the body actually can be conceived of as the effect of the single resultant electric dipole vector from the heart at any given instant may probably be an oversimplification of the processes involved.[27] However, it works fairly well for practical understanding of the ECG as recorded by the traditional surface leads. Nevertheless, the effects of proximity cannot be ignored since some dipoles can only be picked up by the electrodes placed over the heart or over the precordium and not seen in the limb leads.

The Lead System Used in Electrocardiography

The basic principle involved in making diagnosis from the ECG is the ability to recognize the direction of the electrical forces not only the mean direction and preferably also the initial, the mid and the terminal forces as applied to the various parts of the ECG namely the P wave that represents the atrial depolarization, the QRS complex that is formed by the depolarization of the ventricles and the ST-T waves that represent the repolarization of the ventricles. The electrical forces and their spatial orientation, which go to form these P, QRS and ST-T waves, have specific directions in the normal hearts based on the normal anatomic and activation sequence. These will be described in detail in the following section. Prior to that, we need to understand the orientation of the traditional 12 leads that are used to record the ECG. Much of the current knowledge of making a diagnosis based on various ECG characteristics and patterns have been studied and correlated mainly to the 12 leads system, which have been in use for the last several decades. We have already discussed above how the site of the positive electrode of a lead shows the direction of the electric dipole vector and how it is related with the axis of orientation of the lead in relation to the orientation of the spread of excitation.

The next step is the understanding of the lead system that we use in the 12 leads ECG recording and interpretation. More importantly, we need to understand both directions and the orientation of the leads in the three-dimensional space of the human torso where the heart is located. *It is like learning to read a map. In order to understand the locations and directions of specific places of interest on a map, one needs to know how the directions are shown on the map. The lead system is our directions on the map. When we understand the directions they point to in the three-dimensional space, then we can figure out the directions of the different parts of the waves on the ECG. Knowing what the normal activation sequence is and how that shows itself in directions, we will be able to pick out the abnormalities in directions. This is in fact the major part of all diagnoses made from the ECG.*

Luckily we do not even need to dwell in the three-dimensional system of cardiac vector concept. The 12 leads system presents two essential planes, one set of six leads is in the frontal plane and the other set of six leads is in the horizontal plane. We can essentially stick to these two planes and learn all that needs to be learnt from the ECG for cardiac diagnosis.

The 12 leads system consists essentially of ***6 limb leads and 6 precordial leads***. The traditional ***six limb leads*** (the bipolar leads I, II, III and the augmented limb leads aVR, aVL and aVF) essentially have their main orientation ***in the frontal plane*** of the human body (the plane as one observes a standing human body by looking at it from the front). It ***gives essentially four directions*** namely *up (superior) and down (inferior) and anatomic left and right.* The six ***precordial leads*** (the unipolar V1, V2, V3, V4, V5 and V6) on the other hand give an orientation in the ***horizontal plane*** and therefore allow us *to distinguish anterior versus posterior and anterior rightward and antero-lateral.*

The Limb Leads and the Hex-axial System in the Frontal Plane

The bipolar limb leads, lead I, II and III were the first three to be developed and used. They essentially measure the potential difference between the two sites of placement of the two electrodes. The electrode placed on the right leg serves as a ground.

Lead I is a right arm and left arm lead with the positive end on the left arm. Its orientation in the frontal plane is like an X-axis in a geometric diagram with the arrow-head pointing to the left arm.

Lead II is a right arm and left foot lead with the positive end on the left foot. The orientation of this lead in the frontal plane is about 30° tilt to the left from the Y-axis and pointing down. (It is about 60° tilt from the X-axis.)

Lead III is a left arm and left foot lead with the positive end in the left foot. It has approximately 30° tilt to the right from the vertical and down.

These three leads provide three different axes of orientation in the frontal plane (Fig. 12.7A).

When the physiologists wanted more axes to study the cardiac electrical force, the engineers came up with three more leads. This time the voltage on the respective limbs were read against a central terminal (termed the central terminal of Wilson) that essentially was made to register zero voltage.[28] The latter was achieved electronically by bunching the outputs of the three limb electrodes placed on the right arm, the left arm and the left foot through a fixed resistor. The resultant potentials essentially showed zero voltage. The leads placed on the left arm, the right arm and the leg (foot) were made as the exploring (positive) electrodes. The leads were labeled VL, VR and VF, for the left arm, right arm and the leg (foot) respectively. The resultant voltage recorded turned out to be too small. In order to augment the voltage, the limb where the exploring electrode was connected, was disconnected from the central terminal electronically. For instance, when the left arm electrode was made the exploring electrode, then the left arm connection to the central terminal was disconnected. This led to augmentation of the voltage in the recorded tracings. The resultant leads were labeled as augmented VL (aVL) augmented VR (aVR) and augmented VF (aVF). The approximate axes of orientation of these three additional limb leads are shown in Figure 12.7B.

These six limb leads essentially provide six different axes in the frontal plane (Fig. 12.7C). One can actually assign the orientation by assigning them as axes in a circle. The bottom semicircle (0°-180°) starting on the anatomic left side as 0° and going clockwise, by convention is labeled as positive. The top half (the semicircle) is labeled as negative. It is easy to quickly learn the

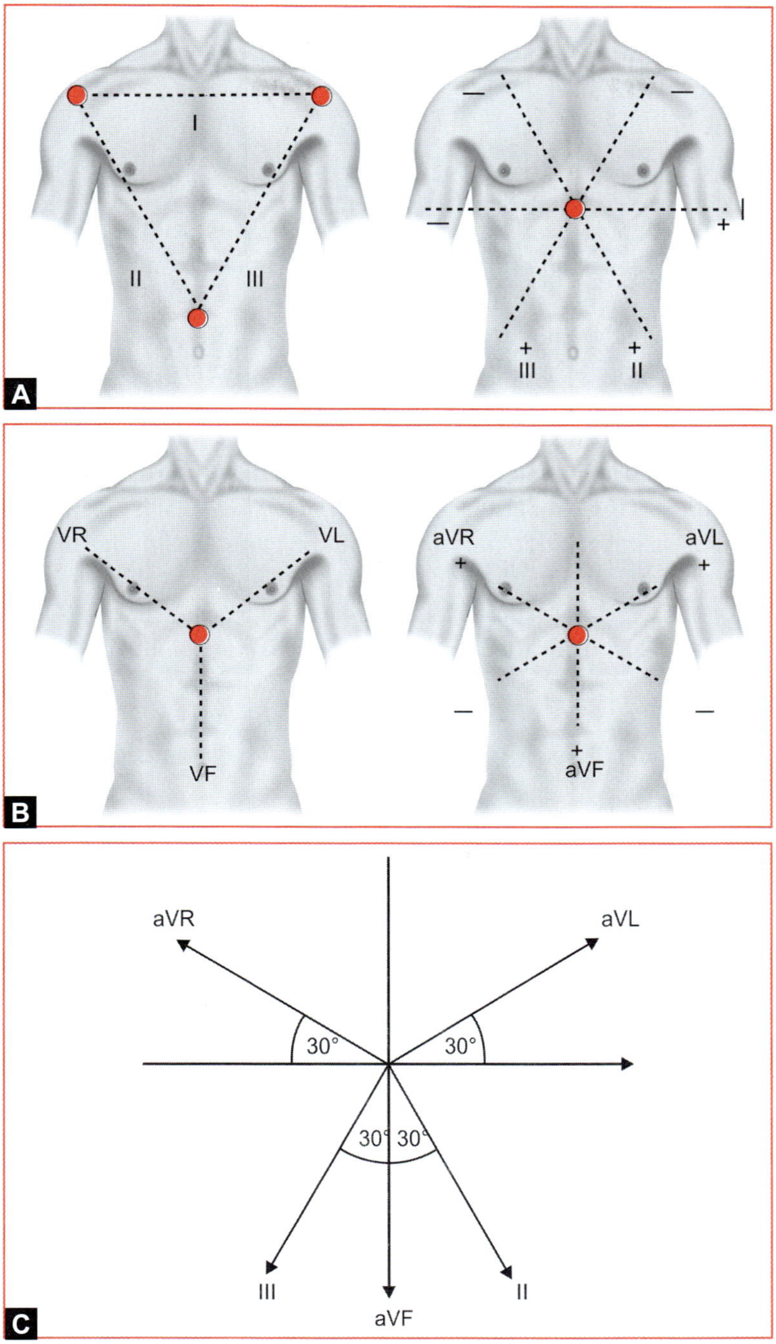

Figs. 12.7A to C: (A) Shows the directions of the three bipolar limb leads in relation to the frontal plane of the human torso. (B) Shows the directions of the augmented limb leads aVR, aVL and aVF in relation to the frontal plane of the human torso. (C) The directions of the six limb leads in the frontal plane showing the hex-axial system of reference. The arrows point toward the positive side.

axes of orientation in the frontal plane. Lead I is like the X-axis of a cross, with positive end pointing to the anatomic left arm and marks the 0°. The lead aVF is at right angles to this (+90°) and is vertical as the Y-axis of a cross. It points to the foot and therefore down anatomically. The leads II and III make about 30° tilts on either side of the vertical aVF also pointing down. The leads aVL and aVR can be thought of being at 30° tilts above the X-axis on either side of the vertical each pointing to the respective arms namely aVR to the anatomic right and aVL to the anatomic left. It is important that beginners learn to draw this hex-axial reference system diagram and label the positive side in solid line and the negative side in dotted line. The tip of the positive end should also be marked with an arrow head to indicate the direction of positivity and mark the degrees that they point to. It is simple to do and easily learned when done a few times from memory (Fig. 12.8A). It becomes obvious that the positive ends of leads ***II, III and aVF*** all point in the inferior direction in the frontal plane. So they are also called ***the inferior leads***. The positive end of lead I points laterally and to the left and can be grouped with the augmented lead aVL that also points laterally. Thus leads I and aVL are sometimes referred to as ***the lateral limb leads.*** It may be argued that aVL is probably high lateral whereas the lead I is strictly lateral. It should be also noted that each of the six limb leads (three bipolar leads I, II and III and the three modified unipolar leads aVR, aVL and aVF) has one other lead at right angles to it, namely lead I (0°) and lead aVF (+90°), lead II (+60°) and lead aVL (-30°), and lead III (+120°) and aVR (-150°).

Deducing the Direction of the Electrical Force from the Frontal Plane Leads

Since each of the six limb leads has a positive and a negative side, it should be clear that when the resultant cardiac electrical force at any instant were to point to the positive hemi-circle subtending the axis of any specific lead, it would record a positive wave. If it were to fall in any direction in the negative hemi-circle subtending the axis of the same lead, it would record a negative wave. The amplitude will depend on the angle of orientation of the cardiac electrical force at that instant in relation to the axis of the lead (Fig. 12.8B). The maximum amplitude will be seen only when the cardiac electrical force is parallel and lines up along the axis of the lead, being positive when pointing toward the positive side and being negative when pointing to the negative and the opposite side. As mentioned earlier, if the cardiac electrical force at any given instant were to be at right angles to any specific lead axis, then that lead will show only equal areas of positive and negative waves (equiphasic complex) or remain isoelectric. This can be learnt by considering the scenario of ECGs taken from two normal subjects using the six limb leads (Figs. 12.9A and B). For the purposes of understanding, we will only pay attention to the

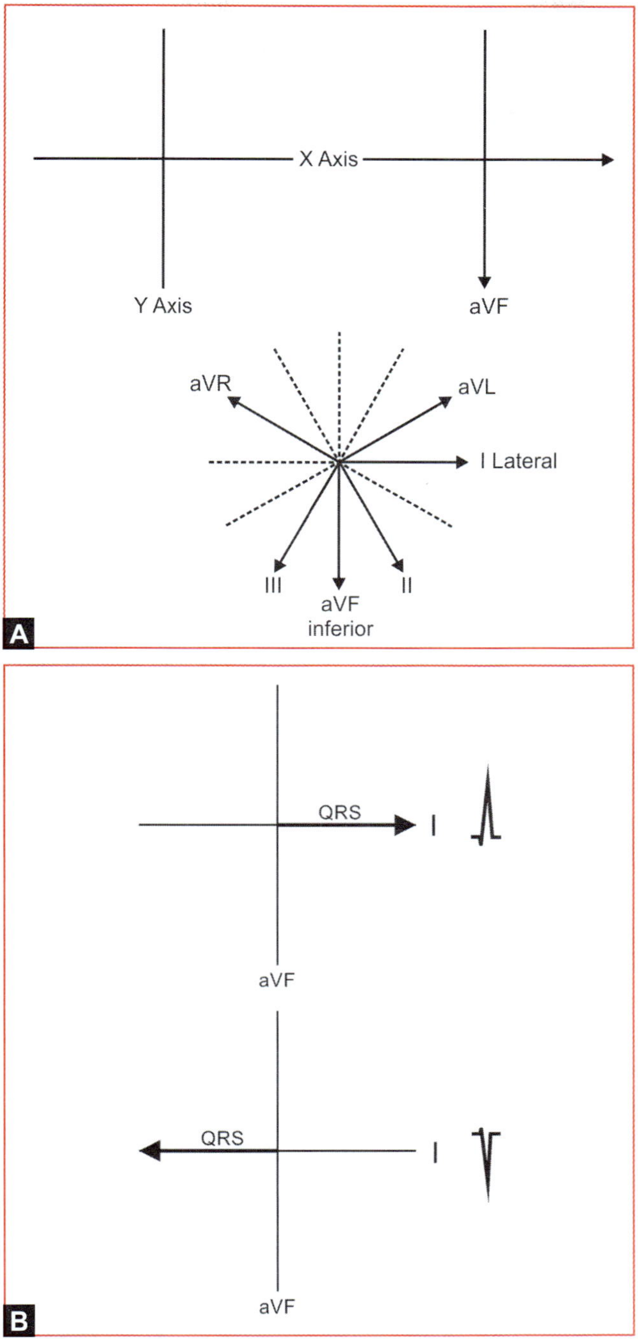

Figs. 12.8A and B: (A) Shows how to draw the six limb lead axes in the frontal plane (see the text). (B) Shows how the amplitude of the cardiac electrical force relates to the axis of the lead. The maximum amplitude is seen by lead I when the direction of the electrical force is parallel to the axis of the lead I (positive when it points toward it and negative when it points away from it).

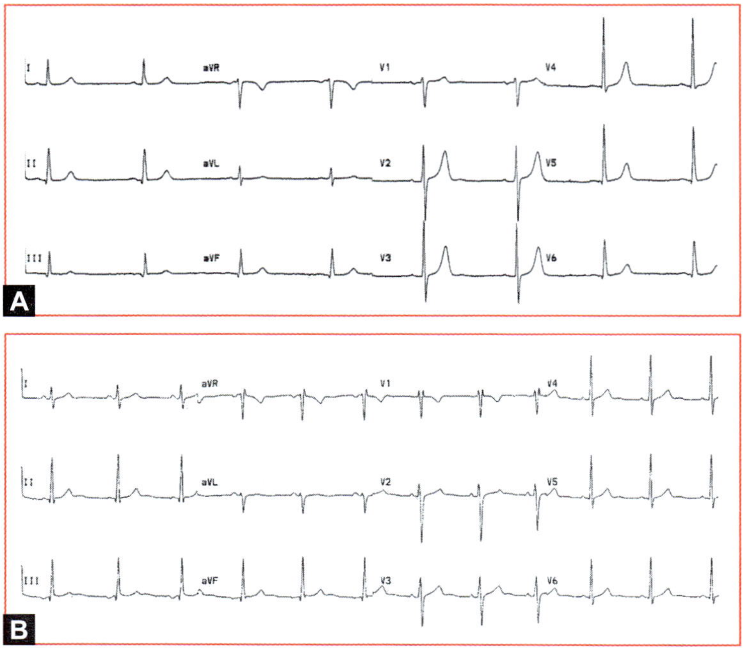

Figs. 12.9A and B: (A) Electrocardiogram from a normal young man. The mean direction of the QRS complex in the frontal plane points toward lead II being maximally positive in this lead. In this and all other ECG illustrations, the 12 leads that are normally used are as labeled. (B) Electrocardiogram from another normal subject. The mean direction of the QRS complex is toward lead aVF and is at right angles to lead I where it is equiphasic. Note the QRS shape in V1 is rSr′. This means that the terminal part of the QRS is positive in V1 indicating that the terminal part of the ventricular activation is finishing in the right ventricle (usually somewhere in the right ventricular outflow tract).

average or more precisely the mean direction of the QRS complex of the ECG in the frontal plane using the hex-axial system. In the ECG shown in Figure 12.9A, the QRS complex has the maximum positivity in lead II, this indicates that for the majority of the time, the electrical force must be lining up along the axis of lead II and pointing toward the positive side of this lead. It must therefore indicate that the mean axis of the electrical (QRS) force must be +60°. If we examine the same ECG, it will be seen that the lead aVL that is at right angles to the lead II, has a biphasic QRS with equal positive and negative areas (in other words has an ***equiphasic complex***). In the second example shown in Figure 12.9B from a different normal subject, the maximum positivity is seen in lead aVF and in lead I that is at right angles to lead aVF, the QRS complex is equiphasic. So we can visualize the mean electrical axis in the frontal plane easily by either choosing *the maximum amplitude QRS (parallel method) or by picking the equiphasic QRS complex perpendicular method.* But we must also understand that if we use the equiphasic

QRS complex method, then we will have to look at least for one more lead to identify the correct direction. This is mainly because the equally positive and negative QRS complex only tells us that the electrical force is half the time toward and half the time away from that lead. This means the mean electrical axis is at right angles to that lead axis. Since there are two possible right angle directions to any given lead axis, one will have to look at least to one more lead to pick the correct right angle. In the ECG shown in Figure 12.9A, lead II serves that purpose. It is positive and therefore the mean QRS axis in the frontal plane is +60°. In the second example (Fig. 12.9B), lead aVF shows the correct direction.

It is also important to realize that in the frontal plane we can only determine four major directions ***right, left, up and down***, the lead that critically distinguishes right and left is lead I. If any part, namely the major or the mean part of the QRS is negative in lead I, then the corresponding component of the QRS force is directed toward the right instead of the left. Later when we have gone over the normal activation sequence, the importance of this will become clear. Similarly the lead that distinguishes clearly up and down (superior versus the inferior) directions is lead aVF. If any part, namely the major or the mean part of the QRS is negative in aVF, then it will immediately show that the corresponding component of the QRS force is directed superiorly. The lead I and the lead aVF axes line up along the X and the Y axes respectively and they are at right angles to each other. They are orthogonal leads and will be shown later to be critical leads.

Later we will show how one can place the silhouette of the heart in this diagram to show the activation sequence and the resulting direction of the normal electrical forces, which are formed.

The Precordial (Unipolar) Leads in the Horizontal Plane

The precordial leads are all recorded with the unipolar exploring electrode V leads with the help of the central terminal of Wilson. The leads are placed at designated sites and labeled as V1, V2, V3, V4, V5 and V6. The six precordial electrodes are placed at the following designated sites. Lead V1 is placed in the fourth intercostal space at the right sternal border. Lead V2 is placed also in the fourth intercostal space but left of the sternal border. Leads V4, V5 and V6 are placed on the fifth left intercostal space along the mid-clavicular line, the anterior axillary and the mid-axillary lines respectively. The V3 lead is placed at a spot in between the V2 and V4. Thus, V4, V5 and V6 leads end up being all placed at the same level. One need not assign actual degrees for their respective axes in the horizontal plane. It suffices to point out that V1 lead points anterior and right of the sternum. The V5 and V6 leads point toward the left lateral part of the chest. Leads V2, V3 and V4 point strictly anterior and tend to overlap the anteroseptal and anterior wall of the left ventricle (Fig. 12.10A). Leads V4 and V5 often overlap the surface of the antero-lateral wall of the left ventricle.

Sometimes, the following terms are used when describing combinations of some of the precordial leads. The term "right precordial leads" is used with reference to leads V1 and V2. The term "mid-precordial leads" refers to the combination of V3 and V4 and the term "left precordial leads" is usually referred to the combination of leads V5 and V6.

It must be also noted that the *designated placing of these precordial electrodes by convention,* also make their orientation in any individual patient to be affected by the location of "the heart" in the chest and more importantly "***the electrical center of the heart***". The latter is defined as a point from where the ventricular activation actually begins. As will be discussed later, this usually corresponds to the upper part of the inter-ventricular septum on its left side where the left bundle begins to divide and arborize into finer branches or fibers. The location of the left precordial leads V4–V6 in some normal subjects may be low enough on the chest in relation to the heart's electrical center that they may actually pick up inferiorly directed forces. This can be easily identified by the fact that in those situations, these left chest leads will look similar to the inferior leads (II, III and aVF) of the frontal plane. When the location of these leads is not too low on the chest and therefore not lower than the electrical center, then typically the QRS complex in V5 and V6 will be similar to what one will see in lead I.

The Scale or the Grid on the ECG Output Paper

The ECG is normally recorded on a paper that has grid markings to measure the height (the amplitude in millivolts) as well as the width (the duration in seconds or ms) of the various waves produced by the depolarization and the repolarization of both the atria and the ventricles. A gain selection button allows the amplification to be adjusted to the desired level of a standard voltage signal. When the recording is done at usual normal standard each mm in height is equal to about 0.1 mv since the standard gain signal produces a signal of 10 mm height to correspond to the 1 mv signal that it produces. The ECG paper output or the display on the oscilloscope can be adjusted with regard to the speed of writing. It is normally recorded on a moving paper at 25 mm/s. It means therefore that each mm in width will correspond to about 0.04 second (or 40 ms). The beginner needs to also familiarize oneself with how a standard signal looks like when the ECG recording is turned on to write and when the standard selection button is pushed. It should produce a rectangular signal with a specific height (10 mm for the normal standard of 1 mv signal) rising and falling sharply if the recording system has acceptable and good frequency response (from 0.14 Hz to about 100 Hz) (Fig. 12.10B).[29] Machines with deterioration of the acceptable frequency response will cause the signal to drag when it falls off. It usually is not a problem with modern ink jet or laser recorders that usually have good frequency response. When one measures the duration of the various waves or the various designated intervals, these must always be measured from the beginning to the end of the particular wave or the interval.

The Language of the ECG

The terminology that is used to describe the various waves seen on an ECG must be also learned as part of learning the basics so that everyone is able to understand as well as visualize what we are talking about. The wave produced by the depolarization of the atria is referred to as the P wave. The wave produced by the depolarization of the ventricles is designated generically as the QRS complex. The waves of repolarization of the ventricles that normally follow the QRS complex are called together ST-T wave. Sometimes, further small wave may follow the T wave called the U wave. It also represents final parts of repolarization waves of the ventricles.

All waves (positive or negative) generally have amplitude (voltage) as well as duration in time. Thus they also have an area enclosed by the height and the width in mm. In addition, the QRS complex produced by the depolarization of the ventricles can take a variety of forms depending on the number of positive and negative areas (waves) that are noted in it. Since the generic term QRS complex does not express the actual shape of the QRS seen on any particular lead, special definitions are given for the individual parts of the QRS complex. The initial or the first negative area of a QRS complex is referred to as a ***Q*** wave. A first positive area of a QRS complex is referred to as an ***R*** wave. A second negative area of a QRS complex is referred to as an ***S*** wave. A second positive area of a QRS complex is referred to as ***R prime*** (***r***′). From this terminology, it follows that the QRS can be described by the waves seen in it. It can take various configurations such as the following ***qR*** (when it has a small ***q*** wave followed by a dominant ***R***), ***qRs*** (when small ***q*** and small ***s*** enclosing a dominant ***R*** in between), ***rS*** (when small ***r*** wave followed by a large ***S*** wave), ***rsR***′ (when a small ***r*** and ***s*** followed by a bigger secondary R wave called ***R***′), ***QS*** (when the entire QRS is negative) or ***R*** (just a single dominant positive ***R*** wave) (Fig. 12.10C).

The Normal Activation Sequence and the Direction of the Normal Electrical Forces

The normal activation sequence of the human heart has been studied in isolated hearts as far back as 1918.[30] The classic study in more recent years is that of Durrer and coworkers. The excitatory process was mapped in isolated human hearts supported by Langendorff perfusion apparatus using 870 intramural terminals.[31] These have demonstrated the following.

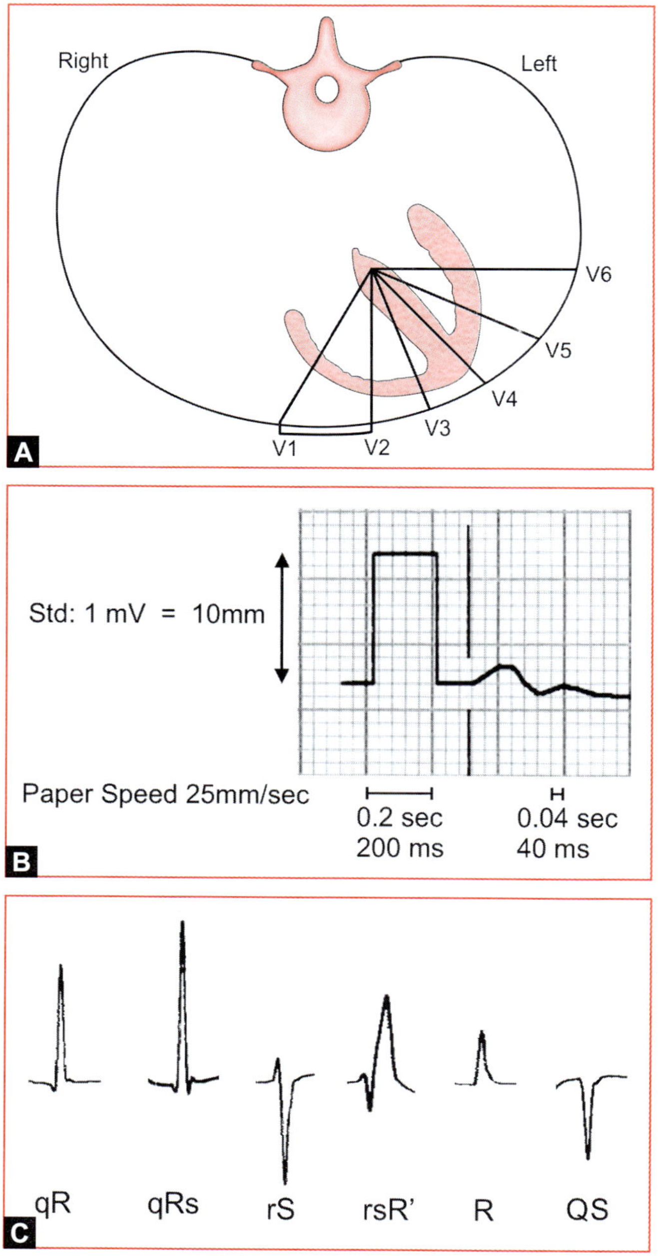

Figs. 12.10A to C: (A) Shows the directions of the unipolar precordial leads V1–V6. V1 is at the fourth intercostal space at the right sternal border. V2 is also at the same level but at the left sternal edge. V4–V6 are all in the left fifth intercostal space, with V4 at the mid-clavicular line, V5 at the anterior axillary line and V6 at the mid-axillary line. V3 is in-between V2 and V4. (B) Shows the scale or the grid of the ECG paper. The grid is marked in mm per small square. Each large square has 5 mm. The standard for amplitude is set at 10 mm equal to 1 mV. The paper speed is usually set at 25 mm/s. At this speed, each mm in width will be 0.04 second or 40 ms. (C) Shapes of different QRS complexes and their nomenclature (*see* the text).

Atrial Activation

Electrical activation appears to spread more or less according to concentric isochronic lines over the atrial surface. Their study did not point to a preferential path of conduction from the right to the left atrium.

The implication of the concentric spread of excitation from about the location of the SA node at the top of the right atrium down to the lower parts of both atria allows the electrical force resulting from the atrial activation that produces the P wave to be oriented toward the left lower quadrant in the hex-axial frontal plane reference system. That will make the SA node originated P wave to be positive in leads I, II and aVF, with the maximum positive amplitude probably in lead II. The precordial lead V1 is directly over the right atrial area being in the fourth intercostal space at the right sternal border. Anatomically the SA node being in the right atrium, the right atrium gets activated before the left atrium that happens to be the most posterior chamber in the heart. The activation toward it must necessarily have to spread in anteroposterior direction. So it is reasonable to ascribe the first part of the P wave to represent predominant right atrial activation and the second half to the left atrial activation. In fact, in many normal subjects it is not uncommon to see a biphasic P wave in lead V1, which is initially positive and terminally negative corresponding to the direction of the spread of excitation within the atria. Initial activation involves the right atrium, which is anterior and the spread is anteriorly directed and the terminal activation is of the left atrium that is posterior in location and therefore posteriorly directed away from lead V1 and is therefore negative (*see* Fig. 12.9A).

The normal P wave usually has a maximum height of 2.5 mm and duration also about 2.5 mm in width (corresponding to about 0.100 second or 100 ms).

Ventricular Activation

Three endocardial sites in the left ventricle get activated first (within 0 to 5 ms after the onset of the left ventricular activity potential) and they increase rapidly in size and become confluent within 15–20 ms. They are located on the anterior paraseptal area just below the attachment of the mitral valve, the central portion of the left surface of the inter-ventricular septum and the posterior paraseptal area. This point therefore can be considered "***the electrical center***" of the heart, from where the ventricular activation begins. The last part of the left ventricle to be activated is usually the posterobasal area. The endocardial activation of the right ventricle starts near the insertion of the anterior papillary muscle also within 0-5 ms after the onset of the left ventricular activity potential. Then rapid extension to the septum and the adjoining free wall of the right ventricle occurs. The spread of excitation

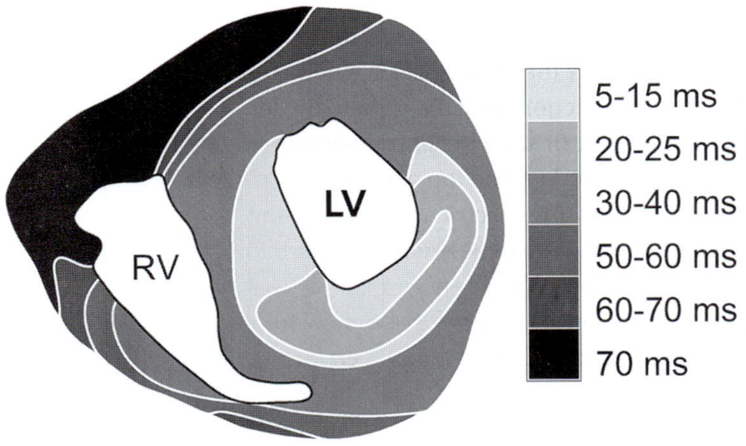

Fig. 12.11: Shows diagrammatic representation of the activation sequence of the ventricles (shown at the mid-ventricular level—cross sectional view). The diagram is adapted from the classic study of Durrer and coworkers in isolated human hearts.[31] (Copyright with permission, Wolters Kluwer Health, 2014). Earliest activation (between 5 and 25 ms) noted in the left side of the inter-ventricular septum. The later part of the activation (60 ms and over) is in the posterobasal part of the left ventricle.

reaches the pulmonary conus and the right ventricular outflow tract last. The epicardial excitation follows generally the intramural excitation fronts (Fig. 12.11). Epicardial excitation of the right ventricle occurs before the epicardial excitation of the left ventricle.

When the exploring electrode is placed directly on the surface of the heart, the spread of excitation from the endocardium to the epicardium will register increasing positivity of the electrical potential. When depolarization is completed under the exploring electrode, then the ECG stylus will return to the base line. When the final downstroke is registered it is termed ***the intrinsic deflection.*** If the exploring electrode is not directly on the heart but on the chest wall, the final downstroke is called the ***intrinsicoid*** deflection. The time taken for the electrical activation of the septum and the spread of excitation from the endocardium to the epicardium is called the ***ventricular activation time*** (Fig. 12.12A).

The total duration of the ventricular depolarization from the beginning to the end in the normal heart usually is about 0.08 second. That means normal QRS duration is about 2 mm in width from the beginning to the end. The measurement must always be made in the lead that shows clearly the beginning and the end of the QRS complex. It is important of course to consider all the leads and choose the one showing the maximum duration.

Based on the activation sequence demonstrated in the isolated human heart, one can formulate the directions of the major resultant electrical force if we divide the activation *into three parts, the initial, the mid and the terminal part of the QRS complex* (Fig. 12.12B). The initial spread of excitation is left to right of the inter-ventricular septum. Although activation of the right ventricle also begins fairly early, since the overall right ventricular wall is much thinner in the normal heart compared to the left ventricle, the left to right septal force dominates for about 20–30 ms. This will result in an initial positive deflection or ***r*** wave in the precordial leads (V1-V3) since the septal spread not only is left to right but also begins to depolarize part of the anterior wall of the left ventricle overlying the inter-ventricular septum. The early and preferential activation of the septum on the left side arises from the fact that the left bundle branch begins to arborize into Purkinje network rather high on the left of the septum as we saw earlier from the anatomic features of the His-Purkinje system. It must also be realized that the same initial force will give rise to a negative area of deflection or ***q*** wave in the left precordial leads. Since the left to right activation can either be up or down going from left to right, in the frontal plane any or all of the limb leads can show an initial negativity or ***q*** wave. It can be visualized easily from drawing various possible directions of an initial left to right force using the diagram of the hex-axial reference system (Fig. 12.12C).

During the major mid-portion of the ventricular activation sequence, the electrical force is oriented along the paths of the two divisions of the left bundle following the endocardial and the intramural course breaking through to the epicardial surface. One of the divisions is antero-superior in orientation and the other is infero-posterior in orientation. The resultant of the two will point toward the direction of the left ventricle (Fig. 12.12B). The mass of the left ventricle being larger than that of the right ventricle, again the electrical forces pointing rightward and anterior toward where the anatomic right ventricle actually is located under the sternum, get overshadowed, by the major electrical forces from the left ventricle turning the major mid-portion of the QRS complex (for about the duration of 40–50 ms) more toward the anatomic left ventricle. The leads that typically face the left ventricle directly are the left precordial leads V5 and V6. So the QRS complex in these leads will be predominantly positive. In the frontal plane the major direction will fall toward the left lower quadrant where the major part of the left ventricle is oriented anatomically.

The third and the final part of the ventricular depolarization can either be along the right ventricular outflow tract and the pulmonary conus or face toward the posterobasal area of the left ventricle. The duration of this terminal force is often short and does not extend beyond 20 ms in the normal subjects. The activation front finishing along the RV outflow tract generally tends to be seen in younger subjects. When this is the case, the terminal portion of the QRS complex will be oriented again rightward away from the left and lateral leads. This may be seen as a small terminal ***s*** wave in leads I and/or V6 and as positive small ***r'*** in V1 or as a terminal ***r*** in aVR (Fig. 12.9B).

When the posterobasal area is activated last, the resultant final force will be directed also toward the left ventricle like the mid or major portion of the QRS described above and this time also turning more posteriorly away

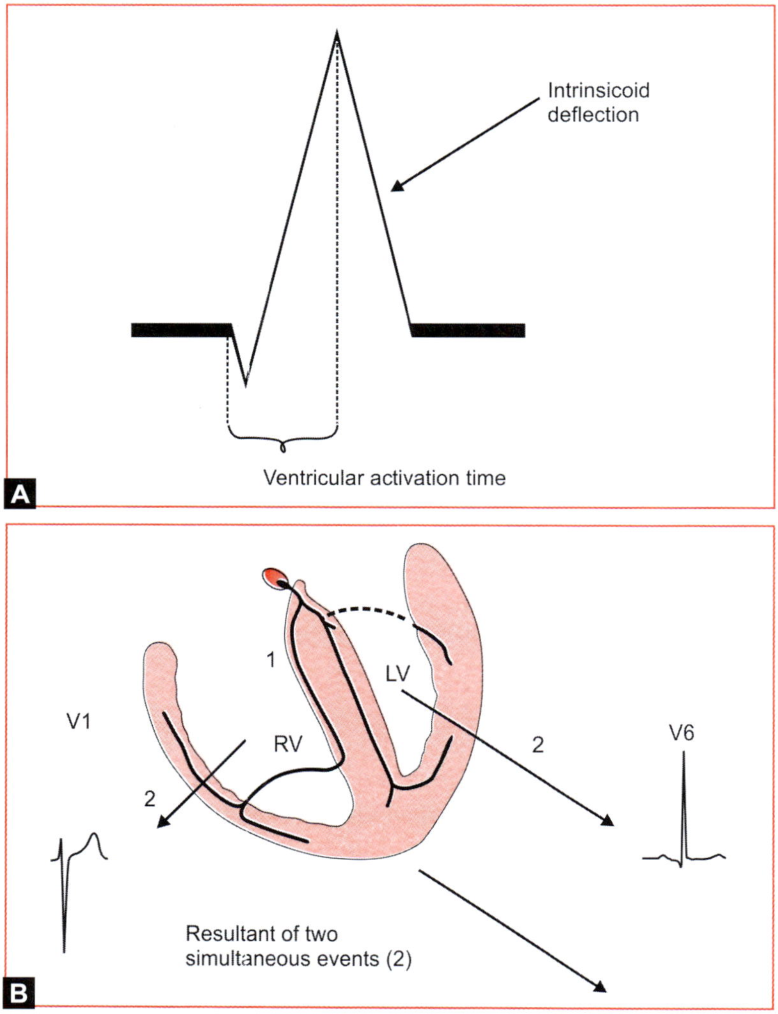

Figs. 12.12A and B: (A) Intrinsicoid deflection as it relates to the ventricular activation (*see* the text) (B) The normal sequence of activation of the ventricles and the resultant wave fronts causing the predominant directions of the QRS forces as seen by the surface leads V1 (right and anterior) and V6 (left and lateral). Arrows indicate the dominant direction of the electrical force from the ventricular activation. The early activation is dominated by left to right septal depolarization.1 (This points toward V1 and away from lead V6 making a septal r in V1 and septal q in V6). The later activation2 has two components, one from the right ventricle and the other from the left ventricle. The left ventricular (LV) mass is bigger and its electrical force is larger (thicker arrow) and therefore it dominates the resultant of these two forces. The resultant, therefore points towards the LV side (making a dominant positive QRS in V6 (R wave) and a negative QRS in V1 (S wave in V1).

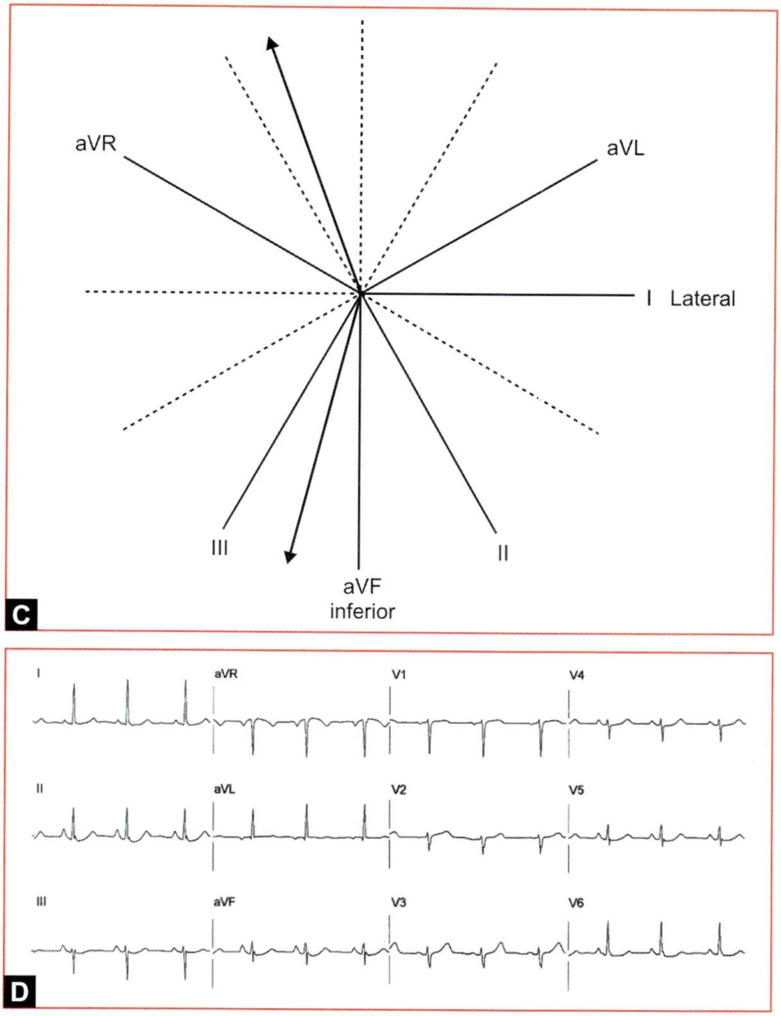

Figs. 12.12C and D: (C) The possible directions of the early left to right septal force in the frontal plane can be anywhere in the hemicircle subtending the negative side of lead I (that is a left lateral lead). Thus the early left to right septal force can result in a q wave in any of the limb leads. (D) The electrocardiogram from a normal patient showing slight ST segment depression starting immediately after the end of the QRS. Atrial repolarization wave (Ta wave) that is often buried in the QRS is suggested as the cause of this early ST segment depression.

from all the right and the mid-precordial leads becoming part of the terminal portion of the ***rS*** complex in these leads and becoming part of the terminal portions of the ***qR*** complex in V5 and/or V6.

Repolarization of the Atria

Atrial repolarization starts right after atrial depolarization and usually the wave form sometimes is referred to as the ***Ta*** wave. This period often overlaps the PR segment (the interval between the P wave and the beginning of the QRS complex) and the ventricular depolarization. The PR segment is usually supposed to be isoelectric but sometimes it is not because of the Ta wave, which can slightly distort the PR segment. It also can be buried in the QRS complex. When the PR interval is short and associated with mild sinus tachycardia, it can also distort the ST segment causing some depression of the ST segment (***J*** point) (Fig. 12.12D).

Repolarization of the Ventricles

The repolarization of the ventricles results in ST- T waves. The repolarization is in many ways different from depolarization. The process is slower and takes much longer than that of normal depolarization. It also is subject to variations in the tone of the autonomic nervous system. The ventricular depolarization is produced in the normal hearts, by the rapid spread of excitation wave through the His-Purkinje system. In the intact heart, mechanical systole takes place with rising intra-ventricular pressures at the time of electrical repolarization. The coronary flow to the sub-endocardial regions is compromised by the actively contracting myocardium squeezing the intra-myocardial branches of the coronary arteries. Although the endocardium is depolarized first, and the spread of excitation wave reaches the epicardium later, the repolarization does not start first in the endocardium because of the contracting ventricle and high intracavitary ventricular pressures and the resulting relative sub-endocardial ischemia. Therefore, it should not be surprising that the epicardium begins to repolarize first and the repolarization spreads slowly to the endocardium, when the mechanical systole has almost ended (Fig. 12.13). In addition, action potential durations are much longer in the regions near the endocardium than those near the epicardium.[32] Multiple types of voltage-gated inward and outward currents have been demonstrated in cardiac cells. The outward K^+ currents are more numerous and diverse than Na^+ and Ca^{2+} inward currents. Many myocytes also express multiple voltage gated and inwardly rectifying K^+ currents. Since repolarization is dependent on these K^+ channels, regional variations in their densities and function also appear to underlie the intramural variations in recovery.[33]

Thus the T wave, which is formed by the repolarization of the ventricles, is slowly inscribed and takes longer time to finish. By definition the T wave comes after the QRS complex. The end of the QRS can often be identified by the sharp junction point (***J*** point), where the rapidly inscribed QRS meets the slowly rising portion of the T wave. This ***J*** point begins the ST segment.

Since repolarization starts on the outer epicardium and spreads slowly to the inner layers of the myocardium and the sub-endocardium, the electric dipoles result from the differences in potentials between partly repolarized

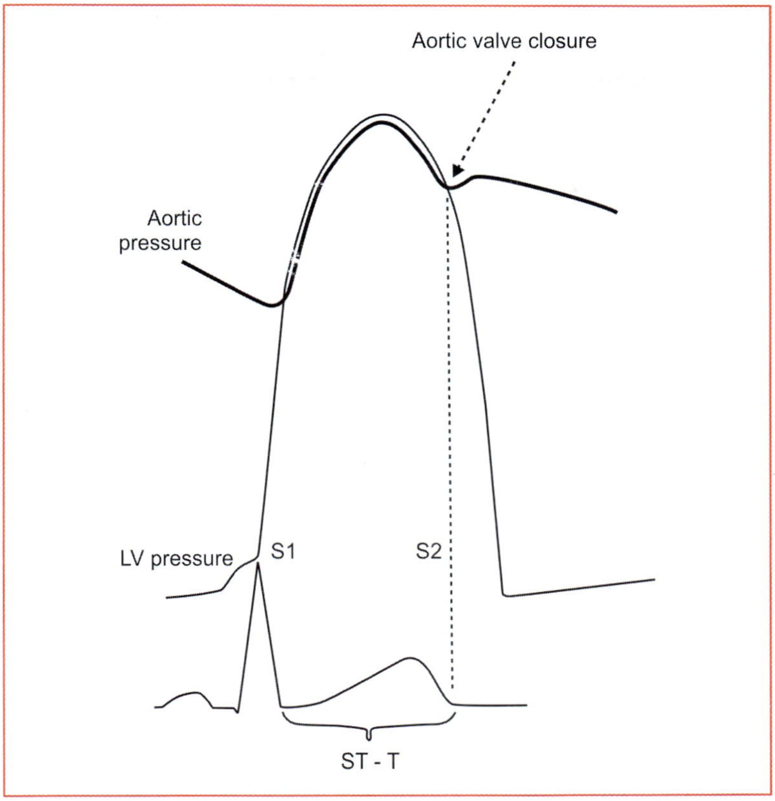

Fig. 12.13: Ventricular repolarization forming the ST segment and the T wave in the intact human heart occurs during mechanical systole as indicated in this diagram (*see* the text).

cells in the epicardium that become positive on the outside as in the resting state and the non-repolarized cells in the endocardial regions that are still negative on the outside due to the persisting depolarized state. The orientation of the electric dipole is again from negatively charged endocardium and toward the positively charged epicardium similar to what happens during depolarization. Thus the T wave points in the same direction as the QRS in the intact normal human hearts as opposed to what is seen in the isolated muscle strips where it points in the reverse direction.

We will recall here, what we have said about the direction of the major QRS electrical force in the normal hearts. The mean electrical axis of the QRS in the normal hearts points toward the anatomic left ventricle that is in the lower left quadrant in the frontal plane. This is mainly because the resultant of the major electrical forces from the simultaneous spread of excitation through the two divisions of the left bundle, depolarizing the left ventricle with a greater muscle mass overshadows the thinner right ventricle. If the electrical forces resulting from repolarization of the ventricles also line up in the same direction as that of the depolarization in the intact normal human heart, then it becomes easy to understand that the T wave in the normal hearts also points in the same direction as the QRS.

QRS-T Angle

The fact that the major and mean QRS force and the major and mean T wave force point in the same direction, means that the axes of the major or the mean QRS electrical force and that of the T wave must not be farther apart from each other. Sometime this relationship is expressed as QRS-T angle, which should be normally <+45°. Obviously, when the T wave points in the opposite direction of the QRS, this angle must become wider and obtuse. When it is almost 180° apart then it will be markedly abnormal. This can be easily visualized by looking at the QRS and the T waves in the same lead and comparing their waveforms. The leads that show maximum positivity of the QRS complex must also show the maximum positivity of the T wave. If those leads, which show maximum positivity of the QRS, were to be accompanied by low amplitude T waves, inverted or negative T waves, then, the QRS-T angle is wide and the T wave will be considered abnormal.

The Ventricular Gradient

This expresses the differences in magnitude between the net area under the QRS complex and ST-T waves. It is dependent on the normal differences in the properties of ventricular activation and recovery.[34]

If the QRS is prolonged as in a bundle branch block (BBB) due to delayed spread of activation, the repolarization also will become abnormal and delayed and cause an abnormal QRS-T angle. However, the ventricular gradient will still remain normal.[35] Since this measurement is hard to plot and time-consuming, it is not used often in electrocardiography.

The Duration of Repolarization and the QT interval

The duration of the repolarization is often expressed by the measurement of QT interval. The QT interval is measured from the onset of the QRS to the end of the T wave.[36] This interval obviously includes the duration of depolarization (QRS) as well. However, when it gets prolonged, it is usually due to prolongation of the repolarization (ST-T waves). The maximum measurement noted is often corrected for the heart rate since repolarization tends to be longer when frequency or the rate of ventricular activation per minute is slower. It is shorter when the heart rate is fast. It also varies slightly depending on the gender as well, being longer in females. The rate corrected QT interval is called the QTc. For the rate correction, the observed QT interval is divided by the square root of the RR interval (Bazett formula).[37] The normal QTc is accepted as equal to or <440 ms.

It can be shown that the duration of the action potential essentially is a function of the recovery period of the cell to regain its resting membrane potential. It actually relates to the frequency of excitation in isolated myocardial cells. When the frequency of excitation is high as in tachycardia or faster heart rates, the action potential duration becomes shorter. When the frequency of excitation is slower (as in bradycardia), the action potential duration becomes longer. The reason for this is that the His-Purkinje system recovers quickly in general and is able to receive another excitation wave as soon as the voltage is recovered back to its normal level. In other words its refractoriness to the next wave of excitation is voltage-dependent. This is termed as voltage-dependent recovery. This can be also shown in the intact hearts by stimulating the ventricle through an electrode catheter placed in the right ventricle. The ventricle can be stimulated to have a 1:1 response even when stimulated directly to a rate of 300/min. The normal AV node offers protection to the ventricles from being stimulated to rapid heart rates. Atrioventricular node responds differently electrophysiologically. Atrioventricular node is usually refractory and will not respond to repeat stimulation even when it has recovered its resting membrane potential until certain time elapses. Its refractory period or recovery is time-dependent and not voltage-dependent. In other words, the His-Purkinje system has voltage-dependent recovery whereas the AV node exhibits time-dependent recovery.[38]

The QT interval not only varies with rate, it also becomes subject to autonomic tone. Sympathetic stimulation lengthens the QT interval and delays recovery and prolongs the T wave duration. In general, normal QT interval is usually <50% of the RR interval. RR interval is measured from the onset of a QRS to the next QRS onset. This interval expresses the rate. If the ECG paper is run at a paper speed of 25 mm/s interval, then using the grid of the ECG paper, one can calculate the heart rate. Since every fifth grid lines are slightly thicker and darker, one can quickly count the number of large squares between two successive QRS complexes and divide 300 by that number to get the approximate heart rate (beats/min). If one counts all of the small squares of the distance between two successive QRS complexes, then 1,500 needs to be divided by the number in mm to get the accurate heart rate. For instance, if the RR interval is roughly four large squares, then the rate will be 75/min. Expressing the same interval as 20 small squares (mm), then dividing 1,500 by 20, one also gets the same rate of 75/min (Fig. 12.14).

It has been shown that the QT interval also tends to vary between the different ECG leads. In normal subjects, this variation may be as high as 50 ms. This has been termed ***QT interval dispersion.***[39] It is thought that the greater the difference between the maximum and the minimum

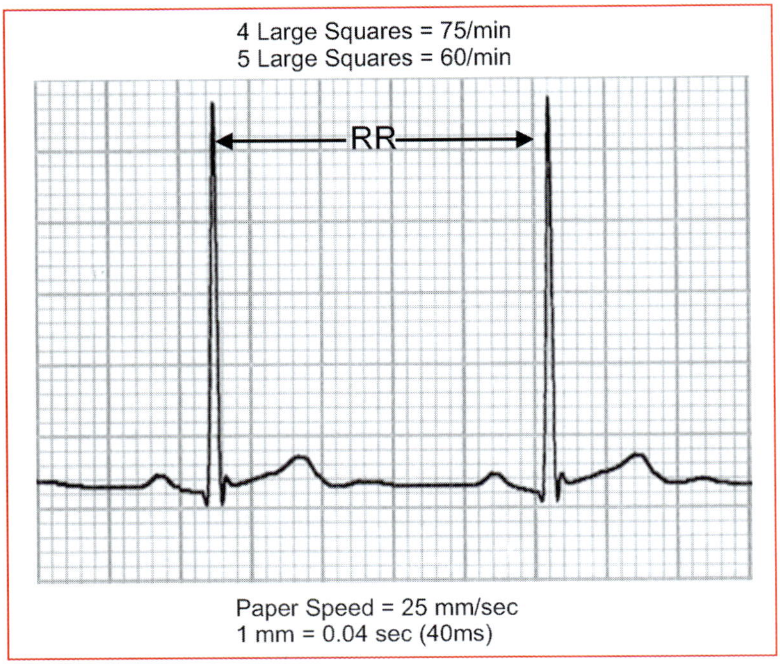

Fig. 12.14: Electrocardiogram scale and grid. The heart rates can be calculated from the duration of the R-R interval knowing the paper speed (normally set at 25 mm/s) (*see* the text).

measured QT interval, the greater is the variations in myocardial repolarization. This may have some importance in acute ischemic syndromes and infarction.

The ECG of Normal Patients

From the foregoing sections, we can summarize the features of the ECG of the normal subject. In the fontal plane, the mean and the major direction of the P wave, the QRS as well as the T waves fall in the lower left quadrant. The left lower quadrant in the frontal plane in the hex-axial reference system points to the anatomic left ventricle in the normal subject. It encompasses the axis of lead I (that marks +0°) and the axis of lead aVF (that marks +90°). This means the following, namely the P wave in normal sinus rhythm is usually positive in the leads that are encompassed by these two axes. So are the QRS and the T waves.

The QRS complex across the precordium will progress from being predominantly negative in the right precordial leads (V1 and V2), to more and more positive going toward the left precordial leads (V5 and V6) that face the left ventricle normally. The left precordial leads will therefore show dominant R waves. The precordial leads will show a progression in the relative heights of the ***r*** wave versus the ***S*** wave. This can be expressed also as

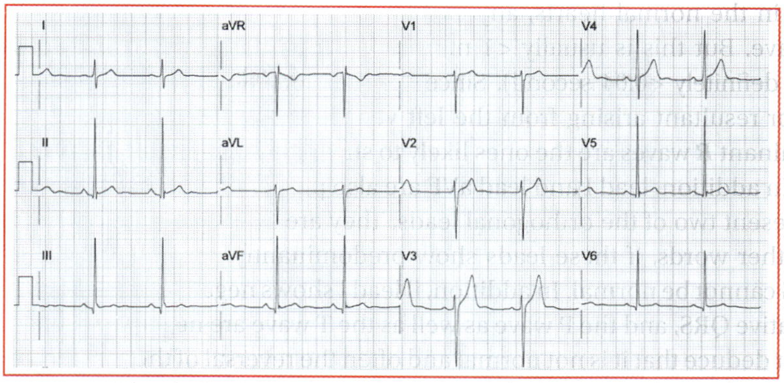

Fig. 12.15: Electrocardiogram from a normal subject who is somewhat lean and tall. In the frontal plane limb leads, the major QRS force is equiphasic in lead I making the mean direction almost vertical pointing toward lead aVF (+90o). The P wave and the T wave directions are also similar and positive in leads II and aVF. The initial septal force shows itself as a small q wave in leads II, III and aVF. Precordial leads show a septal r wave in V1 and a septal q wave in V6. The QRS progresses from a predominantly negative complex in V1–V3 to a predominantly positive QRS in V4–V6. This shows a normal r/s progression.

follows. There is a normal progression of the ***r/S*** ratio across the precordial leads such that the ratio increases across the precordium going from right to left. Also as mentioned earlier, the leads that show dominant ***R*** waves must also show upright T waves if the T waves are normal since the T wave direction follows that of the QRS. It usually means that the T waves are generally upright in the mid and the left precordial leads that show dominant R waves. They may be inverted (negative) in the right precordial leads (V1 and V2).

Since the initial force is caused by the septal depolarization from left to right lasting no more than 30 ms and the major force is right to left toward the left ventricle in the normal hearts, one can expect the initial force to show itself as a small ***q*** wave in leads that show predominant ***R*** waves in the precordium. This generally means leads V5 and V6 may show the septal ***q*** waves, but in some individuals it can extend up to V4. It must be realized that in the right precordial leads, the same septal force will show itself as small initial ***r*** wave (Fig. 12.15).

In the frontal plane, lead I shows the X-axis direction and separates the left from the right. The lead aVF shows the vertical Y-axis direction and separates the superior from the inferior. The left to right normal septal force as mentioned earlier points toward the negative limb of lead I. This means that it can be directed in any direction within the hemicircle (of 180°) subtending the negative limb of lead I. It can be left to right and upward pointing toward the right shoulder (toward the axis of lead aVR) or left to right and pointing inferior toward the axis of lead III. It means therefore that in the normal hearts, any and all of the limb leads may show a small ***q*** wave. But this is usually < 1 mm in width (usually 20-30 ms in duration and definitely < 0.04 second). Since the initial septal force is opposite to the major resultant arising from the left ventricular walls, the leads that show dominant ***R*** waves are the ones likely to show the small initial ***q*** wave.

In addition, lead I and lead aVF are also perpendicular to each other and represent two of the orthogonal leads. They are also called the critical leads. In other words, if these leads show predominantly negative QRS, then the ECG cannot be normal. In addition, if lead I shows negative or predominantly negative QRS, and the P wave as well as the T wave are negative in lead I, one must deduce that it is not normal and often the reversal of the arm lead placement is the main cause of all the waves being negative in lead I. This is not an uncommon technical error (Figs. 12.16A and B).

The Effect of Age and Body Habitus on the Normal ECG

Left ventricle is the dominant chamber in the normal adult and therefore it determines mainly the features of the ECG in the normal adults. In infants and young children, the right ventricle may still be somewhat thicker relative to the thickness of the left ventricular walls. Therefore, it may contribute to some of the features of the normal ECG in these young and normal subjects. The relatively dominant right ventricle in the infants and young children may be therefore associated with increased height of the ***r*** waves in the right precordial leads. The right precordial leads may also show inverted ***T*** waves. The T wave inversion may sometimes extend to the mid-precordial leads, which is usually not the case in the normal adults (Fig. 12.17).

The orientation of the heart in the human torso also can be somewhat affected by the body habitus of the patient. This may also show itself in the normal variations in the mean electrical axis of the QRS. The short and stocky individuals with big abdomen tend to have a raised diaphragm and more horizontal orientation of the heart. The anatomic orientation is such that the mean electrical axis of the QRS in these otherwise normal subjects will be more close to being leftward close to or around +0° (Fig. 12.18). This will be in contrast to the tall and lanky subjects who tend to have a lower diaphragm. The anatomic orientation of the heart in these otherwise normal subjects is more vertical. Therefore, their mean electrical axis of the QRS is usually vertical or rightward close to and around +90° (*see* Fig. 12.15).

Review Exercise

We shall end this section with ECGs from the same patient taken at two different times as an exercise in determining and describing the directions of the mean QRS and the T waves as well as the directions of the initial and the terminal forces of the QRS in each in the frontal plane leads as well as in the precordial leads, namely the horizontal plane (Fig. 12.19). The first ECG is

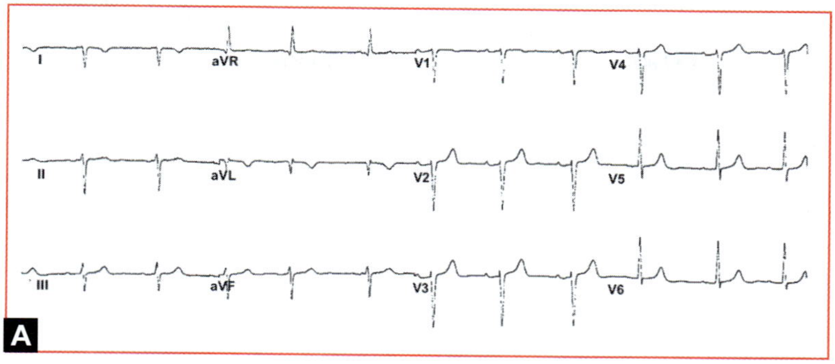

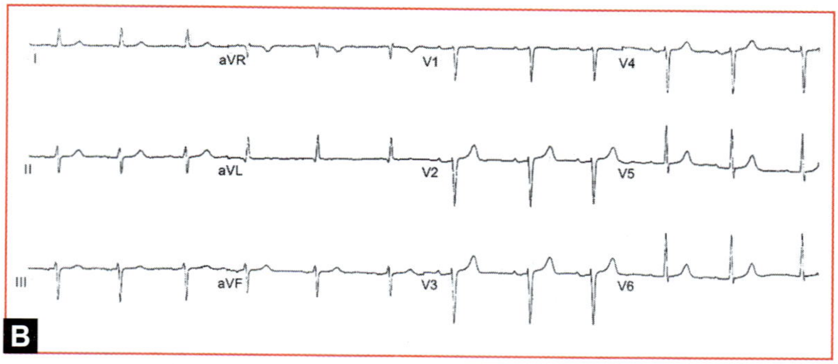

Figs. 12.16A and B: (A) Both electrocardiograms are from the same patient (normal subject). (A) Recording from the patient with the right arm and left arm limb lead reversal. (B) is with normal placement of the limb and the precordial electrodes. The major direction of the QRS force is at right angles to lead II and point toward lead aVL. Note that the precordial leads are similar in both the tracings and show normal r/s progression from V1 to V6. Note P, QRS and T waves all become negative in lead with the right arm and the left arm lead reversal.

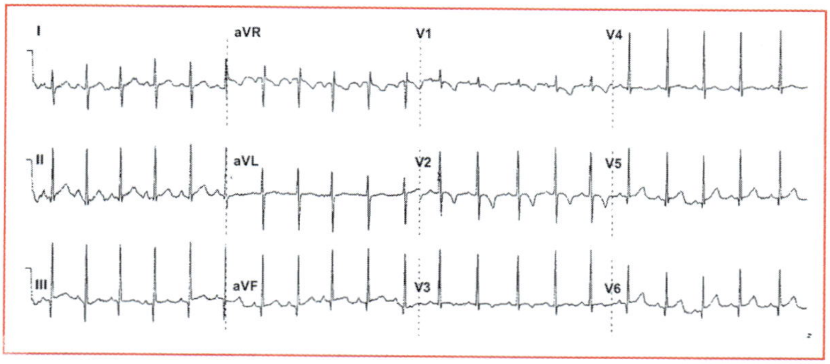

Fig. 12.17: Electrocardiogram from an infant. Note there is a mild sinus tachycardia. The QRS complexes are predominantly positive in V1–V3 with negative T waves.

taken at rest. The second one is taken from the same patient after a short duration of exercise on the treadmill marked under "Peak". The aim here is not only to describe the features but also to conclude from them whether they are normal or abnormal and if abnormal what are the abnormalities.

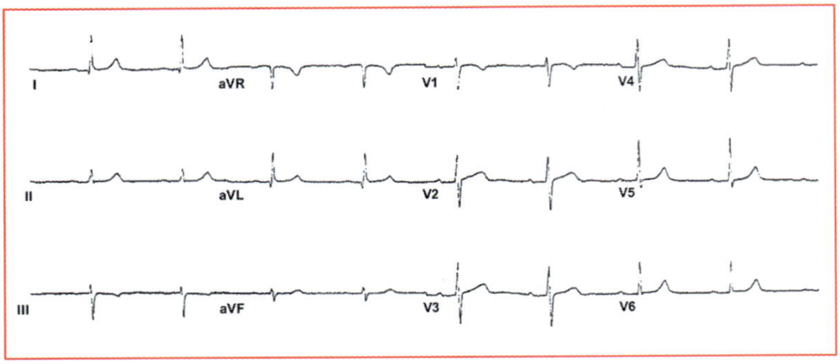

Fig. 12.18: Electrocardiogram from a short and stocky subject who is otherwise normal. The mean QRS axis is close to 0° being equiphasic in aVF.

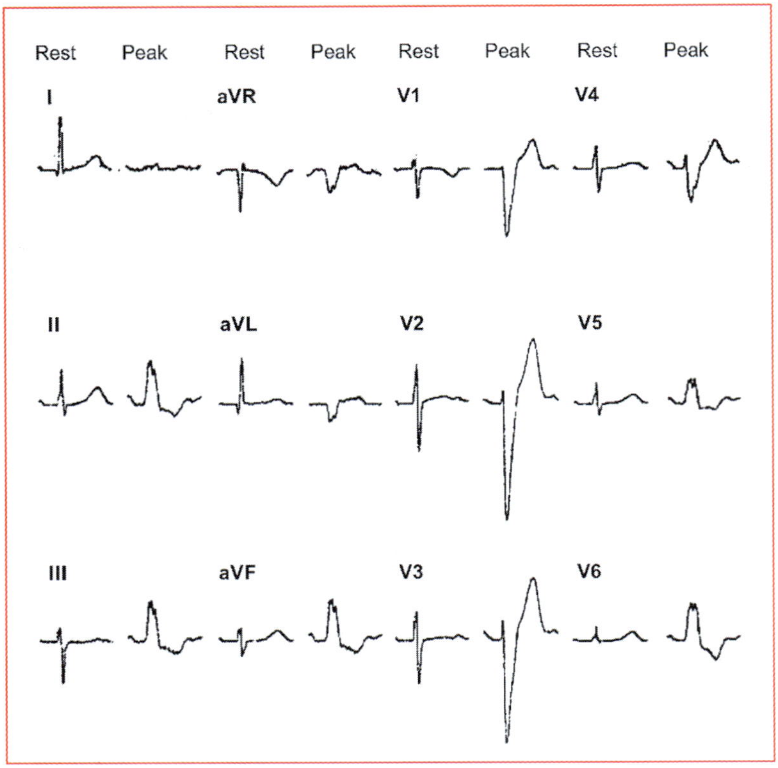

Fig. 12.19: Electrocardiogram (ECG) from a 54-year-old man who is relatively well with mild controlled hypertension. Electrocardiograms both at rest and on exercise (marked as "Peak") are shown next to each other in the respective leads. The resting ECG shows equiphasic QRS in aVF with dominant R in lead I. The T waves also point in the same direction as the QRS. There is normal r/s progression in the precordial leads. With exercise, the QRS complex is wide. The widened QRS is from a left bundle branch block that this patient develops with exercise. The septal q noted in leads I and aVL are not noted in the exercise tracing. In the precordial leads the QRS is all negative in lead V1 and all positive in V6 during the exercise tracing (with the widened QRS). In addition, in the exercise tracing the T waves are pointing away from the major direction of the QRS (compare V1 and V6).

Let us describe these first in the resting ECG. The first observation one can make is that the QRS width is normal at rest. The resting ECG shows an equiphasic complex in aVF thereby showing the mean direction of the QRS to be at right angles to aVF. That will put the mean direction to be still normal pointing to about 0°. The initial QRS force is left to right as shown by a small "***q***" wave in leads I and aVL. The terminal QRS force points toward lead I making the tall R wave in that lead. The T waves are upright and maximally tall in lead II making the direction toward lead II that is about 60° (that is also normal). Please note also that the leads with predominantly upright QRS forces also have upright T waves showing that the QRS-T angle is normal. In the precordial leads, the initial part of the QRS is upright in lead V1 with a small "***r***" wave showing the normal direction of the initial septal force. The QRS progression across the precordial leads is also normal as shown by progressive increase in the ***r/s*** ratio. Please note that it is important that one looks at the progression of this ratio from V1 to V6. Since normal LV dominates the QRS forces, there should be a normal progression of this ratio as one moves from V1 to V6. In this patient's resting ECG, this progression is noted clearly, although the actual amplitude of the R wave appears to diminish comparing V5–V6. However, the ratio is higher in V6 that has no "***s***" wave whereas V5 does. Also, the T wave direction follows the QRS being upright in V5 and V6. In both of these leads the QRS is predominantly positive. One can conclude that the resting ECG is relatively normal.

The second ECG displayed under "Peak" refers to what happened on exercise in the same patient. The first obvious thing one will note is that the QRS width is definitely wider than normal probably occupying three small divisions. This will make the ECG abnormal by itself. It will be shown in the next section that it is characteristic of a BBB. One will also note that the QRS is all positive and tall as well as wide in lead II making the mean direction still in the normal range. One can also note that the initial and the terminal forces also point in the same direction. One cannot detect any sign of the initial left to right septal force or small "***q***" wave. This is also confirmed by the precordial leads that show no initial small "***r***" wave in V1 and no "***q***" wave in V6. The ventricular activation is all proceeding from left to right in one direction as shown by all negative QRS in V1 and all positive QRS in V6. Also, both in the limb leads as well as in the precordial leads, the T waves are negative following predominantly positive QRS complexes. But they are positive following predominantly negative QRS complexes. This will be appreciated if one compares the QRS and the T waves in V2 to those in V6.

The conclusion one can draw is that in this patient the ECG has become abnormal with exercise. The abnormalities include increase in duration of the QRS and absence of the initial left to right septal force. The ventricular activation is all proceeding in one direction and appears to go from right to left. Finally, the repolarization is abnormal and points to the opposite direction of the depolarization. In the next section, it will become obvious that these changes are those that are typically caused by "Left Bundle Branch Block (LBBB)".

SECTION II: AXIS DEVIATIONS AND INTRA-VENTRICULAR CONDUCTION DEFECTS

Determination of Mean Axes and Direction of Normal Axes

Axis can be determined for all waves of the ECG, namely P wave, the QRS and the T wave. The direction of the P wave and the T wave were dealt with in Section I of this Chapter. We will discuss now in detail about the QRS axis normal and abnormal, how to define deviations and identify the causes.

Although the sequence of the normal ventricular depolarization wave fronts has been fully characterized and explained in the previous section,[31] for the purpose of making it easy to understand a simplified method will be used here. In the ventricles, depolarization occurs from the endocardium to the epicardium. Usually the electromotive forces of the waves of depolarization going in opposite directions in opposite walls of the left ventricle cancel each other and the main direction of depolarization therefore goes from base to apex. Therefore, the mean vector of the left ventricle will go in the direction of the position of the left ventricle, which is to the left and down (Fig. 12.20). Similarly, the right ventricular mean vector will be in the direction of where the right ventricle is anatomically located toward the right and under the sternum anteriorly. In a normal intact heart, the right ventricular forces are much smaller compared to the left ventricular forces, because of the marked difference in their respective muscle masses. Since both ventricles depolarize simultaneously, the left ventricular events overshadow

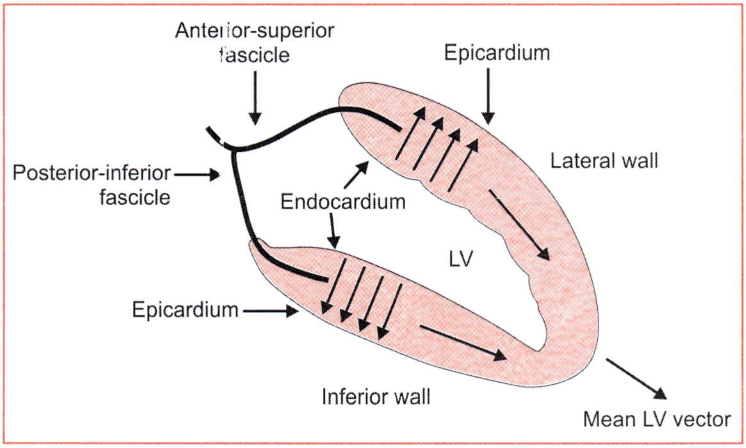

Fig. 12.20: Diagram showing the normal depolarization of the left ventricular (LV) walls from the endocardium to the epicardium through the two fascicles of the left bundle. The mean LV electrical force points toward the lower left quadrant.

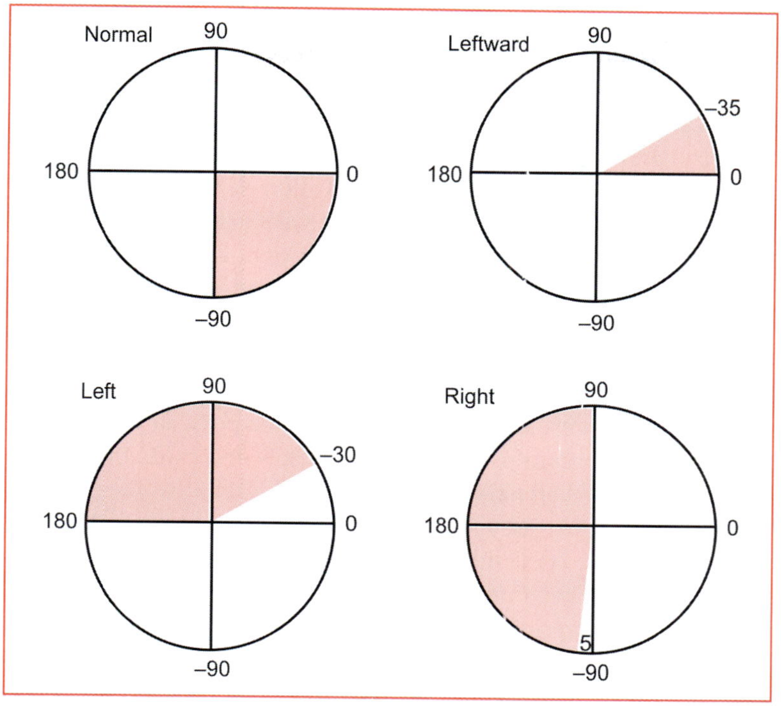

Fig. 12.21: Diagram showing the ranges for the mean QRS axis. Normal and leftward axes are shown at the top half. Left axis deviation and right axis deviation are shown in the bottom half.

any right ventricular forces. Hence, the mean electrical axis of the total heart is mainly driven by the left ventricle and will point to the left lower quadrant (*see* Fig. 12.12B). This means that the QRS will be positive in leads I and aVF. From the hex-axial system previously described, direction of lead I is 0° and the direction of lead aVF is +90°. The normal QRS axis may be anywhere between 0° and +95°-+100° (Fig. 12.21). This depends mostly on the patient's body habitus and age as discussed previously.

Axis Deviations of the QRS

Any deviation of the mean QRS axis from the normal is considered abnormal, and requires determination of the cause. An axis that is between 0° and -30° is called ***leftward axis***. Most of the time, the cause is not clear. Any axis that is superior and to the left, ≥-30° (-30° to -90°) is considered as ***left axis deviation*** (LAD). In both LAD as well as ***leftward axis***, the QRS would be in the left upper quadrant. In both cases, the QRS would be positive in lead I, and negative in lead aVF. To differentiate between the two, one needs to look at lead II with a direction of +60°. In ***leftward axis***, the QRS would still be positive in lead II, whereas in LAD it would be negative in lead II. If lead II is equiphasic (meaning isoelectric), then the axis must be perpendicular to lead II, and therefore toward -30° pointing directly at aVL.

Any axis deviation to the right of +110° (between +110° and +180°) is considered as showing ***right axis deviation*** (RAD). In this case, the QRS would be in the right lower quadrant and it will be therefore negative in lead I and will be positive in lead aVF as well as lead III. Terms such as "no man's land", "extreme right axis", "extreme left axis" are sometimes used to describe that the axis is in the right upper quadrant (between -90° and 180°). We prefer however the following approach. When the QRS axis is in the right upper quadrant, one should look for causes of both right and left axis deviations occurring simultaneously. While this might sound confusing, the logic is as follows. The leftmost axis is 0° that is considered to be a normal axis. Any deviation from 0° is deviation toward the right. What we call left axis deviations is a misnomer. What we really mean to say is "Superior axis deviation". When we think this way then it becomes very much possible to have simultaneous right axis deviations as well as superior axis deviation. But by convention we use the term "***Left axis deviation***" (Fig. 12.21).

Most often textbooks list causes of axis deviations but generally fail to describe the purpose of determining the QRS axis. The purpose of determining the axis as far as the beginners are concerned is to be able to diagnose the "hemi-blocks" [left anterior fascicular block (LAFB) and left posterior fascicular block (LPFB)]. It is true that other conditions also cause axis deviations. In reality, we do not need the axis to make the diagnosis of these conditions. It is important to know all the major causes of axis deviation, because, the diagnosis of the hemi-blocks, which is the purpose of the whole exercise, is made by eliminating the other causes.

Left Axis Deviation

As mentioned above, axis deviation to the superior direction in the hex-axial system to >-30° represents LAD. The purpose of this is to know whether the patient has ***LAFB or hemi-block***. The WHO/ISCF taskforce had specified an axis of -45° to -90° for the diagnosis of LAFB.[40] However, an axis of -30° or more would probably suffice since it will be enough to show the superior orientation. However, different degrees of the conduction disturbance can be clearly observed in patients with intermittent LAFB. Progressive degrees of left axis deviation (superior axis orientation) can sometimes be observed in the same patients bringing the concept of complete or incomplete LAFB. It is more than likely that axis deviation beyond -45° would probably mean more complete involvement of conduction block through the anterior fascicle and lesser degrees of left axis deviation might actually be due to an incomplete involvement.

In adults, four important causes of LAD should be considered as follows:

i. Left anterior fascicular or hemi-block
ii. Inferior infarction
iii. Chronic obstructive pulmonary disease (COPD)
iv. Wolf-Parkinson-White pre-excitation (WPW)

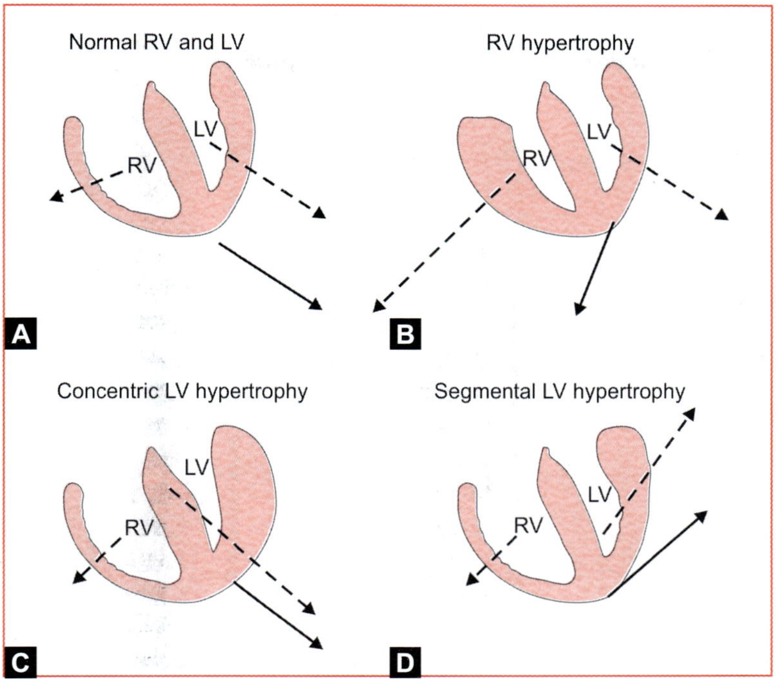

Figs. 12.22A to D: Diagram showing the resultant direction of the QRS force (shown by solid arrow) in the normals (A), in the presence of right ventricular hypertrophy (B), in concentric left ventricular hypertrophy (C) and in segmental LV hypertrophy involving the upper antero-lateral wall (D).

It is very common to see a longer list in some textbooks. Often included in this list is "left ventricular hypertrophy" that requires some comments. It is true that right ventricular hypertrophy (RVH) can cause right axis deviation, but LVH by itself should not cause left axis deviation. But LAD is sometimes associated in patients with LVH as well as many patients with LVH do not have signs of LAD. In RVH, the rightward forces are increased due to increased muscle mass of the right ventricle. The left ventricle can no longer overshadow the rightventricular forces and the axis gradually shifts toward the right, as the RVH gets worse (Figs. 12.22A to D). But in LVH the same cannot occur. The forces may go somewhat leftward and turn posteriorly in the horizontal plane since LV is to the left in the frontal plane but also a posterior chamber. But the leftward forces are usually not enough to put the axis in the left upper quadrant. The left ventricle, although very thick, is still in the same location. The voltage will increase markedly but still in the normal direction (Fig. 12.23).

However, long-standing LVH can be associated with fibrosis that can sometimes involve the anterior fascicle. In these patients LAD will be present. Theoretically marked localized hypertrophy of the antero-lateral wall could shift the axis superiorly but this is not a common finding even in patients

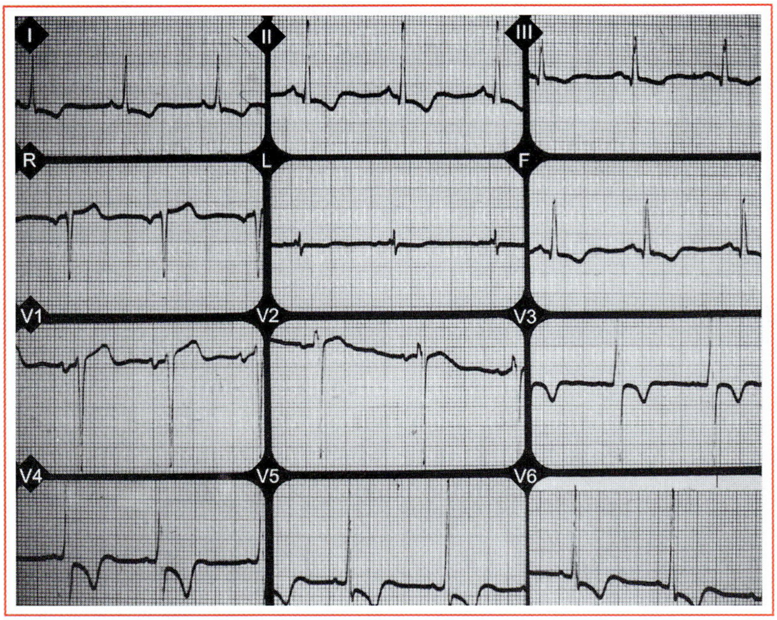

Fig. 12.23: Electrocardiogram showing left ventricular hypertrophy with voltage and strain pattern of ST-T waves as well as P wave with features of left atrial overload. The mean QRS axis is within normal range.

with hypertrophic cardiomyopathy (HCM) who invariably show concomitant marked septal hypertrophy, which is often the characteristic finding in this disorder (Fig. 12.22D).

The diagnosis of the fascicular blocks can be made by eliminating other causes of axis shift. We do not require the axis to make these other diagnoses.

The LAD associated with inferior infarct is caused by abnormally wide and/or deep ***Q*** wave. This is relatively easy to recognize. As mentioned above, the ventricular depolarization spreads endocardium to the epicardium. When there is an inferior infarct, the muscle mass inferiorly is reduced; hence, the electrical forces spreading upward are no longer balanced by equal forces going down. Therefore, the initial forces will be superiorly directed. If the infarct is large enough most of the forces may be superiorly directed giving rise to only a deep ***Q*** wave in the inferior leads (Figs. 12.24A and B). This presents a totally different picture than the LAD of ***LAFB***, where the axis shift is due to an ***S*** wave and not a ***Q*** wave. The anterior fascicle is also the superior fascicle, therefore when it is blocked the initial depolarization will be through the inferior division of the left bundle spreading in the inferior wall from the endocardium to the epicardium. This will result in an initial force, which is directed downward causing an initial ***r*** wave in the inferior leads. The wave front will then swing upward in the latter half of the ventricular depolarization (the second or the terminal part of the QRS) resulting in

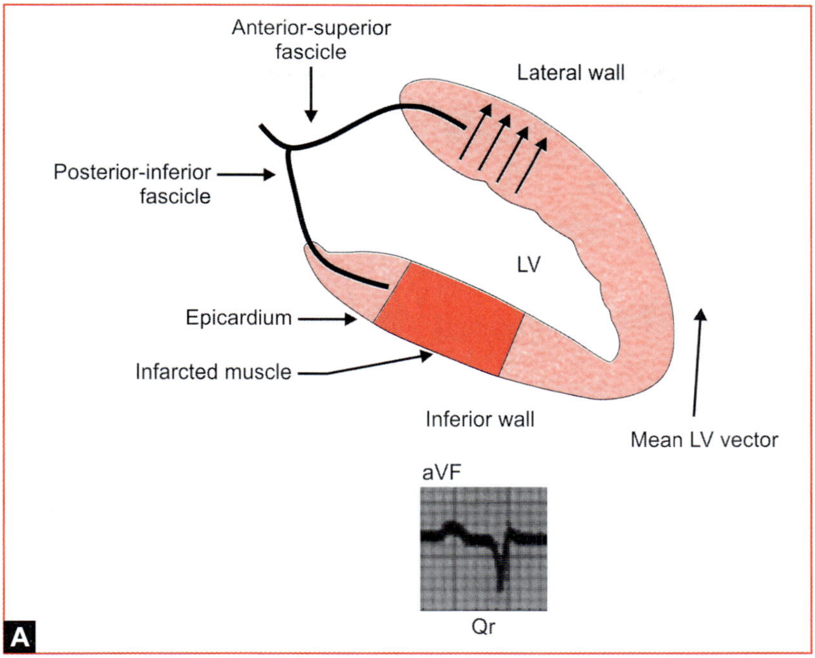

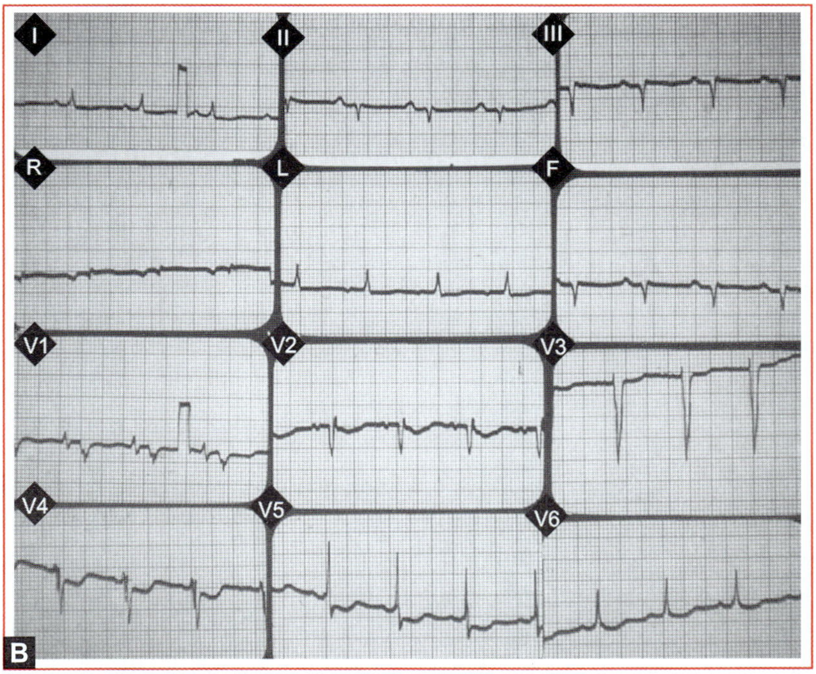

Figs. 12.24A and B: (A) Diagram showing the unbalancing of the opposing forces from the inferior and the lateral wall of the LV in inferior infarct resulting in superior orientation of the initial force and the Q waves in the inferior leads. Electrocardiogram with left axis deviation as a result of an inferior infarct with deep Q waves in the inferior leads is shown in (B).

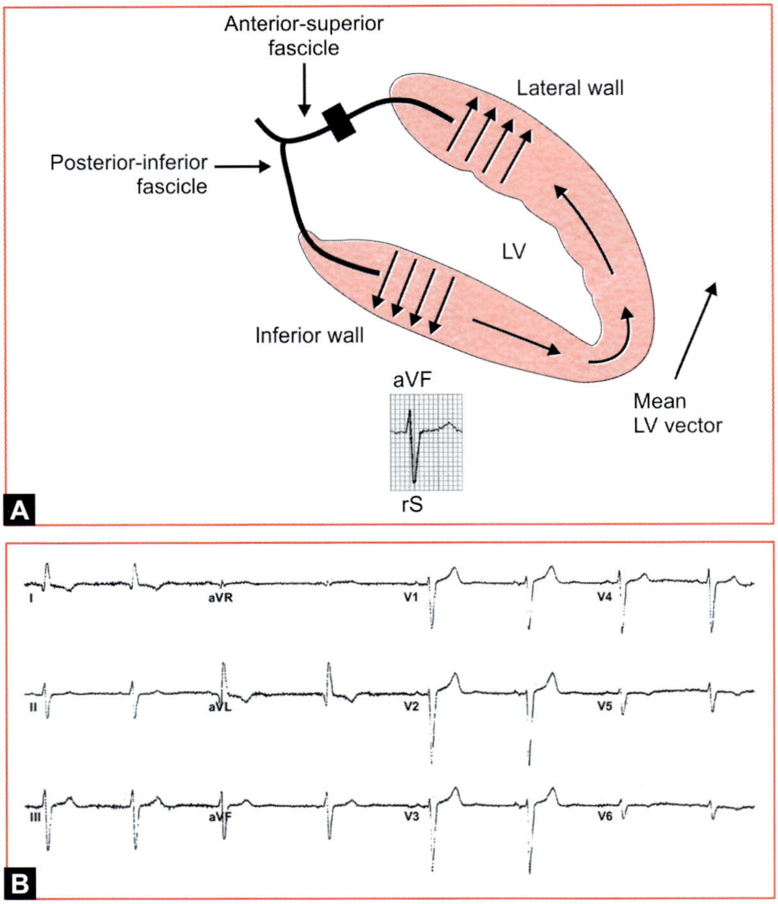

Figs. 12.25A and B: (A) Diagram showing the effect of block in the anterior-superior fascicle of the left bundle. The initial force results from the unopposed activation of the inferior-posterior wall. The wave front swings upward in the latter half of the ventricular depolarization resulting in activation of the antero-superior region of the left ventricle (initially not activated due to the block). The net effect is left axis deviation with an rS pattern in lead II shown in electrocardiogram (B).

depolarization of the antero-superior region of the left ventricle, which could not be depolarized initially due to the block in the superior fascicle. This gives rise to an ***rS*** pattern of the QRS in the inferior leads (II, aVF and III) (Figs. 12.25A and B).

The ECG is recorded at the surface of the body, but the electrical dipoles are in the heart. As already mentioned in part I of this chapter, the electromotive forces have to travel to the surface of the body to be recorded. Intervening tissues to some degree will change these forces and will attenuate them in some directions where there is air, which is a poor conductor of electromotive force. In some other directions they will be facilitated because of tissue, which represents a soup of electrolytes conducive in transmitting electromotive forces. In patients with COPD the normal anatomy is changed. Excess air spaces as in bullae or emphysema will alter the recordings at the surface of the body, whereas they may be completely normal at the level of the heart. Therefore, in COPD the axis shift can actually be in any direction meaning right, left or indeterminate (perpendicular to the frontal plane). Chronic obstructive pulmonary disease will also cause a QRS that will have an ***rS*** pattern in leads aVF in the presence of LAD. The same also applies to RAD, where the axis shift will be due to a QRS with an ***rS*** pattern in lead I. This cause of axis shift may be the most difficult to rule out of all the other causes. Typical changes include also alteration in QRS voltage, P wave direction and posterior displacement of the electrical forces in the horizontal plane.[41,42] These sometimes will result in tall peaked P waves in the inferior leads. P wave direction is usually to the right causing a negative P wave in aVL. This together with significant decrease in QRS voltage particularly due to attenuation of electrical forces oriented in the X-axis direction due to overlapping over aerated left lung and the low position of the diaphragm and persistent ***S*** in leads V5 and V6 makes it easier to attribute the axis shift to COPD. To eliminate axis shift due to COPD, one therefore has to carefully examine the whole ECG. The presence of low voltage QRS in general and in lead I in particular, the presence of an inverted P in aVL and persistent S in V5 and V6 should alert the interpreter to the presence of COPD (Fig. 12.26).

The diagnosis of WPW pre-excitation (discussed in some more detail in Section V) is relatively easy because of the presence of the ***delta*** wave and the short PR interval as well as the prolonged QRS duration. Due to the congenital presence of an accessory pathway of conduction (abnormal bundle called "Kent bundle") that connects the atrium to the ventricle, the ventricle will get depolarized without the impulse being delayed in the AV node causing a short PR interval. Because the Kent bundle inserts into the "working class myocardium" instead of the Purkinje system, the initial wave of depolarization is slower and the forces are inscribed slowly giving rise to the initial slurred ***delta*** wave that is seen in this condition. Although the Kent bundle can be located anywhere around the circumference of the AV sulcus, in some patients they are located posteriorly. When their insertion point is low in the infero-posterior portion of the LV, the LV will start depolarization at that point, there can only be one direction for that wave of depolarization to go and that is superiorly (since there is no heart inferior to it), thus causing a LAD (Figs. 12.27A and B). Thus easily recognizing or eliminating the three other causes of LAD through other ECG findings as described above should help to diagnose LAFB.

In addition, by vectorcardiography (VCG), the spread of excitation is not only superiorly directed, but it is also oriented in a ***"counter clockwise"*** fashion that is often considered as the characteristic feature of LAFB. This of

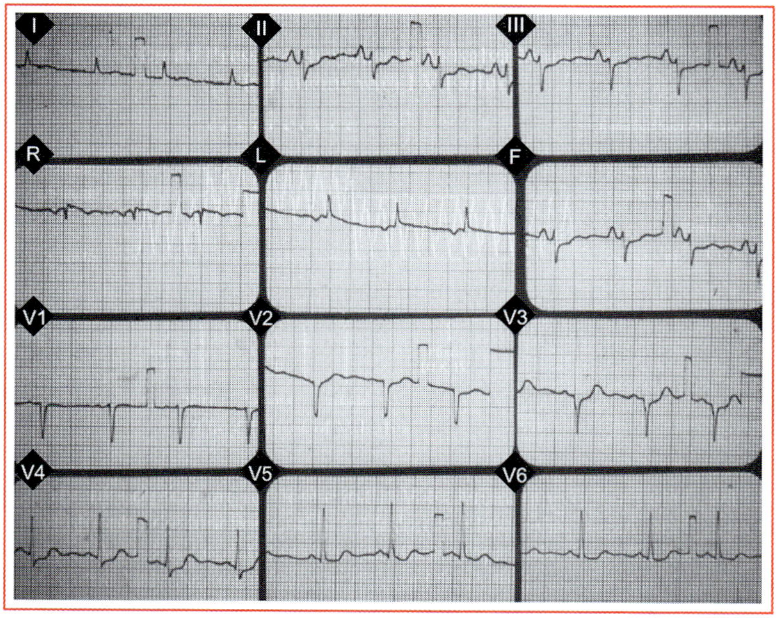

Fig. 12.26: Electrocardiogram of a patient with chronic obstructive pulmonary disease (COPD) showing left axis deviation. The features of COPD are noted including the low voltage QRS in lead I, negative P wave in aVL, delayed r/s progression in the precordial leads.

course is understandable, since the spread of excitation starts at the most inferior point in the frontal plane and swings around the apex to the base along the antero-lateral wall. The late QRS forces are often superiorly oriented enough to cause an ***R*** wave in aVL as well as in aVR. Careful examination of the simultaneously recorded three leads aVL, aVF and aVR will show that the peak of the terminal ***R*** in aVR to occur later than the terminal R in aVL, confirming the counterclockwise spread.[43]

Left Axis Deviation Associated with Congenital Heart Lesions

Left axis deviation associated with some of the congenital heart lesions such as ostium primum-type atrial septal defect is of clinical interest. Most patients with this defect or complete forms of the common AV canal show the superior QRS axis in the frontal plane. It has been demonstrated to be due to early activation of the posterobasal part of the left ventricle, resulting from an abnormal anatomic structure of the conduction system.[44] The bundle is inferiorly displaced and the anterior fascicle of the left bundle is hypoplastic.[45,46] Thus it mimics LAFB and may be considered as "congenital" form of LAFB. Other congenital heart lesions that are also associated with superior axis deviation include tricuspid atresia, common ventricle with transposition of the great vessels, corrected transposition of the great vessels when the

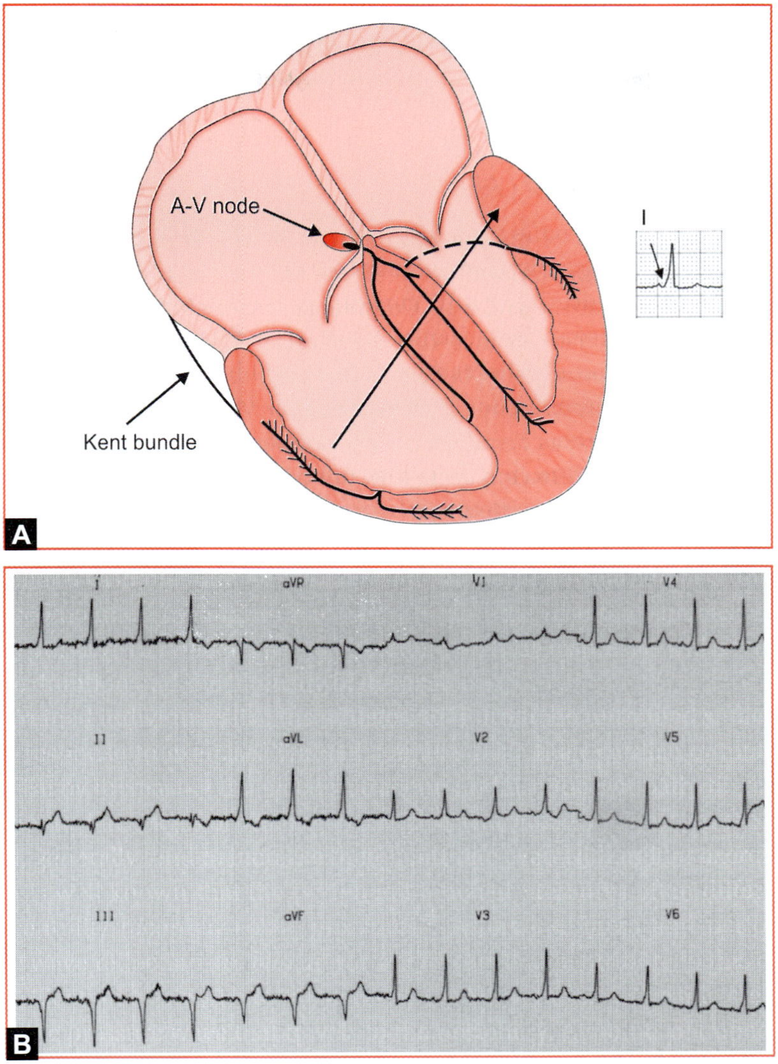

Figs. 12.27A and B: (A) Diagram showing left axis deviation (LAD) as a result of an accessory pathway (Kent bundle) activation of the basal portion of the infero-posterior left ventricular wall. Electrocardiogram from a patient with Wolf-Parkinson-White pre-excitation showing LAD is shown in (B). Typical features of delta wave (initial slurring of the QRS seen well in the precordial leads), short PR and slight QRS prolongation. The delta waves and the QRS complexes are negative in the inferior leads resulting in LAD.

arterial ventricle is dominant.[47] In congenitally corrected transposition, since the ventricles are reversed, the conduction system is also reversed. The "left" bundle lies on the right side of the inter-ventricular septum. The initial septal depolarization is from right to left. This results in the absence of the normal septal ***q*** waves in the left precordial leads. In addition, the plane of the inter-ventricular septum is not parallel to the chest wall like in the normals. It is perpendicular to the chest wall with the left side of the septum facing upward. The right to left septal depolarization causes the initial QRS forces to have a left and superior direction forming ***q*** waves in the inferior leads.

Clinical Significance of LAFB

The anterior division of the left bundle may be involved in diseases that involve the left ventricular outflow tract, the anterior half of the ventricular septum and the antero-lateral wall. Conditions that might be associated with it include idiopathic fibrosis involving the cardiac skeleton (Lev's disease) or the distal conduction system (Lenegre's disease), cardiomyopathies, hypertension, spontaneous and surgical closure of a ventricular septal defect, other cardiac surgeries such as Tetralogy of Fallot correction. In the general population at large the incidence is quite low. In hospital population, LAFB is not uncommonly associated with hypertension and coronary artery disease.[15,48]

Right Axis Deviation

As indicated previously an axis between +110° and +180° constitutes ***right axis deviation***. The purpose of this is to be able to make diagnosis of ***left posterior fascicular or hemi-block (LPFB)***.

The important causes of right axis deviation in adults are listed below. It is well known that infants normally have right axis deviation that can easily persist sometime up to the age of five. Also not included in this list is the rare condition of "***mirror image dextrocardia***" (Figs. 12.28A and B), which can cause RAD, since the left ventricle is on the right side. In these patients, the P waves are also inverted in lead I, since the right atrium is on the left side and the spread of excitation from the sinus node will move left to right instead of right to left as in the normal patients. This is not considered "true axis deviation" since the axis is normal for the position of their heart. One, seeing both the P and the QRS to be negative in lead I, however may easily make a mistake in assuming that the arm leads may have been reversed (Figs. 12.16A and B). If the position of the heart is normal, when the arm leads are reversed, the left precordial leads will show normal ***R/S*** progression. In "mirror image dextrocardia" however, in the precordial leads as one moves from V1 to V6, the ***R*** wave will be seen to diminish gradually and become small, instead of increasing in size as in the normal. Recording of the right precordial leads however will confirm increasing R wave amplitude toward V5R and V6R.

In most adults however, causes of RAD that need to be considered are four in number:

i. Left posterior fascicular or hemi-block
ii. Lateral infarction
iii. Chronic obstructive pulmonary disease
iv. Right ventricular hypertrophy

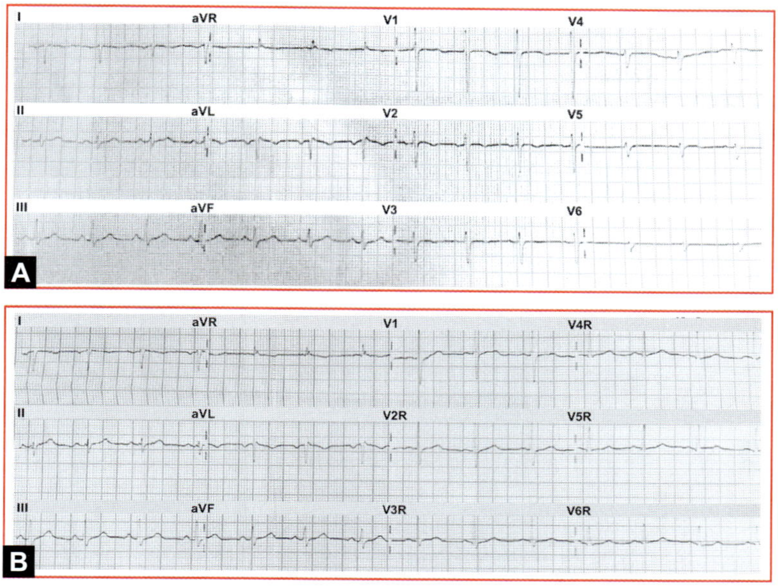

Figs. 12.28A and B: Electrocardiogram (ECG) from a patient with "mirror-image dextrocardia" with normal placement of the leads shown in (A). Electrocardiogram from the same patient with placement of right-sided precordial leads (V2R–V6R) shown in (B). Note the negative P, QRS and T waves in lead I. Diminishing R waves in the left precordial leads, Normal r/s progression noted when the precordial leads are recorded on the right side.

It is however quite rare to see LPFB, because the posterior division of the left bundle is a very thick fascicle with widely radiating fibers and it would take extensive disease process to cause a block in this fascicle.

The diagnosis of ***LPFB*** can be made by exclusion. The RAD caused by a lateral infarct will also be due to an abnormal ***Q*** wave. When the muscle mass in the lateral wall is significantly decreased due to an infarct, the electrical forces spreading from the endocardium to the epicardium going rightward are no longer balanced by opposite forces from the antero-lateral wall (Figs. 12.29A and B). The initial forces therefore will be directed rightward causing a ***Q*** wave in the lateral leads I and aVL. If the infarct is large enough, the QRS could be almost all negative instead of a ***QR*** pattern. This would be easy to differentiate from LPFB because the latter will show an ***rS*** pattern of QRS in the lateral leads I and aVL. Because of the block in the left posterior fascicle, the depolarization has to spread initially through the unaffected anterior fascicle. Depolarization will spread superiorly, anteriorly and laterally going from the endocardium to the epicardium resulting in an ***r*** wave in leads I and aVL. It will then swing around rightward and inferiorly producing an ***S*** wave in lead I (Figs. 12.30A and B). The spread of excitation is exactly opposite of the ***LAFB*** and it is clockwise (instead of counterclockwise) by VCG.

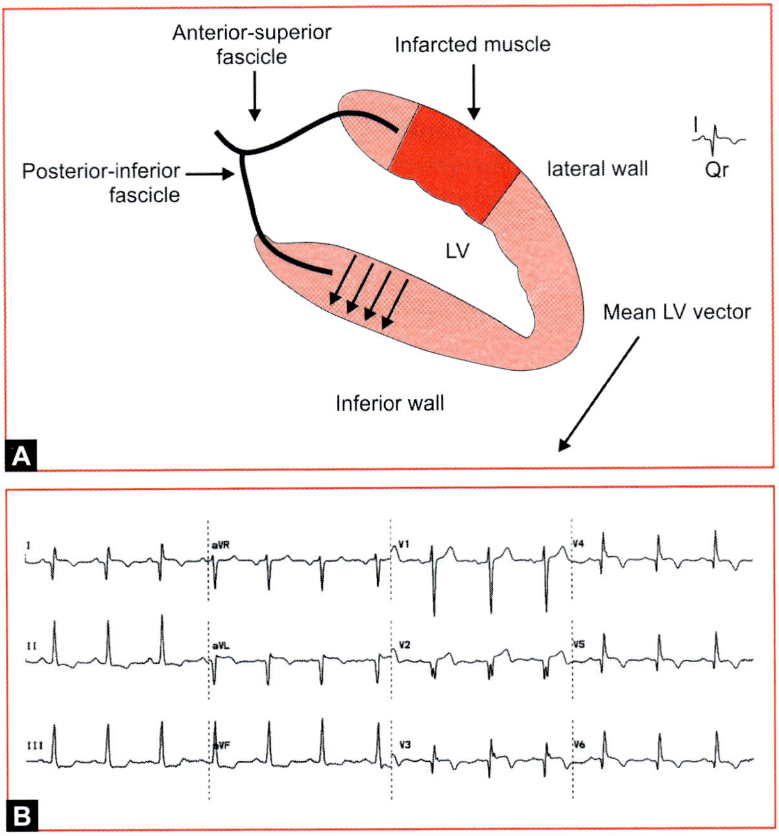

Figs. 12.29A and B: Diagram showing the unbalancing of the opposing forces from the inferior and the lateral wall of the left ventricular in lateral infarct resulting in inferior and rightward direction of the initial force and the Q waves in the lateral leads. Electrocardiogram with right axis deviation as a result of a lateral infarct with deep Q waves in the leads I and aVL is shown in (B). Q waves also noted in the precordial leads V2–V6, suggesting anterior wall involvement.

Right axis deviation secondary to COPD is different from RAD due to RVH, although RVH can occur in some patients with COPD.

Right ventricular hypertrophy will also cause RAD with a QRS that will produce an ***rS*** pattern in the lateral leads I and aVL (Figs. 12.22B and 12.31). The way to differentiate this from LPFB is to look at leads V1 or V2. In the presence of RVH, these leads will show tall R waves and associated ST-T changes. The right ventricle is not only located to the right, but also anteriorly under the sternum. As RV hypertrophies, the anterior forces will also increase and cause the tall R waves. In patients with LPFB alone, on the other hand, leads V1 and V2 will be completely normal.

Thus having eliminated the three other causes of RAD through other ECG findings, and if we are still left with unexplained RAD, then the cause must be considered to be LPFB.

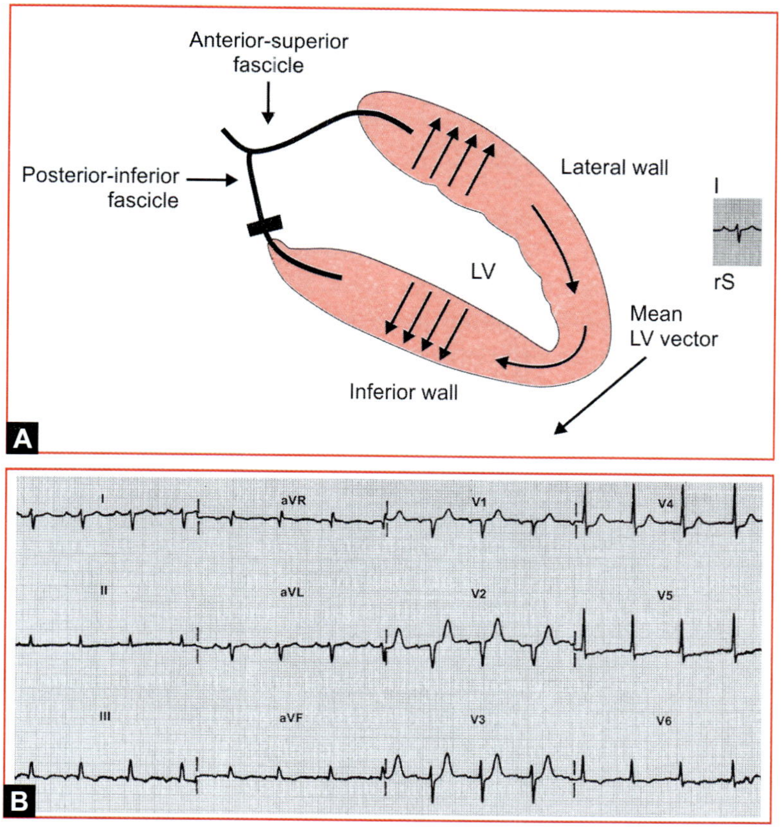

Figs. 12.30A and B: (A) Diagram showing the effect of block in the posteroinferior fascicle of the left bundle. The initial force results from the unopposed activation of the antero-lateral wall through the antero-superior fascicle. The wave front swings around rightward and inferiorly in the latter half of the ventricular depolarization resulting in depolarization of the inferior wall (not activated initially due to block). The net effect is right axis deviation with an rS pattern in lead I shown in electrocardiogram (B).

Diagnosis of Fascicular Blocks in the Presence of an Infarct

It is important to realize that the anterior-superior fascicle may become involved secondary to an anteroseptal and/or antero-lateral infarction resulting in LAFB associated with the infarction (Fig. 12.32A). Similarly, the infero-posterior fascicle may also become involved in infero-posterior infarction and result in LPFB associated with the infarction.

In the case of inferior infarct in lead aVF, and in the case of lateral infarct in lead I, if the infarct is large enough and the ECG shows only a deep negative ***QS*** complex without any ***R*** wave at all, it would be impossible to also make an additional diagnosis of a fascicular block causing the same type of axis shift, despite the fact that it may be present (Fig. 12.32B). In the case of inferior infarct if the abnormal Q waves in the inferior leads are followed by

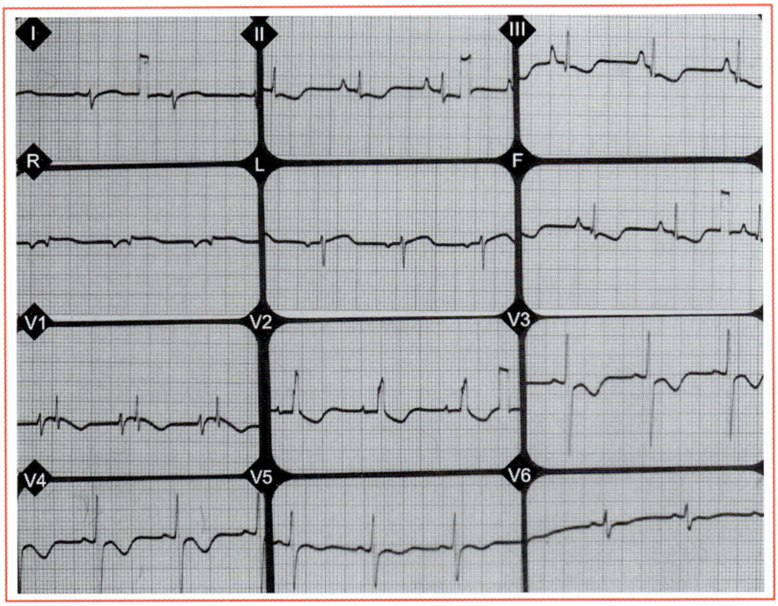

Fig. 12.31: Electrocardiogram from a patient with right ventricular hypertrophy (RVH) showing right axis deviation with an rS pattern in lead I. The typical features of RVH include the dominant R waves in V1 and V2 with negative T waves in the same leads. In addition, P wave features of right atrial overload are also noted.

a terminal R, it will negate the presence of a concomitant LAFB (Fig. 12.33). Similarly, in the case of lateral infarct, if the Q waves were followed by a terminal R in the lateral leads, it will also negate a concomitant LPFB (*see* Fig. 12.30B). On the other hand, the presence of a ***W*** pattern of the QRS (a small ***r*** wave in the middle preceded by a ***Q*** wave and followed by ***S*** wave) will indicate the presence of both the infarct and the fascicular block. The initial portion of the ***"W"*** represents the negative ***Q*** wave of the infarct and the terminal portion of the ***"W"*** represents the ***S*** wave of the fascicular block. This ***"W"*** pattern of the QRS in lead I would indicate the presence of a lateral infarct and LPFB (Fig. 12.34). Whereas the same pattern of QRS in leads aVF and II would indicate the presence of an inferior infarct and LAFB (Fig. 12.35).

When the axis is in the right upper quadrant, one should consider possible presence of two different axis shifts. For instance, this could occur as a result of large lateral infarction with a Qr pattern in lead I in combination with rS pattern in leads II and aVF indicating the presence of LAFB. Similarly, a large inferior infarct with Qr in aVF and the rS pattern in lead I indicating the presence of LPFB could also cause the axis to be in the right upper quadrant. It is also possible for a patient to have a lateral infarct as well as an inferior infarct causing a similar axis with ***Qr*** waves in both leads I and aVF.

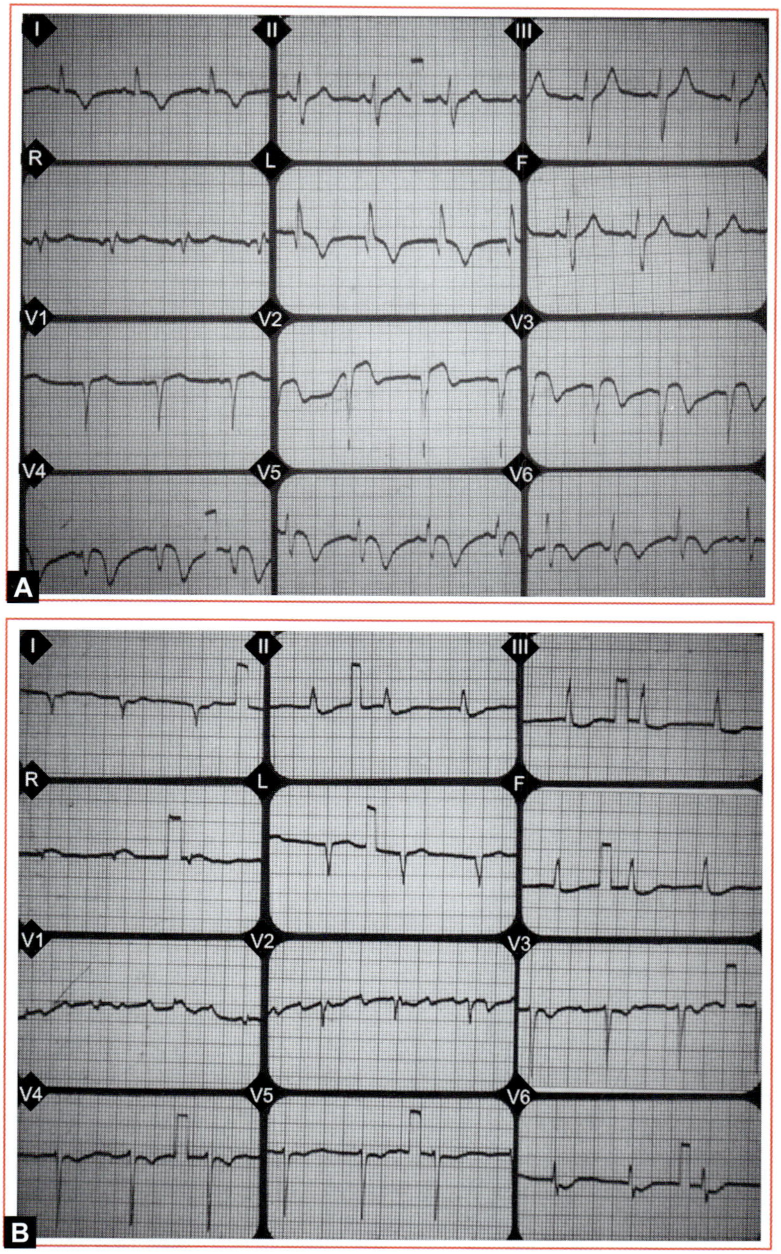

Figs. 12.32A and B: (A) Electrocardiogram (ECG) from a patient with anteroseptal and lateral infarct showing the associated anterior fascicular block with r/S pattern in lead II. Note the features of the infarct with QS complexes in leads V1–V3 with inverted T waves in the antero-lateral leads and abnormal Q in aVL with inverted T waves in leads I and aVL. (B) Electrocardiogram from pt suggestive of possible lateral infarct and coexistent left posterior fascicular block with right axis deviation. However QS complexes in leads I and aVL make it difficult to be sure.

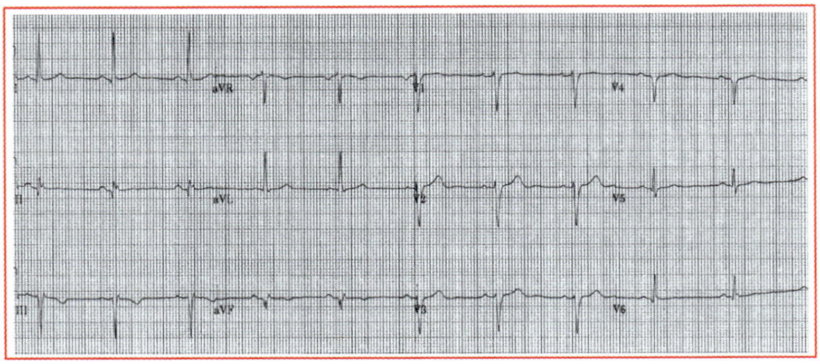

Fig. 12.33: Electrocardiogram from a patient with inferior infarct and left axis deviation with QR in leads II and aVF. Excludes associated left anterior fascicular block.

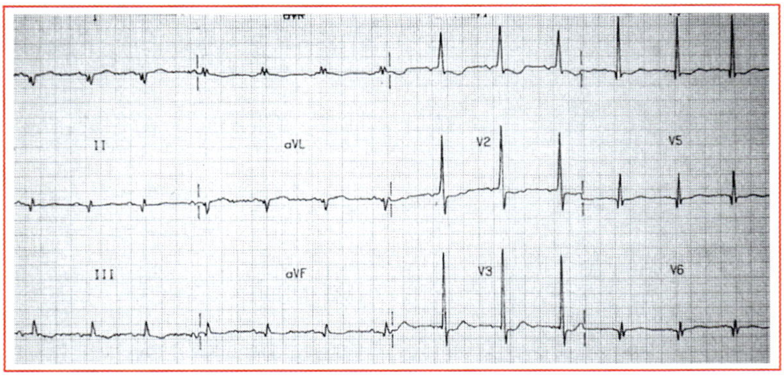

Fig. 12.34: Electrocardiogram from a patient with lateral infarct showing "W" pattern in leads I and aVL with right axis deviation. The terminal force is also directed rightward indicating the co-existing left posterior fascicular block with the lateral infarct.

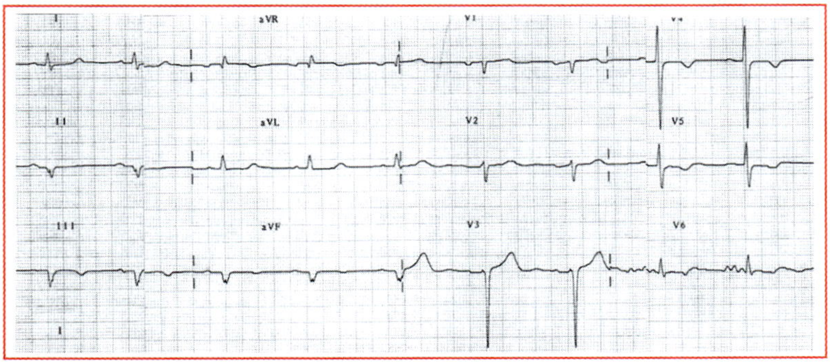

Fig. 12.35: Electrocardiogram from a patient with inferior infarct with "W" pattern in leads II and aVF. This is therefore very suggestive of inferior infarct with co-existing left anterior fascicular block (LAFB). Note a small s wave in leads I and V6 raising the question of possible terminal force arising from the right ventricular outflow tract as in incomplete right bundle branch block pattern. However, the terminal force is not pointing toward V1 (no r′). Also note the peak of the R wave in aVL is clearly inscribed before the peak of the R wave in aVR in these simultaneously recorded leads indicating a counter-clockwise spread of activation (that is also characteristic of LAFB).

Blocks in the Conduction System

Blocks in the conduction system represent an impediment to the electrical conduction. Delayed conduction or failure of conduction can occur at any level of the conduction system from the SA node to the level of the distal Purkinje system and even in the "working myocardial cells of the ventricles". Delayed conduction and blocks can be generally classified into the following three types according to the severity.

First Degree Block

Implies delayed conduction. All the impulses are conducted but conducted slower with increased conduction time.

Second Degree Block

Is intermittent failure of conduction followed by recovery. This is of two Types.

Type I, 2° block (Wenckebach conduction)

Is progressive increase in delay in conduction, with eventual failure of conduction, followed by recovery.

Type II, 2° block

Is sudden unexpected intermittent failure of conduction with no warning or preceding delay in conduction, followed by recovery.

Third degree block

Implies complete failure of conduction.

Bundle Branch Blocks

The normal duration of conduction from the time the Bundle of His is depolarized to the time of the ventricular activation and the onset of the QRS is about 45 ms as explained in Section I. Thus, if for any reason, the conduction through one of the bundle branches gets delayed even slightly (first degree block), the ventricular depolarization will start at the opposite ventricle through its Purkinje fibers. The resulting alteration in the depolarization sequence will end up producing the typical QRS morphology of the BBB matching the side of the delay. Thus although the term "bundle branch block" may convey the idea to the beginner that the bundle branch is totally blocked, it does not have to be. Mere delay in conduction would be sufficient to produce the BBB.

Normal Intra-ventricular Conduction

Normal intra-ventricular conduction is dependent on the integrity of the conduction system from the top of the inter-ventricular septum where the Bundle of His divides into two main bundle branches, the right and the left and the sub-divisions of the left bundle branch into the two main fascicles as well as the septal branch that may in fact be responsible for the initial left to right septal activation (*see* Fig. 12.12B).

For a clear understanding of the QRS formation, we will consider two separate phases of the ventricular depolarization and call them Events #1 and #2.

Event 1 is the initial wave of depolarization, which starts on the left side of the septum and propagates toward the right and remains dominant for a short period of time (20–30 ms) and not totally opposed by other waves of depolarization. This initial force will be directed rightward. Just looking at the leads V1 (a right-sided lead) and lead V6 (a left-sided lead), one will see an initial positive deflection of the QRS in lead V1, initial ***r*** wave (the septal ***r***). In lead V6, the opposite occurs and the same left to right force will produce a small ***q*** wave (the septal ***q***).

Event 2 is the depolarization of the free walls of the ventricles that occur simultaneously. The right ventricular forces will tend to be rightward directed. The left ventricular forces will be directed leftward. Since both ventricles depolarize simultaneously, this comprises actually of two simultaneous forces. The left ventricular muscle mass being larger, the left ventricular force will dominate and the resultant force will be directed to the left. This will therefore point away from lead V1 resulting in a negative deflection, the ***S*** wave in the QRS of lead V1. Since it points to the left and toward lead V6, it will produce a positive ***R*** wave after the initial small septal ***q*** (*see* Fig. 12.15).

Right Bundle Branch Block (RBBB)

In RBBB, the initial septal depolarization is not dependent on the right bundle branch and therefore Event 1 will be the same as before.

During Event 2, the left ventricular depolarization is also undisturbed and will occur as before, but the right ventricular portion cannot occur, because the impulse cannot reach the right ventricle simultaneously. The wave of depolarization has to take a separate route to reach the right ventricle, through the "working class myocardium" and distal Purkinje system. Therefore, during Event 2, there will be a rightward current through the tissues common to both ventricles trying to reach the right ventricle, as the left ventricle is depolarizing. The forces of Event 2 are still driven by the muscle mass of the free wall of the left ventricle and the resultant will be directed leftward. This of course will result in an ***S*** wave following the initial ***r*** in lead V1 and an ***R*** wave following the initial septal ***q*** in lead V6, as seen in the normal conduction. Eventually the wave of depolarization will reach the distal Purkinje system on the right side and depolarize the right ventricle. The right ventricular forces as before will be directed rightward. Since they are no longer simultaneous with the left ventricle, they are not overshadowed by the LV muscle mass and will express their existence. This expression becomes Event 3. Thus there are three events in succession instead of the original two events. The QRS would be wider since the part of the conduction has to go through the working myocardial cells. Event 3 forces are directed toward the right, therefore will register a positive deflection in lead V1. This gives rise to the secondary R, termed the ***R'***. The QRS in V1 thus will end up having the morphology of ***rSR'***. In V6, once again the opposite is seen and a negative deflection ***S*** wave is recorded. The terminal portion of the QRS representing the Event 3 is inscribed slowly and causes the total QRS duration to be prolonged. When the delay is significant enough then it will result in prolongation of the QRS to 0.12 second from the normal of 0.08 second. The terminal ***R'*** in V1 and the terminal ***S*** wave in V6 as well as lead I (that is also a left-sided lead in the frontal plane) will be typically wide (Figs. 12.36A and B).

From the point of view of clear understanding, the following needs to be emphasized again. The direction of the terminal force shows which part of the heart is activated the last and where the delay or block is. The rule is: *"The terminal force points toward the site of delay or block in the intra-ventricular conduction".* In RBBB, it points to the right and anteriorly where the RV is located. It was the same with the fascicular blocks, which we discussed previously. In the case of the superior (anterior) fascicular block (LAFB), the terminal force points superiorly and to the left and in the inferior (posterior) fascicular block (LPFB), it points inferiorly and to the right. The diagnosis of RBBB is therefore made by the terminal ***R*** in V1 and (terminal wide ***S*** in V6 and I). The pattern need not be ***rSR'*** pattern. Even if the QRS in V1 showed a ***qR*** pattern (as may happen with a prior septal infarct), and the QRS was wide and the ***terminal R*** was wide, then it would indicate RBBB (*see* Fig. 12.36C).

From the descriptive point of view of the QRS duration, terms such as "***complete***" and "***incomplete***" are used in BBB. This is applicable also to LBBB. If the BBB results in a QRS width of 0.12 second or greater, it is termed "complete" or simply RBBB or LBBB as the case may be. If the delay is such that it only produces increase in QRS duration from the normal of 0.08-0.10 second and the pattern or morphology of the QRS is otherwise typical for the BBB, then the adjective "***incomplete***" is used before the terms RBBB or LBBB (Fig. 12.37). In the case of RBBB, sometimes in many normal young subjects, one may see the pattern of ***rSr'*** in V1 without any QRS prolongation. It can be termed as "incomplete RBBB pattern" that will simply indicate that the terminal force or the last part of the heart to be activated in such subjects is probably the outflow tract of the RV. As discussed in Section I, this is not an uncommon occurrence (*see* Fig. 12.9B).

Left Bundle Branch Block (LBBB)

A strategically placed lesion at the short stem of the left bundle before it divides into the fascicles can cause LBBB. When LBBB is present, the

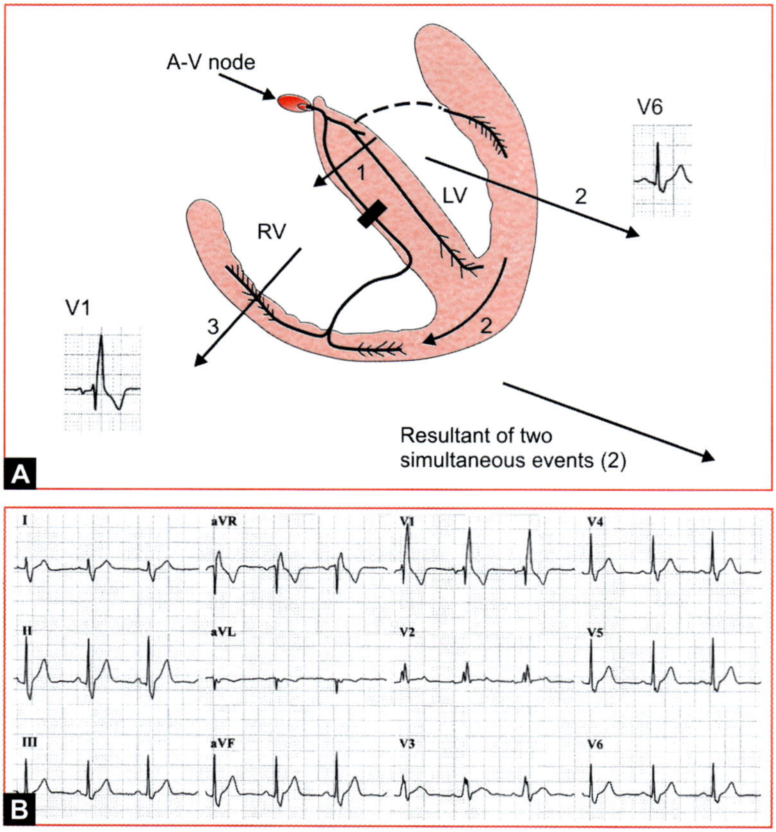

Figs. 12.36A and B: Diagram showing the effect of right bundle branch block on the QRS. Three successive events during depolarization of the ventricles depicted with numbers and arrows showing major direction of the electrical force from the respective events. The resulting QRS configurations are shown as seen from the right-sided lead V1 and the left-sided lead V6.
Event 11 is the normal initial left to right septal depolarization (unaffected by the block in the right bundle). Results in small initial r wave in V1 and small q wave in V6. Event 2 consists of two wave fronts, one causing the normal depolarization of the LV and the second trying to reach the RV through the common areas of the myocardium shared by both the ventricles. The resultant of the two is dominated by the left ventricle (LV) and is toward the LV. The result of this produces the S wave to follow the initial r in V1. The corresponding configuration of the QRS is the qR in V6.
Event 3 is the final and terminal activation of the right ventricle (RV) spreading through the working myocardial cells resulting in prolongation of the QRS duration. The terminal force is directed toward the area of the block, therefore toward the RV. It is therefore rightward and anterior. This causes the terminal portion of the QRS to be wide and slurred. It results in the terminal R or R′ in V1. The same terminal force is seen as S wave in V6 (also in lead I, another left-sided lead).
The electrocardiogram from a patient with RBBB is shown in part (B).

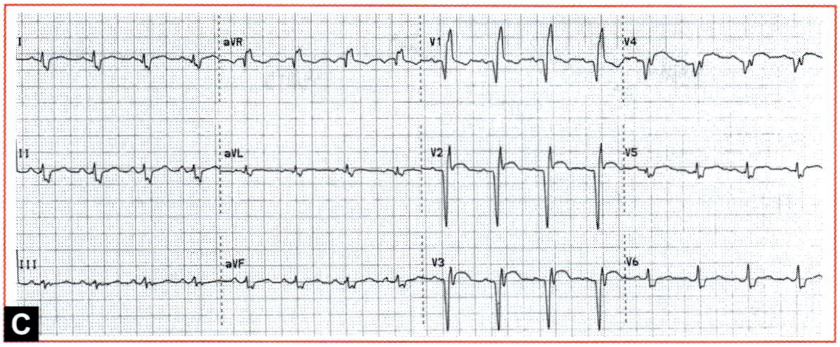

Fig. 12.36: (C). Electrocardiogram from a patient with anteroseptal infarct and associated right bundle branch block. Abnormal Q waves are noted in V1–V4, suggestive of anteroseptal infarct. The QRS duration is prolonged to 0.12 seconds suggesting the presence of a bundle branch block. Note the pattern in V1 is QR. The wide terminal R corresponds to the wide terminal S in lead I and lead V6, features of RBBB.

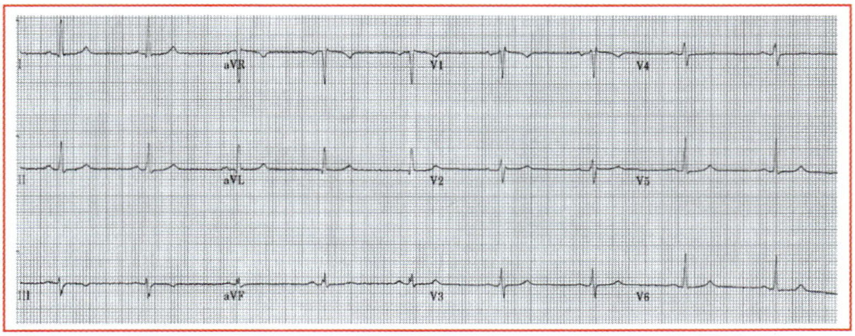

Fig. 12.37: ECG from a patient with rSr′ pattern in V1 but the QRS duration is only slightly prolonged. Therefore this represents incomplete right bundle branch block.

normal septal depolarization cannot occur since the latter is dependent on the integrity of the left bundle. The septum is therefore depolarized on the right side slightly further down from the right bundle. Hence, the wave of depolarization of the septum will travel from the right to the left. This indicates that the forces of Event 1 are changed and are opposite of the normal. This will result in an initial force pointing toward lead V6 and away from lead V1.

The right ventricular portion of Event 2 will be the same as the normal and is rightward directed. However, the left ventricle cannot depolarize as expected during Event 2. The wave of depolarization will try to reach the left ventricle through the common myocardium during this Event 2. Eventually as the depolarization reaches the left side of the distal Purkinje system, the left ventricle will also begin to depolarize. The left ventricular depolarization not being simultaneous with the RV depolarization, will become the Event 3 which is also directed to the left. During Event 2, there are two opposing forces at work. The one is the normal RV depolarization directed rightward and the other is the wave front trying to reach the left ventricle directed leftward. Since the muscle mass of the common area to both ventricles is still greater than the muscle mass of the free walls of the RV, the resultant force of Event 2 will still be directed leftward. *Thus during all the three successive events, the QRS force is essentially directed in one direction, namely from the right toward the left.* This will therefore result in a wide and all negative QRS, namely ***QS*** in V1, and in V6 it will be all upright ***R*** wave (Figs. 12.38A and B). In addition, the QRS duration will be prolonged due to three events instead of two. The mid-portion of the QRS, which represents the Event 2, will have the maximum delay and is inscribed slowly, because of the wave of depolarization, tries to go through "the working myocardial cells". Thus the upright QRS in V6 (also in lead I that is left-sided as well) is not only wide and will be notched in the middle indicating the ***mid-portion delay***. When the QRS duration is 0.12 second or more, then the LBBB is considered complete. When the QRS duration is prolonged slightly (0.10 second), and the pattern is otherwise of the LBBB, then the term used to describe is "incomplete LBBB" (Fig. 12.38C).

Secondary ST-T Wave Changes in BBB

When the BBB is complete and the QRS is prolonged, whether it is RBBB or LBBB, the depolarization sequence is abnormal. Since the depolarization is abnormal, the repolarization also tends to become abnormal. Thus the ST-T waves no longer point in the same direction as the QRS as in the normal heart. Often the ST-T vectors point generally opposite to the direction of the delayed portion of the QRS.

In RBBB, the delay essentially affects the terminal portion of the QRS. It is seen in lead V1 that has upright terminal ***wide R or R'*** to be followed by slightly ***negative ST-T waves.*** In leads V6 and I, since the terminal delay of the QRS shows as a ***wide S*** wave, this will be followed by an ***upright ST-T wave*** (*see* Fig. 12.36B).

In LBBB, the QRS is wide and notched in the middle. It is all negative in V1 and all positive in V6, therefore in V1, the ***QS*** complex will be followed by slightly ***elevated ST with upright T waves.*** In leads V6 and I, the notched wide R will therefore be followed by ***depressed ST and negative T waves*** (Fig. 12.38B).

These are the expected ST-T wave changes, which are ***secondary*** to the abnormal sequence of depolarization. So if the T waves happen to be positive when it is expected to be negative in a specific lead (for instance V6 and I with LBBB), then one must consider some ***primary repolarization abnormality,*** the cause of which would have to be sorted out since it will be unrelated to the BBB (Fig. 12.39).

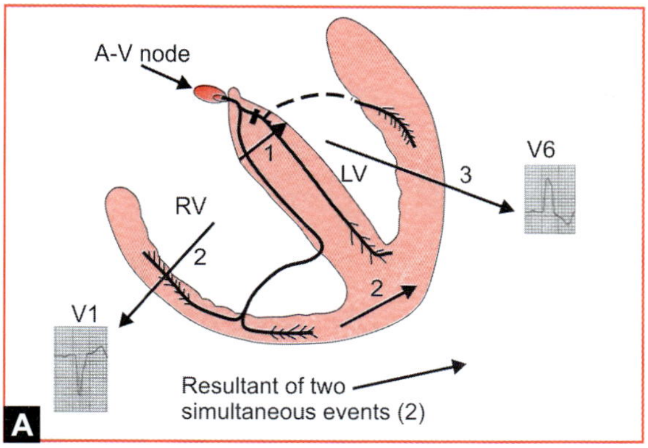

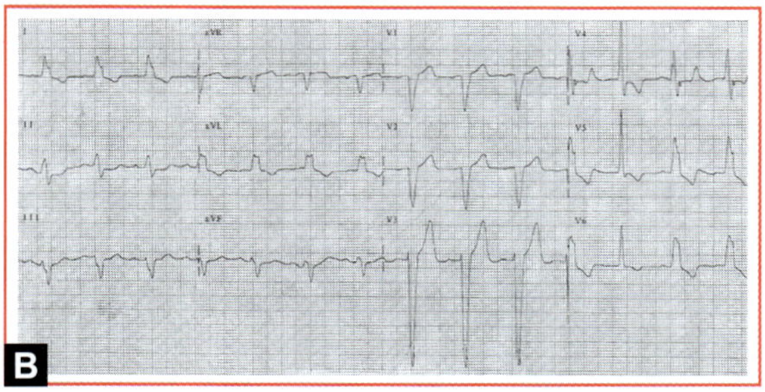

Figs. 12.38A and B: (A) Diagram showing the depolarization of the ventricles in the presence of block in the left bundle (proximal) to the septal branch. Three successive events are marked by the numbers 1, 2 and 3. Directions of the electrical forces of the events are shown by the arrows. Event one (1) is abnormal and is from right to left septal activation instead of the normal left to right direction (due to the block). This will result in loss of the normal initial septal r in V1 and septal q in V6. Event two (2) consists of two wave fronts, one resulting from depolarization of right ventricle (RV). This is opposed by slow spread of excitation through the working myocardial cells of the common areas of the two ventricles. Since the common area of the myocardium is thicker than the RV walls, the resultant points toward the left. Event three (3) the final spread of activation of the free walls of the left ventricle also is toward the left. Since all events are directed right to left, the resulting QRS is all negative in V1 and all positive in V6 with prolongation of the QRS duration. Electrocardiogram from a patient with left bundle branch block (LBBB) is shown in (B). Diagram showing the depolarization of the ventricles in the presence of block in the left bundle (proximal) to the septal branch. Three successive events are marked by the numbers 1, 2 and 3. Directions of the electrical forces of the events are shown by the arrows. Event one1 is abnormal and is from right to left septal activation instead of the normal left to right direction (due to the block). This will result in loss of the normal initial septal r in V1 and septal q in V6. Event two2 consists of two wave fronts, one resulting from depolarization of right ventricle (RV). This is opposed by slow spread of excitation through the working myocardial cells of the common areas of the two ventricles. Since the common area of the myocardium is thicker than the RV walls, the resultant points toward the left. Event three3 the final spread of activation of the free walls of the left ventricle also is toward the left. Since all events are directed right to left, the resulting QRS is all negative in V1 and all positive in V6 with prolongation of the QRS duration. Electrocardiogram from a patient with left bundle branch block (LBBB) is shown in (B). Note wide QS complex in V1 and wide notched R in V6. Since depolarization is abnormal, the repolarization is also abnormal. T waves point opposite to the direction of the QRS. V1 has upright T waves and V6 has negative T waves.

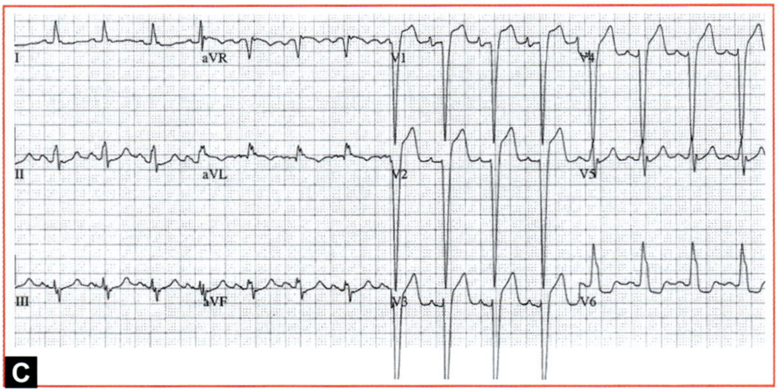

Fig. 12.38C: (C) Electrocardiogram shows incomplete LBBB with similar configuration to complete LBBB except the QRS duration is only about 0.10 second.

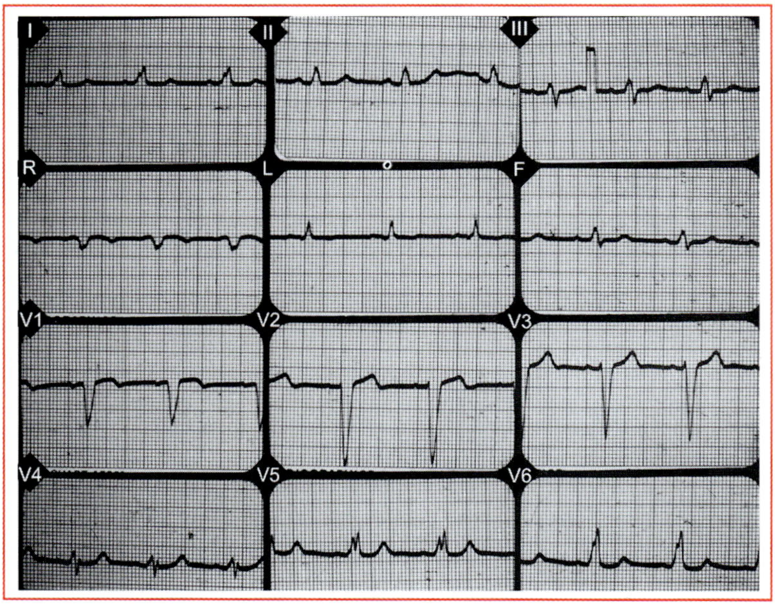

Fig. 12.39: Electrocardiogram showing left bundle branch block configuration. However T waves are upright in leads I and V6 instead of being inverted. This therefore is suggestive of primary repolarization abnormality.

Axis Determination in the Presence of RBBB and Bifascicular Blocks

Sometimes, RBBB can occur with concomitant fascicular block such as the LAFB or LPFB. It will be important to know how to recognize the same, since it would be suggestive of block in two of the three fascicles of the intraventricular conduction. It is sometimes known as ***Bifascicular block***. It can also mean sub-clinical disease in the third fascicle that is yet to manifest it self self and can do so suddenly and without warning with higher degrees of block and/or syncope. Since fascicular blocks classically alter the direction of the mean left ventricular forces superiorly to the left (in LAFB) and inferior and to the right in LPFB, the exercise consists in identifying the mean direction of the left ventricular portion of the QRS in RBBB. In RBBB, we have three events in succession. The RV depolarization is no longer overshadowed by the LV events and exerts its force as Event 3. Since the aim is to determine the LV mean axis, Event 3 (the terminal part of the QRS) should be ignored. The QRS width in complete RBBB is 0.12 second and the first two-thirds of the QRS, namely the first 0.08 second can be considered mainly due to the normal left ventricular activation since normal QRS width is about 0.08 second. The last one-third can therefore be considered due to late and delayed activation of the left ventricular. Sometimes, one can actually recognize a notch at the beginning of the delayed portion of the QRS. We should use the initial portion of the QRS up to that notch to determine the axis. If the axis is LAD, LAFB will be suggested if the second half of that 0.08 second QRS points superiorly and to the left (Fig. 12.40). One can also go through the elimination process of diagnosis as was pointed out under fascicular blocks and axis deviation previously. It might be important to mention that in this situation RVH no longer becomes a cause of RAD. Since there is already RBBB, the right ventricular forces are part of the terminal delayed portion of the QRS.

It is important however to recognize that the diagnosis of co-existing fascicular block will not be possible if the ECG shows incomplete RBBB or incomplete RBBB pattern. In such an instance, the terminal portion of the QRS will have an S in lead I indicating the rightward direction. Often the terminal force will also be anterior and directed toward V1, thereby producing a terminal R or R′ in V1. Occasionally however the terminal force in V1 may not be positive enough to make an R wave but may be seen to distort the S wave in V1 making it a shallow S wave. The underlying problem is overlapping terminal activation of both the left ventricle and the right ventricle (often of the RV outflow tract or the conus). The same terminal force may also be somewhat superiorly oriented enough to cause terminal dominant S waves in the inferior leads. The resultant superior orientation may mimic LAFB but may in fact be due to the terminal RV activation. In any case, the diagnosis of LAFB in such situations will unlikely to be correct (Figs. 12.41A and B).

It is more common to see bifascicular block in the form of RBBB plus LAFB than RBBB plus LPFB, since LAFB is more common than LPFB (Fig. 12.42).

Clinical Significance of RBBB

Histopathologic studies have indeed confirmed the anatomic correlation of ECG findings of RBBB with lesions in the right bundle branch.[49,50] It is well known that RBBB is a common finding following certain types of cardiac

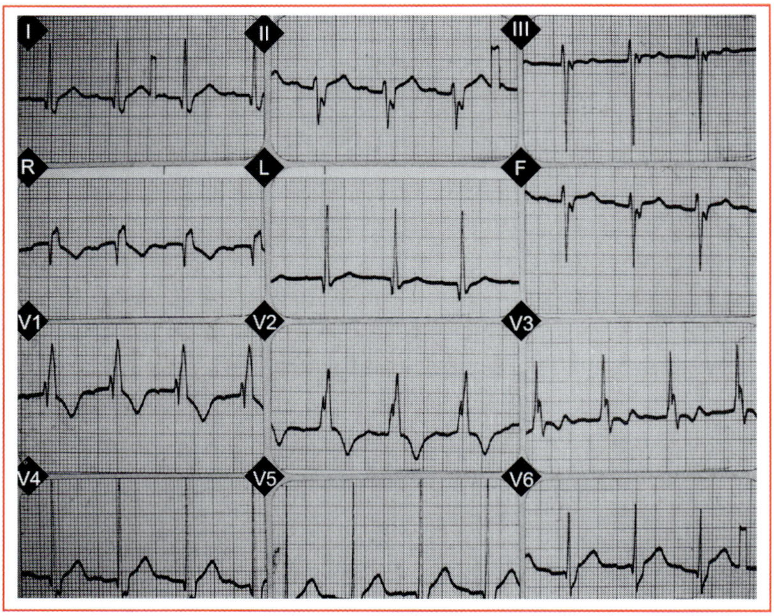

Fig. 12.40: Electrocardiogram showing features of bifascicular block with right bundle branch block (RBBB) and left anterior fascicular block (LAFB). The RBBB is clearly seen with prolonged QRS width to 0.12 second with rSR′ in V1. However the axis of the left ventricular forces (first two-thirds of the QRS) is definitely superior. One can easily see a notch in the S wave in lead II where the right bundle branch delay begins. The S wave before the notch is clearly deep diagnostic of the terminal LV force oriented superiorly as in LAFB.

surgery such as repair of a ventricular septal defect through the tricuspid valve, repair of Tetralogy of Fallot, and following any right ventriculotomy irrespective of the length of the incision. Electrophysiologic studies in the post-operative patients favor the concept that ECG changes of RBBB may be caused by lesions at three levels, the proximal part, the distal part as well as the peripheral ramifications.[51] Right bundle branch block is seen often in patients with large atrial septal defect of both the secundum and an A-V cushion defect, in coarctation of the aorta as well as in patients with Ebstein's anomaly. The latter patients may also have a WPW. The combination of WPW and RBBB is almost diagnostic of Ebstein's anomaly. Right bundle branch block can occur merely from right ventricular distension, sometimes even acutely from a pulmonary embolism.

In many patients among the general population, however, RBBB is not associated with any heart disease. Right bundle branch block developing in association with an acute myocardial infarction (MI) often resolves spontaneously and may however persist in about 15% of the patients. The patients who have persistent new onset RBBB with an acute infarct have been known

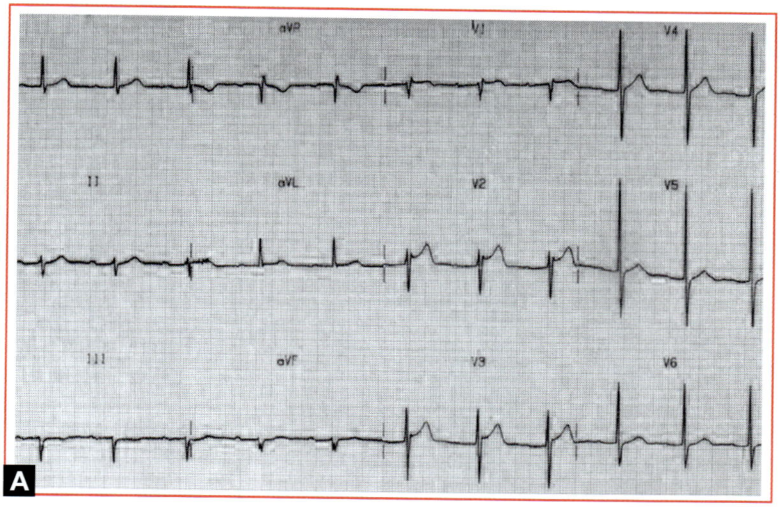

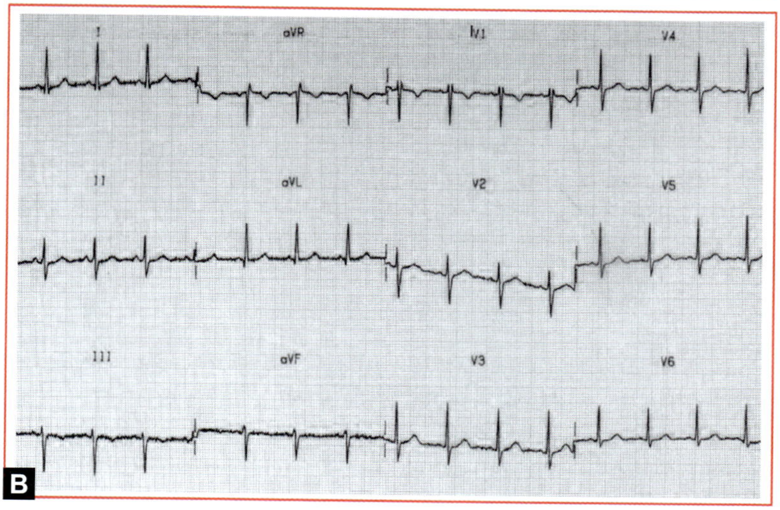

Figs. 12.41A and B: Electrocardiograms both showing features somewhat similar one with incomplete right bundle branch block (RBBB) (A) and the other with incomplete RBBB pattern(B). Both show terminal r′ in V1 and s wave in lead I indicating terminal force is right and anterior. Note the terminal force is also quite superior with deep S in lead II with rS pattern. This demonstrates clearly that in incomplete RBBB as well as incomplete RBBB pattern, the terminal force can be oriented superiorly enough to cause left axis deviation. Therefore in the presence of incomplete RBBB or incomplete RBBB pattern, the diagnosis of associated left anterior fascicular block cannot be made and is likely to be incorrect.

to have an increased 1 year mortality rate.[52] Right bundle branch block is also noted in about 40% of patients with RV infarction.[53]

Right bundle branch block occurs frequently in patients with arrhythmogenic right ventricular dysplasia. Characteristic distortion of the terminal portion of the QRS complex known as the ***epsilon wave*** may be seen in

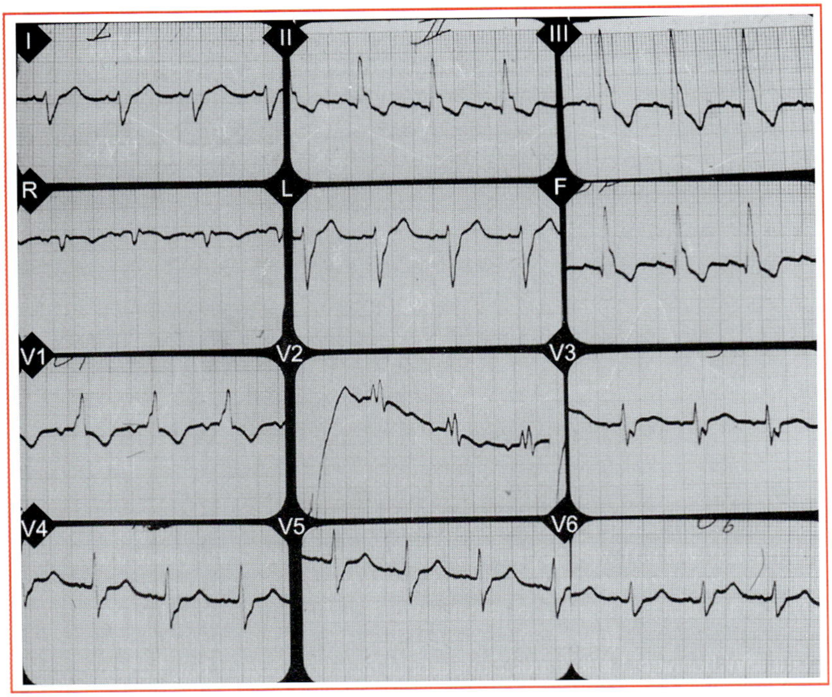

Fig. 12.42: Electrocardiogram showing right bundle branch block with associated left posterior fascicular block. The rS pattern of the first two-thirds of the QRS clearly seen in lead I where a slight notch can be noted with the onset of the right bundle delay. The notch is also seen well in lead II.

these patients[54] The pattern of RBBB with ST elevation associated with sudden cardiac death or ventricular fibrillation (VF) is known as the ***Brugada syndrome***. This will be further discussed in Section VI.

The prognosis of the patients with RBBB is usually related to the underlying heart disease if any present and not dependent on the conduction defect itself.

Clinical Significance of LBBB

The block is often thought of as both predivisional (proximal) and postdivisional (distal). Histopathologic studies have shown that LBBB is often caused by lesions in the proximal part of the left bundle close to the bifurcation of the Bundle of His. Lesions may result from ischemia or mechanical encroachment from sclerosis and calcification of the cardiac skeleton (Lev's disease).[55] Left bundle branch block is often seen in association with structural heart disease. The underlying etiologic factors of the myocardial disease can be from hypertension, ischemic heart disease as well as cardiomyopathies. Occasionally, it may be associated with advanced valvular disease.

It is seen not uncommonly in patients with aortic stenosis.[53] It can also be produced by primary degenerative disease of the conduction system (Lenegre's). Prevalence increases with age. Even in the absence of ischemic heart disease or infarction and myocardial disease, LBBB itself due to asynchronous activation of the ventricle can be associated with wall motion abnormalities with areas of hypokinesis or akinesis involving the anteroseptal wall or the apex. In acute myocardial infarction, the presence of concomitant LBBB is often associated with increased mortality.[56]

Patients with LBBB and predominant superior axis generally tend to be older and often associated with ischemic heart disease, hypertension, cardiomegaly and heart failure and seem to have higher mortality.[57]

Some patients with LBBB may have an initial ***r*** wave in V1. This may be due to unopposed RV free wall forces due to delayed septal activation or septal infarct. It may also be due to the fact that the block in the left bundle branch may be post-divisional and distal in location (Figs. 12.43A and B). In a study of 40 consecutive patients with LBBB seen in the hospital population, we tried to assess the significance of the presence of the ***r*** in V1 in terms of left ventricular function and wall motion abnormality by two-dimensional echocardiography as well as by Thallium scintigraphic studies to define areas of non-reversible defects using resting and exercise as well as delayed imaging. There were no differences in the incidence of septal scars or septal wall motion abnormality and the overall incidence of moderate to severe left ventricular dysfunction between those who had no ***r*** in V1 (23 patients) versus those who had the ***r*** in V1 (17 patients). It was of interest however, that 11 of 23 patients (48%) without ***r*** in V1 had Grade I–II left ventricular function compared to only six of 17 patients (35%) in the group with ***r*** in V1. The lesser incidence of near normal left ventricular function in patients with preserved ***r*** in V1 with LBBB is of interest. This may in fact indirectly suggest that the block may in fact be distal and post-divisional.[58]

Trifascicular Disease

The presence of trifascicular disease is of special importance since it may cause sudden complete AV block and symptoms of syncope and/or cardiac arrest. Trifascicular disease may present in different ways. Complete AV block may occur as a result of AV nodal blocks. The AV nodal block usually presents as type I second degree block and eventually progress to 2:1 block and then higher degrees of block. Complete AV block may also result from intra His disease. The properties of the His bundle and the bundle branches are such that they usually present with type II second degree block and may go on to develop complete block without warning. However, classical type I block can also be present in the His-Purkinje system. Bifascicular blocks in

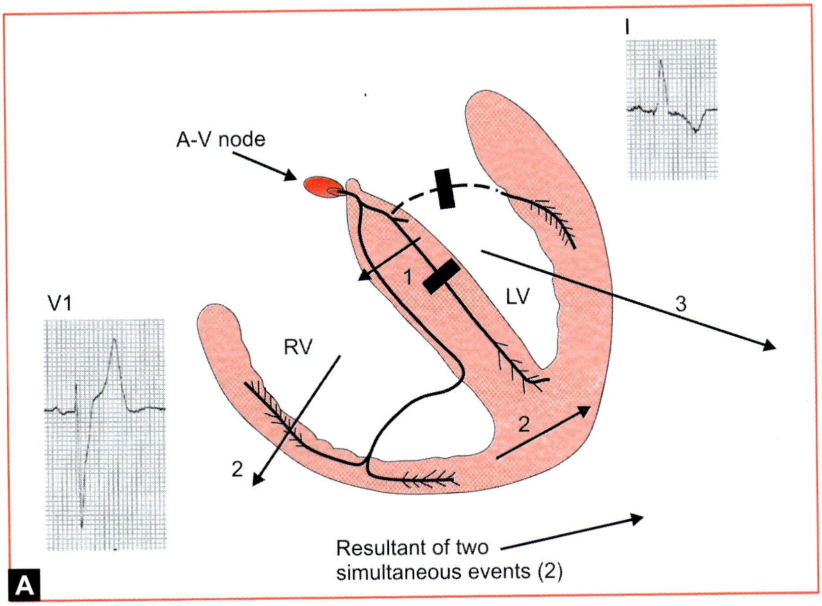

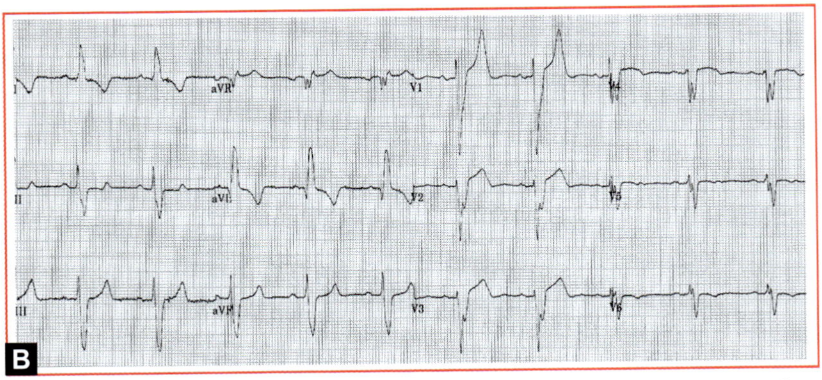

Figs. 12.43A and B: Diagram showing depolarization events in the presence of post-divisional left bundle branch block (distal LBBB). The septal activation Event 1 may be normal and may be the cause of the initial r wave sometimes seen in V1 in patients with electrocardiogram otherwise showing features of LBBB (B). Other reasons for the preservation of the initial r wave may be unopposed right ventricular wall activation due to delayed septal activation or septal infarct.

the form of RBBB plus LAFB, RBBB plus LPFB or LBBB have been discussed. Presence of delayed conduction through the third fascicle would indicate trifascicular disease and may become the cause of complete AV block. Fortunately, most BBBs and fascicular blocks are not complete and patients with bifascicular blocks do not always get into higher degrees of symptomatic block. Electrocardiogram depicting patients with trifascicular disease are shown in Figures 12.44A and B. The ECG in Figure 12.44A shows RBBB with second degree AV block with 3:2 AV conduction. In conducted beats

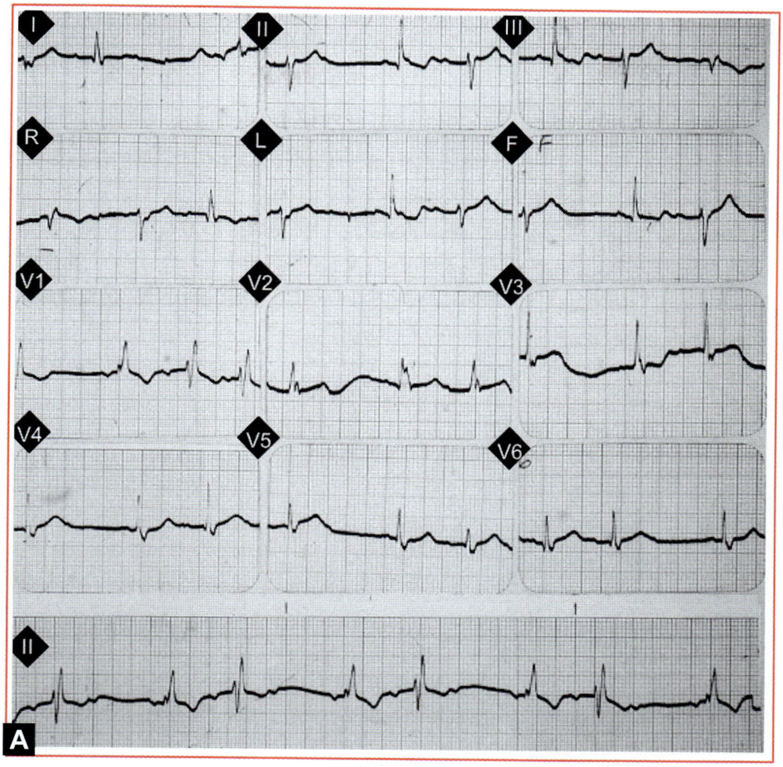

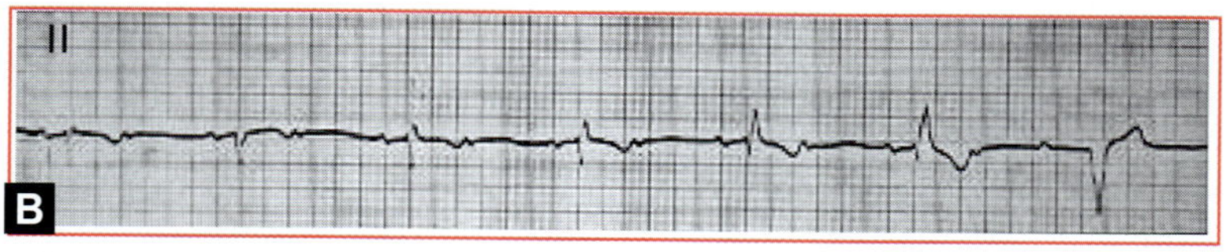

Figs. 12.44A and B: (A) Electrocardiogram with features of trifascicular disease. Right bundle branch block (RBBB) is noted with second degree atrioventricular (AV) block and 3:2 AV conduction. In conducted beats, prolongation of the PR interval is associated with shift in QRS axis from right to left in the frontal plane leads, indicating change from left posterior fascicular block to left anterior fascicular block (LAFB) conduction. The longer PR interval during LAFB and superior axis is probably the result of delayed conduction through the posterior fascicle. (B) Electrocardiogram with features of trisfascicular disease. Shows a rhythm strip with second degree AV block. There is progressive widening of the QRS showing various degrees of RBBB. In addition, when the conduction has the configuration of light bundle branch block, it is associated with lengthening of the PR interval. This is very suggestive and diagnostic of delay in the His-Purkinje system and not at the AV node.

with longer PR interval, the frontal plane limb leads show shift in axis to superior direction indicating co-existing LAFB. This indicates also most likely the prolongation of the PR interval may in fact be due to delayed conduction through the infero-posterior fascicle. This will therefore indicate the presence of trifascicular disease. The rhythm strip in Figure 12.44B demonstrates second degree AV block (could be due to intra His disease, likely type II although not certain). In addition, there is a type I RBBB shown by progressive widening of the R′ and the QRS in the conducted beats with RBBB configuration. When the conduction changes from RBBB to LBBB following a dropped beat, the associated long PR interval during LBBB type conduction confirms the delay in the right bundle.[59] What appears to be complete RBBB, obviously is not. Nevertheless, there is evidence of conduction defect involving both the right and the left bundle (in essence trifascicular disease). When a clear diagnosis is made of trifascicular disease with symptoms, the treatment would require a permanent pacemaker implant.

SECTION III: CHAMBER ENLARGEMENT, HYPERTROPHY, OVERLOADS

Normal heart has four chambers: two atria and two ventricles. They can be affected secondarily by congenital lesions and/or acquired conditions. The type of hemodynamic burden will depend on whether the chamber receives and ejects normal or increased volume of blood and/or whether it has to work against normal resistance or high resistance. When the right or the left ventricles receive a larger than normal volume of blood in diastole and therefore eject an increased stroke volume, the hemodynamic burden is termed as volume overload. When the ejection of stroke volume (normal or increased) occurs against an increased resistance, then the hemodynamic burden is described as pressure overload. The primary physiologic adaptation of the ventricles faced with volume overload states is to dilate or enlarge in size (dimension). Hypertrophy of the eccentric type will occur secondarily. The physiologic adaptation to pressure overload of the ventricle results in concentric hypertrophy. In late stages of chronic pressure overload the ventricles may also undergo dilatation. Generally this usually entails decompensation. Similar issues of pressure or volume overloads can also affect the atria depending on the hemodynamic changes resulting from the underlying lesion or condition.

Electrocardiogram is not a good tool to identify specific cardiac chamber dilatation or enlargements. These are best assessed with imaging techniques. Chest Radiographs were popular six decades ago but in more modern days, the two-dimensional echocardiography has become the preferred method for this. Increased cardiac muscle mass associated with hypertrophy affecting either the right or the left ventricle can be expected to produce increased electrical voltages and/or affect the direction of the electrical forces associated with ventricular depolarization (QRS complex). Similarly, atrial hypertrophy and/or enlargement may also alter the electrical forces associated with the atrial depolarization (P waves).

Atrial Enlargement/Hypertrophy (Overloads)

Electrical abnormalities associated with atrial enlargement/hypertrophy (overloads) will be dealt with first. Since it is hard to specifically distinguish enlarged atrium from hypertrophy of the atrium by ECG, the preferred term for P wave abnormalities associated with them is "***Atrial overload or Abnormalities***" (right or left as the case may be).

Right Atrial Overload/Abnormalities

The normal P wave results from depolarization of both the right and the left atria. The SA node is on the upper part of the right atrium close to the superior vena cava. The initial part of the P wave represents the right atrial activation and the terminal part of the P wave represents the left atrium. The right atrial activation spreads downward from the upper part of the right atrium toward the lower part. The left atrial activation spreads leftward in the frontal plane and front to back in the horizontal plane since the left atrium is predominantly a posterior chamber. The normal direction of the P wave in the frontal plane is therefore leftward and inferior. The amplitude of the normal P wave usually does not exceed 2.5 mm and the upper normal P wave duration is also about 100 ms (2.5 mm width).

When the right atrium is dilated or hypertrophied or both, it will result in alteration of the initial part of the P wave force. The direction of the P wave force is often not significantly altered. But the amplitude of the P wave may in fact be increased. The increased voltage may cause tall peaked P waves in the inferior leads. The right atrium is located anteriorly in the heart and anatomically close to the precordial lead V1. The abnormal initial P wave force may cause a sharp peaked P wave or show as a peaked initial part of a biphasic P wave in lead V1 (Fig. 12.45).

The duration of the P wave force is not usually increased. The axis of the P wave may sometimes be more inferiorly directed (>+60°) seen usually in COPD. The P wave may therefore be negative in aVL.[60] Since there is no correlation of this finding to the degree of cor-pulmonale or RVH that is noted in such patients, the reason for this is considered to be due to the attenuation of the electrical vectors in the X-axis by the overlying lungs that surround the heart and the low diaphragms. In COPD, the QRS axis also tends to be oriented more vertically superiorly and left or inferiorly and rightward (*see* Section II—Axis Deviations and Intra-ventricular Conduction Defects).

The criteria for diagnosing right atrial overload/abnormalities

- Tall peaked P waves in the inferior leads (3 mm or more) (termed ***P-pulmonale*** in the older literature) (Fig. 12.45).
- Sharp peaked P wave in lead V1 or sharp peaked initial part of a biphasic P in lead V1.

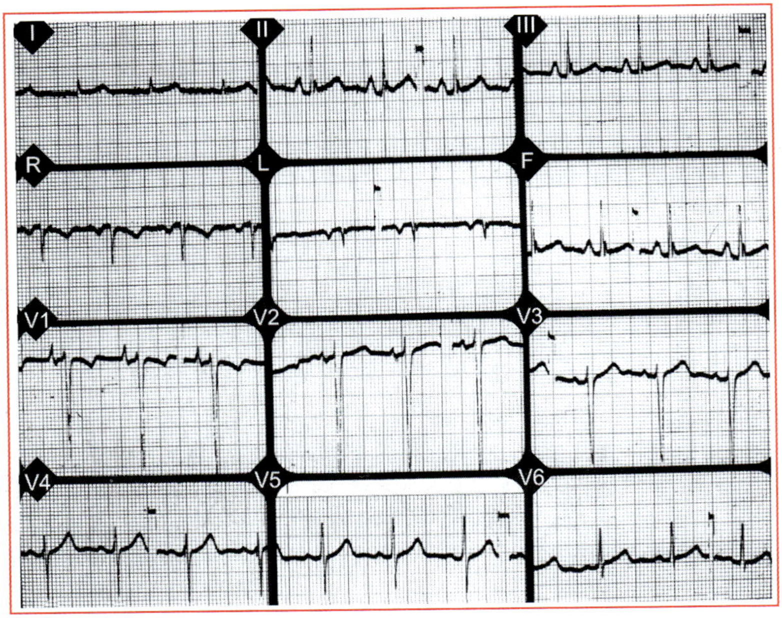

Fig. 12.45: Electrocardiogram with features of right atrial overload/ abnormality. Tall P waves in lead II. Initial component is sharp and peaked and lead V1.

- Occasionally, the P wave in V1 can be totally negative or markedly negative terminally in some patients with marked right atrial enlargement.
- A ***qR*** pattern in V1 when the right atrium is dilated with associated significant RVH that may actually result in the septum being anatomically rotated clockwise viewed from the apex, becoming more parallel to the frontal plane.[61,62] Lead V1 in such patients may almost become similar to an electrode placed on the right atrium due to proximity effect.

The P waves in the inferior leads can be tall and peaked in states of excess sympathetic stimulation with sinus tachycardia (e.g. hypoxic states). This may be due to synchronous activation of both atria and overlapping right and left atrial forces. Tall inferior P waves may be seen in some normal tall thin patients.

Electrocardiogram signs of right atrial overload may be seen in patients with severe pulmonary stenosis, significant pulmonary hypertension and in pulmonary embolism (in the latter condition, the signs may actually develop with the acute episode).

Certain congenital lesions may be associated with very large and tall P waves (sometimes termed ***giant P*** waves, amplitude > 6 mm). Notable lesions are Ebstein's anomaly (where part of the right ventricle is atrialized with an abnormal tricuspid valve that is displaced downward), total anomalous pulmonary venous connection, severe pulmonary stenosis and tricuspid atresia.[63]

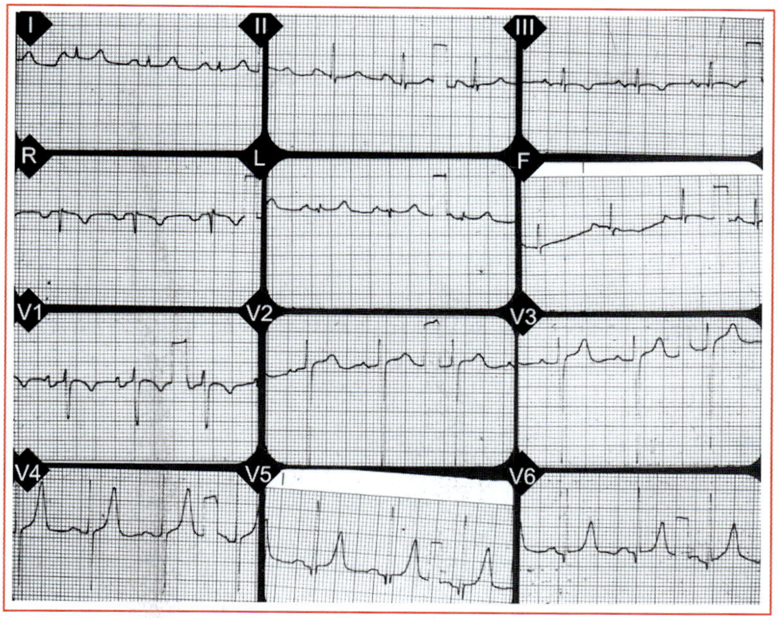

Fig. 12.46: Electrocardiogram features of left atrial overload/abnormality. P wave in V1 is biphasic with broad and deep (0.04 second duration and 1 mm depth) negative terminal force.

Left Atrial Overload/Abnormalities

Left atrial abnormality usually prolongs the atrial activation time and thus the P wave duration is often increased. The delayed activation results in notched or double peaked P wave as a result of asynchronous activation of the right and the left atria. Since the latter is a posterior chamber, activation of the left atrium turns the terminal electrical force of the P wave leftward as well as posterior. This is usually evident in lead V1, where the P wave is not only biphasic but will also show a wide and deep terminal negativity. The area of terminal negativity of the P wave in V1 is considered abnormal and indicative of left atrial overload if it is equal to 1 mm in depth and 1 mm (0.04 second) in width (Fig. 12.46).[64]

Prolongation of activation of the atrium (total duration of 120 ms or more) commonly accompanies left atrial overload or abnormality. Prolonged duration of the P wave may also be due to a delay in conduction through the interatrial pathway (Bachmann's bundle).[65] If the two peaks of the P waves are separated by about 0.04 second, then a definite interatrial block is probably present.

In patients with atrial fibrillation, the presence of coarse fibrillatory waves in lead V1 has also been shown to be indicative of left atrial overload or abnormality.[66]

The criteria for diagnosing left atrial overload/abnormality

i. Increased P wave duration of 120 ms or more
ii. Terminal negativity of P wave in lead V1 of about 1 mm (depth-amplitude) and about 0.04 second duration.

The wide notched P wave of left atrial abnormality has been referred to as ***P-mitrale*** (an old term) since it is seen in rheumatic heart disease, classically in mitral stenosis.[67] This term is no longer used since it can be caused by other conditions that cause left atrial overload.[68]

Increased terminal negativity of P wave may be seen in some patients with emphysema and COPD. Due to the low position of the diaphragms, the heart is often anatomically too low and vertical and the normal placement of the V leads may be too high in relation to the electrical center and therefore the P forces tend to point away from the electrodes. Pectus excavatum may also distort the apex of the heart more posteriorly. This tilt may cause the upper part of the right atrium to be more anterior and cause its activation to point posteriorly increasing the P negativity in V1.

P wave changes of left atrial overload/abnormalities can be seen in hypertensive and ischemic heart disease as well as in cardiomyopathies especially when accompanied by left ventricular dysfunction and elevated left atrial pressures. In acute myocardial infarction, it can be seen in patients with acute pulmonary edema, as well as in those with left ventricular dysfunction accompanied by papillary muscle dysfunction and mitral regurgitation.[68-71] It can also be seen in aortic valve disease especially in the presence of significant aortic stenosis.

Pathophysiology of P Wave Abnormalities in Atrial Overloads

It must be understood that left atrium can be secondarily involved in all conditions that affect the left ventricle just as the right atrium gets secondarily involved in conditions that affect the right ventricle such as pulmonary hypertension and pulmonary stenosis. The reason of course is that during diastole, the AV valves (mitral valve on the left side and the tricuspid valve on the right side) are open, both the atrium and the ventricle act as though they are one chamber. If the ventricles are involved in any disease process that leads to altered myocardial structure or function such as caused by hypertrophy, infiltration, ischemia, scarring or fibrosis, then its compliance will be decreased due to impaired relaxation as well as increased stiffness. This will lead to increased diastolic filling pressures in the ventricles, which will be transmitted to the atria since they form one chamber in diastole. In addition to these if there were any degree of AV valve regurgitation (e.g. mitral regurgitation on the left side and tricuspid regurgitation on the right side) it will further add to volume and pressure overloading of the corresponding atrium. The increased atrial pressures and/or volume will evoke strong atrial contraction due to Starling mechanism and will over a period of time eventually lead to atrial hypertrophy and/or enlargement with resultant P wave abnormalities discussed above.

Ventricular Hypertrophy (Enlargement)

Left Ventricular Hypertrophy

Hypertrophied ventricles by virtue of increased muscle mass that is often associated with the process, can be expected to increase electrical voltages of the QRS. Left ventricular hypertrophy (LVH) results when the left ventricle handles increased hemodynamic burden over a prolonged period of time as in systemic hypertension and/or aortic outflow obstruction (aortic stenosis). The increased systolic pressure will cause raised systolic wall tension (stress). Concentric hypertrophy is a basic adaptive mechanism for this type of increased work load, since increased wall thickness will tend to reduce the wall tension (by Laplace relationship). The criteria that have been developed over the years to diagnose left ventricular hypertrophy most often use measurements of QRS voltages derived either from the frontal plane leads and/or the precordial leads. Some of the criteria have been correlated to autopsy data.[72-74] More recent studies have used echocardiographically derived left ventricular mass for correlations.[75] The point score system[76] incorporates in addition to voltage criteria, other secondary abnormalities in QRS axis, QRS duration, QRS onset to peak time as well as P wave and ST-T abnormalities.

The important thing to realize is that the overall sensitivity of the various ECG criteria of diagnosis of LVH is generally low (<50%) although the specificity is usually high (about 85-90%).[77] In addition, the various criteria have different positive and negative predictive values in different populations.[78]

The criteria for the diagnosis of LVH are:

A. The (primary) voltage criteria
B. The various secondary criteria

The Voltage Criteria

It is imperative to understand that the QRS voltages can vary and be influenced by many other factors including, age, gender, race and body habitus. In addition to sites of electrode placement, the nature of intervening tissues between the heart and the electrodes also can affect the QRS voltages.

The commonly used QRS voltage criteria generally apply to adults older than 35 years of age.[77] In younger patients using voltage criteria alone will likely result in false positive diagnosis. Normal values of QRS voltages are higher in African-Americans. Women have a slightly lower upper limit of normal as well. Although obesity is associated with increased left ventricular muscle mass, the precordial voltages often do not reflect this and in fact the excess adipose tissue will in general decrease the voltages. The precordial voltages will often be exaggerated in patients with left mastectomy.[79]

Low limb lead voltages particularly in lead I (<5 mm) can be seen as a normal variant. They also can occur in COPD and mitral stenosis. The residual lung volume is increased in COPD as well as in mitral stenosis, which will tend to attenuate the X-axis electrical vectors.[80] In addition, low limb voltages can result from other causes of generalized decrease in QRS voltage as seen in pericardial diseases (with effusion or chronic constrictive process, infiltrative disorders such as amyloidosis and myxedema and cachectic states as seen in advanced malignancies.

The QRS amplitude in ECG is usually expressed in mm rather than millivolts. Under normal standardization, 10 mm equals 1 mV (meaning 1 mm equals 0.1 mV).

Some of the most commonly used voltage criteria are generally derived using combination of two leads, one closer to the left ventricle and the other far from the left ventricle. The ***R*** and ***S*** amplitudes in leads I and III are used in the index of Lewis,[72] and the index of Ungerleider.[73] The ***S*** in V1 and ***R*** in V5 or V6 are used in the index of Sokolow and Lyon.[74] The more recent Cornell voltage criteria use combination of both the frontal plane lead aVL and the horizontal plane lead V3 (Figs. 12.47A to C).[75]

The limb leads criteria are:

i. Index of Lewis: The net positivity in lead I plus the net negativity of lead III is 17 mm or more. This means that the opposite deflections in each lead need to be subtracted. If there is a q in lead I, the amplitude of the q is subtracted from the amplitude of the R wave to get the net positivity. If lead III has an rS complex, then the r wave amplitude is subtracted from the S wave amplitude to get the net negativity. Sometimes, one may get a deep Q followed by small r in lead III. In such a case, the amplitude of the r wave is subtracted from the amplitude of the Q to get the net negativity.

ii. Index of Ungerleider:
The ***R*** in lead I plus ***S*** in lead III equals to 25 mm or more.

iii. ***R*** in aVL > 11 mm.

iv. ***R*** in aVF > 20 mm.

The precordial leads criteria are:

i. ***Index of Sokolow and Lyon:***
The ***S*** in V1 plus ***R*** in V5 or V6 equals to 35 mm or more.
S in V2 can be used with ***R*** in V6 to make a modified index of Sokolow[21] (Fig. 12.47C).

ii. ***Index of McPhie:***
Any ***R*** plus any ***S*** in the precordium equals to 45 mm or more (Fig. 12.47D).

The Combination Voltage Criteria (Cornell)

S in V3 plus ***R*** in aVL equals to 28 mm or more (for men) and 20 mm or more (women)

The specificity of LVH diagnosis is increased when QRS voltage criteria are met in both the frontal and the horizontal planes. The accuracy is also enhanced when the presence of voltage criteria is accompanied by certain secondary criteria.

The secondary criteria

1. ***P wave of Left atrial overload/abnormality*** (Fig. 12.47D).
2. ***A delayed intrinsicoid deflection*** (ventricular activation time of 50 ms or more in leads with predominant R waves). The onset of the intrinsicoid deflection (also known as R wave peak time) usually corresponds to the peak of the R wave in the left precordial leads. The ventricular activation is the time from the onset of the QRS to the peak of the R wave in the left precordial leads. (Normal ventricular activation time is about 0.045 second or 45 ms). The delayed intrinsicoid deflection reflects the

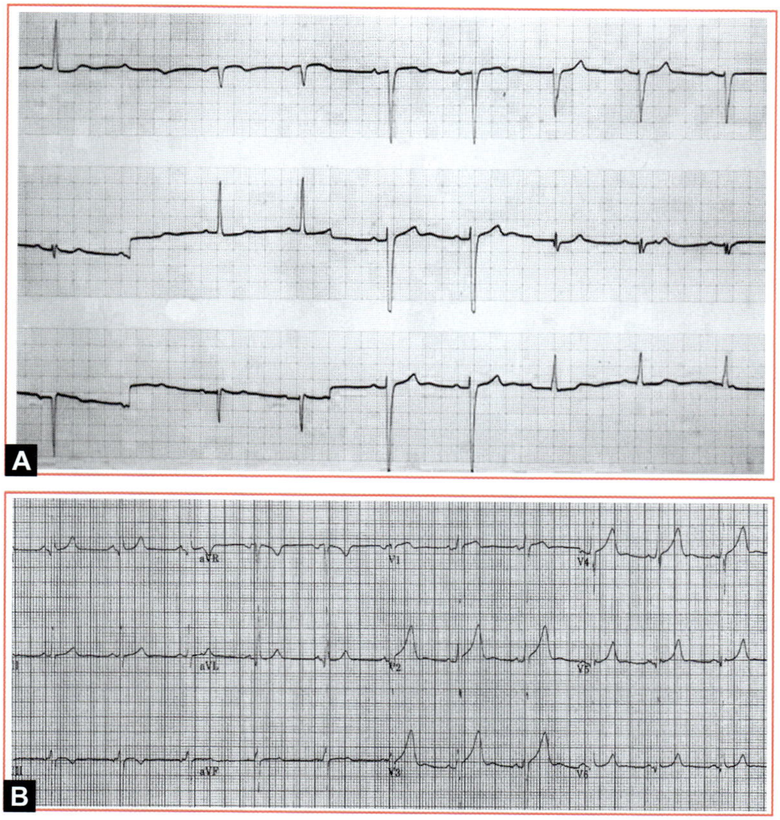

Figs. 12.47A and B: Electrocardiograms with features of left ventricular hypertrophy. Index of Lewis and combination voltage criteria (Cornell) are met in (A). Index of Lewis and Index of Sokolow and Lyon are met in a patient with moderately severe aortic regurgitation (B).

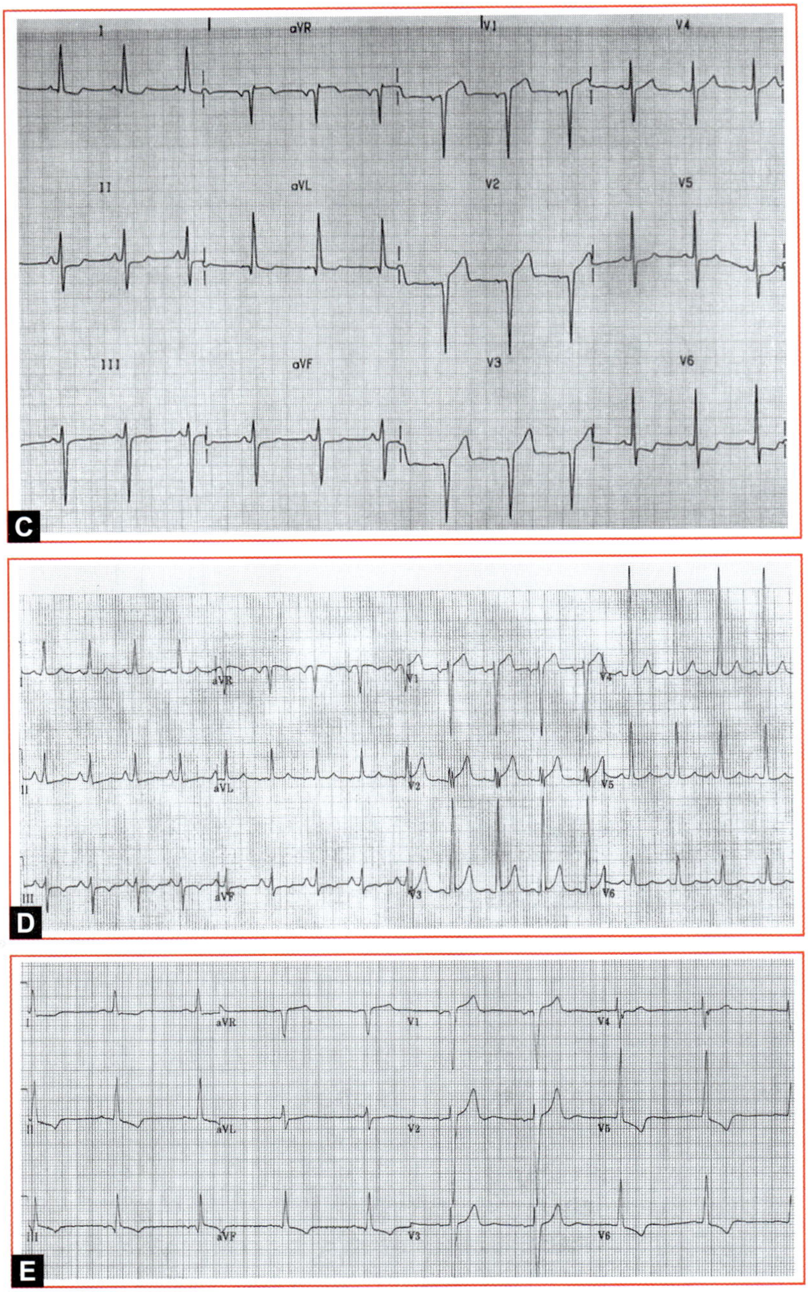

Figs. 12.47C to E: (C) Electrocardiogram with LVH. Modified Index of Sokolow and Lyon are met in this ECG. Left axis deviation secondary to left anterior fascicular block, a strong secondary criterion also present. (D) Electrocardiogram with LVH. Index of McPhie is met (any R plus any S in the precordium equals 45 mm or more). Also shows P wave of left atrial overload in V1. (E) Electrocardiogram with LVH. Loss of r wave in V1. Some slurring of the upstroke in V5 (inc left bundle branch block pattern).

increased time taken for the spread of excitation from the endocardium to the epicardium due to the increased ventricular wall thickness.

3. Initial right to left conduction resulting in ***the loss of the septal r wave in V1***. This may or may not be accompanied by prolongation of the QRS. In addition, it may be accompanied by some slurring of the upstroke of the R wave in the left ventricular leads (leads with predominant R waves, generally the left precordial leads) in the absence of LBBB or pre-excitation. These changes are similar to incomplete LBBB, without prolongation of the QRS. It can be simply termed as "incomplete LBBB pattern". These changes are usually due to septal scarring unbalancing the initial forces.[81] Invariably LVH is always present in such patients (Fig. 12.47E).
4. ***Leftward axis or left axis deviation/anterior fascicular block:*** Left ventricular hypertrophy per se may only contribute to some leftward axis but still within the normal range. In congenital aortic stenosis, the axis tends to be inferiorly oriented. This is seen most commonly without any associated right ventricular overload.[82]

   Abnormal left axis deviation may also be seen in association with LVH. When found with other LVH criteria, it probably represents a co-existing anterior fascicular block. Presence of anterior fascicular block is a strong secondary criterion for the diagnosis of LVH. Left ventricular hypertrophy in patients with hypertension often shows fibrosis in the upper part of the septum. In hypertrophic cardiomyopathy (HCM), left axis deviation has been shown to be present in about 10% of patients[83] (Fig. 12.47C).
5. ***Secondary ST- T wave abnormalities and abnormal QRS-T angle:*** It has been pointed out earlier that repolarization is a difficult process even in the normals since it takes place during mechanical systole when the intra-ventricular pressure is high and the endocardium is deprived of coronary flow. Since conditions that lead to LVH are usually associated with abnormal intra-ventricular systolic pressure as in systemic hypertension, aortic stenosis and others, repolarization in such states must be even more difficult. In addition, long-standing hypertrophy leads to decreased left ventricular compliance and increased stiffness. This will lead to increased filling pressures in diastole. This will further compromise sub-endocardial flow. Chronic sub-endocardial ischemia will lead to areas of myocyte necrosis and scarring and fibrosis. This will further increase the diastolic filling pressures making it a vicious cycle. Thus it will not be surprising to realize that the repolarization will significantly be altered when LVH is significant or present for prolonged periods. This can therefore result in various degrees of abnormality of ST-T waves. The T wave, which represents repolarization, tends to turn away from the QRS instead of being directed in the same direction as in normal patients. The QRS-T angle widens. This can be seen in the precordial leads in the early stages as lowish T wave in the left precordial leads. Normal T wave height

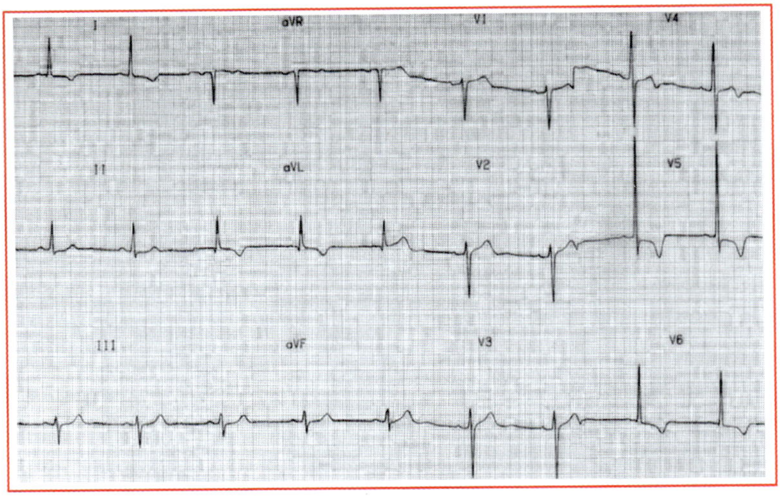

Fig. 12.48: Electrocardiogram with left ventricular hypertrophy (LVH) showing the LVH strain pattern seen in the left ventricular leads with predominant R waves (leads I and V6). ST segment has an upward convex long descending limb followed by a short ascending limb with asymmetrical inversion of the T waves.

in V6 is at least 10% of the R wave in the same lead. If the T wave height is <10% of the R wave in V6, it will represent a low T wave. In such cases the T wave in V1 will be taller than T wave in V6.[84]

As the LVH progresses, the T wave turns more and more anteriorly and away from the QRS and becoming inverted in the left precordial leads. Eventually, when fully developed, it results in the characteristic ST-T wave abnormalities termed as the ***"LVH strain pattern".*** This pattern of ST-T wave abnormality is seen typically in the left ventricular leads (leads with predominant R waves like the left precordial leads V5 and V6 and leads I and aVL). The ST segment is depressed at the ***J*** point with long descending limb that is upward convex and is followed by inverted T wave with a sharp ascending limb. The T wave inversion is asymmetric so that if one were to split the T wave into two halves by drawing a line through its nadir, the T wave inversion will be clearly seen to be asymmetric. This of course is unlike ischemic T waves that are often symmetrically inverted. The LVH strain pattern is quite specific for LVH even when the voltage criteria are not fully met[85,86] (Fig. 12.48). When the abnormal ST-T waves are seen in leads in the mid-precordial leads without predominant R waves, then it is no longer typical of LVH strain pattern. Ischemia will have to be clearly considered in such situations.

Diagnosis of LVH in the Presence of Bundle Branch Blocks

Anatomic LVH often coexists in patients with LBBB. Strict definitions of LBBB that require mid-ventricular slowing as shown by plateau topped or notched R waves in leads I, aVL, V5 and V6 show low sensitivity for LVH criteria.[87] If

QRS prolongation alone is present without significant notching of the QRS, then the voltage criteria will probably apply without leading to over diagnosis of LVH. A co-existing left atrial P wave abnormality/overload will also point to the co-existing LVH.[88]

The RBBB reduces the ***S*** wave in the precordial leads thereby reducing the sensitivity of the LVH criteria. The associated presence of left atrial overload and anterior divisional block will be helpful in the diagnosis of LVH.[89]

Left Ventricular Hypertrophy (LVH) in Hypertrophic Cardiomyopathy (HCM)

In this disorder, the LVH is an integral part of the clinical spectrum. Left ventricular hypertrophy with both voltage criteria and characteristic LVH strain pattern of ST-T abnormalities may be noted with and without obstruction (Fig. 12.49). The marked septal hypertrophy may actually cause deep septal ***Q*** waves in the left precordial leads and prominent septal ***R*** waves in the right precordial leads. With disease progression, development of an incomplete LBBB pattern and slurred upstroke of the R wave have been noted and pathologically this has been observed to be due to the development of septal scarring.[90] Occasionally, LVH may be absent in some patients without resting obstruction across the aortic outflow tract and no mitral regurgitation. In patients without obstructive component, the QRS tends to be more anterior with early R wave transition with negative T waves in the mid-precordium.[91] Sometimes, symmetrical T wave inversions have also been noted instead of the classic strain pattern.

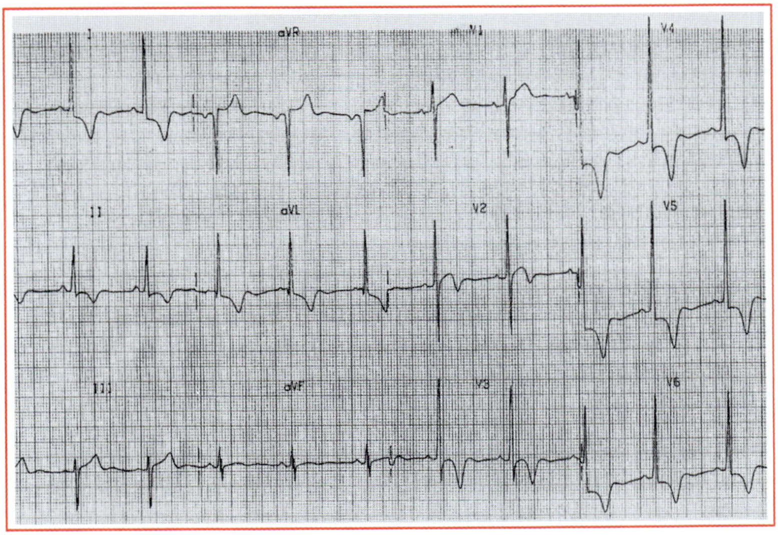

Fig. 12.49: Patient with non-obstructive hypertrophic cardiomyopathy with Electrocardiogram showing marked left ventricular hypertrophy (LVH) with typical ST-T abnormalities of LVH strain pattern noted on the left-sided leads.

Systolic (Pressure) and Diastolic (Volume) Overload of the Left Ventricle

These terms were first introduced by Cabrera and Monroy.[92,93] The typical ECG pattern of left ventricular systolic (pressure overload) are the features of LVH with the classical LVH strain pattern of ST-T waves described above under the secondary criteria. It is usually seen in systemic hypertension, aortic stenosis and coarctation of aorta. In these conditions, the left ventricle faces increased impedance to ejection that results in higher intra-ventricular systolic pressures. The increased intra-ventricular pressures result in concentric hypertrophy and when it becomes significant is typically associated with the secondary ST-T waves of the LVH strain pattern. In contrast, in conditions such as aortic regurgitation, mitral regurgitation, ventricular septal defect and persistent ductus arteriosus, the left ventricle ends up receiving more volume during diastole due to regurgitation or due to the left to right shunt. This will result in volume overload. This usually results in ventricular dilatation and sub-sequent eccentric hypertrophy as mentioned earlier. The ECG pattern typical of diastolic overload of the left ventricle consists of tall R waves in the left precordial leads, together with prominent septal ***q*** waves and with slight ST segment elevation and prominent upright T wave (*see* Fig. 12.47B).

The concept while of interest in understanding the hemodynamic burden in the various states, its application for diagnosis particularly in adult patients with acquired heart diseases is quite problematic and not clearly useful. This is because ST-T abnormalities may occur for a variety of causes including myocardial damage with and without ischemic heart disease. In young patients with congenital heart disease, it may be slightly more helpful.

Right Ventricular Hypertrophy

Electrical activation of the normal right ventricle is overshadowed by the thicker left ventricle and its contribution to the normal QRS complex is minimal and not easily seen except when late activation of the right ventricular outflow tract and pulmonary conus is present as in some normal subjects. The latter is recognized by the fact that the terminal portion of the QRS forces turns anterior and rightward showing positivity in leads V1 and aVR (with a terminal ***r*** or ***r'***) and away from the lateral leads (leads I and V6 showing terminal ***s*** instead). However, when significant RVH does occur, as in significant pulmonary stenosis and/or primary pulmonary hypertension, then the increased right ventricular muscle mass will tend to turn the mean electrical QRS forces toward the right in the frontal plane and anteriorly in the horizontal plane. This will result in a deep ***S*** wave in lead I and a prominent ***R*** in lead III as well as a dominant ***R*** in the right precordial leads together with deep S waves in the V6. The increased ventricular activation time may cause delayed

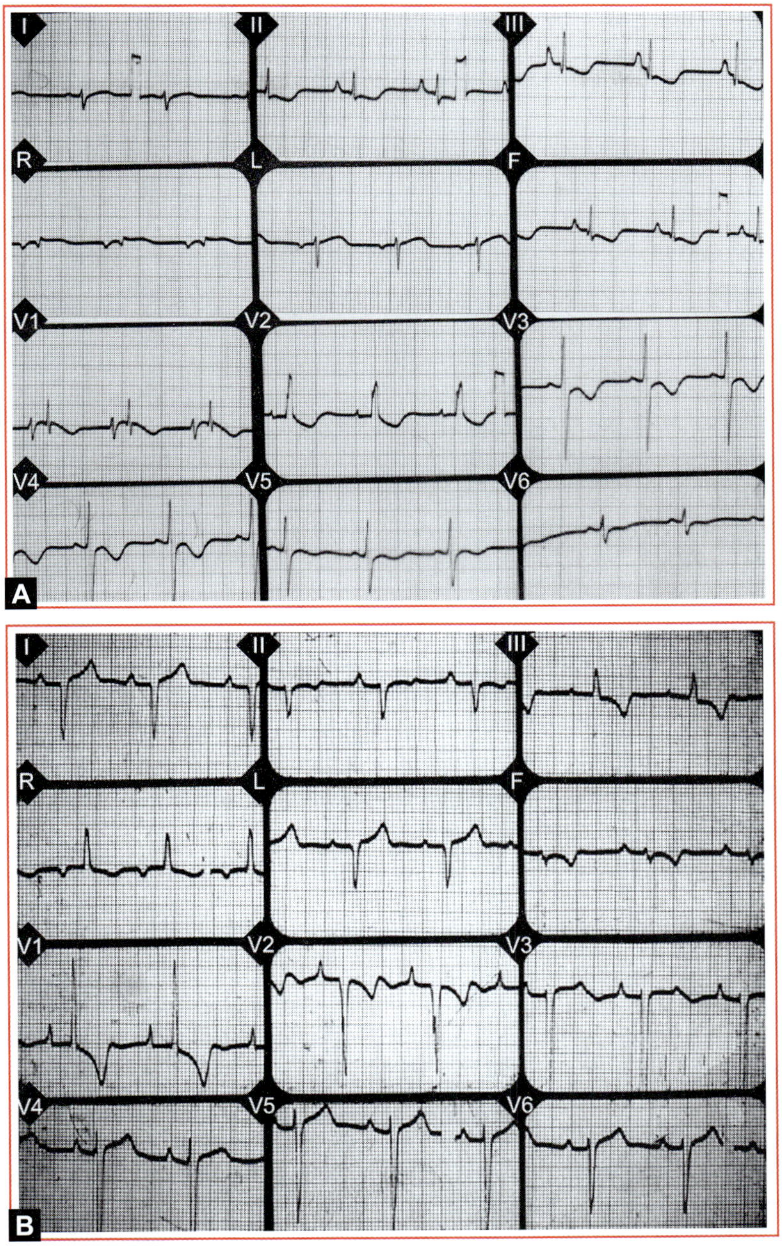

Figs. 12.50A and B: Electrocardiogram features of right ventricular hypertrophy (RVH) dominant R waves with negative T waves noted in leads V1 and V2 with sharp peaked initial component of P wave in V1 as with right atrial overload (A). Marked RVH noted with right axis deviation and dominant R waves in leads V1 and V2 with classic strain pattern of ST-T waves. Also noted right atrial overload P wave in V1 (B).

R wave peak in the right precordial leads. However, the delay is usually not pronounced to be of diagnostic value[94] (Figs.12.22B and 12.50A).

When the RVH is significant, eventually the repolarization forces will also become altered resulting in wide QRS-T angle similar to what is observed, in late stages of LVH. The secondary ST-T changes of RVH would result in ST depression with asymmetric T wave inversion as in LVH strain pattern except these will be seen in the right precordial leads that will have the predominant R waves due to hypertrophied right ventricle (Fig. 12.50B).

ST-T abnormalities may also be noted in the inferior leads. If the T waves are biphasic in the right precordial leads, the configuration associated with RVH is usually of the type that is negative followed by positive.

T wave may remain upright however in infants and children with RVH. In normal infant, T wave remains upright in the right precordium for about a week after birth. After that period, it normally becomes negative and remains so until early adulthood and is called the juvenile T pattern. A T wave, which remains or becomes positive in V1 (or V3R) during infancy, will be suggestive of RVH.

Several criteria derived from the amplitude of the ***R*** and ***S*** waves in leads I, III, V1 and V6 have been proposed. Some of them have been based on autopsy data, and some based on clinical and hemodynamic data consistent with increased right ventricular workload.[77,95-99]

The limb lead criteria that is similar to the index of Lewis, is ***S*** in I plus ***R*** in lead III equals to 15 mm or more (subtracting the opposite deflections). The horizontal plane voltage criterion (the index of Sokolow for RVH) is ***R*** in V1 plus ***S*** in V5 or V6 equals to 11 mm or more.[100]

The combination of the following criteria is quite specific for RVH:

1. Right axis deviation 100° or more
2. ***qR*** in V1 (or V3R, i.e. V3 placed to the right of the sternum instead the left) and
3. R/S ratio in V1 > 1

In the presence of incomplete RBBB with QRS duration <0.12 second, an R/S or R′/S ratio > 1 with R′ in V1 > 5 mm with a mean QRS axis of +110° has been suggested as indicative of RVH.[101] Predicted RVH was correct in 24 of their 32 autopsy confirmed cases. Although the sensitivity of the electrocardiographic criteria is low, some criteria have high specificity. The variations in sensitivity are mainly due to differences in the patient categories studied. In addition, acquired RVH such as in mitral stenosis and chronic obstructive pulmonary disease is less striking than RVH associated with thromboembolic pulmonary hypertension or congenital lesions such as isolated pulmonary valvular stenosis and tetralogy of Fallot.

Right Ventricular Systolic and Diastolic Overload

Right ventricular systolic overload pattern is classically seen in conditions such as isolated severe pulmonary valvular stenosis and severe Tetralogy of Fallot (with resting right to left shunt due to severe right ventricular outflow tract obstruction) and in significant pulmonary hypertension. It usually is accompanied by an ***R*** wave in V1 with a small ***s*** or tiny ***q*** before it. The T wave is usually negative with ST-T configuration as in Strain pattern described under LVH except that it is noted in lead V1.

With diastolic overload as seen in atrial septal defect, where the right ventricle receives more volume during diastole (the normal venous return plus the additional flow as a result of the left to right shunt through the atrial septum), the right ventricular gets enlarged and the hypertrophy seems to involve mainly the crista supraventericularis in the right ventricular outflow tract.[102] This results in the classic ***rSR′*** pattern in V1. It is seen in atrial septal defect, partial anomalous pulmonary venous return or tricuspid regurgitation. It may be sometimes associated with some QRS prolongation enough to cause ***R′*** in V1, and the terminal ***S*** in leads I and V6 to be slightly wider as in incomplete RBBB. It is conceivable that RV enlargement may in fact cause some stretching of the right bundle and produce the electrical delay in such situations (*see* Fig. 12.37).

The clinical application of this concept of systolic and diastolic overloads has limitations particularly in acquired heart conditions. The correlation to the hemodynamic burden is better in congenital heart disease.[47]

Specific Clinical Conditions

1. ***Congenital pulmonary valvular stenosis and Tetralogy of Fallot and primary pulmonary hypertension:*** The RVH when significant in these conditions would reflect the underlying abnormal hemodynamic burden on the right ventricle. The resultant ECG changes include typical RAD, ***qR*** in V1 (or V3R) and ***R/S*** ratio > 1 in V1 (accompanied by ***R/S*** ratio in V6 < 1). In severe pulmonary stenosis, the QRS–T angles particularly in the horizontal plane are usually wide and > 100°.[103]
2. ***Chronic obstructive pulmonary disease:*** The ECG changes accompanying chronic obstructive pulmonary disease (COPD) are ascribed to the poorly conducting overinflated lungs with low diaphragms. The QRS forces are oriented often superiorly and posteriorly, the axis of the P wave is usually 60° or more.[42] The P wave in lead aVL is usually negative and often accompanied by low QRS voltage in general and especially in lead I (Fig. 12.51). Recognition of co-existing RVH in patients with COPD is often difficult. However, if the QRS axis is 110° or more, with a classic RVH pattern in V1, then concomitant RVH must be present. In patients with O_2 saturation <85%, often ECG might show slight tachycardia, T wave inversion in the right precordial leads and ST segment depression in the inferior leads. In severe cases of cor-pulmonale, prominent R waves develop in the right precordium as well.
3. ***Pulmonary hypertension in mitral stenosis***: Patients with mitral stenosis who show ECG evidence of RVH with dominant ***R*** in V1 with abnormal ***R/S*** ratio in V1 and RAD often tend to have elevated pulmonary arterial pressures.[104]

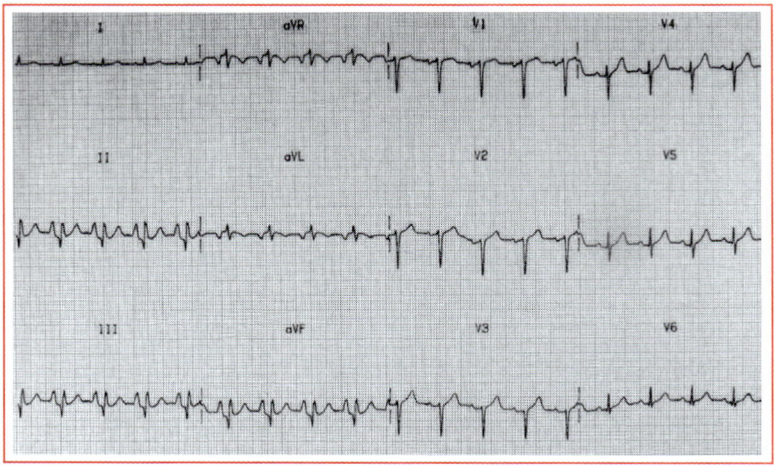

Fig. 12.51: Electrocardiogram of patient with chronic obstructive pulmonary disease (COPD). Tall P waves in the inferior leads, low voltage in lead I and negative P in aVL, typical features of COPD noted.

4. ***Right ventricular hypertrophy and pulmonary embolism:*** Acute pulmonary embolism tends to produce sudden rise in pulmonary outflow resistance. As a consequence, the pulmonary arterial and the RV systolic pressures rise. Right ventricle unable to deal with acute rise in pulmonary arterial pressures ends up also being dilated. Often there is hypoxemia that develops which also leads to sympathetic stimulation and tachycardia. Sudden dilatation of the RV will end up stretching the right bundle branch that courses through the moderator band. It may result in the development of RBBB. Besides sinus tachycardia, the sudden rise in RV pressure may also cause right atrial overload. The P wave may become tall and peaked in the inferior leads (Figs. 12.52A and B). It may also precipitate atrial arrhythmias, atrial flutter in particular and also atrial fibrillation.

The frontal plane QRS axis may shift classically to the right or sometime also to the left. The initial part of the QRS often turns superiorly causing a ***Q*** wave in the inferior leads (leads III and aVF). The terminal portion of the QRS often turns rightward and inferior resulting in ***S*** in leads aVL and I. In addition to the RBBB, anterior and even posterior divisional blocks may develop as a result of massive pulmonary embolism. The divisional blocks if they develop, are thought to be caused by dilatation of the part of the septum through which the anterior or the posterior fascicles of the left bundle course through.[105-108] The T wave may turn away from the RV toward the left causing negative T waves in the inferior leads, often called "S1,Q3,T3" for short. It is part of the so-called ***McGinn-White Syndrome*** that in addition includes symptoms and signs of massive pulmonary embolus (tachycardia, tachypnea, hypoxemia and hypotension with or without collapse), depressed

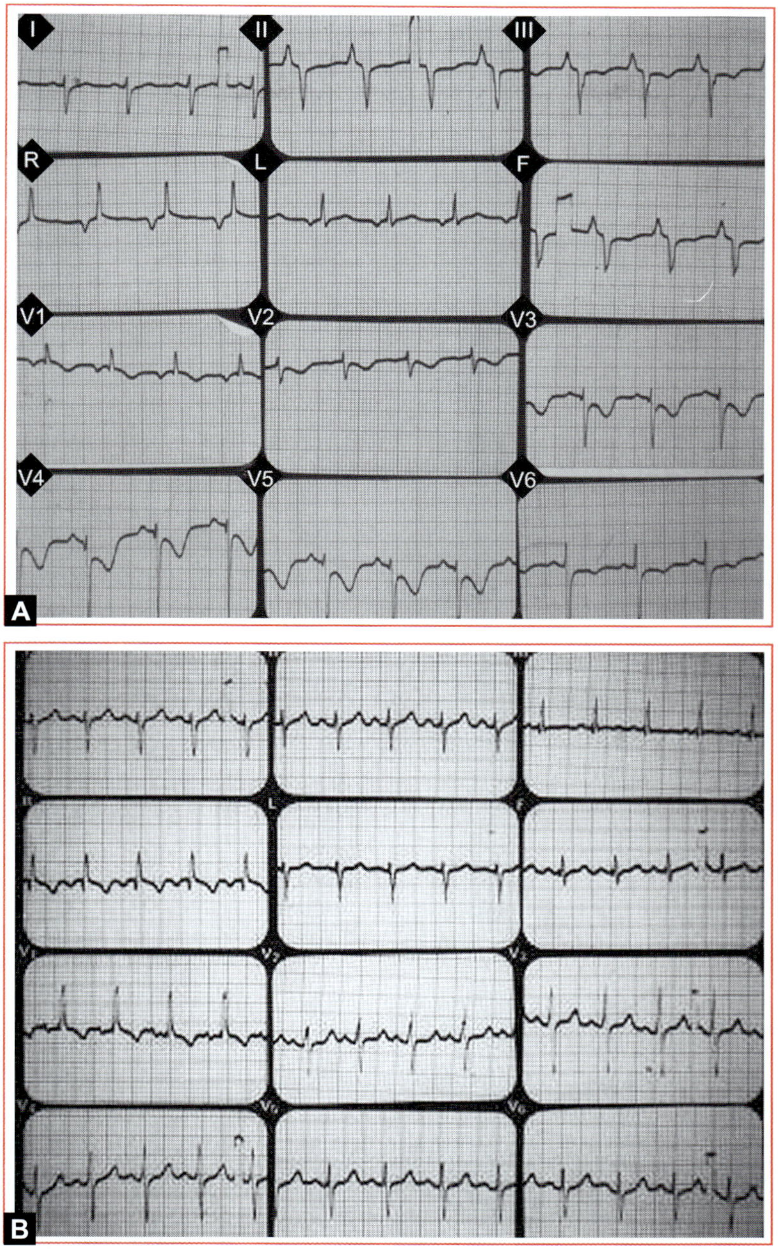

Figs. 12.52A and B: Patient with acute pulmonary embolism. Electrocardiogram showing right axis deviation, P waves as with right atrial overload. Dominant R waves in lead V1 with negative T waves in the right precordial leads (A).
Electrocardiogram from another patient with thromboembolic pulmonary hypertension showing mild sinus tachycardia, RAD and dominant R in V1 with negative T waves.

ST segment in lead II and ***J*** point depression in lead I and terminal T wave inversion in lead III.

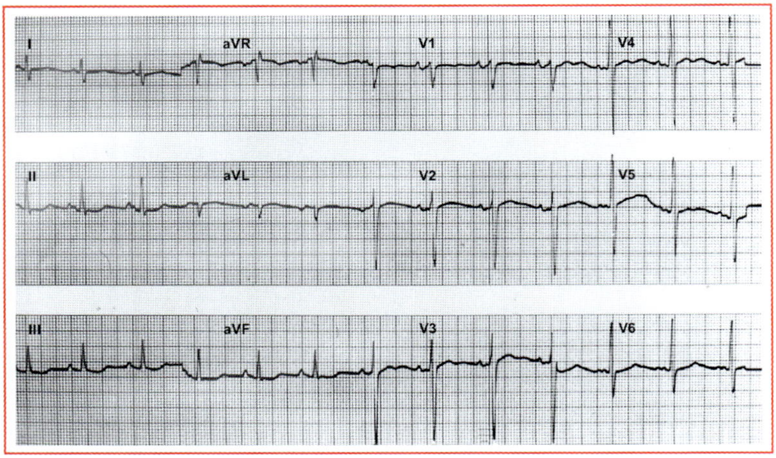

Fig. 12.53: Electrocardiogram showing vertical axis and large biphasic QRS complexes in the precordial leads suggestive of biventricular hypertrophy.

Combined Ventricular Overload/Hypertrophy

Biventricular hypertrophy is suggested when in the presence of ECG criteria of LVH, if the following[109,110] are noted:

i. Prominent ***S*** waves in V5 or V6
ii. Right axis deviation with LVH voltage in the chest leads (except in the case of congenital aortic stenosis)
iii. Tall biphasic ***R/S*** complexes are noted in the mid-precordial leads (typically seen in patients with ventricular septal defect, termed as ***Katz-Wachtel*** phenomenon)[111] (Fig. 12.53)
iv. Presence of both right and left atrial overload are suggested

SECTION IV: MYOCARDIAL INFARCTION

Definition and Diagnostic Criteria

The term myocardial infarction implies cardiomyocyte necrosis. The mechanisms for such pathological consequence are known to be multiple. It can be from atherosclerotic plaque rupture in the coronary vessels that initiates cascading processes that lead to platelet adhesion, clumping and formation of an occluding thrombus that results in total interruption of flow in a coronary artery. The latter will lead to ischemia of the cardiac muscle cells perfused by the affected coronary artery and when the ischemia has been maintained long enough without spontaneous or therapeutic clot lysis and re-establishment of flow will lead to myocardial cell death. This will be reflected in rising levels of biomarkers such as the cardiac enzymes or more specifically cardiac troponin (cTn*)* (the I or the T fraction) within several minutes (as little as 20 minutes) to a few hours (2–4 hours) of the ischemic injury.[112,113] The same result can occur in situations where demand in myocardial oxygen exceeds supply with or without the presence of coronary artery disease. The supply-demand imbalance can occur in a variety of clinical situations such as severe tachy or brady arrhythmias, aortic dissection, severe aortic valve disease, HCM, shock syndromes (septic, cardiac and others), states of hypoxia (respiratory failure), severe anemia, severe hypertension, coronary spasm, coronary embolism, vasculitis, coronary endothelial dysfunction without coronary artery disease. Myocardial injury can also result unrelated to ischemia from direct myocardial involvement such as chest trauma, defibrillator shocks, myocarditis with or without associated pericarditis and cardiotoxic agents such as anthracyclines.[114] Recent development of sensitive markers of myocardial necrosis and their application in diagnosis in critically ill patients as well as those related to percutaneous coronary interventions and after cardiac surgery had led to the development of an expert consensus document called the "third universal definition of myocardial infarction". It was developed jointly by the European Society of Cardiology (ESC), the American College of Cardiology Foundation (ACCF), the American Heart Association (AHA) and the World Heart Federation (WHF). The definition establishes the troponin levels required to make a diagnosis of MI in various clinical situations.[115] An increased cTn concentration is defined as a value exceeding the 95th percentile of a normal reference population (upper reference limit). Myocardial infarction is determined by the specific cTn value and at least one of the following five criteria*:*

i. Symptoms of ischemia
ii. New (or presumably new) significant ST-T wave changes or left bundle branch block
iii. Development of pathological ***Q*** waves on ECG
iv. Imaging evidence of new loss of viable myocardium or regional wall-motion abnormality
v. Identification of intracoronary thrombus by angiography or autopsy

Symptoms of Ischemia

Symptoms related to acute coronary syndromes and more specifically to acute myocardial infarction include typical central chest tightness, with or without radiation to neck, throat or the arms. Discomfort can be vague in description and character and can also be in other locations including the jaw, epigastrium, in the back or in the arms or the hands. The episode may or may not be provoked or associated with physical or mental stress. The discomfort associated with a myocardial infarction usually will last more than 20 minutes. It is important to realize that sometimes there may not be any discomfort or pain but patient may simply present with ischemic equivalent symptoms of dyspnea, tiredness, fatigue or syncope. Sometimes, there may be associated symptoms such as nausea vomiting or sweating. Finally, MI may be entirely silent without any symptoms or present with symptoms of palpitation or cardiac arrest.

Clinical Types of Myocardial Infarction

The modern era of thrombolysis and percutaneous interventions of the occluded coronary vessel to re-establish flow on an urgent basis to preserve myocardial function has also improved the clinical outcome of patients with acute MI. For the sake of reperfusion therapy, the practice dictates that patients presenting with suspected or confirmed MI be classified into two main types, namely:

i. Those who have typical diagnostic ST segment elevation (*see* below under ECG Changes of MI) called ***"ST elevation MI" (STEMI)***.

ii. Those who do not show ST segment elevation called ***"non-ST elevation MI" (NSTEMI)***

Many patients with MI may develop pathological ***Q*** waves but some may not.

ECG Changes of Myocardial Infarction

The changes in the electrical force caused by an Myocardial Infarction include:

- The initial part of the QRS often tends to turn away from the site of an infarction
- The terminal part of the QRS usually points to the site of the infarction
- ST segment vector points also toward the site of infarction when the infarction is truly transmural meaning both sub-epicardial and sub-endocardial
- The T wave often points away from the site of the infarction after the hyperacute phase.

However, in the very early phase ***(hyperacute)***, the T wave points to the site of the infarct. It must be noted that acute myocardial infarction being a clinical diagnosis aided by ECG changes as well as confirmation with elevated biomarkers, not all or any of the ECG changes need to be present in al instances. Often combination of changes may be found. Sometimes, infarction could occur without any ECG changes as well. This is more frequently seen in cases of circumflex vessel occlusion. The outcomes of MI, in patients with or without the development of Q waves, were thought to be similar. However, in the current era of early thrombolysis, the outcome seems to be somewhat better when the Q waves do not develop.[116]

Temporal Sequence of Changes

In experimental coronary occlusion in animal models such as the dog, the first effect of occlusion with a clamp will be to cause T wave inversion, which will reverse if the artery is unclamped immediately. If the coronary artery is occluded more than a minute, ST segment will be elevated due to what is known as the ***"current of injury"*** in leads overlying the infarcted area. If coronary occlusion is maintained for 45 minutes or more, abnormally wider ***Q*** waves will develop. The ***Q*** waves may or may not regress completely with unclamping.[117] In experimental studies in monkeys as well as in humans, the first change with an acute MI is ST segment elevation due to injury current in leads facing the infarcted area.[118] Sometimes, this may be accompanied by tall upright T waves called the ***hyper acute T waves***. If infarction results in pathological ***Q*** waves they usually appear about 2 hours after the onset of symptoms and often fully develop within 12 hours[119] By the time the ***Q*** waves develop, the T waves become inverted in the same leads that show the ***Q*** waves. The T wave inversion can persist for variable periods of time ranging from several days to several weeks or more. Electrocardiograms may return to normal in 20% of patients after 4 years. However if ***Q*** waves develop with infarction, only in about 5% of patients, it is likely to become normal.[120] We shall discuss the various changes mentioned above in the order of the sequence of their development.

Changes in the ST Segment

Vector of Infarction—Current of Injury

The current of injury is recognized in the ECG by the presence of abnormal ST segment elevation in two or more contiguous leads among the standard 12 leads (except lead aVR). The definition requires that the elevation of the ST segment at the ***J*** point be >2 mm with standard calibration in leads V1,V2 and V3 and > 1 mm in all other leads.[121] The ***junctional "J" point*** (where the QRS ends and the ST segment begins) is used to determine the magnitude of the ST segment shift. New or presumed new ***J*** point elevation of >1 mm (> 0.1 mV) is required in all leads other than V2 and V3. In healthy men under age 40, ***J*** point elevation can be as much as 0.25 mV in leads V2 and V3. It decreases with increasing age. In healthy women, the ***J*** point elevation is less than in men. ***"Contiguous leads"*** refers to lead groups such as ***anterior leads*** (leads V1–V6), ***inferior leads*** (leads II, III, aVF) or ***lateral leads*** (leads I and aVL).

Small potential differences normally may occur across the myocardial cells briefly just at the end of depolarization and this may cause deviation of the junctional (***J***) point of the ST segment (where the QRS ends and the ST segment begins) but not the distal plateau phase of the ST segment. Ischemic injury however can lead to generation of currents both during electrical systole and electrical diastole for the following reasons:

i. Shortening and decreased amplitude of the action potentials of the affected myocardial cells
ii. In addition, during the diastolic phase (the TP segment from the end of the T wave to the next P wave), the injured cells will remain in a depolarized state (less negative resting membrane potential)

The former will result in shift of the ST segment while the latter will displace the baseline.[122,123] With epicardial injury, the resultant effect is elevation of the ST segment in leads facing the affected area. With endocardial injury, the effect will be to cause ST segment depression (Fig. 12.54).

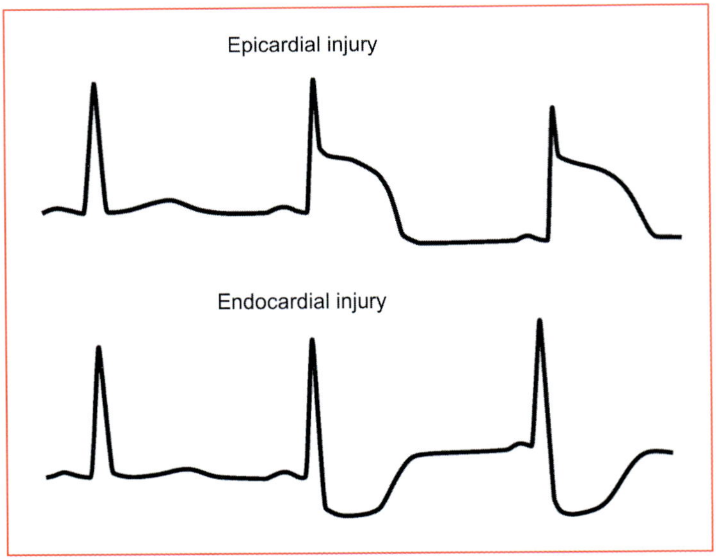

Fig. 12.54: Diagram showing the effect of epicardial and endocardial injury on ST segment. Epicardial injury results in ST segment elevation and endocardial injury results in ST segment depression in leads facing the affected area of the heart. Arrows indicate flow of currents shifting the ST segment and the baseline. (Adapted from Surawicz and Saito (1978).

Correlation of ST Segment Elevation and Depression to the Anatomic Region of the Heart and the Coronary Artery Involved

The affected region of the heart usually corresponds to the position of the leads on the body surface that shows the ST segment elevation. The correlations of the ST segment elevation to the actual culprit coronary lesion have also been carried out during coronary angiographic studies performed in patients presenting with acute MI.[53,124,125]

Some of the salient points of these Correlations are as follows:

A. ***Anterior wall ischemia/infarction:*** Anterior wall ischemia/infarction is usually due to occlusion of the left anterior descending coronary artery. The ST segment vector is usually directed to the left and laterally resulting ST segment elevation in some of the leads V1–V6. Whether the occlusion is proximal or distal can be discerned by the specific leads that show the ST segment elevation and or reciprocal depression due to the resulting ST vector direction.

   i. ***Proximal LAD occlusion (before the first septal and the first diagonal branch):*** This will result in infarction of the anterior and lateral walls and the inter-ventricular septum. The ST segment vector will be directed superiorly and to the left. This will result in ST segment elevation in V1–V4 and aVL (Fig. 12.55).

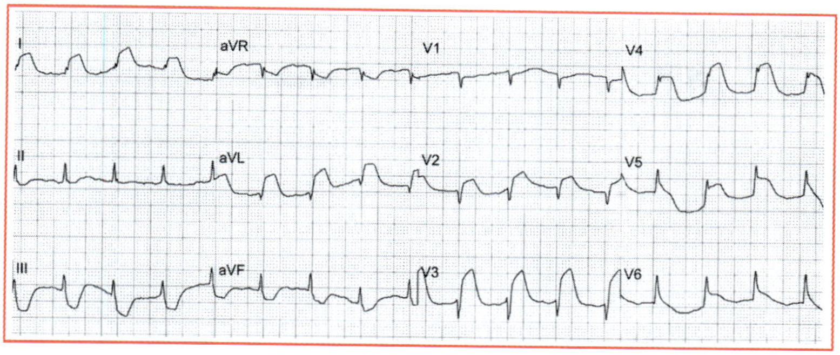

Fig. 12.55: Acute ST elevation myocardial infarction with ST segment elevations in leads V2–V5 and aVL. Suggestive of proximal occlusion of left axis deviation before the first septal and first diagonal branch.

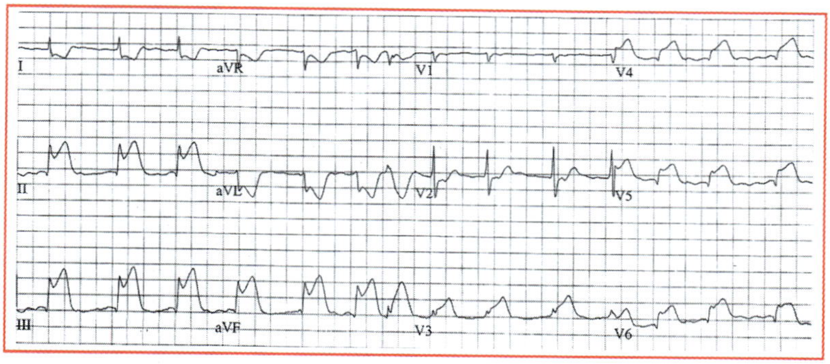

Fig. 12.56: Acute ST elevation myocardial infarction with ST elevations in the inferior leads and leads V3–V6. Suggestive of distal left axis deviation occlusion (distal to the first septal and the first diagonal branch).

ii. ***LAD occlusion between the first septal and the first diagonal:*** The basal inter-ventricular septum will be spared. ST segment in V1 will not be elevated. ST segment vector will be directed toward lead aVL. Lead III will show reciprocal depression.

iii. ***Distal LAD occlusion (distal to the first septal and the first diagonal):*** This will spare the basal part of the left ventricle. ST segment vector will be directed more inferiorly. The ST segment will not be elevated in aVL or aVR. There will be ST segment elevation in the inferior leads as well as in leads V3–V6. This likely indicates a large LAD that goes around the apex. ST segment elevation will be less prominent in V2 unlike in the proximal occlusions[126] (Fig. 12.56).

B. ***Inferior wall infarction***: Inferior infarction is associated with ST segment elevation in the inferior leads II, III and aVF only. It may be caused by occlusion of either the right coronary artery (RCA) or the left circumflex (LCx) depending on which vessel is dominant and provides the posterior descending branch (Fig. 12.57).

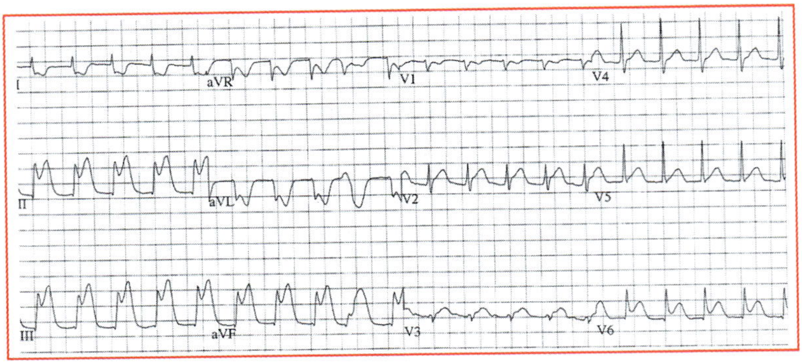

Fig. 12.57: Acute inferior myocardial infarction. ST segment elevations in the inferior leads. Occlusion of right coronary artery or the left circumflex depending on the dominant vessel.

i. ***RCA occlusion:*** This causes ST vector to be directed more to the right than when the LCx is the culprit artery. ST segment elevation will be more in lead III than in lead II and will be associated with reciprocal depression in lead aVL and less so in lead I.[127]

ii. ***Proximal RCA occlusion and RV involvement:*** When the RCA is occluded quite proximally, RV ischemia or infarction may result. ST segment vector will be directed to the right, anteriorly and inferiorly. ST segment elevation will therefore be seen in right anterior chest leads in positions referred to as V3R and V4R. It is important to realize that ST elevation in the right chest leads associated with RV involvement is often transient and may not be seen after symptoms abate.[124]

C. ***ST segment depression in leads V1–V3 in inferior infarction:*** When inferior infarction with typical ST segment elevation in the inferior leads is associated with ST segment depression in the precordial leads V1–V3 with subsequent development of abnormally tall and/or wide R waves in the same leads, it has been traditionally attributed to posterior or postero-lateral ischemia or infarction. These have been based on pathologic correlations.[128,129] However, recent studies using magnetic resonance imaging (MRI) have demonstrated that the wall that truly corresponds to the traditional posterior wall to be actually lateral. It has therefore been suggested that it be replaced by the term lateral[130] (Figs. 12.58A and B).

D. ***Inferior infarction due to LCx occlusion:*** The ST segment vector in this instance will be directed more to the left than right and the ST segment elevation will be more in lead II than in lead III and likely to show ST to be isoelectric or elevated also in leads I and aVL.[131]

E. ***ST segment depression in more than one discrete region (not reciprocal):*** In the absence of ST elevation in the inferior leads, Leads I and aVL and V2–V6, if ST segment depression is noted and is seen in all of the

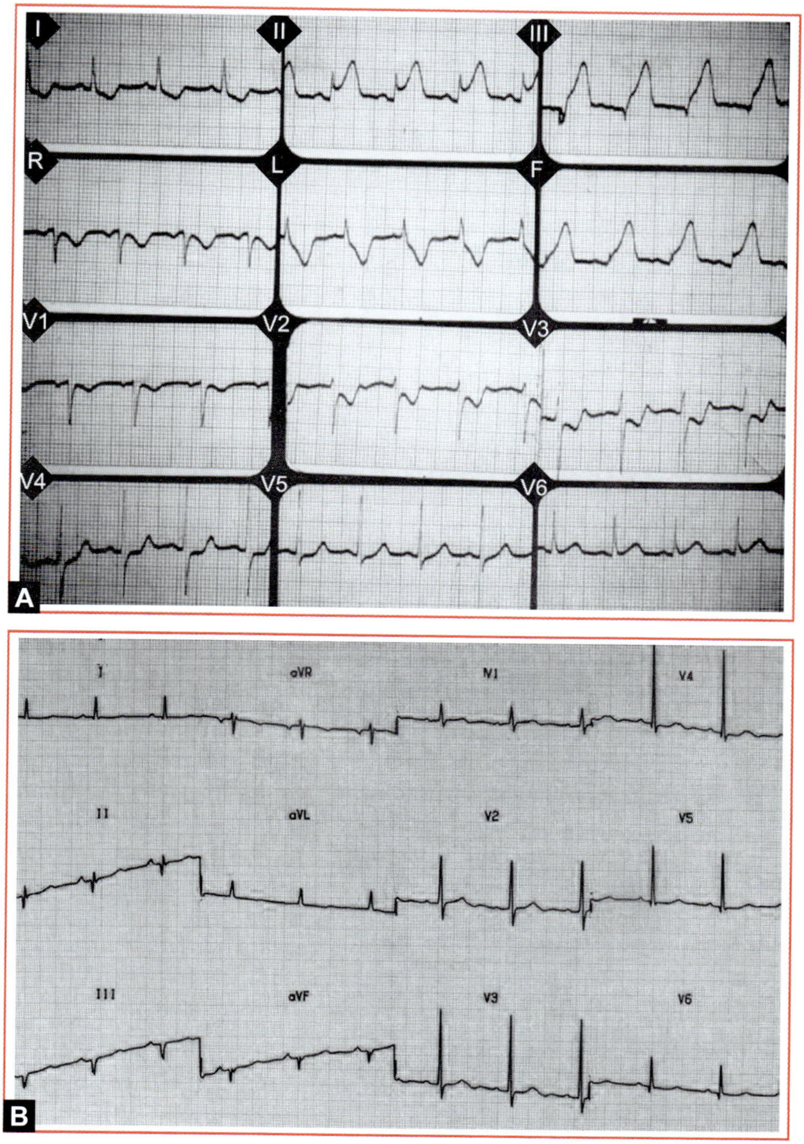

Figs. 12.58A and B: Electrocardiogram from pt with ST elevation myocardial infarction inferior wall with ST segment depression in the right precordial leads in the acute phase (A). Electrocardiogram from the late phase of similar infarction, with development of Q waves in the inferior leads accompanied by dominant R waves in V1 and V2 confirming posterior wall involvement (B).

leads except aVR and V1, this will mean that the current of injury is directed toward the cavity of the left ventricular chamber and away from the epicardial surface. In this situation, leads aVR and V1 may in fact show ST elevation indicating that the current of injury is pointing rightward

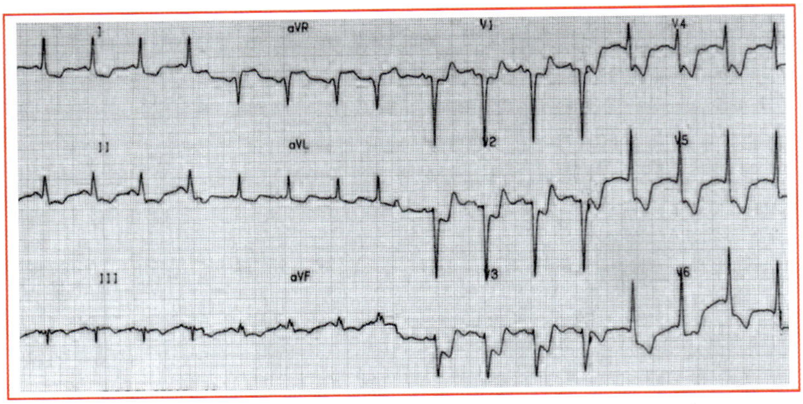

Fig. 12.59: Patient with acute coronary syndrome with marked ST segment depression in leads I and aVL and V2–V6 indicating possible sub-endocardial infarction (may indicate multivessel or left main coronary stenosis).

and superiorly away from the main body of the left ventricle. This usually means non-transmural (sub-endocardial) ischemia if brought on during stress test. If it occurs in the setting of symptoms of acute coronary syndromes, it usually implies multivessel disease or left main stenosis[124,132] (Fig. 12.59).

Other causes of ST segment elevation include the following:[53,133]

- ST segment elevation in more than one discrete region is characteristic of pericarditis involving large areas of the epicardial surface.[53] (*see* Section V: Ventricular Pre-excitation/Pericarditis)
- Elevated serum potassium
- Osborne (***J***) waves of hypothermia
- Acute myocarditis
- Certain cardiac tumors
- Normal variant referred to as early repolarization (ER)
- Pulmonary embolism and acute cor-pulmonale usually lead III
- Pancreatitis
- Brugada syndrome
- Arrhythmogenic right ventricular dysplasia

Resolution of and Persistence of ST Segment Elevation after an Acute MI: With the advent of thrombolytic and other reperfusion therapy including percutaneous intervention, it has become clear that regression of ST segment elevation is a good sign of successful recanalization.[134,135] Incomplete resolution often implies increased early mortality.[136] Persistence of ST segment elevation appears to correlate better with dyskinesia rather than a true ventricular aneurysm (that usually has a scar in its wall that tends to have a bulge both during systole and diastole).[137]

Evaluation of ST Segment Elevation in the Setting of Intra-ventricular Conduction Defect

ST segment elevation associated with an acute MI is not affected by the presence of fascicular blocks and/or right bundle branch block. They are however affected by the presence of left bundle branch block because of the presence of more pronounced secondary ST-T wave changes associated with the conduction defect. Criteria for infarction in the presence of LBBB have been put forth from a retrospective analysis of patients enrolled in the thrombolysis GUSTO I trial.[138] These include concordant ST elevation of 1 mm or more in leads with positive QRS and ST segment depression of 1 mm or more in leads with dominant S wave. The third criterion is discordant ST segment elevation of 5 mm or more in leads with negative QRS complex. The concordant ST changes have been reported to have high specificity but low sensitivity.

Changes in the T Waves Direction Due to Infarction

T wave after an infarction is formed by the resultant of the normal myocardial repolarization as well as the repolarization from the ischemic and injured myocardium. Often after an ischemic event following ST segment elevation, T waves become inverted in leads with previous ST segment elevation. This reflects the fact that the T wave direction points away from the site of the infarction. T waves may remain inverted for several days and occasionally persist for a long time (Fig. 12.60). Sometimes, tall pointed or deeply negative T waves associated with prolonged QT interval may occur either before or after regression of ST segment elevation begins. The peaked T waves that appear quite early in the infarction are termed the ***hyperacute T waves***.

Patients with deeply inverted T waves (>5 mm or 0.5 mV) in the precordial leads V2, V3, V4 and occasionally in V5 with long QT interval after an episode

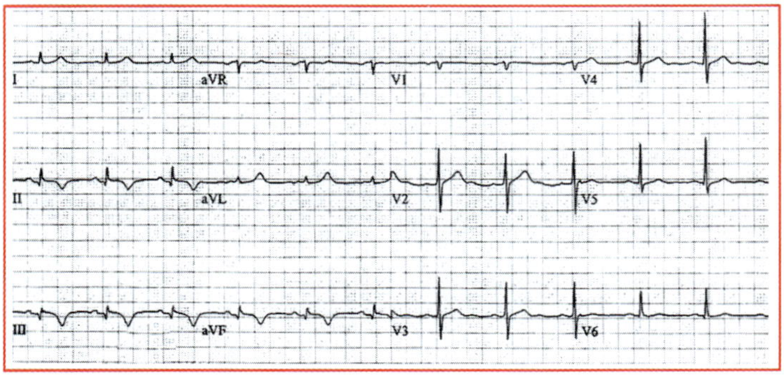

Fig. 12.60: Electrocardiogram from a patient with recent inferior myocardial infarction (MI). T waves inverted in the inferior leads. T waves after an acute MI point away from the site of infarction. May remain inverted for several days and occasionally persist for a long time.

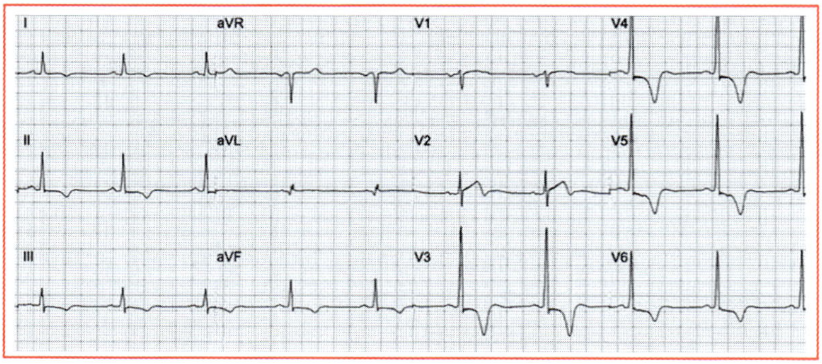

Fig. 12.61: Electrocardiogram from a patient with apical hypertrophic cardiomyopathy showing marked T wave inversions in the left precordial leads.

of chest discomfort but with no further evidence of evolving MI or unremitting ischemia form a distinct group which needs to be recognized. Similar ECG pattern can occur after an intracranial hemorrhage [cerebrovascular accident (CVA)] and in some forms of apical cardiomyopathy[53] (Fig. 12.61). It has been associated with hypertrophic cardiomyopathy of the apical type and Takotsubo cardiomyopathy characterized by transient apical ballooning that is often seen in post-menopausal women. The latter patients may present also with symptoms of MI and ST segment elevation in the precordial leads.[139,140] When other causes such as CVA and cardiomyopathies have been excluded, patients presenting with these ECG features should be evaluated for coronary artery disease. Often severe stenosis in the proximal LAD is found in coronary angiography and if untreated will suffer the consequences of the proximal LAD occlusion.[141]

Patients with normalization of T waves in the healing phase of infarction appear to have smaller infarcts with good functional recovery of the myocardium.[142]

Changes in the Initial QRS Force Due to Infarction

Infarction with associated loss of myocardial cells will be expected to shift the balance of the electrical forces since the infarcted myocardium will be electrically non-functional and this will result in slow conduction and/or loss of voltage. The new resultant of the electrical forces will be such that the initial activation will be oriented toward the uninfarcted region and away from the infarcted region. This results in the formation of the ***Q*** waves in leads facing the infarct. Since normal septal activation spreads from the left side of the septum to the right side, the initial event in ventricular activation also can result in initial negativity or ***q*** waves in all the limb leads. The infarct-related ***Q*** waves (***the pathologic Q waves***) need to be distinguished from these ***physiologic septal q waves***. Since the duration of the normal septal

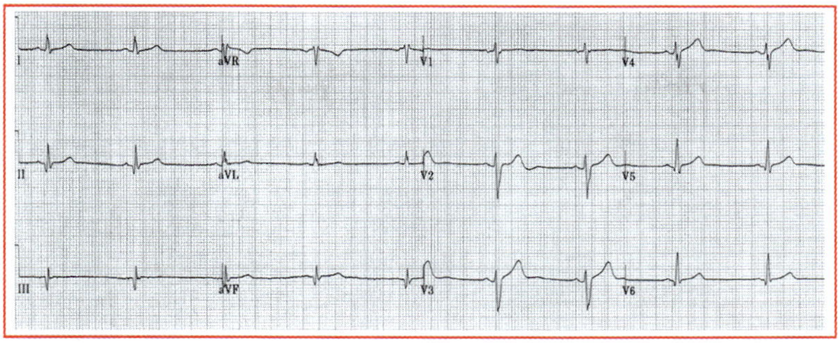

Fig. 12.62: Relatively deep Q wave (>30% of the R wave height) in lead aVF indicating an inferior infarct.

q waves usually is no more than 20–30 ms, and since the infarct related pathologic ***Q*** waves are often wider, the duration of the ***Q*** wave becomes an important feature in differentiation. Thus the infarct ***Q*** waves need to be >30 ms and must be 0.04 second wide. This definition of wide pathologic ***Q*** waves does not however apply to lead aVR, which faces the ventricular cavity.

In addition, the depth of the ***Q*** wave in relation to the height of the ***R*** wave has also been found to be a useful distinguishing feature. ***Q*** waves in the limb leads exceeding 30% of the ***R*** wave height have also been considered abnormal.[21] This feature is particularly useful in the two orthogonal limb leads, namely lead aVF and lead I (that face the inferior and the lateral wall respectively) (Fig. 12.62). Relatively deep ***Q*** waves in lead III and again in aVR, by themselves are not of particular value. In lead III, deep ***Q*** wave is often seen in LVH alone without infarct.

In the precordial leads, all the leads to the right of the transitional zone usually have a septal ***r*** wave. The septal ***q*** wave occurs only in leads with dominant ***R*** waves. These are the leads that are situated to the left of the transition. The normal transitional zone where the ***R*** begins to exceed the ***S*** wave in the precordium is usually V4. Normal septal ***q*** wave may often be seen therefore in V5 and/or V6. So in the precordium, the location of the ***q*** wave becomes more important than its duration. Thus ***q*** waves of any duration and depth seen in leads right of the transition zone (before the ***R*** wave exceeds the ***S*** wave) will be considered abnormal initial vector of infarct or a scar (Fig. 12.63). By vectorcardiography (VCG), it has been shown that in anterior MI, the initial anterior forces must not exceed 0.1 mv in maximal anterior amplitude and must not exceed 24 ms in duration.[143] This will mean that the ***r*** wave in V2 with amplitude <1 mm and width <20 ms will be abnormal and indicative of anterior MI. Vectorcardiographic loops are found to be superior to ECG in many studies for diagnosing old infarct. The VCGs are recorded at 2.5 ms intervals; this makes the duration of the forces accurate to within 1 ms. Also, VCGs are recorded with reference to the planes of orientation. However,

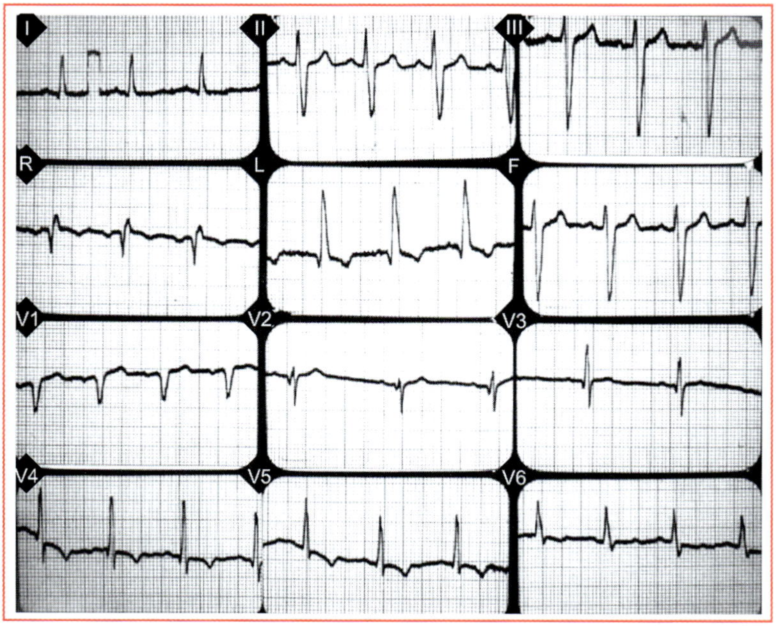

Fig. 12.63: Electrocardiogram (ECG) of a patient with old anterior infarct or scar. Small q noted in V2 right of the transition zone in the precordium. Transition is between V3 and V4 in this ECG.

in precordial leads, ***loss of septal r or delayed r/s progression*** alone can be caused by multiple factors. ***The most important factor contributing to this is the position of the electrode in relation to the electrical center of the heart.*** This typically occurs in chronic pulmonary disease and other situations with low diaphragms. Sometimes, the initial septal force is oriented at right angles to the right precordial leads resulting in "***isolectric r waves***". Other causes include initial right to left activation caused by incomplete or complete LBBB, LVH, dextrocardia or corrected transposition of the great vessels.[53]

Correlation of Q Waves to the Site of Infarction

Classic ***Q*** waves of MI are formed only when the infarct is at least 3–4 cm in diameter and 5–7 mm thick, involving about 50% of the thickness of the walls. In addition, it should be located in sites that are activated during the initial half of the depolarization.[144] Also, presence of previous infarcts can cause cancellation of the effect of the new infarct.

Anterior Infarct

Q waves when present in leads V2 and V3 or V2–V4, the infarction usually involves the anterior wall. If ***Q*** wave is also noted in aVL, then the infarct is

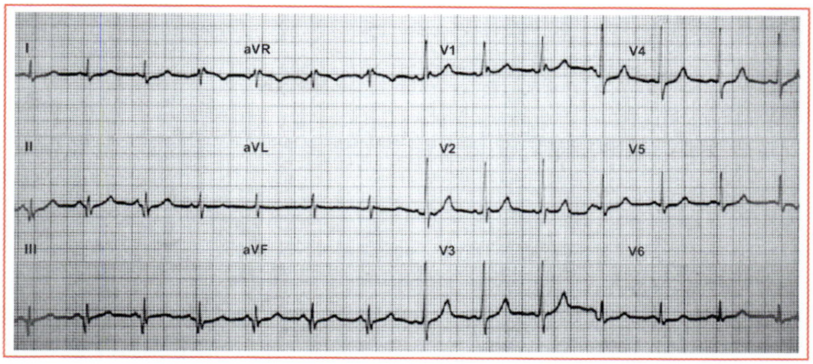

Fig. 12.64: Electrocardiogram from a patient with previous inferior-posterior infarction. Note the relatively deep Q wave in aVF consistent with inferior infarct. The dominant R wave in V1 and V2 with upright T waves suggest associated posterior wall involvement.

called ***antero-superior***. If ***Q*** waves are present in addition in leads V5–V6, then it is termed ***antero-lateral***.

Antero-septal infarct usually is a large anterior infarct with abnormalities of both antero-superior and ***antero-lateral*** infarct. When the LAD supplies also the apex, its occlusion will often result in changes consistent with anterior and inferior infarction. The term ***high lateral*** infarction has been applied to ***Q*** waves confined to leads I and aVL.

Posterior and Postero-lateral Infarct

In ***posterior or postero-lateral*** infarct, the initial QRS forces will be directed anteriorly and to the right. This will result in increased ***R*** wave in the right precordial leads and ***Q*** wave in aVL, V5 or V6. When posterior infarction occurs in association with an inferior infarction, the abnormal Q waves can be seen in the inferior leads (Fig. 12.64). In the absence of ***Q*** waves in these leads, it will be difficult to diagnose posterior infarct mainly on the basis of prominent R waves alone in the right precordial leads. The latter can occur due to other causes including RVH, septal hypertrophy, RBBB, Wolff-Parkinson-White pattern and also can be a normal variant.[145] If RVH and RBBB are excluded, broad ***R*** waves (>50 ms in duration in V2) in these right precordial leads and ***R/S*** >1.0 together with upright T waves, will be highly suggestive of postero-lateral infarct.[146] As pointed out with regard to ST segment depression in these leads, broad ***R*** with ***R/S*** pattern with dominance of ***R*** in V1, in studies using MRI correspond to lateral rather than true posterior. It has been suggested that the term posterior be eliminated.[147] This new terminology has not been universally accepted including us. It has also been shown that in some patients the inferobasal segment of the left ventricle may actually swing up to some degree and form a true posterior wall.

The term ***high lateral infarct*** is used when the ***Q*** wave is confined to aVL.

Inferior Infarct

In inferior infarction, the initial forces are directed superiorly forming ***Q*** waves in the inferior leads II, III and aVF. The classical criteria using aVF requires the QRS amplitude to be at least 0.5 mV (5 mm) and ***Q*** wave duration of at least 0.03 second from onset to nadir, and the ***Q:R*** ratio to be at least 1:4. If QRS amplitude and ***Q:R*** ratio do not meet these criteria, then the ***Q*** wave must be 0.04 second wide. In correlative studies, these ECG criteria have been found to have high specificity (98%) but less sensitivity (34%).

The VCG loops are found to be superior to ECG in many studies for diagnosing old inferior infarct. Typically in inferior infarction, the VCG loop will show initial forces to be superiorly oriented for at least 20 ms with a clockwise rotation.[148] In addition, the VCGs had high specificity as well as high sensitivity. In anterior fascicular block also, the QRS forces are directed superiorly. But this superior direction more typically involves the terminal forces. However, the spread of excitation to the blocked superior antero-lateral wall of the left ventricle must come from the uninvolved infero-posterior fascicle, in the direction from apex to the base in a counterclockwise spread. The QRS loop in a VCG will typically show this counterclockwise rotation in anterior fascicular block. When both an inferior infarct and anterior fascicular block coexist, the ECG will show initial and terminal negativity in the inferior leads. The initial force will be superior and clockwise as is usually the case in inferior infarction. Since the terminal force is due to the fascicular block, it will be directed superiorly but will be seen to move counterclockwise. It may be recognized using the modern ECG machines that give display of three simultaneous leads. Since the terminal force is superior, it will show a terminal ***R*** wave in both aVR and aVL. However, the peak of the ***R*** wave in lead aVR will be later than the peak of the ***R*** wave in the lead aVL indicating that the terminal force is not only directed superiorly to produce these R waves in these two leads but also they are moving in a counterclockwise fashion[43] (Fig. 12.65A). This can be appreciated if one visualizes the direction of the fontal plane leads in the hex-axial system.

Right Ventricular Infarction

Isolated right ventricular infarction is very rare. But right ventricular infarction can occur in the presence of an inferior or infero-posterior infarction.[149] An old right ventricular infarct is not diagnosable due to lack of specific ECG changes and the ST segment elevation in the right chest leads from right ventricular infarction is often transient. Lead V4R is most useful for evaluation in the acute stage of the infarction.[150]

Reliability of the Q Waves

The ECG criteria of the various infarcts have been established originally by correlative studies to the autopsy findings.[151-155] Modern diagnostic imaging modalities have allowed direct visualization of previous scars and infarcts more accurately using the delayed enhancement (DE) magnetic resonance imaging MRI.[156] This method (DE-MRI) has been used to quantify the post-infarct scar, identify regression of scar, scar burden to predict arrhythmic outcomes,[157,158] as well as image edema to identify myocardium at risk.[159] The question of reliability of the ***Q*** waves as defined to identify old infarcts in the ECGs has in fact been answered by correlative studies using MRI.[160] In this study, classic ***Q*** waves were correlated with infarct size. Patients with ***Q*** wave myocardial infarction (QWMI) had larger infarcts, lower left ventricular ejection fraction (LVEF). ***Q*** wave regression was noted in 40% of the patients with QWMI and correlated with improvement in LVEF. This in fact confirms that the ECG identification of ***Q*** waves of infarct not only is reliable but also allows useful information in clinical follow up of patients.

Changes in the Mid and Late QRS Forces Caused by Infarction

Changes in the mid and late portions of the QRS can be caused by infarction due to changes in sequence of activation or slow activation in and around the infarcted area. The latter often causes in addition some prolongation of the QRS duration. The term ***"Peri-infarction block"*** was used to describe ECG changes with pathologic ***Q*** waves together with slow terminal portion.[161] The QRS axis shift that comes with late half of the QRS pointing toward the site of infarction is thought to be due to a fascicular block. Classically the LAD due to the anterior fascicular block will be associated with the presence of an antero-lateral or a lateral infarct (with ***Q*** waves in leads I and aVL) and the infero-posterior fascicular block with an inferior infarct (***Q*** waves in leads II, III and aVF) (Figs. 12.65B and C).

If the QRS is prolonged, it appears that the conduction is probably prolonged in the myocardium as opposed to in the conduction system.[162] Signal averaging has shown high frequency components of low amplitude in the QRS of patients with infarcts. This has been attributed to fragmentation of the wave front in the scar together with the decrease in the electrical force.[163]

The sequential changes of myocardial infarction presented above are often considered in interpreting the date of an infarct seen on the ECG of any given patient. When the diagnosis is based on the ST elevation, the infarction is described as acute. When the diagnosis is made purely on the basis of abnormal Q waves, the infarction is described as old. But when the ECG shows abnormal Q waves associated with T wave inversion, then the term "infarction of undetermined age" must be used, bearing in mind that the T wave changes begin to occur fairly early after the onset of infarction but however can persist for a variable period of time ranging from a few weeks to many months and may even be permanent.

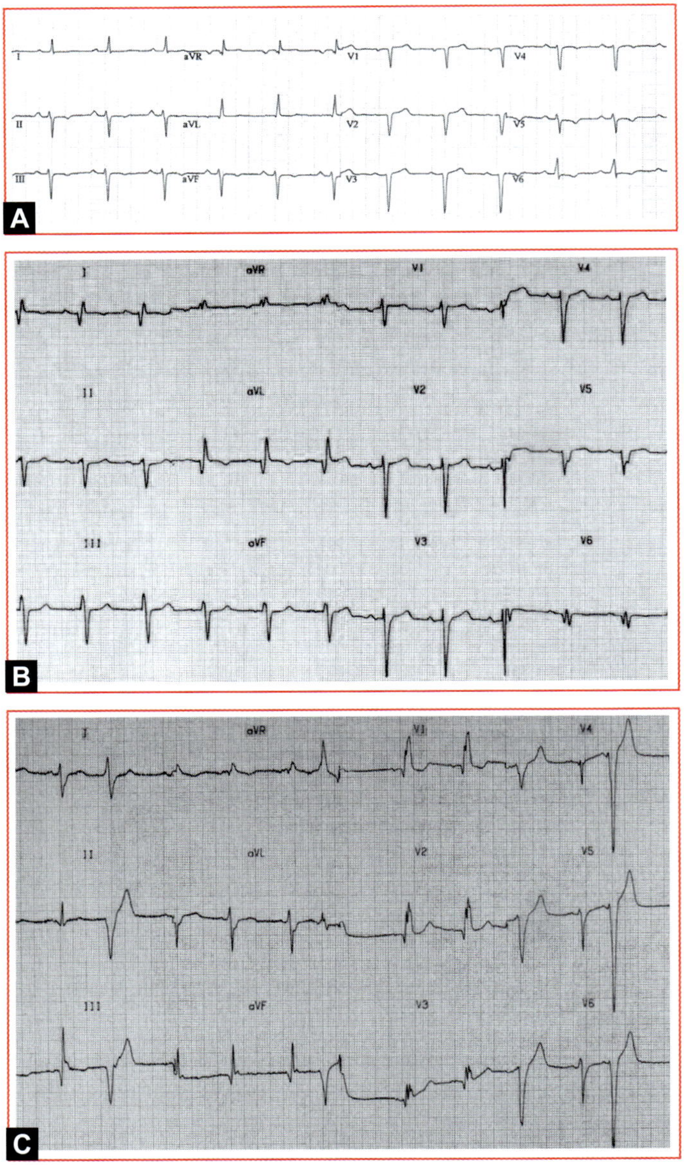

Figs. 12.65A to C: (A) Electrocardiogram from a patient with anteroseptal infarction with associated anterior fascicular block (LAFB). Note the peak of the terminal R wave in aVL is inscribed before the peak of the R wave in aVR indicating the counterclockwise direction of the superior terminal force. (B) Electrocardiogram from a patient with antero-lateral infarction (poor r/s progression V1–V6 with Q waves in V6, I and aVL. Note the associated left axis deviation due to LAFB (deep S in leads II and aVF). (C) Electrocardiogram from a patient with old inferior infarct (abn Q waves in aVF) in the presence of right bundle branch block (terminal wide R in V1). Note also the associated right axis deviation of the left ventricular portion of the QRS (r/S pattern in lead I) indicating the associated posterior fascicular block. Need to look at the sinus beats only ignoring the ventricular ectopic beats (that form the second complex in lead I–III, the first and the last complexes in V4–V6).

Ventricular Aneurysm

Persistent ST segment elevation after a myocardial infarction can be a useful sign of ventricular aneurysm. It may also indicate areas of myocardial asynergy in left ventricular wall motion.[164,165]

Ventricular Rupture

Patients with ventricular rupture had higher incidence of pericarditis of myocardial infarction.[166] ST segment elevation in aVL appeared to be a feature predictive of cardiac rupture in one study.[167]

Recognition of Myocardial Infarction in the Presence of Intra-ventricular Conduction Defect

It is important to know how the presence of intra-ventricular conduction defect can affect the QRS changes of MI, and thereby affect the recognition of the infarction. It has been stressed before that the His-Purkinje system is essentially a trifascicular system. The right bundle is one of the three fascicles and the left bundle divides on the left side of the inter-ventricular septum into two major groups of fibers. One is oriented anteriorly and superiorly and can be termed the anterior fascicle. The other larger division of fibers is oriented posteriorly and inferiorly and is termed the posterior fascicle. There are two issues regarding myocardial infarction and intra-ventricular conduction defect or BBB. The MI could cause the conduction defect or it could occur in a patient who has a pre-existing conduction defect. Pre-existing conduction defect could be congenital or acquired. The latter is often caused by some fibrosis in the conduction system that could be idiopathic or associated with an underlying cardiac or systemic condition. For instance, fascicular blocks (both anterior and posterior) are seen not infrequently in patients with hypertension, diabetes, obesity or aortic valve disease.[168,169] In this section, we are focusing only on the recognition of the myocardial infarction in the presence of intraventricular conduction defect in the ECG. The intra-ventricular conduction defect can be in the form of RBBB, anterior fascicular block, posterior fascicular block and combination of the RBBB with one of the two fascicular blocks, LBBB or intra-ventricular delay that does not conform to any of the aforementioned. These will be discussed below.

Infarct Recognition in the Presence of Fascicular Block, RBBB and/orBifascicular block

Recognition of infarction in the presence of a fascicular block should not be difficult if we understand that the fascicular block produces the direction of the terminal half of the QRS force to be directed toward the site of the blocked fascicle. In fascicular blocks, the major portion of the QRS force that arises from the main body of the left ventricle will not be synchronously activated by the two fascicles. In anterior fascicular block, the initial activation will be directed inferiorly and posteriorly along the unaffected posterior division and terminally directed anteriorly and superiorly. This will shift the mean QRS axis superiorly and to the left and will produce terminal R in aVL and aVR and deep S wave in the inferior leads. The QRS force will follow the spread of excitation from the apex to the base moving anteriorly and superiorly in a counter clockwise manner. The terminal R in lead aVR will occur after the terminal R in lead aVL. The opposite sequence will occur with posterior fascicular block. The latter will cause initial force to be oriented superiorly and leftward and terminal force will be directed toward the site of blocked division, namely inferiorly and rightward. The spread of excitation is clockwise and will produce qR complexes in the inferior leads with small r and deep S in leads I and aVL. When the fascicular block is caused by fibrosis alone in general, the QRS will not be prolonged. But when fascicular block is caused by infarction or associated with dilated and hypertrophied ventricle it may often be associated with prolonged duration of QRS.[169] Since the initial force is unaffected by the blocked fascicle, the initial QRS changes of infarction, namely the pathologic Q waves will be unaffected. If the infarction were to cause the fascicular block, the terminal force will be similar to the terminal force of the fascicular block. The block will also be likely associated with QRS prolongation. When the terminal force has the features of a fascicular block, it used to be referred to as a peri-infarction block. Instead, it is preferable to state the location of the infarct and describe the fascicular block seen as either anterior or posterior fascicular blocks. Anterior fascicular block due to an infarct requires the infarction to be antero-superior in location and the posterior fascicular block may result from an inferior infarction.

In RBBB, the QRS is prolonged to about 0.12 second due to late activation of the right ventricle turning the terminal force away from the left side and toward the right and anterior direction since the right ventricle is an anterior chamber and lies under the sternum. This results in the typical slurred ***S*** wave in leads I and V6 and terminal ***R*** prime in the lead V1. The prolonged QRS of 0.12 second can be analysed by dividing it into three parts of 0.04 second. The first two-thirds of the QRS (0.08 second of the QRS) are due to the normal left ventricular activation sequence. It is therefore unaltered. This means that the initial left to right septal force is normal, therefore the initial QRS changes of the infarction, which produce the pathologic ***Q*** waves, would not be hidden by the presence of RBBB (whether the RBBB was pre-existing or caused by the infarction) (Fig. 12.66). In addition, the ST-T changes of infarction will dominate the secondary ST-T changes, which are normally associated with the RBBB. Thus in the acute stage of infarction, the ST elevation will be recognized and also subsequent progression of the ST-T waves of the infarction would be largely unaffected.

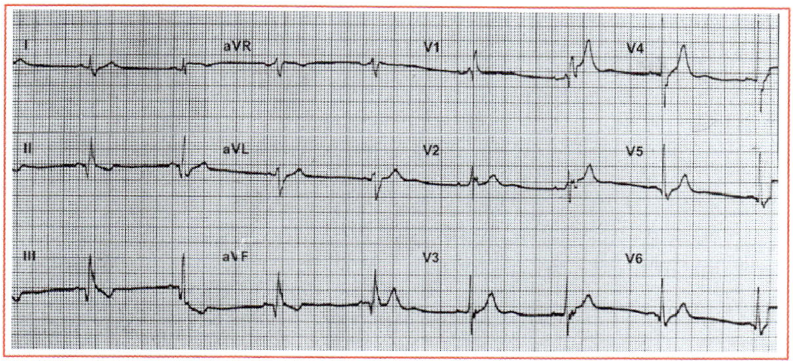

Fig. 12.66: Electrocardiogram from a patient with inferior infarction of undetermined age. Note the abnormal Q waves in the inferior leads with T wave inversion. The co-existing right bundle branch block (rsR′ in V1 with prolonged QRS to 0.12 second) does not hide the infarction.

The second third of the QRS in RBBB, which also pertains only to the left ventricular activation, is unaltered. Thus, if a bifascicular block such as RBBB with anterior fascicular block or RBBB with posterior fascicular block were present, it would be recognized as such (Fig. 12.65C). The ST-T wave changes of infarction again will dominate the ECG features rather than the ST-T abnormalities secondary to the conduction defect.

Infarct Recognition in the Presence of LBBB

In LBBB, the left ventricular activation is totally altered from the beginning. The activation begins on the right and spreads leftward and posteriorly. The normal septal ***q*** in the lateral leads I, V6 and septal ***r*** in V1 and V2 are not usually present. In addition, ST-T abnormalities develop secondary to the abnormal depolarization sequence. The ST-T waves are usually directed opposite to the main QRS force. The leads with positive ***R*** waves (leads I, V6 and aVL) show ST depression with negative T waves. Leads with negative QRS (V1–V3) show elevated ST and upright T waves. Since the initial force is abnormal in LBBB, old infarction will be difficult to identify.[170-172] Sometimes, the loss of ***R*** in leads expected to have only ***R*** may be an indicator of an old infarct, but its specificity is poor and difficult to differentiate from non-specific intraventricular conduction delay.

In acute infarction however ST segment changes may be seen to occur in unexpected leads. If ST segment deviation is opposite to the expected ST-T wave direction as related to the QRS configuration, it would be abnormal and indicate ischemia/infarction. These are referred to as concordant (primary) ST segment changes. For instance, if one finds ST segment elevation instead of the expected ST depression with negative T waves in the lateral leads (leads I and aVL), it would suggest lateral infarction. If leads V1-V3 in LBBB which are expected to show some ST elevation and upright

T waves, show inverted T waves then it would be suggestive of anterior ischemia. Discordant ST segment changes are exaggerations of the expected level of ST segment deviation in the leads as related to the QRS polarity. These were referred to under ST changes of infarction. Despite the difficulties of identifying old infarction in the presence of LBBB some atypical features of the LBBB have been correlated to infarction.[53,173-175] These include the following:

1. Q waves in V5 or V6 and abnormal wide ***Q*** waves in lead I or lead aVL
2. Notching of the ***S*** wave in leads V3–V5 (Cabrera's sign) and tiny notches deforming the terminal QRS
3. Notching of the ***R*** wave upstroke in leads I, aVL, V5 and V6
4. ***Q*** waves in the inferior leads III and aVF[174]

ECG Changes Simulating Infarction

Other conditions with initial QRS changes simulating infarction include the following:[53]

- Left ventricular hypertrophy:
  Marked LVH as seen in significant aortic valve disease or hypertension may sometimes show poor ***r*** waves in the right and mid-precordial leads. In addition, there could be abnormal ***Q*** waves in the precordium right of the transition zone. Also, the secondary ST-T wave abnormalities of LVH might be atypical and simulate ischemic ST-T waves. These changes might occur in the absence of coronary disease. It might actually be due to some patchy fibrosis[176] (Figs. 12.67A and B).
- Myocarditis
- Myocardial contusion
- Scleroderma
- Amyloidosis
- Primary and metastatic tumors
- Septal hypertrophy in hypertrophic cardiomyopathy
- Initial QRS changes of pre-excitation as in Wolff-Parkinson-White
- Duchenne-type muscular dystrophy (typically simulates postero-lateral infarct with tall R waves in the right precordial leads and abnormal Q waves in the lateral leads)[177]
- Anomalous coronary artery arising from the pulmonary artery. In this condition, ischemia and infarction can occur affecting the lateral wall with abnormal Q waves in leads I and aVL that can be quite deep and/or broad. The uninvolved posterobasal portion of the left ventricle supplied by the right coronary artery may be often hypertrophied unlike the rest of the myocardium which may be thin and fibrotic. The terminal portion of the QRS may be superiorly oriented causing deep S waves in the inferior leads.[178]

Terminology of Left Ventricular Walls and Location of Myocardial Infarcts

Although standardized terminology applied to the LV walls have been reported, there exists differences among the terms used by pathologists, electrocardiologists, cardiac imagers and clinicians. The wall that lies on the diaphragm has been originally called the ***posterior*** wall several decades ago. Later on, it was changed and considered to be the ***inferior*** wall. The infarction involving the basal most part of this wall was termed ***true posterior*** wall.[10,13]

A consensus document of the cardiac imaging committee of the AHA suggested that the LV be divided into four walls: septal, anterior, lateral and inferior. The walls were in turn divided into 17 segments, six basal, six mid

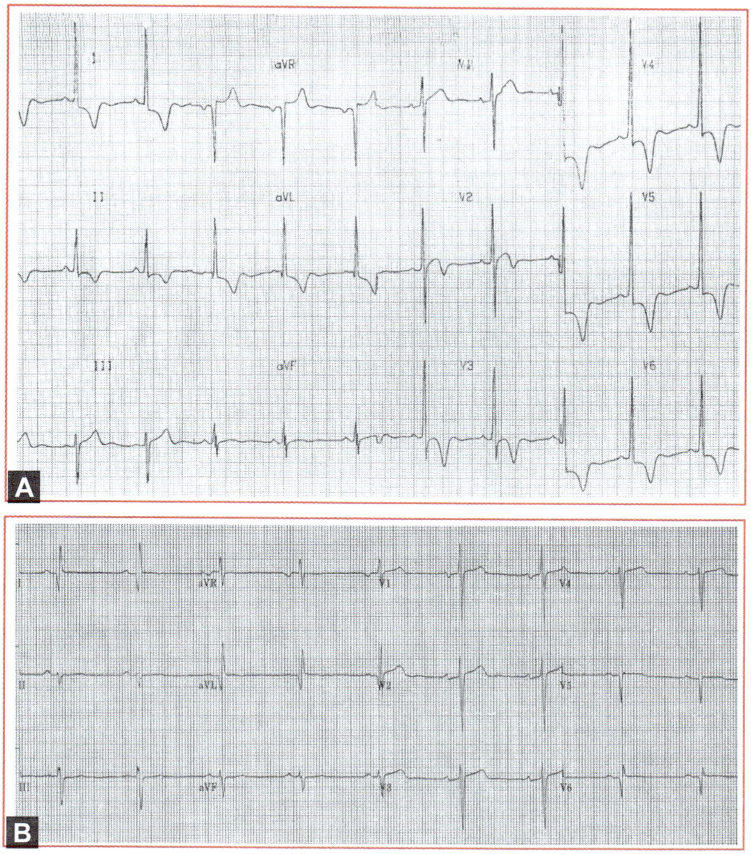

Figs. 12.67A and B: (A) Electrocardiograms taken at age 30 years [shown in (A)] from a male patient with non-obstructive hypertrophic cardiomyopathy with normal coronary arteries. Note the marked left ventricular hypertrophy with abnormal ST-T waves in the left-sided leads. The ECG from the same patient taken at age 44 years [shown in (B)] shows abnormal deep Q waves in leads I, aVL, V5 and V6 with non-reversible defects in perfusion scans indicating antero-lateral scar.

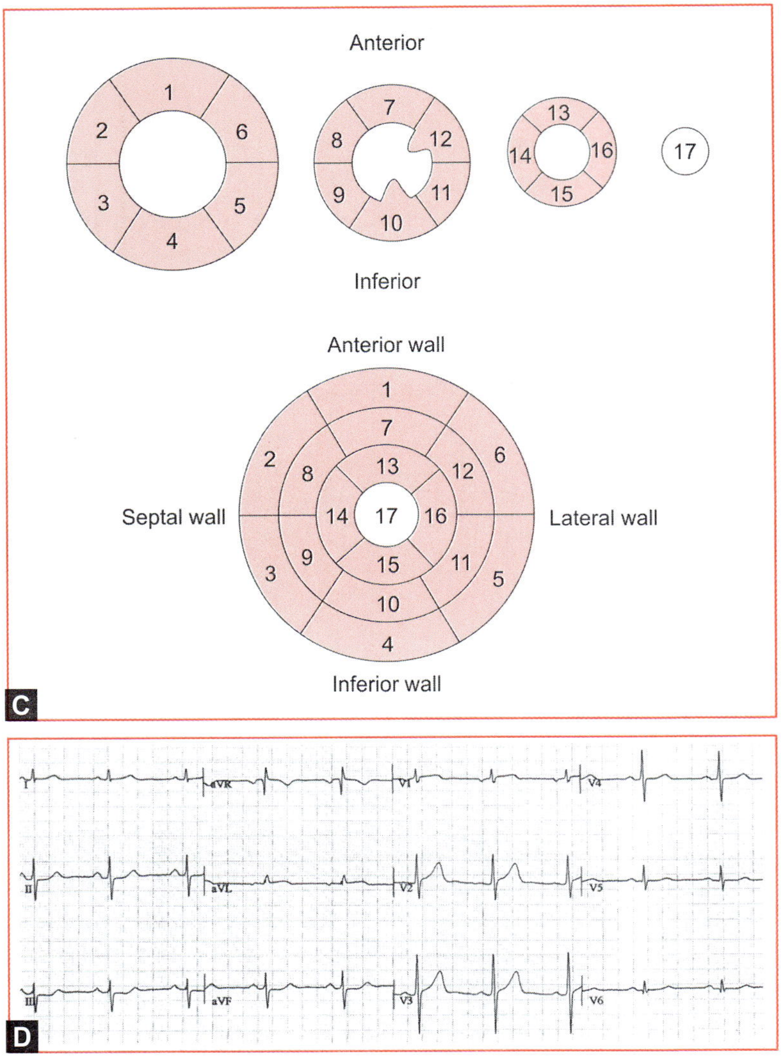

Figs. 12.67C to D: (C) Diagram of the segmental model of the left ventricle adopted by the cardiac imaging committee of the American Heart Association. Left ventricle is divided into four walls, septal, anterior, lateral and inferior. The walls are divided into 17 segments, six basal, six mid, four apical and one segment, the apex. (DE) Electrocardiogram from a 63-year-old man with a prior history of myocardial infarction. Electrocardiogram (D) shows superior axis with dominant R in V1 and V2 with upright T waves suspicious of a posterior scar. The nuclear perfusion scan with persantine infusion.

and four apical and one segment being the apex.[130] The same consensus document suggested that the infero-posterior be called "inferior" and segment 4 should be called inferobasal instead of posterior. This 17 segments model has generally been adopted in echocardiography and in nuclear cardiology (Fig. 12.67C).

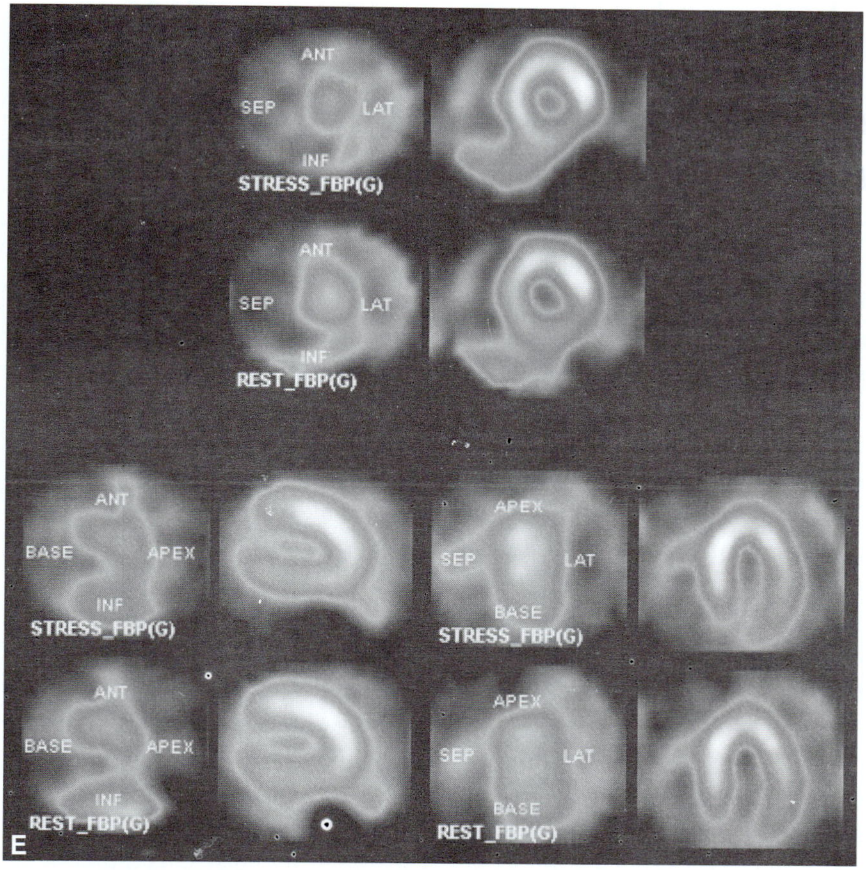

Fig. 12.67E: (E) shows a fixed infero-lateral defect from base to apex.

Delayed enhancement MRI (DE-MRI) is emerging as a gold standard for precise location of infarctions in vivo.[156,157] Cardiac MRI studies have demonstrated that the LV is cone-shaped and lies obliquely in the chest.[179] The basal segment of the inferior wall, in MRI studies, has been shown to be in a straight line with the rest of the segments of this wall in two-thirds of the patients. In some patients, however, it appears to bend upward. The four cardiac walls (septal, anterior, lateral and posterior) are clearly seen in the horizontal plane only when the inferior wall bends upward. In correlative studies of electrocardiographic patterns and infarction location using MRI, the dominant ***R*** in lead V1 was related to lateral MI and Q waves confined to lead aVL to mid-anterior and mid-lateral MI. Therefore, it has been suggested that the terms ***posterior*** and ***high lateral*** infarction be changed to ***lateral wall*** and ***limited antero-lateral*** infarct.[147,179] However, this has not been universally adopted including ourselves[180] (Figs. 12.67D and E) (these two are from BCD patient ECG and nuclear image).

SECTION V: VENTRICULAR PRE-EXCITATION/PERICARDITIS

Initial QRS Abnormalities of Ventricular Pre-excitation

Definition and Diagnostic Criteria

The syndrome of paroxysmal tachycardia in patients with short PR interval and abnormal QRS was first described in 1930, by Wolff, Parkinson and White.[181] The syndrome came to be termed after their names as the ***WPW syndrome*** and the ECG pattern alone without symptoms has been referred to as ***WPW pattern***. This pattern which is characterized by the following: short PR interval (< 0.12 second), abnormally wide QRS with a duration of 0.11 second or more, the presence of initial slurring of the QRS complex called the ***delta*** wave (named because the initial slurred upstroke of the QRS makes the QRS complex look somewhat like the Greek letter "***delta***") and secondary ST-T wave changes. The WPW pattern cannot be diagnosed without the delta wave (Fig. 12.68).

In WPW pattern, the ventricular activation is initiated through often an accessory AV connection or pathway and completed by the normal AV nodal His-Purkinje system. The QRS is essentially a fusion complex arising from the two pathways. The AV accessory pathway is like a muscle band and often referred to as "Kent bundle"[182] after the original description of such connections.[183] Accessory pathways have been documented all along the AV sulcus, anteriorly, posteriorly and laterally. In addition to these lateral AV connections or bypass tracts, accessory pathways have been found in the paraseptal region. Since the AV accessory pathway provides a connection that bypasses the normal AV node, the ventricular excitation occurs before

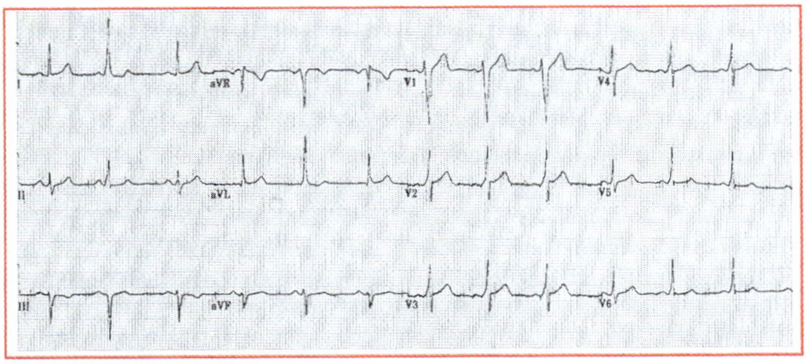

Fig. 12.68: Electrocardiogram from a patient with intermittent Wolf-Parkinson-White pre-excitation (WPW) pattern. "Delta" wave causing the slurring of the upstrike of the R wave can be seen clearly in the second QRS complex in lead I. The delta wave slurring is appreciable in the second and the third QRS complexes in leads V2 and V3 as well. The PR interval is shorter and the QRS duration is prolonged in the beats with WPW-type conduction.

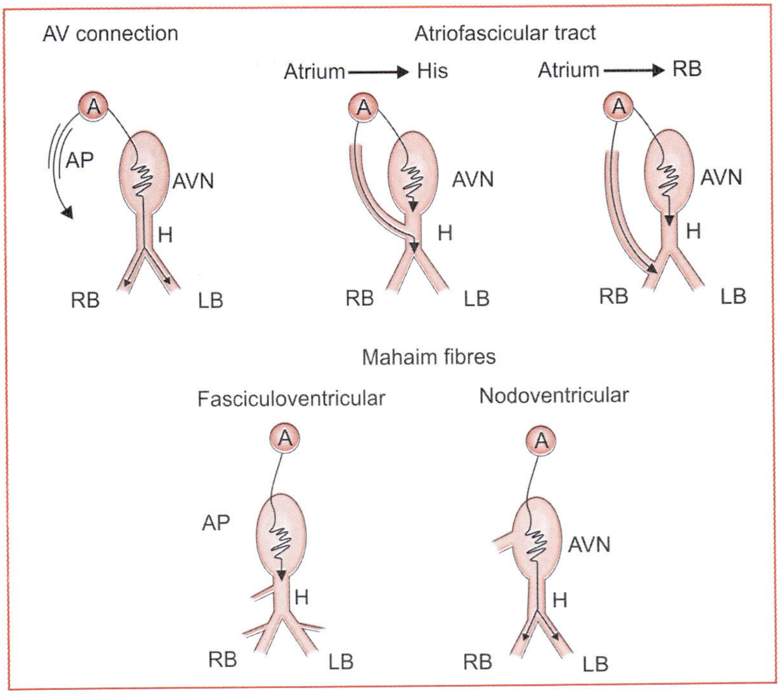

Fig. 12.69: Diagram showing the four types of pathways for ventricular pre-excitation. A, atrium; AVN, atrioventricular (AV) node; H, bundle of His; RB, right bundle branch; LB, left bundle branch. The top panel shows the Kent bundle type AV connection and atriofascicular connection bypasses the AV node and connect to the H or the RB. Accessory pathways arising from the AVN or one of the fascicles form part of the infra-nodal pathways (the bottom panel). Source: Adapted from Prystowsky EN, Miles WM, Heger JJ, Zipes DP. Pre-excitation syndromes: mechanisms and management. Med Clin North Am. 1984;68(4):831-93. (Copyright with permission from Elsevier 2014).

the impulse arrives through the normal pathway. So the ventricle is pre-excited and the condition is referred to as ***ventricular pre-excitation.***

Accessory Pathways

Ventricular pre-excitation can occur through four pathways (Fig. 12.69):[184]

i. Atrioventricular bypass tract (***Kent bundle type*** connection)
ii. These connections can also be atriofascicular: meaning they connect the atrium to the division of the H
iii Nodoventricular connecting the nodal region directly to the ventricle
iv. Fasciculoventricular meaning connecting the His and its division directly to the ventricle

Not included above are the atriohissian connections that are sometimes thought to be associated with short PR and normal QRS complex. These fibers are normally found and described by James, to connect the posterior internodal tract (that is one of the three internodal tracts that connect SA node to the AV node) directly to the H bypassing the upper part of the AV node.[185] Their participation in the so-called ***Lown–Ganong–Levine syndrome***, with tachycardias associated with short PR interval and normal QRS complex is questionable. The connections (iii and iv) are infranodal and sometimes referred to as ***Mahaim fibers/conduction***.

The ventricular activation can either be entirely through the AV node, only through the AV bypass tract or simultaneously through both the normal and the accessory pathways. Thus one can get various degrees of fusion. The impulse if it arrives ahead of the normal pathway through the bypass tract to the ventricle, the initial spread through the bypass as well as through the myocardium will be slow and cause a slurred upstroke (***the delta wave***). With increasing contribution through the bypass tract the QRS will become more prolonged. If the conduction through the AV node is dominant, then the PR will be longer and the QRS will be more normal. Atrial pacing can help to differentiate the pre-excitation from Kent bundle type connection from the infranodal pathways of Mahaim type. Atrial pacing with increasing rate normally causes increased AV nodal delay. With overdrive atrial pacing in patients with Kent bundle type connection, the increasing AV nodal conduction related to increased atrial rate will result in increasing the AH interval (conduction from the atrium to the H that can be measured in recordings obtained through an electrode catheter placed across the tricuspid valve positioned to record the H while pacing the atrium), the bypass tract not delayed like the AV node by increasing atrial rate will pre-excite the ventricle earlier and result in widened QRS with prominent delta waves. The HV interval (interval from His potential to the onset of the ventricular complex) will become shortened and eventually the H potential may be buried entirely inside the ventricular complex because of increasing AV nodal delay (increasing AH interval). The interval from onset of atrial complex to that of the ventricular complex (AV interval) and the PR interval will remain about the same (Fig. 12.70).

In patients with Mahaim type conduction, the sinus impulse may arrive in the upper part of the AV node and has a normal delay and normal PR interval but because of ventricular pre-excitation it could be followed by delta wave. The resulting features are widened QRS and short HV interval. Overdrive atrial pacing in these patients will result in progressive increase in the AV interval (PR interval) in response to increasing atrial rate without affecting the QRS.[186,187] If the accessory pathways insert into the right bundle branch (nodofascicular), then the pre-excitation will result in LBBB pattern. Such conduction can also result from atriofascicular connections, which are found in the right ventricular free wall. They seem to represent a duplication of the AV node and the distal conducting system. Pre-excitation may not be evident during resting sinus rhythm in some patients but may be induced by premature atrial stimulation.

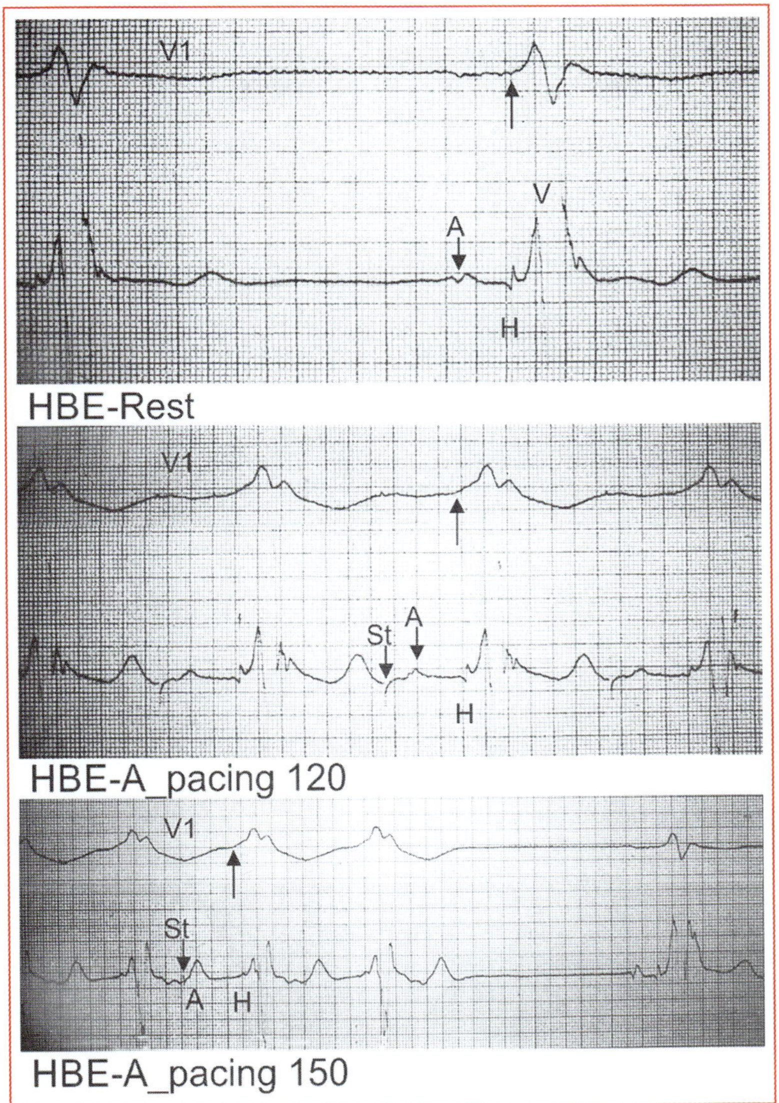

Fig. 12.70: Demonstrates the effect of atrial pacing in a patient with Wolf-Parkinson-White preexcitation (WPW) and Kent bundle type of accessory pathway connection. Electrode catheter recording of the His bundle potential (HBE) with simultaneous surface lead V1 shown in each of the three panels displayed at 100 mm/s. At rest (the top panel) the onset of the QRS complex (surface electrocardiogram) and the timing of the biphasic bundle of His potential (H) in the HBE are almost simultaneous. With atrial pacing at 120 beats/min (the middle panel), the H moves into the QRS since the atrioventricular (AV) nodal conduction is delayed due to the increased heart rate. The delta wave slurring (arrow pointing up) of the QRS begins almost 20 ms before the H. At atrial pacing rate of 150 beats/min (bottom panel), the QRS shows more prominent delta wave (arrow) and begins much earlier than the H. Due to the increased AV nodal conduction, the activation of bundle of His gets delayed and the H gets buried in the ventricular complex (V). St, atrial pacing stimulus; A, atrial complex (P wave).

Delta Wave

A normal septal ***q*** is uncommon in the pre-excited complexes. The delta wave in the WPW pattern can be upright or negative. When it is negative it will resemble abnormal ***Q*** wave of MI. The usual range of directions of the delta wave in the frontal plane is about -30°-+100°. The direction is partly dependent on the location of the accessory pathway and the part of the ventricle that is pre-excited. If it is directed superiorly and to the left toward aVL, then it will imitate inferior infarction by virtue of ***Q*** waves in the inferior leads (Fig. 12.71). If it is directed inferiorly and to the right, then it will imitate lateral infarct. The direction of the delta wave in the horizontal plane is also similar. It means that the V6 will always have an upright delta wave. Therefore, if a septal ***q*** is found in V6, pre-excitation is unlikely.[188] Besides mimicking an infarct, delta waves can hide an infarct. If the accessory pathway activates the right ventricle first, then it can mask RBBB. The altered sequence of ventricular activation in WPW will cause secondary repolarization abnormalities. In general, the ST segment displacement and the T wave direction are opposite to the delta wave and the major deflection of the QRS. In addition, it can also produce false positive ST changes on exercise.[189]

Wolf-Parkinson-White pattern occurs more often in males than the females. About two-thirds of the patients do not have any associated heart disease. It has a higher incidence in patients with hypertrophic obstructive cardiomyopathy. It is also associated with familial type of dilated cardiomyopathy and thyrotoxicosis. It has also been seen in association with mitral valve prolapse syndrome.[53] In congenital heart disease, it is seen most commonly in patients with Ebstein's anomaly. Other associated congenital lesions include atrial septal defect, tricuspid atresia, corrected transposition of the great vessels, ventricular septal defect, tetralogy of Fallot and the coarctation of the aorta.[190,191]

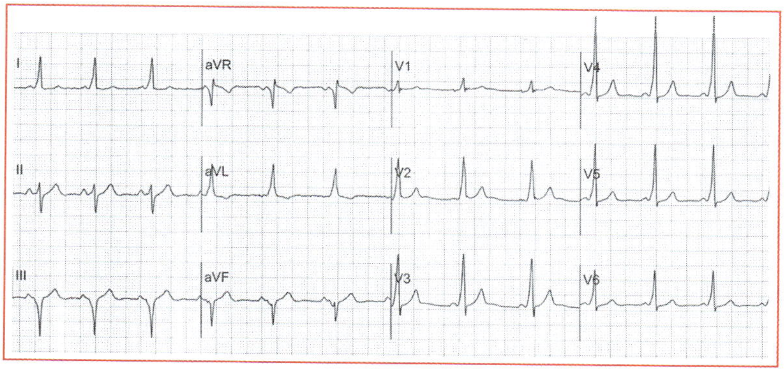

Fig. 12.71: Electrocardiogram from a patient with Wolf-Parkinson-White pre-excitation. The direction of the delta wave is superior and to the left (positive in lead aVL) with Q wave in aVF imitating inferior infarct. Also note the delta wave is positive in V1–V6.

Tachyarrhythmias

The tachyarrhythmias associated with pre-excitation syndrome can be the classical macro re-entry of the circuit-type movement that results in AV re-entrant tachycardia (AVRT). The tachycardia loop in such patients is formed by the atrium, AV node, His-Purkinje system and ventricular myocardium in the anterograde direction. The impulse arrives back into the atrium in the retrograde direction through the accessory pathway. Since anterograde conduction is through the normal pathways, no delta wave will be seen during the tachycardia. The QRS will be narrow. The rate may go up to 250 somewhat faster than the common AV nodal re-entrant tachycardia, which is often in the differential.[192] The retrograde P wave is usually inscribed after the QRS and the P wave is negative in lead I. There can also be electrical alternans due to faster heart rates. If there was transition from bundle branch block to narrow QRS tachycardia with a change in cycle length of the tachycardia, it will also favor the presence of an accessory pathway.[193] If the resting ECG during sinus rhythm shows classic WPW pattern, then the diagnosis of AVRT is also definite. It should be noted that the presence of AV block during tachycardia will rule out participation of a bypass tract.

Intracardiac recordings with electrode catheters from different sites (His bundle, right atrium, coronary sinus proximal and distal) will demonstrate the earliest site of atrial excitation. If the earliest site of atrial excitation is at a distance from the AV node and the Bundle of His, it can help locate the site of the bypass tract. However, paraseptal bypass tracts cannot be located in this way.

Patients with pre-excitation syndromes however can develop other atrial arrhythmia such as atrial flutter or atrial fibrillation, which do not require the accessory pathway for the production of the arrhythmia. These arrhythmias are less common but can pose serious consequences if the accessory pathway has short effective refractory period. In these situations, the atrial impulses are conducted through the accessory pathway. Atrial fibrillation will result in faster heart rates and wide QRS complexes and rarely result in the development of VF with sudden death.[194] In atrial fibrillation and WPW, the ventricular rate often may exceed 200 beats/min. In addition, the gross irregularity will help to rule out ventricular tachycardia. Patients with *intermittent WPW pattern are unlikely to have short effective refractory periods and therefore would not run the risk of developing fast heart rates during atrial fibrillation* (*see* Fig. 12.68).

Localization of the Accessory Pathway

The two major types of WPW patterns were described originally by Rosenbaum into types A and B. The two types were based on the maximum QRS forces in the right precordial leads, whether they were predominantly anterior or posterior.[195] With the advent of ablation therapy of refractory arrhythmias, precise localization of the site of the accessory pathways has become important. Epicardial and endocardial mappings through electrophysiologic techniques as well as catheter ablation therapy have demonstrated that sub-division into major types as to whether they are left-sided (type A) or right-sided (type B) connections is an oversimplification.

Epicardial mapping activation sequence at the time of surgical ablation therapy had demonstrated epicardial pre-excitation at a spectrum of sites over the free wall of the left or right ventricle or in a paraseptal region always adjacent to the AV sulcus.[196] The initial forces in the majority of their patients were directed anteriorly and the epicardial pre-excitation occurred at the base of the heart. This study demonstrated the following:

i. When the initial forces of the ventricular depolarization (20 ms vector) was directed to the right and inferior, the accessory pathway was through the free wall of the left ventricle. The ECG showed negative delta waves in I and aVL and positive delta waves in the inferior leads and V1 and V2.
ii. When the 20 ms vector was to the left and inferior, with positive delta waves in lead I, and aVL as well as II, aVF and III, the epicardial pre-excitation was over either the RV free wall or over the region of the pulmonary outflow tract.
iii. Superior and leftward direction of the initial forces with negative delta waves in the inferior leads, suggested a postero-septal location of the bypass tract.

An ECG algorithm has also been developed and validated prospectively based on correlation of the resting ECG with successful radiofrequency ablation sites.[197]

The surface ECG provides only approximate guide to the location of the anatomic site of the accessory pathway. Other limitations include co-existing ECG abnormalities, degree of pre-excitation and the presence of multiple accessory pathways. Some salient points are as follows:[198]

1. Typical left free wall accessory pathway shows negative delta waves in leads I, aVL or V6 and pseudo RBBB type QRS with ***Rs*** complex in V1
2. Right anteroseptal accessory pathway (earliest activation near the His bundle region) shows positive delta waves in the inferior leads, low ***R:S*** ratio (***QS*** or ***rS***) in V1-V3
3. Postero-septal pathway shows negative or isoelectric delta waves in the inferior leads and rapid transition from V1 to V2 (***rS*** in V1 to ***Rs*** in V2)
4. Right ventricular free wall accessory pathway shows positive delta wave in lead I and LBBB-type morphology of the QRS

ECG Changes of Pericarditis

Acute pericarditis is often in the differential diagnosis of acute chest pain syndromes. Pericarditis can result from a variety of etiologies, including

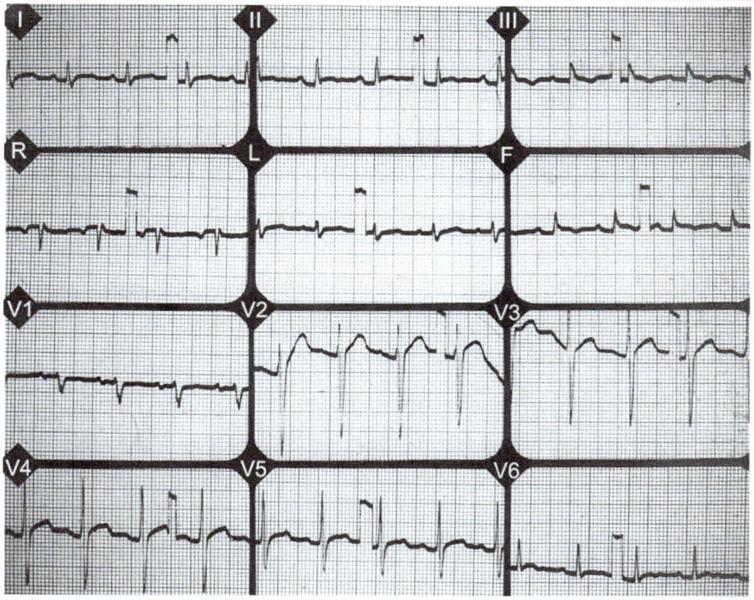

Fig. 12.72: Electrocardiogram from a patient with acute pericarditis. Recording on day 1 of presentation to the hospital. Note mild elevation of ST segments in leads I, II, III, aVF, V2–V6. Also note slight elevation of the PR segment compared to the TP segment in lead aVR.

infective causes (viral, bacterial and others), inflammatory causes, following MI often localized to the area of infarction, renal failure, trauma or post-cardiac surgery and tumor infiltration (most common ovarian tumors followed by breast and lung tumors). The most common variety is often idiopathic and probably caused by unrecognized viral infection. The characteristic changes in the electrocardiogram involve the ST segments, PR segments and the T waves. In addition, these changes evolve in a typical sequential fashion.[199-203]

ST Segment and T Wave Changes

When pericarditis is generalized as in the idiopathic variety, it usually produces ST segment elevation in leads that face the epicardial surface of the ventricles. This is often the first to occur. Typically ST segment vector parallels the QRS vector. It is elevated in leads that show upright QRS. ST segment elevation therefore is noted in leads I, II, V5 and V6. It may also be seen in leads III, aVF, aVL, V2–V4. ST depression (reciprocal) will be seen mostly in leads aVR and V1. ST elevation is related to the underlying myocarditis, which is often superficial and involves the epicardium. However, the changes may also reflect pressure-induced changes if there is significant pericardial effusion.[204] It is therefore not very pronounced as in acute MI. In addition, the elevated ST segment is concave. The changes evolve more slowly unlike in MI (Fig. 12.72).

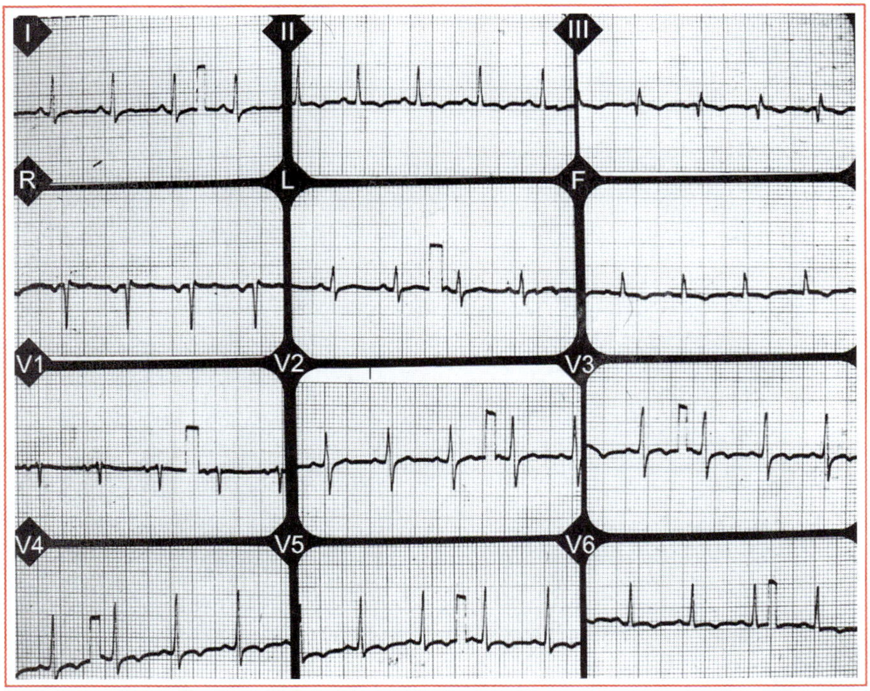

Fig. 12.73: Electrocardiogram from the same patient on day 20 following presentation to the hospital. The ST segments are back to normal. But the T wave is terminally inverted (seen best in leads II, aVF and V3–V6).

During the second stage, the ST segment tends to return to the baseline. At this stage, the amplitude of the T waves may decrease. During the third stage, the T waves will begin to be inverted. The T waves become inverted generally in leads that have upright T waves. T wave inversion is also incomplete and involves the terminal part more than the initial part that may remain positive. Sometimes, the T wave may be notched (Fig. 12.73).

The fourth and the last stage is the resolution of these changes. There could be a variable interval (average about 2–3 days), between the second stage when the ST segments return to the baseline and the third stage when the T waves become inverted. During this interval, the ECG may even appear quite close to being normal. This type of evolution is not seen in acute infarction.

It must be noted that the QTc intervals usually remain normal in pericarditis even when the T waves are inverted excepting post-operative pericarditis following cardiac surgery where the QTc interval may however be prolonged due to multiple factors.[53] In acute MI however, the QTc interval is usually prolonged. In addition, T wave inversion in acute infarction occurs early on, even when the ST segments are still significantly elevated.

PR Segment Changes

Not infrequently also in pericarditis, the PR segment may also show a shift.[201-203] It usually is depressed in all leads except aVR where it will show elevation. It may be more pronounced in leads II, aVF, V5 and V6 (Fig. 12.72). Since the pericardium covers most of the atria except the most posterior surface, the elevation of the PR segment can be thought of as due to atrial current of injury. It may often be noted early on in the clinical course along with ST segment elevation as well as when the ST segments have returned to the baseline and before the T waves become inverted. The shift in PR segment needs to be assessed in relation to the TP segment.

ECG Changes with Pericardial Effusion

When pericarditis results in significant pericardial effusion, the ECG may be affected because of the effusion. The voltage may drop significantly due to the short circuiting effect of the fluid on the electrical current. The predominant change will be in the QRS amplitude, the P wave amplitude may not be that affected. Low voltage is commonly defined as QRS amplitude of <0.5 mV (5 mm) in the limb leads and <1.0 mV (10 mm) in the precordial leads. Generally, pericardiocentesis will result in increase in voltage except when significant fibrin deposits are present.[205]

Low voltage can occur in chronic constrictive pericarditis. It will also be present in other cardiac as well as extracardiac conditions. The cardiac conditions include diffuse myocardial involvement such as in hypothyroidism (myxedema heart), amyloidosis and scleroderma, neoplastic conditions, and sometimes also in chronic ischemic heart disease with fibrosis and scars. The extracardiac conditions include large pleural effusion, pneumothorax, COPD and sometimes increased epicardial fat.

When the pericardial effusion is large, there could be significant pendular oscillatory motion of the heart that can lead to cyclic changes in QRS amplitude that may resemble "electrical alternans."[206] Total electrical alternans involving the P wave, QRS and T waves is rare and will be very suggestive of cardiac tamponade in patients with pericardial effusion (Fig. 12.74).[207,208]

Arrhythmias Associated With Pericarditis

It is not uncommon to see primarily some atrial or supraventricular arrhythmias with acute pericarditis. These may include atrial flutter, atrial fibrillation and even junctional tachycardia. Often sinus node may be secondarily involved in the inflammatory process due to the epicardial location of the sinus node in the right atrium.[209] This may also predispose to the development of the atrial arrhythmias. Atrial fibrillation is commonly seen in patients with chronic constrictive pericarditis.

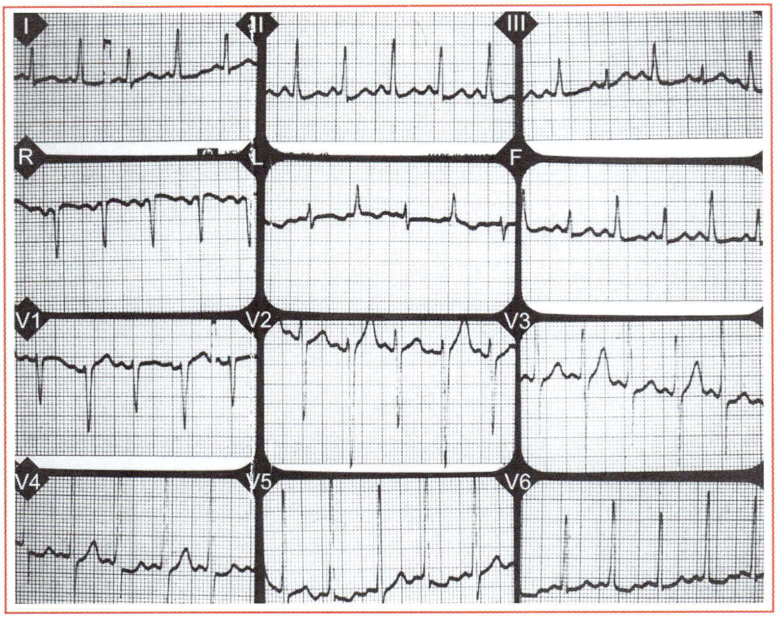

Fig. 12.74: Electrocardiogram showing clearly the electrical alternans of the QRS with alternating large and smaller amplitudes of the QRS.

SECTION VI: ABNORMALITIES OF ST-T WAVES/QT INTERVALS/ST SEGMENT DEVIATIONS/T WAVES

ST-T Abnormalities

Basic Physiology—Correlates

Although some of the mechanisms have been covered in Section I, it may be prudent to have a short review before discussing the abnormalities during the ST interval. The total electrical activity of the ventricles is represented by the QT interval. Electrical diastole in the heart follows the depolarization of the heart (electrical systole). The electrical diastole is comprised of the ST interval, which includes the ST segment and the T wave. In some cases, the T wave may be followed by a U wave (*see* Fig. 12.15).

In the myocardial cell, the resting membrane potential is around -90 mV. When depolarization occurs, there is a rapid shift in the voltage to close to 0 potential over a short period, giving rise to the QRS. After this depolarization, the transmembrane potential remains around +10 to -10 mV without much change. This corresponds to the plateau of the action potential (phase 2). During this period, since there is no net current flow, there is no dipole to register a voltage; hence, the ST segment remains flat. During phase 3 of the action potential repolarization takes place. During this period once again a current flow is generated, therefore a waveform is recorded on the surface ECG. This wave is called the T wave. Under normal circumstances, one would expect the T wave to point in the opposite direction to the QRS as it does in the isolated muscle strip. For reasons explained earlier in Section I, while the depolarization sequence is from the endocardium to the epicardium, repolarization sequence begins at the epicardium. This changes the direction of the T wave that now lines up along the QRS. In addition, there is much asynchrony both spatially and temporally during repolarization. The action potentials are also non-homogeneous in that they are shorter in the epicardium and longer in the endocardium. The combination of the above causes, prevent the wave of repolarization from being a sharp and narrow wave as the QRS. Instead, the T wave is of lower voltage and broader.

U Wave

The interval following the T wave until the next sinus P is known as the T-P interval. At times, at the onset of the TP interval, another small wave is noticed called the U wave. The U wave occurs after the depolarization has ended. The exact cause of the U wave is still somewhat controversial, but it is thought to correspond to an "electric-mechanical" event.[210] The end of the mechanical systole corresponds to the end of the electrical diastole, namely end of the T wave. It is well known that after systole ends, during the rapid filling phase of the ventricles, there is active relaxation of the myocardium. It is possible that this may be associated with some weak currents that can be recorded in some individuals and more so in some circumstances, when they become more prominent. During the periods when there is no significant net current flow across the cell membranes, namely during phase 2 and phase 4 of the action potential the ECG registers a flat line at the same level. At times, the U wave may merge with the T wave and mimic QT prolongation. U waves also tend to be more common during bradycardia as well as in patients with hypokalemia, on certain psychotropic drugs and also while on digitalis.[21,211]

Non-specific ST-T Abnormalities

ST-T changes occur as a result of abnormal voltage gradients during phases 2 and 3 of the action potential. They may also be related to changes in the sequence of repolarization. When considering the causes of these changes, one needs to consider anatomical, pathological, physiological and pharmacological events.[210] Although some of the well-defined ST-T abnormalities will be discussed separately, none of the changes can be attributed to a definite cause all the time. At times, the specificity and the sensitivity of some of the changes can improve but never perfect. Most changes are difficult to sort out as to the cause, because so many variables are operative that they are simply reported as "***non-specific ST-T abnormalities***". When the patient's history and physical findings are known, the sensitivity and specificity of the changes may improve. Also *see* section of "ST depression" and "T wave".

Primary and Secondary ST-T Changes

When the depolarization sequence is abnormal, it stands to reason that the repolarization will also change and will become abnormal. Abnormalities in the ST-T waves arising from this are known as "***Secondary ST-T changes***". Secondary ST-T changes are commonly seen when the QRS is also abnormal as in BBB (Fig. 12.38B), WPW type pre-excitation (Fig. 12.68), ectopic beats and paced rhythms. The secondary ST-T changes are not associated with changes in the action potentials of the individual myocytes. The expected secondary changes of ST-T waves can be easily appreciated by looking at the direction of the QRS and that of the T wave. *In most instances, T wave will point in the opposite direction of the delayed portion of the QRS.* These changes will persist as long as the depolarization abnormality is present. When the latter disappears, the secondary ST-T changes also disappear and revert back to normal most of the time. Sometimes, secondary ST-T changes may persist long after the depolarization abnormality has reverted back to normal. ST-T changes caused by an electronic pacemaker-induced rhythms may persist even when the patient is not being paced.

When the ST-T changes are associated with changes in the action potentials at the individual cell level, they are known as ***"Primary ST-T changes"***. These changes may be localized or diffuse. Primary ST-T changes may occur as a result of ischemia, infarction (Fig. 12.60), myocarditis, pericarditis, drugs, toxins, electrolyte imbalances (specifically Ca^{2+} and K^{+}), changes in heart rate, hyperventilation, catecholamines, changes in function of sympathetic outflow (stellate ganglia) and changes in body temperature.

Sometimes, it is possible to have both primary and secondary ST-T abnormalities in the same patient. As a result of an abnormal QRS, if the expected secondary ST-T wave abnormality were not present, then one would have to consider a concomitant primary ST-T change. For instance in a patient with classical LBBB type QRS, one expects to see depressed ST with inverted T waves following the predominantly upright QRS in leads I and V6. If the T waves in these leads were upright instead, then it would suggest a primary T wave abnormality (Fig. 12.39).

In some situations, both Primary and Secondary ST-T wave changes may be present as a result of the diseased state. This is classically noted in LVH. The repolarization abnormalities accompanying LVH are due to both primary and secondary causes. Primary causes include often the associated fibrosis secondary to relative sub-endocardial ischemia as a result of increased wall tension. Secondary causes occur as a result of the changes in the QRS, namely the increased QRS voltage and duration (Fig. 12.48).

Duration of the Action Potential (QT Interval)

The total duration of the action potential as seen on the surface ECG is represented by the QT interval. As mentioned earlier in Section I, the duration of the QT interval varies with the patient's heart rate (longer QT with slower heart rates); it has to be standardized by correcting the QT interval for the patient's heart rate. The heart rate corrected QT is depicted by QTc. A QTc >440 ms is considered to be prolonged. In females, QTc is usually longer than in males by 20 ms.

If the QT interval is prolonged due to prolongation of the QRS duration as in BBB, it is to be expected. But if the QT interval is prolonged despite a normal duration of the QRS, it would indicate prolongation of the ST interval. This type of QT prolongation needs careful attention. The serious problem of significant QT prolongation is often the associated rapid ventricular tachyarrhythmia or fibrillation that could be fatal. This usually results from non-homogeneity during the phase of repolarization, facilitating re-entrant ventricular tachyarrhythmias.

When the QRS is normal, the QT interval (QRS duration plus the ST interval) may be prolonged as a result of prolongation of the ST segment or as a result of prolongation of the T wave, or a combination of the two. For instance, in ***hypocalcemia,*** which affects the phase 2 of the action potential, the ST segment is prolonged and not the T wave width (Figs. 12.75A and B). In myocardial ischemia on the other hand, QT interval is prolonged as a result of abnormal wide T waves due probably to increased calcium inside the injured cells and less in the extracellular medium (Fig. 12.76).[212]

Although, catecholamine effect generally causes tachycardia and therefore should shorten the QT interval, intense catecholamine surge actually causes significant QT prolongation. The abnormal T waves and QT prolongation of sub-arachnoid hemorrhage are thought to be due to this mechanism (Fig. 12.77). The intense catecholamine may cause diffuse pre-capillary vasoconstriction in the coronary circulation and therefore the mechanism could be similar to that of ischemia.[213] The QT interval may also be variable as a result of the outflows from the two sides of the stellate ganglia. The effects of the right and the left stellate ganglia are opposite to each other. Hence, the QT interval change in intracerebral injury due to hemorrhage or infarct may also be dependent on the location of the injury.[214] QT intervals are also influenced by drug effects such as the psychotropic drugs as well as some of the newer antibiotics. It is well known that class I anti-arrhythmic drugs such as quinidine and procainamide prolong the QT interval as well as sotalol and amiodarone. Occasionally, while some of these drugs may be tolerated by some patients, when inadvertently another medication is added to the therapeutic regimen, the combination may prove serious. In addition to these acquired causes, there are also inherited familial causes of the prolonged QT intervals that may be associated with fatal ventricular arrhythmias and sudden death. The most typical form of ventricular tachyarrhythmia associated with prolonged QT intervals is the ***torsade de pointes*** type. The wide QRS complexes of this arrhythmia are typically seen to twist around the baseline changing directions (Figs. 12.78A and B). The risk of this is increased with increasing QTc intervals and in the presence of complicating

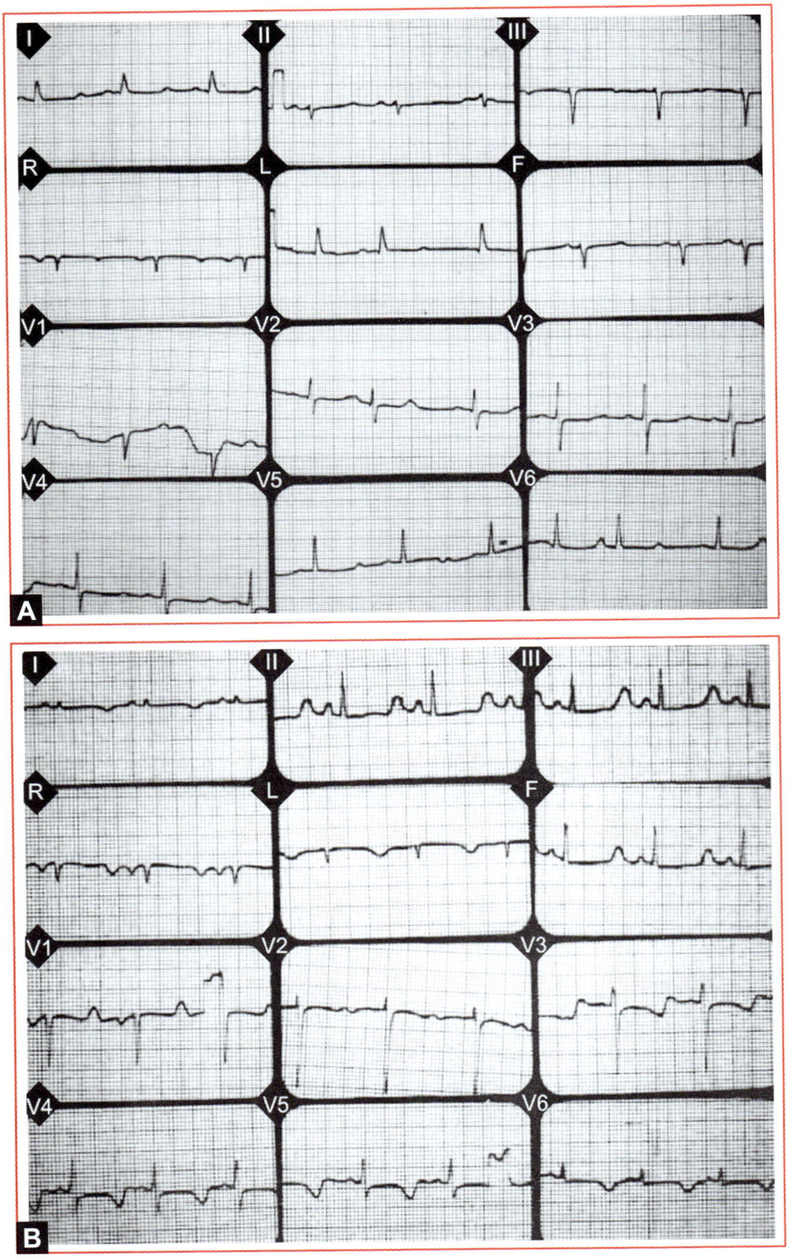

Figs. 12.75A and B: Electrocardiograms (ECGs) from two patients with hypocalcemia. The ST segment is long with upright T wave seen clearly in (A). In ECG from a different patient, the duration of the action potential interval is significantly prolonged at the expense of the ST segment suggestive of hypocalcemia.

hypokalemia, hypomagnesemia, left ventricular dysfunction, serious bradycardia, early coupled premature ventricular beats with an R-on-T pattern as well as in female patients.[53]

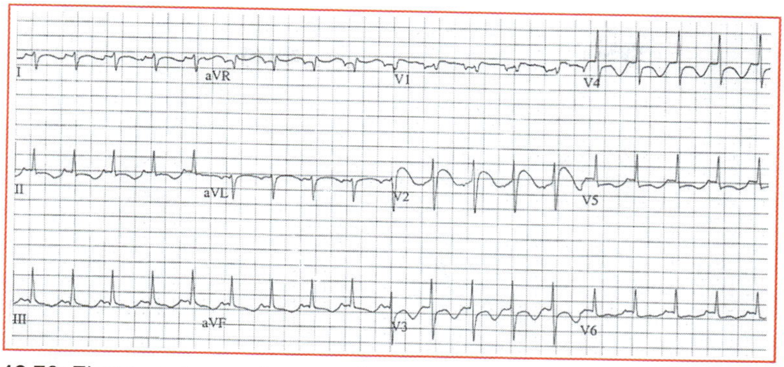

Fig. 12.76: Electrocardiogram from a patient with myocardial ischemia. Note the abnormal inverted T waves with prolongation of the duration of the action potential interval.

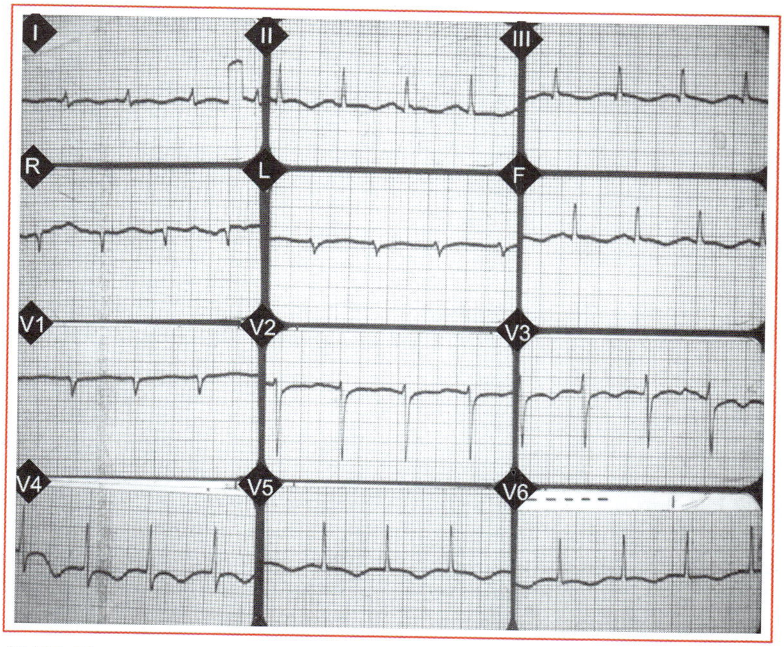

Fig. 12.77: Electrocardiogram from a patient with catecholamine excess causing prolonged duration of the action potential interval with abnormal T waves.

Some of the inherited causes affecting the QT interval will be discussed below.

Inherited Long QT Syndromes (LQTS)

There are three basic "***channelopathies***" recognized that lead to prolonged QT intervals.[215] Types I and II are related to reduction of K^+ transport out of the myocardial cells during the phase 3 of the action potential. The two types represent mutations in different genes. Both types prolong the phase 3 of the

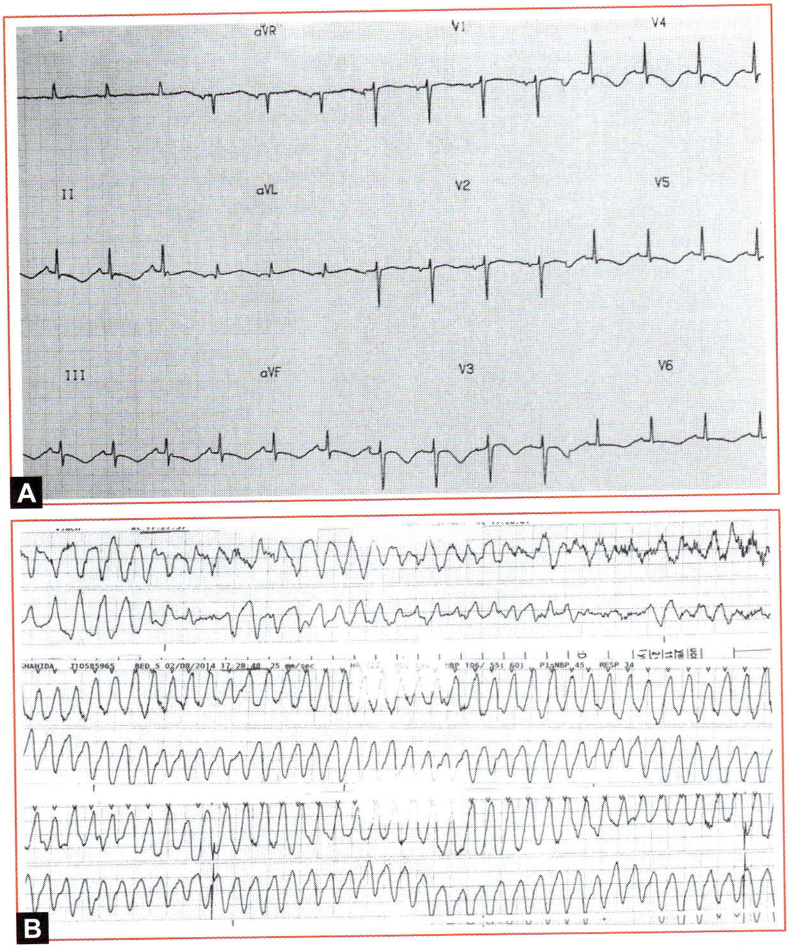

Figs. 12.78A and B: Electrocardiogram from a patient with prolonged duration of the action potential interval secondary to overdose of a psychotropic agent. The rhythm strips obtained in the CCU during sub-sequent cardiac arrest (B) demonstrates the typical features of the polymorphic ventricular tachycardia of the Torsade de pointes type. The wide QRS tachycardia with changing direction twisting around the baseline. Courtesy: By courtesy of Dr. M. Fisher of St. Joseph's Health Centre, Toronto.

action potential. The type III is related to defective inactivation of the Na^+ pump, which allows continued Na^+ influx into the cell during phase 2 of the action potential.

The type I usually shows a short or non-existent ST segment with a tall wide T wave. In these patients, lethal arrhythmias may occur during exercise in 68% of cases, emotional stress in 14% of cases, during sleep in 9% of cases and 19% at other times. The type II is associated with an ECG showing almost normal ST segment with a wide T wave, which may even be bifid. In these patients, lethal arrhythmias have been noted to occur with exercise in 29%

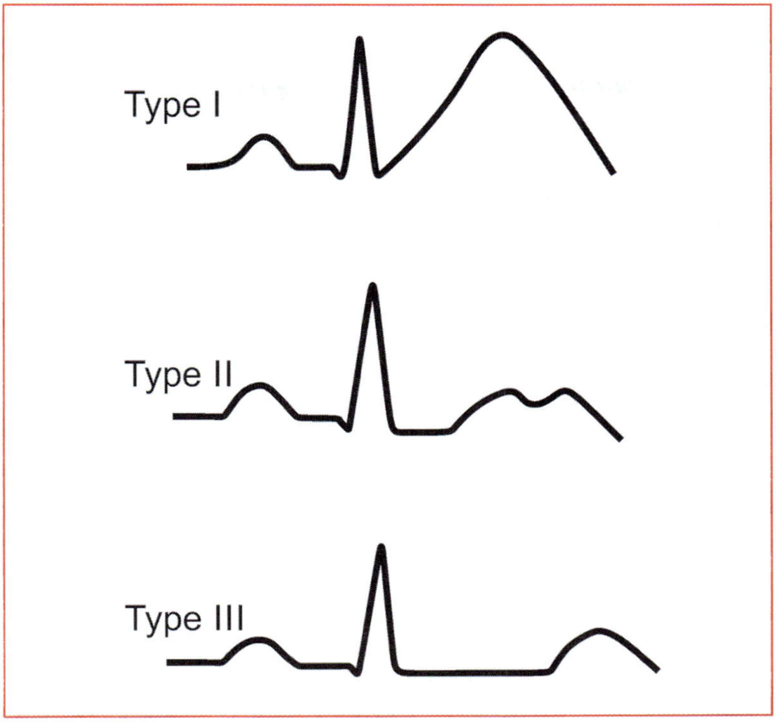

Fig. 12.79: Diagram showing the the three types of the inherited Long duration of the action potential syndrome. Type I with very little or no ST segment and tall wide T waves. Type II with normal ST segment with a wide abnormal T wave. Type III with long ST segment with normal T wave.

of the time, with emotional stress in 49% of the time and during sleep in 22% of the time. The type III is associated with a long ST segment and a normal T wave (Fig. 12.79). Sudden death in these patients tends to occur mostly during sleep when the heart rate is slow (64% of the time). Only 4% may have a fatal arrhythmia during exercise and 12% during emotional stress. Twenty percent occur at other times.[216-218]

The QTc measurement on the 12 lead ECG in assessing the presence of prolongation has 90% specificity and 81% sensitivity when one uses 440 ms as the cut-off.[219] When one considers the limit as 460 ms for females, the specificity increases to 96% but sensitivity drops to 71%. In patients with LQTS, if prolonged QTc is defined as >450 ms, 11% of positive cases will be falsely diagnosed as having the condition when they do not.[220] In some of these patients, resting ECGs may be completely normal; therefore, when there is an unexplained syncope or an episode of cardiac arrest in a patient that has been successfully resuscitated a full history should be obtained with careful attention to the family history. A family history of sudden death or infant death as well as unexplained epilepsy or a history of congenital deafness should alert the clinician to the possibility of the presence of LQTS. This should prompt appropriate investigation, which should include a resting ECG in the supine and standing positions. If the QT interval is still normal, an exercise test should be carried out and the QT measured during exercise as well as during the recovery phase. In some patients, QT may prolong during exercise or only during the postexercise phase. A postexercise paradoxical QTc increase (QTc > 460 ms) makes a diagnosis of LQTS with 90% sensitivity and 92% specificity.[221] These QTc changes are not affected by β-blockers. If this fails and the suspicion is high, one should carry out epinephrine infusion test. Normally, QT should shorten with catecholamines, but in these patients it tends to lengthen.[222]

When low dose epinephrine is infused, a paradoxical QT prolongation by more than 30 ms has 92% sensitivity and 86% specificity in making a diagnosis of LQTS. The positive predictive value of the test is 75% and the negative predictive value 96%. Once a clinical diagnosis is made with certainty, genetic testing may be done for confirmation.[223,224]

Short QT Interval

The QT interval is considered short when the QTc is below 350 ms.[225] Some others may consider the QTc to be short when it is <330 ms.[53] There are many causes of shortened QT, the most common being tachycardia. Among drugs, digitalis is known to shorten the QT interval. Both hyperkalemia and hypercalcemia will shorten the QT interval. Most patients with short QT intervals have no serious consequences. In recent years however, there has been a genetic mutation recognized that causes short QT that has been associated with sudden death.

Inherited Short QT Syndrome (SQTS)

This is a rare condition and the diagnosis requires a full family history and not merely the presence of a short QTc. In these patients, typically the QTc interval is between 220 and 360 ms. In a study of families with history of sudden death reported that the QTc did not exceed 280 ms[226] (Fig. 12.80). Often the patients have structurally normal hearts, but with a tendency of developing atrial fibrillation and ventricular tachycardia or fibrillation. When the resting heart rate is <100, the measured QT interval need not even be corrected for the heart rate in these patients since their QT intervals are much less heart rate-responsive. Genetically, it is a heterogeneous disease and has been associated with mutations in five different genes so far. It may be a cause of sudden infant death. Patients with this condition are at risk throughout their lives. Sixty-two percent of these patients will remain asymptomatic. Of reported symptoms, cardiac arrest was the most common (34%) followed by palpitations (31%) and syncope (24%). Atrial fibrillation occurred

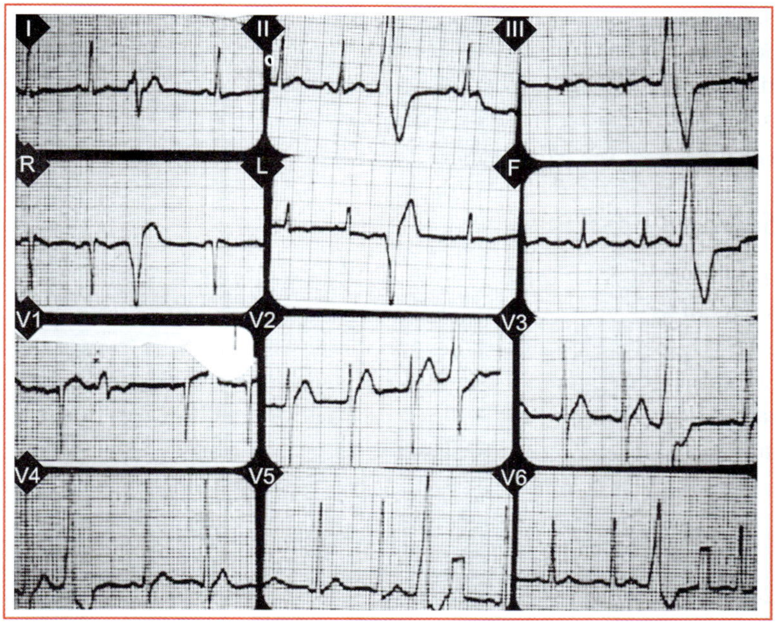

Fig. 12.80: Electrocardiogram from a patient with short corrected duration of the action potential interval.

in 17% of cases as the first presenting symptom.[225] The genetic abnormality may decrease the inward depolarizing Na^+ and Ca^{2+} currents, or increase the repolarizing outward K^+ currents or cause both. This will shorten the action potential duration. This shortening is also heterogeneous between the endocardium and the epicardium. This will result in unidirectional blocks, dispersion of repolarization and refractoriness, setting the stage for re-entry and giving rise to polymorphic ventricular tachycardia. Quinidine being a blocker of K^+ channels appears to be the most effective drug to correct the abnormality.[227] However symptomatic patients are best protected by an ICD implant.

ST Segment

As has been mentioned previously in Section I, the ST segment starts from the ***J*** point (at the end of the QRS) and ends at the onset of the T wave (*see* Fig. 12.15). The ST segment, in the normal patients, is isoelectric on the surface ECG and is located at the same level as the T-P segment. In some normal patients and in certain pathological states, the ST segment may be deviated up (ST elevation) or down (ST depression). There are many causes that can produce deviation of the ST segment. It appears that any myocardial damage at the endocardial or sub-endocardial region causes ST segment depression, whereas, damage to the epicardial myocardium causes

ST segment elevation (Fig. 12.54). ST segment deviations associated with myocardial infarctions and pericarditis have been discussed in detail in Sections IV and V. In some patients at the junction of the QRS and the ST segment, a small "wave" may be seen at the end of the QRS, in the same direction as the QRS known as the ***J*** wave.

ST Segment Elevation

Some degree of ST elevation is considered to be normal in leads V1-V3. This type of ST elevation is somewhat less common among women and the elderly. When the elevation is >2 mm, then it is more likely to be pathological. In some young patients, in the "left ventricular leads" one may see ST elevation even >2 mm, usually associated with a small ***J*** wave. This is known as early repolarization (Figs. 12.81A and B).

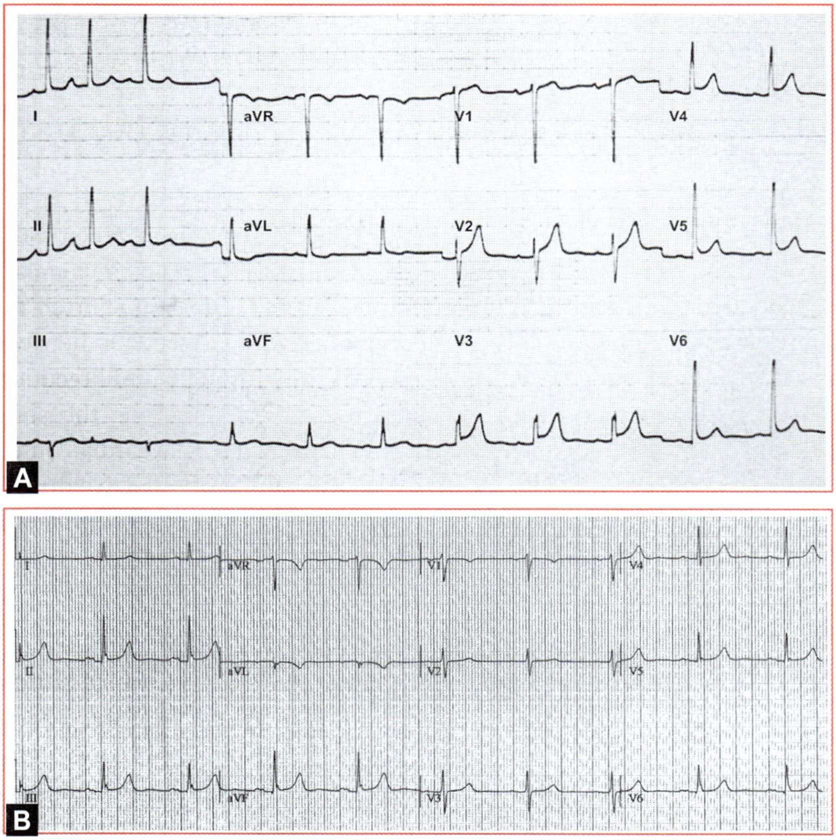

Figs. 12.81A and B: Electrocardiograms from two different patients with normal ST segment elevation of the early repolarization. J point elevation clearly seen followed by upward concave ST segments in leads V3̃V6 (A). In the second patient (B), the J point elevation is noted in the inferior leads followed by the ascending ST segment.

ST Segment Elevation-Normal Variant/Early Repolarization

The ECG features of "early repolarization" (ER) have been known for the last several decades. It has been considered as a benign and normal variant of ST segment and T waves for a long time.[53,228,229] It will be discussed because it is characterized by ST segment elevation and may be part of a differential in acute chest pain syndromes caused by conditions such as pericarditis.[230]

The Classical ECG Features

The ST segment is elevated with an upward concavity most commonly seen in the mid-to-lateral precordial leads (V2–V4) together with positive tall peaked T waves in the same leads. Often the ***J*** point is also elevated before the ST segment. The downstroke of the ***R*** wave close to the ***J*** point may be slurred or the ***J*** point may have a positive hump or notch sometimes termed ***J wave.*** There will be often a reciprocal ST depression in aVR. The changes may also wax and wane over time. The pattern is more commonly seen in young males and athletes, and the pattern is equally common in all races[228,231–233] (Figs. 12.81A and B).

Concept of Benign Versus Malignant ST Segment Morphology in ER

Some recent studies have suggested that the ER might not be entirely benign. It has been recognized for some time now that ER might be prone to serious arrhythmias in isolated case reports.[234] Some of the features of ER are similar to those of the ***Brugada syndrome*** that has been known to be associated with serious ventricular arrhythmias including VF. In experimental models, the ECG features of ER have also been shown to be convertible to that of the Brugada syndrome. While the ST segment elevation in patients with ER is usually localized to leads V2-V5 and is accompanied by a notched J point and a positive T wave, showing an upward concavity, in Brugada, the ***J*** point elevation is prominent in the right precordial leads V1-V3 followed by a larger ***J*** wave and a down sloping ST segment and negative T wave.[235] Autonomic and pharmacologic modulation of ST segment magnitude are also similar in both of these conditions.[236] Slowing of the heart rate exaggerates the ST segment elevation and increase in heart rate by exercise and/or isoproterenol decreases the ST segment elevation in both conditions. Sodium channel blockers can unmask the Brugada syndrome and they can increase the ST segment elevation in ER. Sympathetic stimulation normalizes the ST segment elevation whereas β-blockers augment the ST segment elevation. High cervical cord injury at the level of C5 and C6 completely interrupts cardiac sympathetic activity and is known to cause multilead ST segment elevation.[237]

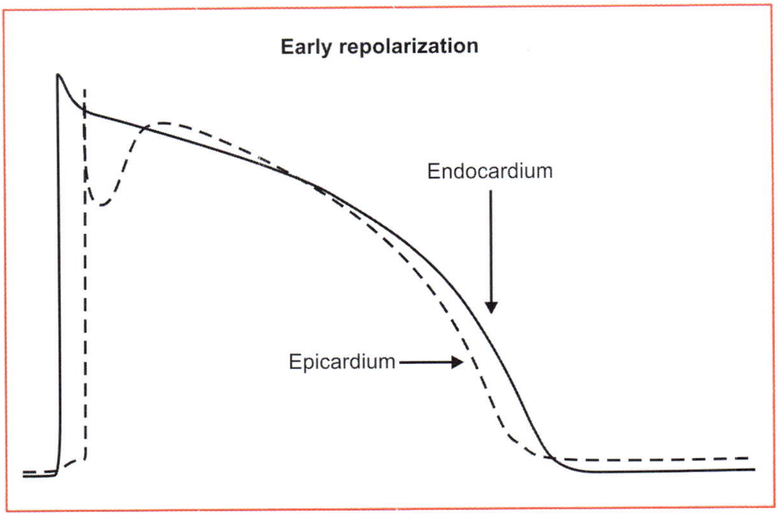

Fig. 12.82: Diagram of the transmembrane action potential in early repolarization syndrome. In experimental studies, a small transmural voltage gradient has been shown to develop between the epicardium and the endocardium caused by the depression of the entire epicardial action potential during the plateau phase of repolarization.[235]

Basic electrophysiologic mechanisms responsible for the ***J*** deflection and ST segment elevation are not clearly understood. It is felt that there is transmural voltage gradient between the epicardium and the endocardium secondary to depression of the action potential plateau of ventricular epicardium but not endocardium (Fig. 12.82) due to early repolarization of epicardium but not endocardium. The Ca^{2+} independent 4-aminopyridine sensitive transient outward current (***Ito***) is a rapidly activating and inactivating potassium current that is responsible for the phase 1 of the action potential (*see* Fig. 12.3). A prominent ***Ito*** gives the epicardial and mid-myocardial cell (M cell) action potentials a notched or a ***spike and dome*** morphology. These features are shown to be lacking in the endocardium due to low tissue density of that current in the endocardium.[236] This manifests itself as ***J*** wave and ST segment elevation.[238]

Recently in case-controlled studies, it has been shown that ER is associated with idiopathic VF.[239-241] It has been recognized that the contour of the ST segment morphology in young male athletic type subjects with benign long-term outcome is different from those who have been found to develop idiopathic VF.[242] The ST segment of this "***benign form***" is of the rapidly ascending type blending with the T wave. The ST segment of the "***malignant form***" remains flat, horizontal or even descends toward the T wave (Fig. 12.83).[243] The latter association has also been noted in a few other studies.[244] It must however be noted that the incidence of ER in population-based studies varies from 5% to 13%. The most prevalent form is of the horizontal type in large unselected population studies and in adults, the incidence is about 65%-73%.[244] The risk of sudden death is reported to be

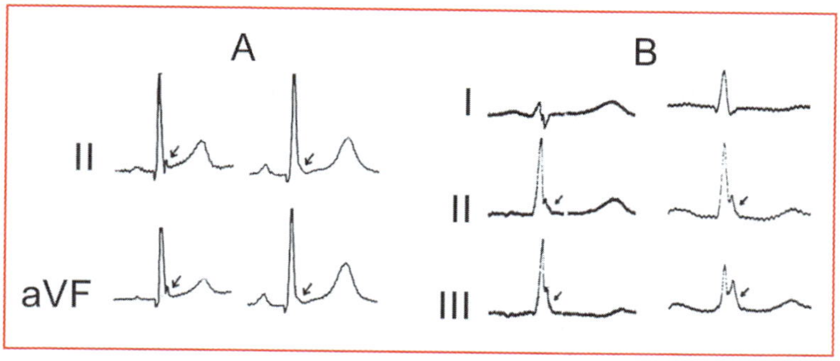

Fig. 12.83: Diagram showing the two different types of ST segment elevation in the inferior leads described.[242] The "benign" type has the rapidly ascending ST segment morphology after the J wave [shown in (A)]. The "malignant form" associated with the risk of idiopathic ventricular fibrillation has a flat, horizontal and even descending ST segment morphology [shown in (B)]. Adapted from: Tikkanen JT, Junttila MJ, Anttonen O, Aro AL, Luttinen S, Kerola T, et al. Early repolarization: electrocardiographic phenotypes associated with favorable long-term outcome. Circulation. 2011;123(23):2666-73. (Copyright with permission-Wolters Kluwer Health, 2014).

..7-fold higher if the horizontal ER is recorded in the inferior leads.[242] In the most recent study the risk of cardiac mortality was found to be five fold higher.[245]

A few recent studies have also suggested that patients with ER seem to have increased risk of having ischemic VF.[246,247] Early repolarization of the horizontal type appeared to be associated also with increased risk of arrhythmic events during ischemia in vasospastic angina.[248]

The true nature of "ER" pattern is yet to be resolved from the electrophysiologic standpoint. The terms early and late repolarization are synonymous with phases 2 and 3 of the transmembrane action potential.[249] In the ECG, they correspond to ST segment and T wave. It must be taken primarily as describing the type of ST segment morphology.

Clinical Perspective

The increased risk associated with the junctional changes in the QRS-ST with the horizontal type ST segment morphology of ER must be taken and used in proper perspective with reference to the clinical context as to whether the patient is symptomatic or asymptomatic. The risk of VF in an asymptomatic young adult with ER is only 1 in 3,000, far lower than in an asymptomatic "Brugada" patient.[244] In the clinical context of ventricular tachyarrhythmias and syncope, efforts must be made to rule out ischemic and non-ischemic causes including the LQTS, the SQTS, the Brugada syndrome and arrhythmogenic right ventricular dysplasia. Once these have been excluded, then the ECG signs described above with regard to the malignant form of ER may be considered also as a diagnostic clue especially in men with a history of unexplained syncope or a familial incidence of sudden death at young age.[250]

J Wave

J waves appear to be deflections of the terminal portion of the QRS in the same direction as the QRS. Small ***J*** wave in relation to early repolarization was already discussed. Most of those are benign and some are pathological in that they are associated with sudden death as already discussed. Large ***J*** waves can be congenital or acquired as well and are always pathological.

Congenital ST Elevation and Large J Wave (Brugada Syndrome)

This is an inherited familial "channelopathy" that is associated with sudden death. It is associated with mutations at three different gene locations. These mutations may result in reduced Na^+ current flow inward (20%), reduced Ca^{2+} current flow inward or increased transient fast K^+ current flow outward during phase 1 of the action potential. In a normal situation, after rapid Na^+ inflow during phase 0 of the action potential, with effective depolarization the cell potential overshoots into being positively charged. The transient K^+ current is rapidly activated during phase 1 of the action potential and reduces the potential closer to zero. In patients with Brugada syndrome, the balance between the inward (Na^+ and Ca^{2+}) and outward K^+ current is disturbed. This transient K^+ current may be exaggerated and may last longer, causing partial repolarization in phase 1 that encroaches on phase 2 causing what appears to be a dip in phase 2 of the action potential. This presents itself as ST elevation (***J*** point elevation >2 mm) on the surface electrocardiogram, seen particularly in leads V1 and V2. The changes are seen in these leads mainly because the loss of action potential dome is more limited to the epicardium of the right ventricle. This results in transmural and epicardial dispersion of repolarization. The transmural dispersion causes the ST elevation, the epicardial dispersion results in the re-entry phenomenon. The combination of the two makes the patient vulnerable for ventricular tachycardia or fibrillation. Vagal stimulation will worsen the condition, whereas adrenergic stimulation will improve it. Usually faster heart rates are associated with less ST elevation and slower heart rates with more ST elevation. This is likely the cause of sudden death commonly noted to occur during sleep in this disorder[251] (Fig. 12.84A).

This may also be associated with what appears to be a RBBB conduction pattern. In fact, there is no RBBB. What mimics as the ***R′*** is a ***large J*** wave.

Three different types of ECG findings are noted (Fig. 12.84B):

Type I: shows an elevated ***J*** point with a large ***J*** wave, a coved ST segment that gradually descends to a negative T wave in V1 and V2.

Type II: shows also elevated ***J*** point (at least 2 mm) with a smaller ***J*** wave, mid and terminal ST elevation (>1 mm) and upright or biphasic T wave.

Type III: is similar to type II, but both ***J*** point as well as the mid and terminal ST elevations are less impressive (<1 mm). This last type may also be a normal variant.[251]

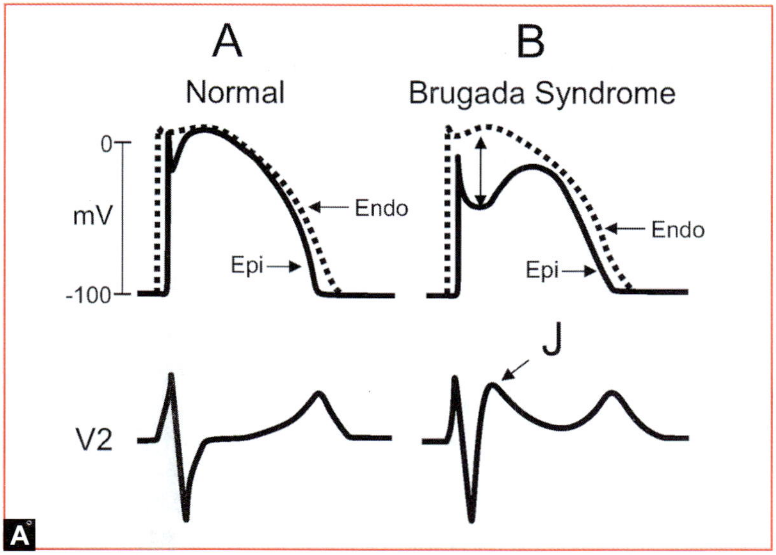

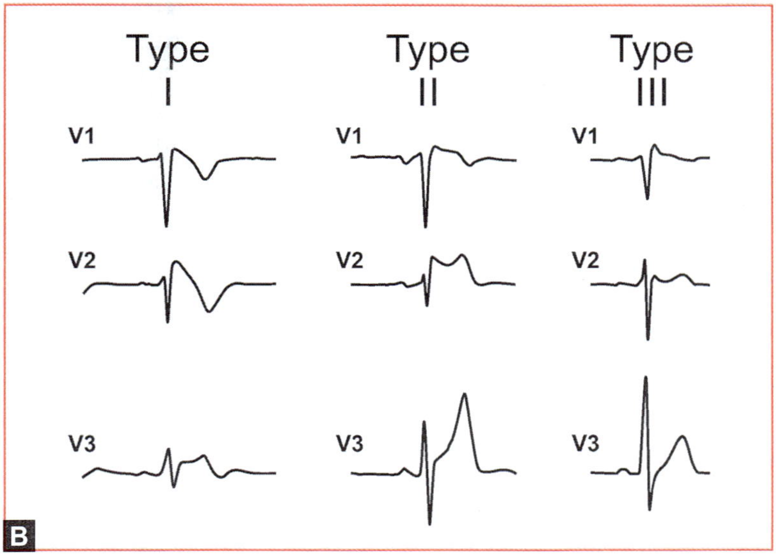

Figs. 12.84A and B: (A) Diagram of the transmembrane action potential in Brugada syndrome (B) compared to the normal (A) with surface electrocardiogram (ECG) lead V1 at the bottom. In patients with Brugada syndrome, the balance between the inward (Na+ and Ca2+) and outward K+ current is disturbed. The transient outward K+ is exaggerated. This may result in partial repolarization in phase 1 encroaching on phase 2 causing what appears to be a dip in phase 2. The loss of action potential dome is more limited to the epicardium of the right ventricle. The transmural voltage gradient results in ST segment elevation. The right precordial leads V1 and V2 show J wave and ST segment elevation.[235,250] (B) Diagram showing the three types of ECG findings noted in the right precordial leads of patients with Brugada syndrome. Type I has elevated J point, large J wave and a coved ST segment descending to a negative T wave. Type II elevated J point, smaller J wave, mid and terminal ST elevation and upright or biphasic T waves. Type III is similar to Type II except the elevations of ST segments are less.

Evaluation of a Suspected Patient

This will require family history, a resting ECG and exercise testing as with LQTS. In addition, it is also important to get high (third interspace) chest leads V1 and V2 as well, since ST segment elevation may only be seen one interspace higher in some patients.[252-256] High precordial leads improve the sensitivity of pharmacologic testing with procainamide (by 35%) and produce better yield in diagnosis during family screening.[257] The presenting symptoms may include syncope or previous unexpected cardiac arrest that the patient has survived or simply sudden death that appears to be more common during sleep.

Ambulatory monitoring is also needed in the suspected cases. The typical ECG findings may not be present at all times. They may be seen during sleep, post-prandially, with low serum potassium and during febrile states. There is no drug therapy for this condition. The antiarrhythmic drugs (class Ia, Ic, III) all increase the ST elevation. In patients who have had documented serious arrhythmias such as ventricular tachycardia or have had syncope, defibrillator implant (ICD) is recommended. In patients who get frequent episodes of VF requiring frequent ICD shocks, quinidine has been used in conjunction with an ICD to decrease the episodes of VF. The asymptomatic patients should be advised to avoid aggravating situations. These include fever control during viral or bacterial illnesses. Other precautions will include avoidance of excessive exercise. Normal amount of exercise by increasing sympathetic tone improves the condition, but excessive exercise becomes detrimental because of the excess body heat it generates. These patients should avoid drugs that block the Na^+ channels (a full drug list is available at brugadadrugs.org).

Arrhythmogenic Right Ventricular Dysplasia/Cardiomyopathy (ARVD/ARVC)

This is an inherited disorder with familial occurrence, transmitted in an autosomal dominant pattern with various degrees of clinical expression.[258-261] A variant of the disease has been described with a recessive mode of transmission as well. Morphologically the characteristic feature is fatty replacement of the epicardium and mid-myocardium of the RV free wall. The endocardium and the septum are spared. In advanced cases, the LV may also get affected. Focal thinning of the RV wall is typical. Typical onset of symptoms occurs in the young adults between 12 and 45 years of age. Symptoms include palpitations, syncope, heart failure or sudden death. It is estimated that 3-4% of sudden deaths during sports and about 17% of all sudden deaths in young patients may be related to this disorder. The propensity of ventricular tachyarrhythmias arising from the RV free wall in these patients almost always is of the LBBB morphology. The ECG during sinus rhythm often shows the following features:[262-265]

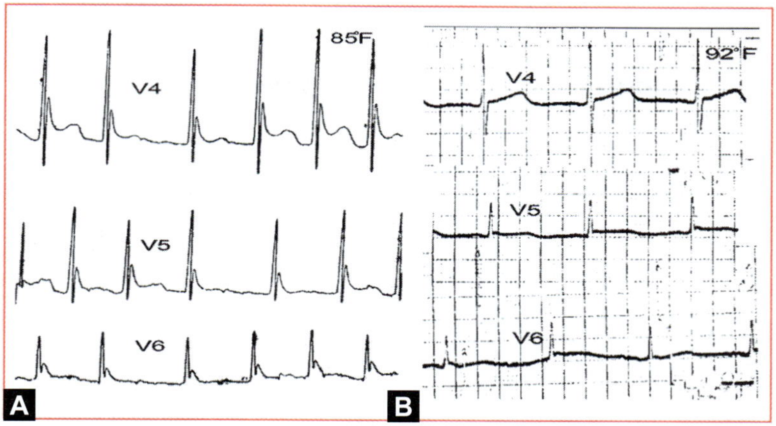

Figs. 12.85A and B: Electrocardiogram from a patient admitted with hypothermia showing large J waves also known as Osborn waves (A). Rhythm may be atrial fibrillation as well. With rewarming, the large J wave is no longer noted (B). Rhythm more regular and probably sinus.

i. QRS morphology will show focal delay resembling incomplete or complete RBBB due to slow conduction through the Purkinje system of the RV free wall, known as "parietal block". The terminal delay is seen best in the right precordial leads V1-V3 and not likely appreciated in other leads.
ii. In some patients, the delayed depolarization does not resemble ***r'***. Instead, it looks like the Greek letter "epsilon." Late potentials by signal averaging method have been demonstrated corresponding to the "epsilon" waves.
iii. T wave inversion in the right and the mid-precordial leads.
iv. In one study, ST segment elevation was induced by exercise in 11 of 17 patients with severe RV asynergy in this disorder.

Acquired Large J wave (Osborn Wave of Hypothermia)

During hypothermia, it is thought that myocardial damage causes a current of injury during phase 1 of the action potential that results in the formation of the ***large J wave*** known as ***Osborn wave***. The size (amplitude) of the ***J*** wave is inversely proportional to the body temperature (degree of hypothermia). The Osborn wave is usually present below body temperatures of 25°C[266] (Figs. 12.85A and B). The excitability at the junction of the QRS and the ST segment during hypothermia is increased by 80 times, at least in dog experiments.[267] During rapid blood transfusion in patients during surgical hypothermia, one also notices T wave alternans.[268]

ST Segment Depression

What constitutes ST depression is a depression of 1 mm or more of the ***J*** point. The ST segment following a depressed ***J*** point can be described as being

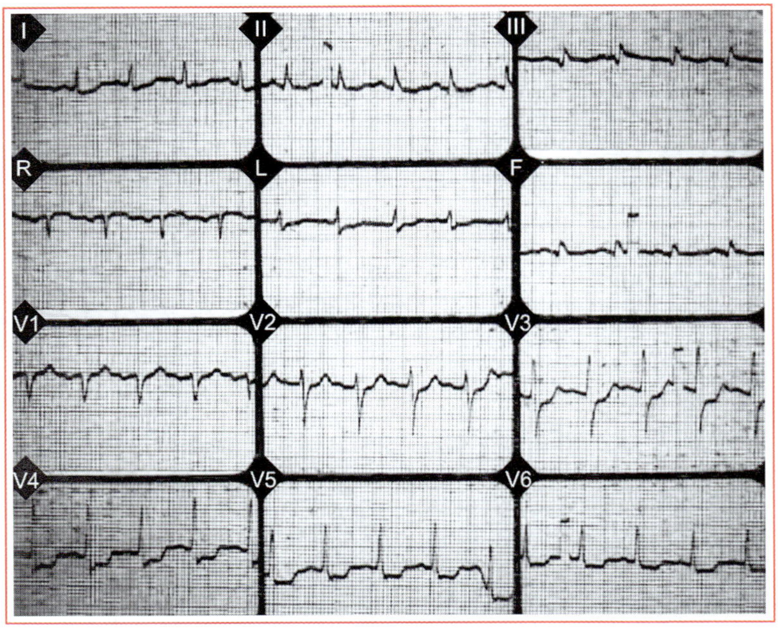

Fig. 12.86: Electrocardiogram from a patient with known ischemic heart disease. Shows horizontal type ST segment depression starting at the J point, about 2 mm in depth in leads V4 and V5 noted during exercise stress test together with symptoms of chest discomfort, which resolved following cessation of exercise. This will be diagnostic of ischemia.

upsloping, horizontal or downsloping. Horizontal or downsloping ST segments are much more significant in making a diagnosis of ischemia or sub-endocardial infarct (Fig. 12.86). In certain circumstances such as during exercise testing a significant ST depression indicating the presence of ischemia (or positive test) is considered to be at least 1 mm depression below the TP level measured 80 ms after the ***J*** point. Transmural hence, epicardial infarct will cause ST elevation whereas myocardial ischemia and/or sub-endocardial infarct will cause ST depression. ST depression may also be present as a result of reciprocal changes in the opposite leads to an ST elevation infarct. Leads that are positioned at 180° to each other may show this phenomenon. False interpretation of "reciprocal changes" would result if the leads are not diametrically opposite. For instance, sometimes in inferior infarct with ST elevation in lead aVF, one may see also ST depression and/or T wave inversion in lead I, which should not be interpreted as reciprocal changes, since in fact they would represent lateral wall ischemia in addition to the inferior infarct. Obviously, the error can be avoided if one realizes that lead I is at right angles to aVF and therefore will not show reciprocal changes. Sometimes, we rely on reciprocal ST segment depression to make diagnosis of a true posterior wall infarction since we do not put leads in the back of the chest. In this situation the reciprocal changes are used to

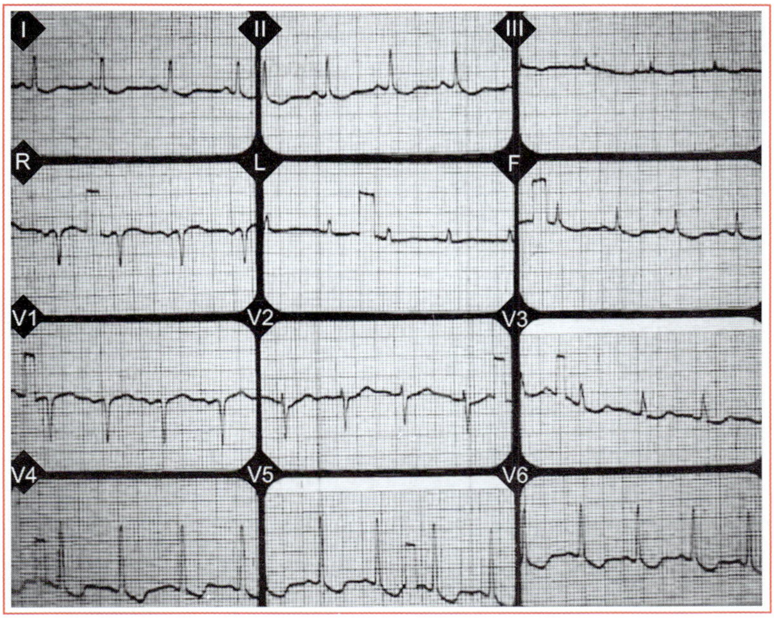

Fig. 12.87: Electrocardiogram from a patient showing ST segment changes (sagging and "hockey stick" appearance) consistent with digitalis effect.

make the diagnosis. Diametrically opposite to the true posterior wall are the anterior chest leads V1 and V2. These would show ST depression, upright tall T waves and broad R wave (usually >50 ms in duration) in lead V2 (*see* Figs. 12.58A and B).

Besides ischemia or infarction, there are other causes that can result in ST segment depression. These include hypertrophy, cardioactive drugs and electrolyte abnormalities, especially hypokalemia.

ST Segment Changes of Digitalis

Along with shortening the QT interval, digitalis will flatten and shorten the T wave. It causes ST depression, which has been described as "scooping," "hockey stick appearance" or "sagging." The J point depression is usually slight but the ST segment is concave[269] (Fig. 12.87).

Electrolyte imbalances such as hypokalemia can also cause ST depression and low T waves. They may be missed and read as "non-specific ST-T changes" if the history and laboratory data are not known[270] (Fig. 12.88).

The T Wave

Abnormalities in the T waves can be exaggerated tall peaked T waves, low voltage T waves, flat T waves, bifid (notched) T waves, inverted T waves and inverted giant T waves. T waves may also be of normal duration (width)

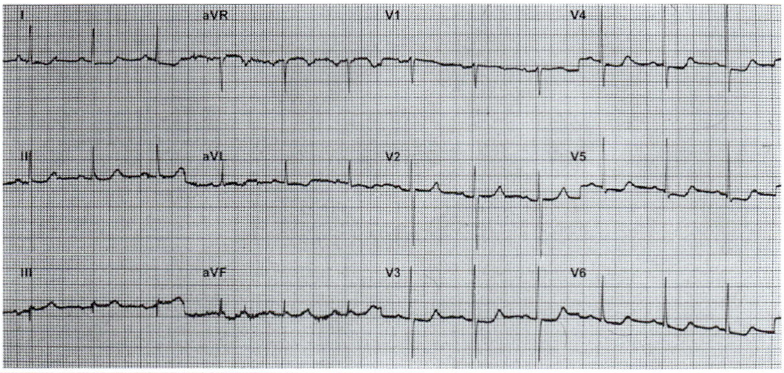

Fig. 12.88: Electrocardiogram from a patient showing non-specific ST-T abnormalities with low T waves and mild ST segment depression. Electrolyte disturbances and hypokalemia could cause similar changes.

short or broad. An abnormal T wave is extremely common and highly sensitive to physiological, pharmacological and pathological changes. It is usually very difficult to make any specific diagnosis based on the T wave abnormalities. Because of this, over 50% of abnormal ECGs are reported as "non-specific ST-T abnormalities.[271] An abnormality in the T wave becomes somewhat more specific when associated with other findings such as ST depression or elevation and changes in QT intervals. T waves may change even in normal hearts due to simple physiological variations such as standing, or even drinking a glass of cold water.[272] Various degrees of T inversions may be produced by hyperventilation.[273,274] T wave abnormalities in leads I and II have been noted in schizophrenia but the mechanism does not appear to be clear.[275] Any type of myocardial infiltrate such as primary or secondary tumors as well as other forms of infiltrates such as amyloid, sarcoid or iron will also cause T wave changes.

Inverted and Low T Waves

T waves are normally always inverted in lead aVR, and may be upright or inverted in leads III and aVL. It is also common to see inverted T in lead V1. This may persist sometimes up to lead V3. Normally, a negative T in V1 should gradually progress toward a positive T in sub-sequent consecutive chest leads, becoming less negative, biphasic or flat to becoming positive. Sometimes, negative T waves persist from V1 up to V4 in the very young and this is known as "juvenile pattern." In the very young, the relative dominance of the right ventricle would be responsible for this. For some reason in some individuals it persists to young adult life. In some females, inverted T waves in the anterior chest leads may be a normal variant (Fig. 12.89).

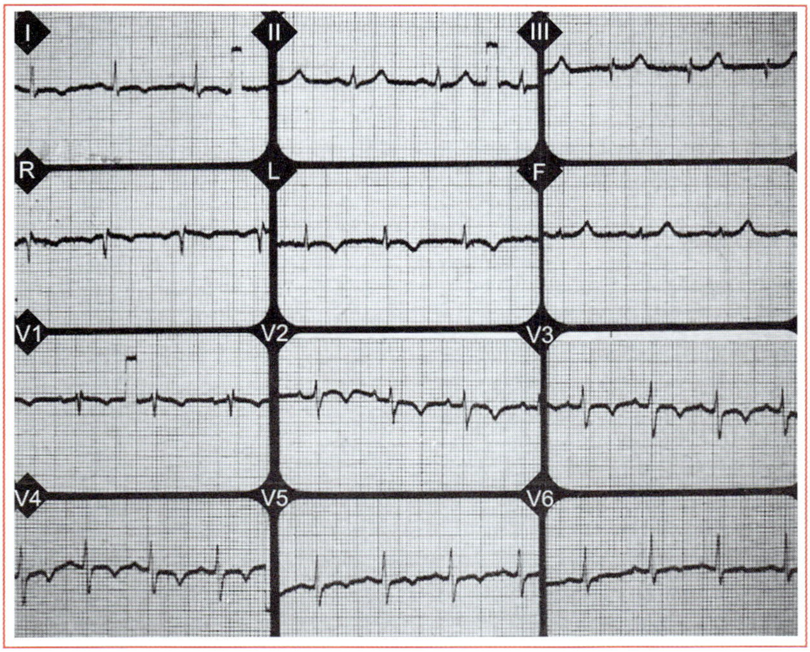

Fig. 12.89: Electrocardiogram from a 32-year-old female patient with atypical symptoms and normal coronary arteries showing incomplete right bundle branch block pattern with minor T wave inversion in leads I, aVL, V2–V5.

In African-Americans also, inverted or biphasic T waves with terminal inversion in the anterior leads may be a normal variant.[276] An anterior T inversion is considered abnormal when the lead to the right shows a more positive T wave or less negativity of the T wave. Sometimes, an isolated anterior lead terminal T wave negativity may revert to normal upright T just by taking a deep breath.

T waves in the inferior leads are also susceptible to non-pathological changes. Inverted T in lead aVF is considered normal when there is left axis deviation. In this situation the QRS-T angle would be narrow. This would be considered as a secondary T change.

Inferior T wave inversions may occur just by standing. Twenty-five percent to 50% of normal people will exhibit at least a biphasic T wave just by standing. Increased sympathetic tone may also cause T waves to change.[277] These can be reversed by β-blockers. The right sympathetic pathways supply the anterior part of the LV and the left pathways the posterior part of the LV. Stimulation of the right stellate ganglion or ablation of the left stellate ganglion will cause T inversion.[214] The reverse will cause upright T waves. These changes can be reversed by isoproterenol infusion. It would not however reverse ischemic T wave changes, which may also look similar.[278]

Mitral valve prolapse has also been associated with inverted or biphasic T waves in the inferior leads.[279] Hyperthyroidism may be associated with notched T wave. Hypothyroidism may show inverted T with a wide (obtuse) QRS-T angle. An athletic heart can also exhibit inverted T in the inferior leads as well as in the left ventricular leads (with predominant R waves usually leads I, V5 and V6).

Tall T Waves

T waves can be tall when the QRS is tall. In young patients with early repolarization, T waves are usually tall and peaked. This is considered to be a normal variant. Increased vagotonia in athletes without heart disease can be associated with tall peaked T waves as well.[280] Although alcoholism will usually cause notched or low T waves as a result of associated hypokalemia, occasionally may be associated with tall T waves. This is felt to be related to low magnesium levels.[281,282] Tall T waves are also seen in patients with hyperkalemia.

T wave alternans without QRS change is rare. It tends to be present during tachycardia or when there are sudden changes in heart rate. In the absence of these two associated findings it may indicate underlying severe myocardial disease. It has also been noted in alcoholics with severe hypomagnesemia[283,284] as well as during severe hyperkalemia. T wave alternans may also be present as a result of electrical alternans with the QRS, seen in cardiac tamponade. In the absence of tamponade, electrical alternans is highly indicative of a re-entrant arrhythmia using a retrograde accessory pathway. It is also possible to have second degree block in one of the left-sided fascicles that causes what appears to be electrical alternans.

Certain Specific Causes of T Wave Abnormalities

Myocardial ischemia or infarction will cause T wave inversion. The T wave inversion of ischemic disease is symmetrical. When a vertical line is drawn through the nadir of the T wave, one will end up with two equal halves of the T wave area. This is unlike the LVH strain pattern discussed in detail in Section V. Ischemic T inversions are often associated with QT prolongation as well. Marked QT prolongation with deeply inverted T waves may represent ischemia or infarct, but can also be associated with some CNS catastrophe such as a sub-arachnoid hemorrhage (*see* Fig. 12.77).

Sometimes, deep perhaps more symmetrical T inversions are also noted in hypertrophic cardiomyopathy with or without associated ST changes. Deep T wave inversions have been found to be associated with the apical type hypertrophic cardiomyopathy in patients seen in Japan.[139]

ECG Changes of Hypokalemia

Hypokalemia will cause several changes on the ECG. This is most commonly seen as a result of diuretics that tend to cause renal loss of potassium. The

ST segment may be sagging and the T waves will be low with prominence of the U wave. It is rare however to see T wave inversion due to hypokalemia. The QT interval is usually unaffected. In some rare instances tall P waves have also been noted as a result of hypokalemia. Hypokalemia makes the myocardium more prone to serious ventricular arrhythmias, especially when associated with other pathology.

ECG Changes of Hyperkalemia

These are best described as early and late changes. Hyperkalemia is noted mostly in patients with poor renal function. Rarely, it may be associated with inadvertent excess intravenous potassium infusion. With use of several classes of drugs (β-blockers, ACE inhibitors, Angiotensin receptor blockers, aldosterone antagonists and other potassium sparing diuretics) that may increase or interfere with the elimination of K^+, milder forms of hyperkalemia and sometimes even severe forms of hyperkalemia are noted in patients with minimal renal impairment, especially when coupled with excess potassium intake either in diet or as a supplement. Hyperkalemia may also be seen in severe acute trauma or hemolysis, where associated with cell death, large amounts of intracellular K^+ are suddenly released into the circulation.

When the hyperkalemia is relatively mild, it will shorten the QT interval and cause a peaked and tall T wave. The T wave will tend to be symmetrical. U waves are never seen with hyperkalemia. When the K^+ level increases further, it will produce abnormalities in conduction. The PR interval will usually lengthen causing first degree AV block. The sinus node will be affected causing some bradycardia. Eventually the atrial myocardium becomes refractory and the patient will go into atrial standstill. The sinus node will keep generating impulses that are transmitted to the AV node through the three internodal tracts. Although the patient may actually still be in sinus rhythm, one would not know this because there would be no P waves visible (Fig. 12.90A). It will appear as though the patient is in a junctional or idioventricular rhythm. Eventually blocks in the intra-ventricular conduction will also develop leading to changes in axis, widening of the QRS of a non-specific type. Finally, with very high levels of K^+, the QRS will be markedly widened with some decreased voltage and tall peaked T waves (Fig. 12.90B) that will give the appearance of a "***sine wave***". This usually is a preterminal ECG finding and when seen requires immediate treatment if the patient is to survive. Sodium bicarbonate and calcium chloride infusions may be life-saving measures before excess K^+ can be removed through dialysis.

ECG Changes of Hypo and Hypercalcemia

The ECG changes of hypocalcemia are relatively simple. Changes in the Ca^{2+} levels affects phase 2 of the action potential, and has no effect on phase 3.

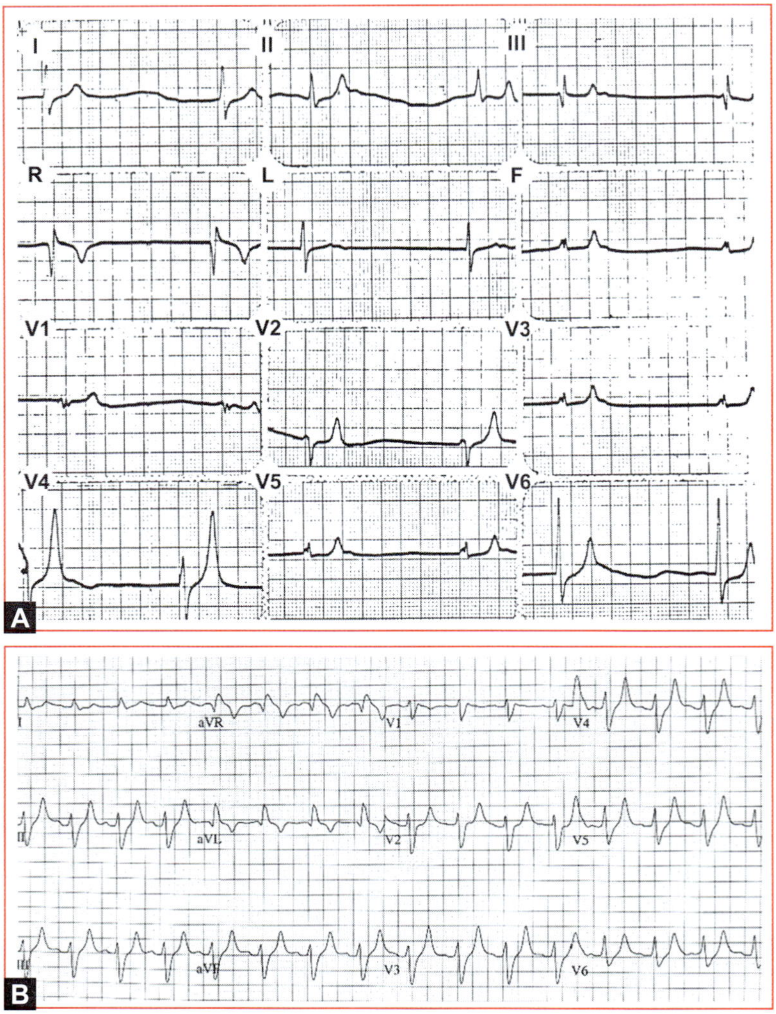

Figs. 12.90A and B: Electrocardiograms from patients with hyperkalemia. The ECG in (A) shows bradycardia with relatively narrow QRS complexes with no P waves and peaked T waves. The atrial standstill with the absence of P waves is one of the characteristic features of hyperkalemia. The rhythm may still be in fact sinus in origin. Part (B) shows widened QRS complexes with peaked T waves typical of hyperkalemia as well.

Low Ca^{2+} levels therefore will not change the T wave but it will prolong the ST segment. This tends to result in an upright T isolated far from the QRS with a long ST segment before it and a long TP segment after it. This appearance is sometimes referred to as the ***"tent in the desert"***[285] (*see* Figs. 12.75A and B).

Hypercalcemia, on the other hand, also affecting phase 2 of the action potential will shorten the QT interval.[285] Because in renal failure it may commonly be associated with hyperkalemia it may also exhibit tall T wave.

This T wave change however is not caused by the Ca^{2+} abnormality. Hypercalcemia in some cases may be associated with a prominent ***J*** wave, at times almost as prominent as in hypothermia.[286]

Hypomagnesemia cannot be recognized by any ECG changes. On the other hand, hypermagnesemia that does not affect the ST segment level may cause some shortening of the QT interval and lengthening of P wave, PR interval and QRS duration.

APPENDIX

Sinoatrial conduction time can be measured if an ECG rhythm strip happens to show an atrial premature beat ***(P′)*** with an underlying sinus rhythm. Since the premature beat ***(P′)*** originates outside the sinus node in the atrium, the wave of depolarization will travel not only down through the AV node and produce the QRS complex, it will also travel into the sinus node and in doing so will reset it. The next sinus impulse will then emerge out of the sinus node and produce the next P wave. The measured interval between the two basic sinus P waves before the atrial premature beat is termed as the P-P interval. This interval will be related to the rate of sinus node discharge. If one were to measure the interval from the ***P′ (premature P wave)*** to the next sinus P wave, this interval is termed ***P′-P*** interval. This will include the basic sinus cycle length as well as the time it takes for the premature atrial depolarization to enter the sinus node and also for the next sinus impulse to come out to produce the normal P wave. If we assume that from the resetting of the sinus node it takes more or less the same time to fire again as the original sinus rate, then by subtracting "***P-P interval***" from "***P′-P interval***", we actually measure the time it took for the impulse to go in and to come out of the sinus node. Any time >240 ms (six small squares on ECG paper at 25 mm/s paper speed) is considered abnormal. If we assume, that time to go in is similar to time to come out, then SA conduction should not be in excess of 120 ms.

REFERENCES

1. Waller A. Demonstration on man of electromotive changes accompanying the heart's beat. J Physiol. 1887;8:229-34.
2. Einthoven W. De galvanometrische registrirung des menschlichen elektrokardiogramms. Zugleich eine Beurteilung der Anwendung des Capillar-Elektrometers in der Physiologie. Pflugers Arch. 1903;99.
3. Lewis T. The Mechanism and Graphic Registration of the Heart Beat (Preface). London: Shaw and Sons; 1920.
4. Wiggers CJ. Principles and Practice of Electrocardiography. St. Louis: CV Mosby; 1929.
5. Wilson FN, MacLeod AG, Barker PS, Johnston FD. The determination and the significance of the areas of the ventricular deflections of the electrocardiogram. Am Heart J. 1934;10:46-61.

6. Wilson F (Ed). Foreword. In: Barker JM. The Unipolar Electrogram: A Clinical Interpretation. New York: Appleton-Century-Crofts, Inc; 1952.
7. Goldberger E. Unipolar Lead Electrocardiography and Vectorcardiography, 3rd edition. Philadelphia, PA: Lea & Febiger; 1953.
8. Johnston FD (Ed). Selected Papers of Dr. Frank N. Wilson. Ann Arbor, MI: Edwards Brothers, Inc. ; 1954.
9. Sodi-Pallares D, Calder RM. New Bases of Electrocardiography. St. Louis: The CV Mosby Co.; 1956.
10. Grant RP. Clinical Electrocardiography: The Spatial Vector Approach. The Blakiston Division, Inc, New York, Toronto, London: McGraw-Hill Book Company; 1957.
11. Burch GE, Depasquale NP. A History of Electrocardiography. Chicago: Year Book Medical Publishers; 1964.
12. Wellens HJ. Bishop lecture. The electrocardiogram 80 years after Einthoven. J Am Coll Cardiol. Historical Article Review. 1986;7(3):484-91.
13. Massie E, Walsh TJ. Clinical Vectorcardiography and Electrocardiography. Chicago, IL: Year Book Publishers Inc; 1960.
14. Sodi Pallares D, Bisteni A, Medrano G, et al. Electrocardiography and Vectorcardiography. New York, NY: Grune and Stratton; 1960.
15. Rosenbaum MB, Elizari M, Lazzari JO (Eds). The Hemiblocks. New Concepts of Intraventricular Conduction Based on Human Anatomical, Physiological and Clinical Studies. Oldsmar, FL; 1970.
16. Sodi-Pallares D, Medrano GA, Bisteni A, et al. Deductive and Polyparametric Electrocardiography. Mexico: Instituto National Cardiologia Mexico; 1970.
17. Lipman BS, Massie E, Kleiger RE. Clinical Scalar Electrocardiography, 6th edition. Chicago, IL: Year Book Medical Publishers, Inc; 1972.
18. Chou T. Electrocardiography in Clinical Practice. New York, NY: Grune and Stratton; 1979.
19. Marriott H. Practical Electrocardiography, 7th edition. Baltimore, MD: The Williams and Wilkins Company; 1983.
20. Schamroth L. The Electrocardiology of Coronary Artery Disease, 2nd edition. Oxford: Blackwell Scientific Publications Ltd; 1984.
21. Constant J. Learning Electrocardiography. A Complete Course, 3rd edition. Boston, Toronto, London: Little Brown and Company; 1987.
22. James TN. Anatomy of the conducting system of the heart. Heart Bull. 1963; 12:21-5.
23. James TN. The connecting pathways between the sinus node and A-V node and between the right and the left atrium in the human heart. Am Heart J. 1963;66:498-508.
24. James TN. Anatomy of the Coronary Arteries. New York: Hoeber Medical Division, Harper & Row; 1961.
25. Gensini GF. Coronary Arteriography. New York: Futura Publications; 1975.
26. Grant AO. Cardiac ion channels. Circ Arrhythm Electrophysiol. [Review]. 2009;2(2):185-94.
27. Geselowitz DB. Dipole theory in electrocardiography. Am J Cardiol. 1964;14: 301-6.
28. Bryant JM, Johnston FD, Wilson FN. Unipolar electrocardiographic leads; effects produced by eliminating the resistors between the limb electrodes and the central terminal. Am Heart J. 1949;37(3):321-32.

29. Kossman CE, Brody DA, Burch GE, et al. Recommendations for standardization of leads and of specifications for instruments in electrocardiography and vectorcardiography. Circulation. 1967;35:583-601.
30. Scher AM. Newer data on myocardial excitation. In: Taccardi B, Marchetti G (Eds). Electrophysiology of the Heart. New York: Pergamon Press; 1965.
31. Durrer D, van Dam RT, Freud GE, et al. Total excitation of the isolated human heart. Circulation. 1970;41(6):899-912.
32. Abildskov JA. The sequence of normal recovery of excitability in the dog heart. Circulation. [Research Support, U.S. Gov't, P.H.S.]. 1975;52(3):442-6.
33. Nerbonne JM, Kass RS. Molecular physiology of cardiac repolarization. Physiol Rev. [Research Support, N.I.H., Extramural Research Support, U.S. Gov't, P.H.S. Review]. 2005 Oct;85(4):1205-53.
34. Ashman R, Byer E. The normal ventricular gradient. Am Heart J. 1943;25:16.
35. Pantridge JF. Observations on the electrocardiogram and ventricular gradient in complete left bundle branch block. Circulation. 1951;3(4):589-99.
36. Bednar MM, Harrigan EP, Anziano RJ, et al. The QT interval. Prog Cardiovasc Dis. [Review]. 2001;43(5 Suppl 1):1-45.
37. Bazett HC. An analysis of the time relations of the electrocardiograms. Heart. 1920;7:353-70.
38. Myerburg RJ, Lazzara R. Electrophysiologic basis of cardiac arrhythmias and conduction disturbances. Cardiovasc Clin. [Review]. 1973;5(3):1-19.
39. Franz MR, Zabel M. Electrophysiological basis of QT dispersion measurements. Prog Cardiovasc Dis. [Comparative Study Research Support, Non-U.S. Gov't Research Support, U.S. Gov't, Non-P.H.S. Review]. 2000;42(5):311-24.
40. Willems JL, Robles de Medina EO, Bernard R, et al. Criteria for intraventricular conduction disturbances and preexcitation. World Health Organizational/ International Society and Federation for Cardiology Task Force Ad Hoc. J Am Coll Cardiol. [Research Support, Non-U.S. Gov't Review]. 1985;5(6):1261-75.
41. Shmock CL, Pomerantz B, Mitchell RS, et al. The electrocardiogram in emphysema with and without chronic airways obstruction. Chest. 1971;60(4):328-34.
42. Selvester RH, Rubin HB. New criteria for the electrocardiographic diagnosis of emphysema and cor pulmonale. Am Heart J. 1965;69:437-47.
43. Warner RA, Hill NE, Mookherjee S, et al. Electrocardiographic criteria for the diagnosis of combined inferior myocardial infarction and left anterior hemiblock. Am J Cardiol. 1983;51(5):718-22.
44. Durrer D, Roos JP, van Dam RT. The genesis of the electrocardiogram of patients with ostium primum defects (ventral atrial septal defects). Am Heart J. [Case Reports]. 1966;71(5):642-50.
45. Borkon AM, Pieroni DR, Varghese PJ, et al. The superior QRS axis in ostium primum ASD: a proposed mechanism. Am Heart J. 1975;90(2):215-21.
46. Feldt RH, DuShane JW, Titus JL. The atrioventricular conduction system in persistent common atrioventricular canal defect: correlations with electrocardiogram. Circulation. 1970;42(3):437-44.
47. Burch GE, Depasquale NP. Electrocardiography in the Diagnosis of Congenital Heart Disease. Philadelphia, PA: Lea & Febiger; 1967.
48. Elizari MV, Acunzo RS, Ferreiro M. Hemiblocks revisited. Circulation. [Research Support, Non-U.S. Gov't Review]. 2007;115(9):1154-63.
49. Lev M, Unger PN, Lesser ME, et al. Pathology of the conduction system in acquired heart disease. Complete right bundle branch block. Am Heart J. 1961; 61:593-614.

50. Lenegre J. Contribution a l'Etude des Blocs de Branche. Paris: JB Bailliere; 1958.
51. Horowitz LN, Alexander JA, Edmunds LH, Jr. Post-operative right bundle branch block: identification of three levels of block. Circulation. [Research Support, U.S. Gov't, P.H.S.]. 1980;62(2):319-28.
52. Moreno AM, Alberola AG, Tomas JG, et al. Incidence and prognostic significance of right bundle branch block in patients with acute myocardial infarction receiving thrombolytic therapy. Int J Cardiol. 1997;61(2):135-41.
53. Surawicz B, Knilans T. Chou's Electrocardiography in Clinical Practice, 6th edition. Philadelphia, PA: Elsevier Saunders; 2008.
54. Angelini P, Springer A, Sulbaran T, et al. Right ventricular myopathy with an unusual intraventricular conduction defect (epsilon potential). Am Heart J. [Case Reports]. 1981;101(5):680-3.
55. Lev M, Unger PN, Rosen KM, et al. The anatomic sub-strate of complete left bundle branch block. Circulation. 1974;50(3):479-86.
56. Hindman MC, Wagner GS, JaRo M, et al. The clinical significance of bundle branch block complicating acute myocardial infarction. 1. Clinical characteristics, hospital mortality, and one-year follow-up. Circulation. [Research Support, U.S. Gov't, P.H.S.]. 1978;58(4):679-88.
57. Dhingra RC, Amat YLF, Wyndham C, et al. Significance of left axis deviation in patients with chronic left bundle branch block. Am J Cardiol. [Research Support, U.S. Gov't, Non-P.H.S. Research Support, U.S. Gov't, P.H.S.]. 1978;42(4):551-6.
58. Ramlall H, Sivaciyan V, Ranganathan N. Significance of R wave in V1 in patients with Left Bundle Branch Block—Two Dimensional Echocardiographic and Thallium Scintigraphic Study. Proceedings of the Annual Great Lakes Regional Non-invasive Cardiology Society Meeting -Toronto, Canada; 1993.
59. Ranganathan N, Dhurandhar R, Phillips JH, et al. His bundle electrogram in bundle-branch block. Circulation. 1972;45(2):282-94.
60. Silver HM, Calatayud JB. Evaluation of QRS criteria in patients with chronic obstructive pulmonary disease. Chest. 1971;59(2):153-9.
61. Reeves WC, Hallahan W, Schwiter EJ, et al. Two-dimensional echocardiographic assessment of electrocardiographic criteria for right atrial enlargement. Circulation. 1981;64(2):387-91.
62. Munoz-Armas S, Del Toro A, Sodi-Pallares D, et al. Tetralogy of Fallot and pulmonary stenosis with intact interventricular septum. Anatomic and electrocardiographic study. Am J Cardiol. 1968;21(6):773-84.
63. Anselmi G, Munoz-Armas S, Salazar A, et al. Electrocardiographic patterns of right atrial overloading in some congenital heart conditions. Am J Cardiol. 1968;21(5):628-38.
64. Morris JJ, Jr, Estes EH, Jr, Whalen RE, et al. P-wave analysis in valvular heart disease. Circulation. 1964;29:242-52.
65. Waldo AL, Bush HL, Jr, Gelband H, et al. Effects on the canine P wave of discrete lesions in the specialized atrial tracts. Circ Res. 1971;29(5):452-67.
66. Peter RH, Morris JJ, Jr, McIntosh HD. Relationship of fibrillatory waves and P waves in the electrocardiogram. Circulation. 1966;33(4):599-606.
67. Bekheit S, Murtagh G, Morton P, et al. His bundle electrogram in P mitrale. Br Heart J. 1972;34(10):1057-61.
68. Josephson ME, Kastor JA, Morganroth J. Electrocardiographic left atrial enlargement. Electrophysiologic, echocardiographic and hemodynamic correlates. Am J Cardiol. 1977;39(7):967-71.
69. Chandraratna PA, Hodges M. Electrocardiographic evidence of left atrial hypertension in acute myocardial infarction. Circulation. 1973;47(3):493-8.

70. Di Bianco R, Gottdiener JS, Fletcher RD, et al. Left atrial overload: a hemodynamic, echocardiographic, electrocardiographic and vectorcardiographic study. Am Heart J. [Research Support, U.S. Gov't, P.H.S.]. 1979;98(4):478-89.
71. Keikkila J, Luomanmaki, K. Value of serial P wave changes in indicating left heart failure in myocardial infarction. Br Heart J. 1970;32(4):510.
72. Lewis T. Observations upon ventricular hypertrophy with special reference to preponderance of one or the other chamber. Heart. 1914;5:367-402.
73. Gubner RS, Ungerleider HE. Electrocardiographic criteria of left ventricular hypertrophy: factors determining the evolution of the electrocardiographic patterns in hypertrophy and bundle branch block. Arch Intern Med. 1943;72: 196-209.
74. Sokolow M, Lyon TP. The ventricular complex in left ventricular hypertrophy as obtained by unipolar precordial and limb leads. Am Heart J. 1949;37(2):161-86.
75. Casale PN, Devereux RB, Kligfield P, et al. Electrocardiographic detection of left ventricular hypertrophy: development and prospective validation of improved criteria. J Am Coll Cardiol. [Comparative Study Research Support, Non-U.S. Gov't Research Support, U.S. Gov't, P.H.S.]. 1985;6(3):572-80.
76. Romhilt DW, Estes EH, Jr. A point-score system for the ECG diagnosis of left ventricular hypertrophy. Am Heart J. 1968;75(6):752-8.
77. Hancock EW, Deal BJ, Mirvis DM, et al. AHA/ACCF/HRS recommendations for the standardization and interpretation of the electrocardiogram: part V: electrocardiogram changes associated with cardiac chamber hypertrophy: a scientific statement from the American Heart Association Electrocardiography and Arrhythmias Committee, Council on Clinical Cardiology; the American College of Cardiology Foundation; and the Heart Rhythm Society. Endorsed by the International Society for Computerized Electrocardiology. J Am Coll Cardiol. [Practice Guideline Review]. 2009;53(11):992-1002.
78. Murphy ML, Thenabadu PN, de Soyza N, et al. Sensitivity of electrocardiographic criteria for left ventricular hypertrophy according to type of cardiac disease. Am J Cardiol. 1985;55(5):545-9.
79. LaMonte CS, Freiman AH. The electrocardiogram after mastectomy. Circulation. 1965;32(5):746-54.
80. Garbagni R, Angelino PF, Brusca A, et al. Residual lung volume in mitral disease. Br Heart J. 1958;20(4):479-82.
81. Amad KH, Brennan JC, Alexander JK. The cardiac pathology of chronic exogenous obesity. Circulation. 1965;32(5):740-5.
82. Postell WN, Rainey RL, Witham AC, et al. Vectorcardiographic and electrocardiographic manifestations of increasing left ventricular pressure overload. Am Heart J. 1969;77(1):33-44.
83. Grayzel J, Neyshaboori M. Left-axis deviation: etiologic factors in one-hundred patients. Am Heart J. 1975;89(4):419-27.
84. Ishikawa K, Berson AS, Pipberger HV. Electrocardiographic changes due to cardiac enlargement. Am Heart J. 1971;81(5):635-43.
85. Griep AH. Pitfalls in the electrocardiographic diagnosis of left ventricular hypertrophy; a correlative study of 200 autopsied patients. Circulation. 1959; 20(1):30-4.
86. Selzer A, Naruse DY, York E, et al. Electrocardiographic findings in concentric and eccentric left ventricular hypertrophy. Am Heart J. 1962;63:320-8.
87. Haskell RJ, Ginzton LE, Laks MM. Electrocardiographic diagnosis of left ventricular hypertrophy in the presence of left bundle branch block. J Electrocardiol. 1987;20(3):227-32.

88. Klein RC, Vera Z, DeMaria AN, et al. Electrocardiographic diagnosis of left ventricular hypertrophy in the presence of left bundle branch block. Am Heart J. 1984;108(3 Pt 1):502-6.
89. Vandenberg B, Sagar K, Paulsen W, et al. Electrocardiographic criteria for diagnosis of left ventricular hypertrophy in the presence of complete right bundle branch block. Am J Cardiol. 1989;63(15):1080-4.
90. Adelman AG, Wigle ED, Ranganathan N, et al. The clinical course in muscular sub-aortic stenosis. A retrospective and prospective study of 60 hemodynamically proved cases. Ann Intern Med. 1972;77(4):515-25.
91. Chen CH, Nobuyoshi M, Kawai C. ECG pattern of left ventricular hypertrophy in non-obstructive hypertrophic cardiomyopathy: the significance of the mid-precordial changes. Am Heart J. [Case Reports]. 1979;97(6):687-95.
92. Cabrera E, Monroy JR. Systolic and diastolic loading of the heart. I. Physiologic and clinical data. Am Heart J. 1952;43(5):661-8.
93. Cabrera E, Monroy JR. Systolic and diastolic loading of the heart. II. Electrocardiographic data. Am Heart J. 1952;43(5):669-86.
94. Wallace AG, Spach MS, Estes EH, et al. Activation of the normal and hypertrophied human right ventricle. Am Heart J. 1968;75(6):728-35.
95. Butler PM, Leggett SI, Howe CM, et al. Identification of electrocardiographic criteria for diagnosis of right ventricular hypertrophy due to mitral stenosis. Am J Cardiol. [Research Support, U.S. Gov't, P.H.S.]. 1986;57(8):639-43.
96. Murphy ML, Hutcheson F. The electrocardiographic diagnosis of right ventricular hypertrophy in chronic obstructive pulmonary disease. Chest. [Comparative Study]. 1974;65(6):622-7.
97. Murphy ML, Thenabadu PN, de Soyza N, et al. Reevaluation of electrocardiographic criteria for left, right and combined cardiac ventricular hypertrophy. Am J Cardiol. 1984;53(8):1140-7.
98. Myers GB, Klein HA, Stofer BE. The electrocardiographic diagnosis of right ventricular hypertrophy. Am Heart J. 1948;35(1):1-40.
99. Scott RC. The electrocardiographic diagnosis of right ventricular hypertrophy: correlation with the anatomic findings. Am Heart J. 1960;60:659-61.
100. Sokolow M, Lyon TP. The ventricular complex in right ventricular hypertrophy as obtained by unipolar precordial and limb leads. Am Heart J. 1949;38(2):273-94.
101. Milnor WR. Electrocardiogram and vectorcardiogram in right ventricular hypertrophy and right bundle-branch block. Circulation. 1957;16(3):348-67.
102. Blount SG, Jr, Munyan EA, Jr, Hoffman MS. Hypertrophy of the right ventricular outflow tract: a concept of the electrocardiographic findings in atrial septal defect. Am J Med. 1957;22(5):784-90.
103. Bassingthwaighte JB, Parkin TW, Dushane JW, et al. The Electrocardiographic and hemodynamic findings in pulmonary stenosis with intact ventricular septum. Circulation. 1963;28:893-905.
104. Fowler NO, Noble WJ, Giarratano SJ, Mannix EP. The clinical estimation of pulmonary hypertension accompanying mitral stenosis. Am Heart J. 1955;49(2):237-49.
105. Kamper D, Chou TC, Fowler NO, et al. The reliability of electrocardiographic criteria of chronic obstructive lung disease. Am Heart J. 1970;80(4):445-52.
106. McGinn S, White PD. Acute cor pulmonale resulting from pulmonary embolism. JAMA. 1935;104:1473.
107. Scott RC. The S1Q3 (McGinn-White) pattern in acute cor pulmonale: a form of transient left posterior hemiblock? Am Heart J. 1971;82(1):135-7.

108. Spodick DH. Electrocardiographic responses to pulmonary embolism. Mechanisms and sources of variability. Am J Cardiol. 1972;30(6):695-9.
109. Nunez BD, Messerli FH, Amodeo C, et al. Biventricular cardiac hypertrophy in essential hypertension. Am Heart J. [Comparative Study]. 1987;114(4 Pt 1): 813-8.
110. Jain A, Chandna H, Silber EN, Clark WA, Denes P. Electrocardiographic patterns of patients with echocardiographically determined biventricular hypertrophy. J Electrocardiol. 1999;32(3):269-73.
111. Katz LN, Wachtel H. The diphasic QRS type of electrocardiogram in congenital heart disease. Am Heart J. 1937;13:202.
112. Jennings RB, Ganote CE. Structural changes in myocardium during acute ischemia. Circ Res. [Review]. 1974;35(Suppl 3):156-72.
113. Thygesen K, Alpert JS, White HD, et al. Universal definition of myocardial infarction. Circulation. [Consensus Development Conference Practice Guideline Research Support, Non-U.S. Gov't]. 2007;116(22):2634-53.
114. Olson RD, Mushlin PS. Doxorubicin cardiotoxicity: analysis of prevailing hypotheses. FASEB J. [Review]. 1990;4(13):3076-86.
115. Thygesen K, Alpert JS, Jaffe AS, et al. Third universal definition of myocardial infarction. J Am Coll Cardiol. [Consensus Development Conference Practice Guideline]. 2012;60(16):1581-98.
116. Barbagelata A, Califf RM, Sgarbossa EB, et al. Thrombolysis and Q wave versus non-Q wave first acute myocardial infarction: a GUSTO-I sub-study. Global utilization of streptokinase and tissue plasminogen activator for occluded arteries investigators. J Am Coll Cardiol. [Comparative Study Research Support, Non-U.S. Gov't]. 1997;29(4):770-7.
117. Bayley RH, LaDue JS. Electrocardiographic changes of impending infarction and the ischemic injury pattern produced in the dog. Am Heart J. 1944;28:54.
118. Hill JD, Malinow MR, McNulty WP, Ochsner AJ, 3rd. Experimental myocardial infarction in unanesthetized monkeys. Am Heart J. 1972;84(1):82-94.
119. Selwyn AP, Fox K, Welman E, et al. Loss of electrically active myocardium during inferior infarction in man. Br Heart J. 1978;40(9):1019-24.
120. Cox CJ. Return to normal of the electrocardiogram after myocardial infarction. Lancet. 1967;1(7501):1194-7.
121. Myocardial infarction redefined—a consensus document of The Joint European Society of Cardiology/American College of Cardiology Committee for the redefinition of myocardial infarction. Eur Heart J. [Consensus Development Conference Review]. 2000;21(18):1502-13.
122. Surawicz B, Saito S. Exercise testing for detection of myocardial ischemia in patients with abnormal electrocardiograms at rest. Am J Cardiol. 1978;41(5): 943-51.
123. Cohen D, Kaufman LA. Magnetic determination of the relationship between the S-T segment shift and the injury current produced by coronary artery occlusion. Circ Res. [Research Support, U.S. Gov't, Non-P.H.S. Research Support, U.S. Gov't, P.H.S.]. 1975;36(3):414-24.
124. Wellens HJJ, Gorgels APM, Doevendans PA. The ECG in Acute Myocardial Infarction and Unstable Angina: Diagnosis and Risk Stratification. Boston, MA: Kluwer Academic Publishers; 2004.
125. Birnbaum Y, Sclarovsky S, Solodky A, Tschori J, Herz I, Sulkes J, et al. Prediction of the level of left anterior descending coronary artery obstruction during anterior wall acute myocardial infarction by the admission electrocardiogram. Am J Cardiol. 1993;72(11):823-6.

126. Engelen DJ, Gorgels AP, Cheriex EC, et al. Value of the electrocardiogram in localizing the occlusion site in the left anterior descending coronary artery in acute anterior myocardial infarction. J Am Coll Cardiol. 1999;34(2):389-95.
127. Zimetbaum PJ, Krishnan S, Gold A, et al. Usefulness of ST segment elevation in lead III exceeding that of lead II for identifying the location of the totally occluded coronary artery in inferior wall myocardial infarction. Am J Cardiol. 1998;81(7):918-9.
128. Perloff JK. The recognition of strictly posterior myocardial infarction by conventional scalar electrocardiography. Circulation. 1964;30:706-18.
129. Horan LG, Flowers NC, Johnson JC. Significance of the diagnostic Q wave of myocardial infarction. Circulation. 1971;43(3):428-36.
130. Cerqueira MD, Weissman NJ, Dilsizian V, et al. Standardized myocardial segmentation and nomenclature for tomographic imaging of the heart. A statement for healthcare professionals from the Cardiac Imaging Committee of the Council on Clinical Cardiology of the American Heart Association. Circulation. [Consensus Development Conference Review]. 2002;105(4):539-42.
131. Bairey CN, Shah PK, Lew AS, et al. Electrocardiographic differentiation of occlusion of the left circumflex versus the right coronary artery as a cause of inferior acute myocardial infarction. Am J Cardiol. 1987;60(7):456-9.
132. Gorgels AP, Vos MA, Mulleneers R, et al. Value of the electrocardiogram in diagnosing the number of severely narrowed coronary arteries in rest angina pectoris. The American journal of cardiology. 1993;72(14):999-1003.
133. Wang K, Asinger RW, Marriott HJ. ST segment elevation in conditions other than acute myocardial infarction. N Engl J Med. [Review]. 2003;349(22):2128-35.
134. Fernandez AR, Sequeira RF, Chakko S, et al. ST segment tracking for rapid determination of patency of the infarct-related artery in acute myocardial infarction. J Am Coll Cardiol. [Clinical Trial Comparative Study]. 1995;26(3):675-83.
135. Andrews J, Straznicky IT, French JK, et al. ST segment recovery adds to the assessment of TIMI 2 and 3 flow in predicting infarct wall motion after thrombolytic therapy. Circulation. [Clinical Trial Randomized Controlled Trial]. 2000;101(18):2138-43.
136. Shah A, Wagner GS, Granger CB, et al. Prognostic implications of TIMI flow grade in the infarct related artery compared with continuous 12-lead ST segment resolution analysis. Reexamining the "gold standard" for myocardial reperfusion assessment. J Am Coll Cardiol. [Clinical Trial Clinical Trial, Phase I Comparative Study Randomized Controlled Trial]. 2000;35(3):666-72.
137. Arvan S, Varat MA. Persistent ST segment elevation and left ventricular wall abnormalities: a 2-dimensional echocardiographic study. Am J Cardiol. 1984;53(11):1542-6.
138. Sgarbossa EB, Pinski SL, Barbagelata A, et al. Electrocardiographic diagnosis of evolving acute myocardial infarction in the presence of left bundle-branch block. GUSTO-1 (Global Utilization of Streptokinase and Tissue Plasminogen Activator for Occluded Coronary Arteries) Investigators. N Engl J Med. [Multicenter Study Research Support, Non-U.S. Gov't]. 1996;334(8):481-7.
139. Keren G, Belhassen B, Sherez J, et al. Apical hypertrophic cardiomyopathy: evaluation by non-invasive and invasive techniques in 23 patients. Circulation. 1985;71(1):45-56.
140. Bybee KA, Kara T, Prasad A, et al. Systematic review: transient left ventricular apical ballooning: a syndrome that mimics ST segment elevation myocardial infarction. Ann Intern Med. [Review]. 2004;141(11):858-65.

141. Simon K, Hackett D, Szelier A, et al. The natural history of post-ischemic T-wave inversion: a predictor of poor short-term prognosis? Coron Artery Dis. [Clinical Trial Comparative Study]. 1994;5(11):937-42.
142. Tamura A, Nagase K, Mikuriya Y, et al. Significance of spontaneous normalization of negative T waves in infarct-related leads during healing of anterior wall acute myocardial infarction. Am J Cardiol. [Comparative Study]. 1999;84 (11):1341-4, A7.
143. Starr JW, Wagner GS, Draffin RM, et al. Vectorcardiographic criteria for the diagnosis of anterior myocardial infarction. Circulation. [Research Support, U.S. Gov't, P.H.S.]. 1976;53(2):229-34.
144. Selvester RH, Wagner GS, Ideker RE. Myocardial infarction. In: MacFarlane PW, Lawrie TD (Eds). Comprehensive Electrocardiography. New York: Pergamon; 1989.
145. Casas RE, Marriott HJ, Glancy DL. Value of leads V7-V9 in diagnosing posterior wall acute myocardial infarction and other causes of tall R waves in V1-V2. Am J Cardiol. 1997;80(4):508-9.
146. Nestico PF, Hakki AH, Iskandrian AS, et al. Electrocardiographic diagnosis of posterior myocardial infarction revisited: a new approach using a multivariate discriminant analysis and thallium-201 myocardial scintigraphy. J Electrocardiol. 1986;19(1):33-40.
147. Bayes de Luna A, Cino JM, Pujadas S, et al. Concordance of electrocardiographic patterns and healed myocardial infarction location detected by cardiovascular magnetic resonance. Am J Cardiol. 2006;97(4):443-51.
148. Hurd HP, 2nd, Starling MR, Crawford MH, et al. Comparative accuracy of electrocardiographic and vectorcardiographic criteria for inferior myocardial infarction. Circulation. [Comparative Study]. 1981;63(5):1025-9.
149. Andersen HR, Falk E, Nielsen D. Right ventricular infarction: frequency, size and topography in coronary heart disease: a prospective study comprising 107 consecutive autopsies from a coronary care unit. J Am Coll Cardiol. [Research Support, Non-U.S. Gov't]. 1987;10(6):1223-32.
150. Candell-Riera J, Figueras J, Valle V, et al. Right ventricular infarction: relationships between ST segment elevation in V4R and hemodynamic, scintigraphic, and echocardiographic findings in patients with acute inferior myocardial infarction. Am Heart J. 1981;101(3):281-7.
151. Myers GB, Klein HA, Hiratzka T. Correlation of electrocardiographic and pathologic findings in post-erolateral infarction. Am Heart J. 1949;38(6):837-62, illust.
152. Myers GB, Klein HA, Hiratzka T. Correlation of electrocardiographic and pathologic findings in posterior infarction. Am Heart J. 1949;38(4):547-92.
153. Myers GB, Klein HA, Hiratzka T. Correlation of electrocardiographic and pathologic findings in infarction of the interventricular septum and right ventricle. Am Heart J. 1949;37(5):720-70.
154. Myers GB, Klein HA, Stofer BE. Correlation of electrocardiographic and pathologic findings in lateral infarction. Am Heart J. 1949;37(3):374-417.
155. Myers GB, Klein HA, Hiratzka T. Correlation of electrocardiographic and pathologic findings in anteroposterior infarction. Am Heart J. 1949;37(2):205-36.
156. Moon JC, De Arenaza DP, Elkington AG, et al. The pathologic basis of Q-wave and non-Q-wave myocardial infarction: a cardiovascular magnetic resonance study. J Am Coll Cardiol. [Research Support, Non-U.S. Gov't]. 2004;44(3):554-60.
157. Kim RJ, Fieno DS, Parrish TB, et al. Relationship of MRI delayed contrast enhancement to irreversible injury, infarct age, and contractile function. Circulation. [Research Support, Non-U.S. Gov't Research Support, U.S. Gov't, P.H.S.]. 1999; 100(19):1992-2002.

158. Scott PA, Morgan JM, Carroll N, et al. The extent of left ventricular scar quantified by late gadolinium enhancement MRI is associated with spontaneous ventricular arrhythmias in patients with coronary artery disease and implantable cardioverter-defibrillators. Circ Arrhythm Electrophysiol. [Comparative Study Research Support, Non-U.S. Gov't]. 2011;4(3):324-30.
159. Raman SV, Simonetti OP, Winner MW, et al. Cardiac magnetic resonance with edema imaging identifies myocardium at risk and predicts worse outcome in patients with non-ST segment elevation acute coronary syndrome. J Am Coll Cardiol. [Comparative Study Research Support, Non-U.S. Gov't]. 2010;55(22):2480-8.
160. Delewi R, Ijff G, van de Hoef TP, et al. Pathological Q waves in myocardial infarction in patients treated by primary PCI. JACC Cardiovasc Imaging. [Comment Multicenter Study]. 2013;6(3):324-31.
161. First SR, Bayley RH, Bedford DR. Peri-infarction block; electrocardiographic abnormality occasionally resembling bundle branch block and local ventricular block of other types. Circulation. 1950;2(1):31-6.
162. Vassallo JA, Cassidy DM, Marchlinski FE, et al. Abnormalities of endocardial activation pattern in patients with previous healed myocardial infarction and ventricular tachycardia. The Am J Cardiol. [Research Support, Non-U.S. Gov't Research Support, U.S. Gov't, P.H.S.]. 1986;58(6):479-84.
163. Goldberger AL, Bhargava V, Froelicher V, et al. Effect of myocardial infarction on high-frequency QRS potentials. Circulation. [Research Support, Non-U.S. Gov't Research Support, U.S. Gov't, Non-P.H.S. Research Support, U.S. Gov't, P.H.S.]. 1981;64(1):34-42.
164. Mills RM, Jr, Young E, Gorlin R, et al. Natural history of S-T segment elevation after acute myocardial infarction. Am J Cardiol. [Research Support, U.S. Gov't, Non-P.H.S.]. 1975;35(5):609-14.
165. Dubnow MH, Burchell HB, Titus JL. Post-infarction ventricular aneurysm. A clinicomorphologic and electrocardiographic study of 80 cases. Am Heart J. 1965;70(6):753-60.
166. Oliva PB, Hammill SC, Edwards WD. Cardiac rupture, a clinically predictable complication of acute myocardial infarction: report of 70 cases with clinicopathologic correlations. J Am Coll Cardiol. [Comparative Study Research Support, Non-U.S. Gov't]. 1993;22(3):720-6.
167. Yoshino H, Yotsukura M, Yano K, et al. Cardiac rupture and admission electrocardiography in acute anterior myocardial infarction: implication of ST elevation in aVL. J Electrocardiol. 2000;33(1):49-54.
168. Pryor R. Fascicular blocks and the bilateral bundle branch block syndrome. Am Heart J. 1972;83(4):441-6.
169. Pryor R. Recognition of Myocardial infarction in the presence of bundle branch block. Cardiovasc Clin 1974; 6(1):255-71.
170. Scott RC. Left bundle branch block—a clinical assessment. I. Am Heart J. [Review]. 1965;70(4):535-66.
171. Scott RC. Left bundle branch block—a clinical assessment. II. Am Heart J. [Case Reports]. 1965;70(5):691-712.
172. Scott RC. Left bundle branch block—a clinical assessment. 3. Am Heart J. [Review]. 1965;70(6):813-29.
173. Barold SS, Falkoff MD, Ong LS, et al. Electrocardiographic diagnosis of myocardial infarction during ventricular pacing. Cardiol Clin. [Review]. 1987;5(3): 403-17.

174. Fesmire FM. ECG diagnosis of acute myocardial infarction in the presence of left bundle-branch block in patients undergoing continuous ECG monitoring. Ann Emerg Med. [Case Reports]. 1995;26(1):69-82.
175. Hands ME, Cook EF, Stone PH, et al. Electrocardiographic diagnosis of myocardial infarction in the presence of complete left bundle branch block. Am Heart J. [Comparative Study Research Support, Non-U.S. Gov't]. 1988;116 (1 Pt 1):23-31.
176. Beamer V AM, Scheuer J. Vectorcardiographic findings simulating myocardial infarction in aortic valve disease. J Electrocardiol. 1970;3(1):71-5.
177. Perloff JK, Roberts WC, de Leon AC, et al. The distinctive electrocardiogram of Duchenne's progressive muscular dystrophy. An electrocardiographic-pathologic correlative study. Am J Med. 1967;42(2):179-88.
178. Burch GE, Depasquale NP. The anomalous left coronary artery: an experiment of nature. Am J Med. 1964;37:159-61.
179. Bayes de Luna A, Wagner G, Birnbaum Y, et al. A new terminology for left ventricular walls and location of myocardial infarcts that present Q wave based on the standard of cardiac magnetic resonance imaging: a statement for healthcare professionals from a committee appointed by the International Society for Holter and Non-invasive Electrocardiography. Circulation. [Research Support, Non-U.S. Gov't Review]. 2006;114(16):1755-60.
180. Wagner GS, Macfarlane P, Wellens H, et al. AHA/ACCF/HRS recommendations for the standardization and interpretation of the electrocardiogram: part VI: acute ischemia/infarction: a scientific statement from the American Heart Association Electrocardiography and Arrhythmias Committee, Council on Clinical Cardiology; the American College of Cardiology Foundation; and the Heart Rhythm Society: endorsed by the International Society for Computerized Electrocardiology. Circulation. [Practice Guideline Review]. 2009;119(10): e262-70.
181. Wolff L, Parkinson J, White PD. Bundle branch block with short PR interval in healthy young people prone to paroxysmal tachycardia. Am Heart J. 1930;5:685.
182. Wolferth CC, Wood FC. The mechanism of production of short P-R intervals and prolonged QRS complexes in patients with presumably undamaged hearts: hypothesis of an accessory pathway of auriculoventricular conduction (bundle of Kent). Am Heart J. 1933;8:297.
183. Kent AFS. Observations on the auriculo-ventricular junction of the mammalian heart. Quart J Exp Physiol. 1913;7:193.
184. Prystowsky EN, Miles WM, Heger JJ, et al. Preexcitation syndromes: mechanisms and management. Med Clin North Am. 1984;68:831.
185. James TN. Morphology of the human atrioventricular node, with remarks pertinent to its electrophysiology. Am Heart J. 1961;62:756-71.
186. Castellanos A, Jr, Castillo CA, Agha AS, et al. His bundle electrograms in patients with short P-R intervals, narrow QRS complexes, and paroxysmal tachycardias. Circulation. 1971;43(5):667-78.
187. Castellanos A, Jr, Chapunoff E, Castillo C, et al. His bundle electrograms in two cases of Wolff-Parkinson-White (preexcitation) syndrome. Circulation. 1970;41(3):399-411.
188. Bogun F, Kalusche D, Li YG, et al. Septal Q waves in surface electrocardiographic lead V6 exclude minimal ventricular preexcitation. Am J Cardiol. 1999; 84(1):101-4, A9.

189. Gazes PC. False-positive exercise test in the presence of the Wolff-Parkinson-White syndrome. Am Heart J. 1969;78(1):13-5.
190. Schiebler GL, Adams P, Jr, Anderson RC. The Wolff-Parkinson-White syndrome in infants and children. A review and a report of 28 cases. Pediatrics. 1959;24: 585-603.
191. Giardina AC, Ehlers KH, Engle MA. Wolff-Parkinson-White syndrome in infants and children. A long-term follow-up study. Br Heart J. 1972;34(8):839-46.
192. Gallagher JJ, Pritchett EL, Sealy WC, et al. The preexcitation syndromes. Prog Cardiovasc Dis. [Research Support, U.S. Gov't, P.H.S. Review]. 1978;20(4): 285-327.
193. Kerr CR, Gallagher JJ, German LD. Changes in ventriculoatrial intervals with bundle branch block aberration during reciprocating tachycardia in patients with accessory atrioventricular pathways. Circulation. [Research Support, Non-U.S. Gov't Research Support, U.S. Gov't, P.H.S.]. 1982;66(1):196-201.
194. Gallagher JJ, Gilbert M, Svenson RH, et al. Wolff-Parkinson-White syndrome. The problem, evaluation, and surgical correction. Circulation. [Research Support, U.S. Gov't, P.H.S.]. 1975;51(5):767-85.
195. Rosenbaum F, Hecht HH, Wilson FN, et al. Potential variations of the thorax and the esophagus in anomalous atrioventricular excitation (Wolff-Parkinson-White syndrome). Am. Heart J. 1945;29:281-94.
196. Tonkin AM, Wagner GS, Gallagher JJ, et al. Initial forces of ventricular depolarization in the Wolff-Parkinson-White syndrome. Analysis based upon localization of the accessory pathway by epicardial mapping. Circulation. [Research Support, U.S. Gov't, P.H.S.]. 1975;52(6):1030-6.
197. Arruda MS, McClelland JH, Wang X, et al. Development and validation of an ECG algorithm for identifying accessory pathway ablation site in Wolff-Parkinson-White syndrome. J Cardiovasc Electrophysiol. [Clinical Trial]. 1998; 9(1):2-12.
198. Prystowsky EN, Yee R, Klein GJ. Wolff-Parkinson-White syndrome. In: Zipes, DP, Jalife J (Eds). Cardiac Electrophysiology from Cell to Bedside, 4th edition. Philadelphia, PA: Saunders; 2004. p. 869.
199. Hull E. The electrocardiogram in pericarditis. Am J Cardiol. 1961;7:21-32.
200. Surawicz B, Lasseter KC. Electrocardiogram in pericarditis. Am J Cardiol. 1970; 26(5):471-4.
201. Spodick DH. Electrocardiogram in acute pericarditis. Distributions of morphologic and axial changes by stages. Am J Cardiol. 1974;33(4):470-4.
202. Spodick DH. Diagnostic electrocardiographic sequences in acute pericarditis. Significance of PR segment and PR vector changes. Circulation. 1973;48(3): 575-80.
203. Spodick DH. Differential diagnosis of acute pericarditis. Prog Cardiovasc Dis. 1971;14(2):192-209.
204. Scott RW, Feil HS, Katz LH. The electrocardiogram in pericardial effusion I. Clinical. Am Heart J. 1930;5:68.
205. Nizet PM, Marriott HJ. The electrocardiogram and pericardial effusion. JAMA. 1966;198(2):169.
206. Mc GM, Baskind E. Electric alternans in pericardial effusion. Circulation. 1955;11(6):837-43.
207. Spodick DH. Electric alternation of the heart. Its relation to the kinetics and physiology of the heart during cardiac tamponade. Am J Cardiol. [Case Reports]. 1962;10:155-65.

208. Niarchos AP. Electrical alternans in cardiac tamponade. Thorax. 1975;30(2): 228-33.
209. James TN. Pericarditis and the sinus node. Arch Intern Med. 1962;110:305-11.
210. Rautaharju PM, Surawicz B, Gettes LS, et al. AHA/ACCF/HRS recommendations for the standardization and interpretation of the electrocardiogram: part IV: the ST segment, T and U waves, and the QT interval: a scientific statement from the American Heart Association Electrocardiography and Arrhythmias Committee, Council on Clinical Cardiology; the American College of Cardiology Foundation; and the Heart Rhythm Society. Endorsed by the International Society for Computerized Electrocardiology. J Am Coll Cardiol. [Practice Guideline Review]. 2009;53(11):982-91.
211. Reddy GV, Schamroth L, Schamroth CL. Tall and peaked U waves in hypokalemia. Chest. [Case Reports]. 1987;91(4):605-7.
212. Doroghazi RM, Childers R. Time-related changes in the Q-T interval in acute myocardial infarction: possible relation to local hypocalcemia. Am J Cardiol. [Research Support, U.S. Gov't, P.H.S.]. 1978;41(4):684-8.
213. Neil-Dwyer G, Walter P, Cruickshank JM, et al. Effect of propranolol and phentolamine on myocardial necrosis after sub-arachnoid haemorrhage. Br Med J. [Clinical Trial Randomized Controlled Trial]. 1978; 2(6143):990-2.
214. Yanowitz F, Preston JB, Abildskov JA. Functional distribution of right and left stellate innervation to the ventricles. Production of neurogenic electrocardiographic changes by unilateral alteration of sympathetic tone. Circ Res. 1966;18(4):416-28.
215. Priori SG. The fifteen years of discoveries that shaped molecular electrophysiology: time for appraisal. Circ Res. [Research Support, Non-U.S. Gov't Review]. 2010;107(4):451-6.
216. Schwartz PJ, Priori SG, Spazzolini C, et al. Genotype-phenotype correlation in the long-QT syndrome: gene-specific triggers for life-threatening arrhythmias. Circulation. [Clinical Trial Research Support, Non-U.S. Gov't Research Support, U.S. Gov't, P.H.S.]. 2001;103(1):89-95.
217. Zhang L, Timothy KW, Vincent GM, et al. Spectrum of ST-T-wave patterns and repolarization parameters in congenital long-QT syndrome: ECG findings identify genotypes. Circulation. 2000;102(23):2849-55.
218. Zareba W. Genotype-specific ECG patterns in long QT syndrome. J Electrocardiol. [Review]. 2006;39(4 Suppl):S101-6.
219. Rossenbacker T, Priori SG. Clinical diagnosis of long QT syndrome: back to the caliper. Eur Heart J. [Comment Editorial]. 2007;28(5):527-8.
220. Medeiros-Domingo A, Iturralde-Torres P, Ackerman MJ. Clinical and genetic characteristics of long QT syndrome. Rev Esp Cardiol. 2007;60(7):739-52.
221. Horner JM, Horner MM, Ackerman MJ. The diagnostic utility of recovery phase QTc during treadmill exercise stress testing in the evaluation of long QT syndrome. Heart Rhythm. [Comparative Study Research Support, Non-U.S. Gov't]. 2011;8(11):1698-704.
222. Kleber AG, Rudy Y. Basic mechanisms of cardiac impulse propagation and associated arrhythmias. Physiol Rev. [Research Support, Non-U.S. Gov't Research Support, U.S. Gov't, P.H.S. Review]. 2004;84(2):431-88.
223. Ackerman MJ, Khositseth A, Tester DJ, et al. Epinephrine-induced QT interval prolongation: a gene-specific paradoxical response in congenital long QT syndrome. Mayo Clin Proc. [Clinical Trial Controlled Clinical Trial Research Support, Non-U.S. Gov't]. 2002;77(5):413-21.

224. Vyas H, Hejlik J, Ackerman MJ. Epinephrine QT stress testing in the evaluation of congenital long-QT syndrome: diagnostic accuracy of the paradoxical QT response. Circulation. [Comparative Study Evaluation Studies Research Support, N.I.H., Extramural Research Support, Non-U.S. Gov't]. 2006;113(11):1385-92.
225. Patel C, Yan GX, Antzelevitch C. Short QT syndrome: from bench to bedside. Circ Arrhythm Electrophysiol. [Research Support, N.I.H., Extramural Research Support, Non-U.S. Gov't Review]. 2010;3(4):401-8.
226. Gaita F, Giustetto C, Bianchi F, et al. Short QT syndrome: a familial cause of sudden death. Circulation. [Clinical Trial]. 2003;108(8):965-70.
227. Wolpert C, Schimpf R, Giustetto C, et al. Further insights into the effect of quinidine in short QT syndrome caused by a mutation in HERG. J Cardiovasc Electrophysiol. [Clinical Trial Controlled Clinical Trial Research Support, Non-U.S. Gov't]. 2005;16(1):54-8.
228. Mehta MC, Jain AC. Early repolarization on scalar electrocardiogram. Am J Med Sci. 1995;309(6):305-11.
229. Kambara H, Phillips J. Long-term evaluation of early repolarization syndrome (normal variant RS-T segment elevation). Am J Cardiol. 1976;38(2):157-61.
230. Spodick DH. Differential characteristics of the electrocardiogram in early repolarization and acute pericarditis. N Engl J Med. 1976;295(10):523-6.
231. Mehta M, Jain AC, Mehta A. Early repolarization. Clin Cardiol. [Comparative Study Review]. 1999;22(2):59-65.
232. Rosso R, Adler A, Halkin A, et al. Risk of sudden death among young individuals with J waves and early repolarization: putting the evidence into perspective. Heart Rhythm. [Review]. 2011;8(6):923-9.
233. Goldman MJ. RS-T segment elevation in mid- and left precordial leads as a normal variant. Am Heart J. 1953;46(6):817-20.
234. Kalla H, Yan GX, Marinchak R. Ventricular fibrillation in a patient with prominent J (Osborn) waves and ST segment elevation in the inferior electrocardiographic leads: a Brugada syndrome variant? J Cardiovasc Electrophysiol. [Case Reports]. 2000;11(1):95-8.
235. Gussak I, Antzelevitch C, Bjerregaard P, et al. The Brugada syndrome: clinical, electrophysiologic and genetic aspects. J Am Coll Cardiol. [Research Support, Non-U.S. Gov't Research Support, U.S. Gov't, P.H.S. Review]. 1999;33(1):5-15.
236. Gussak I, Antzelevitch C. Early repolarization syndrome: clinical characteristics and possible cellular and ionic mechanisms. J Electrocardiol. [Comparative Study Research Support, Non-U.S. Gov't Research Support, U.S. Gov't, P.H.S.]. 2000;33(4):299-309.
237. Lehmann KG, Shandling AH, Yusi AU, et al. Altered ventricular repolarization in central sympathetic dysfunction associated with spinal cord injury. Am J Cardiol. [Research Support, U.S. Gov't, Non-P.H.S.]. 1989;63(20):1498-504.
238. Antzelevitch C, Yan GX, Viskin S. Rationale for the use of the terms J-wave syndromes and early repolarization. J Am Coll Cardiol. [Comment Research Support, N.I.H., Extramural Research Support, Non-U.S. Gov't]. 2011;57(15):1587-90.
239. Haissaguerre M, Derval N, Sacher F, et al. Sudden cardiac arrest associated with early repolarization. N Engl J Med. [Multicenter Study]. 2008;358(19):2016-23.
240. Rosso R, Kogan E, Belhassen B, et al. J-point elevation in survivors of primary ventricular fibrillation and matched control subjects: incidence and clinical significance. J Am Coll Cardiol. [Comparative Study]. 2008;52(15):1231-8.
241. Nam GB, Kim YH, Antzelevitch C. Augmentation of J waves and electrical storms in patients with early repolarization. N Engl J Med. [Letter]. 2008;358(19):2078-9.

242. Tikkanen JT, Junttila MJ, Anttonen O, et al. Early repolarization: electrocardiographic phenotypes associated with favorable long-term outcome. Circulation. [Research Support, Non-U.S. Gov't]. 2011;123(23):2666-73.
243. Tikkanen JT, Anttonen O, Junttila MJ, et al. Long-term outcome associated with early repolarization on electrocardiography. N Engl J Med. [Research Support, Non-U.S. Gov't]. 2009;361(26):2529-37.
244. Adler A, Rosso R, Viskin D, et al. What do we know about the "malignant form" of early repolarization? J Am Coll Cardiol. [Review]. 2013;62(10):863-8.
245. Rollin A, Maury P, Bongard V, Sacher F, Delay M, Duparc A, et al. Prevalence, prognosis, and identification of the malignant form of early repolarization pattern in a population-based study. Am J Cardiol. [Comparative Study]. 2012; 110(9):1302-8.
246. Rudic B, Veltmann C, Kuntz E, et al. Early repolarization pattern is associated with ventricular fibrillation in patients with acute myocardial infarction. Heart Rhythm. 2012;9(8):1295-300.
247. Tikkanen JT, Wichmann V, Junttila MJ, et al. Association of early repolarization and sudden cardiac death during an acute coronary event. Circ Arrhythm Electrophysiol. [Research Support, Non-U.S. Gov't]. 2012;5(4):714-8.
248. Oh CM, Oh J, Shin DH, et al. Early repolarization pattern predicts cardiac death and fatal arrhythmia in patients with vasospastic angina. Int J Cardiol. [Randomized Controlled Trial Research Support, Non-U.S. Gov't]. 2013;167 (4):1181-7.
249. Surawicz B, Macfarlane PW. Inappropriate and confusing electrocardiographic terms: J-wave syndromes and early repolarization. J Am Coll Cardiol. [Review]. 2011;57(15):1584-6.
250. Wellens HJ. Early repolarization revisited. N Engl J Med. [Comment Editorial]. 2008;358(19):2063-5.
251. Benitoa B, Brugadab J, Brugadac R, et al. Brugada syndrome. Rev Esp Cardiol. 2009;62(11):1297-315.
252. Govindan M, Batchvarov VN, Raju H, et al. Utility of high and standard right precordial leads during ajmaline testing for the diagnosis of Brugada syndrome. Heart. [Research Support, Non-U.S. Gov't]. 2010;96(23):1904-8.
253. Shin SC, Ryu HM, Lee JH, et al. Prevalence of the Brugada-type ECG recorded from higher intercostal spaces in healthy Korean males. Circ J. 2005;69(9): 1064-7.
254. Brugada P, Brugada J, Brugada R. Dealing with biological variation in the Brugada syndrome. Eur Heart J. [Comment Editorial]. 2001;22(24):2231-2.
255. Shimeno K, Takagi M, Maeda K, et al. Usefulness of multichannel Holter ECG recording in the third intercostal space for detecting type 1 Brugada ECG: comparison with repeated 12-lead ECGs. J Cardiovasc Electrophysiol. [Comparative Study Evaluation Studies In Vitro]. 2009;20(9):1026-31.
256. Miyamoto K, Yokokawa M, Tanaka K, et al. Diagnostic and prognostic value of a type 1 Brugada electrocardiogram at higher (third or second) V1 to V2 recording in men with Brugada syndrome. Am J Cardiol. [Evaluation Studies Research Support, Non-U.S. Gov't]. 2007;99(1):53-7.
257. Brugada J, Brugada R, Antzelevitch C, et al. Long-term follow-up of individuals with the electrocardiographic pattern of right bundle-branch block and ST segment elevation in precordial leads V1 to V3. Circulation. [Research Support, Non-U.S. Gov't Research Support, U.S. Gov't, P.H.S.]. 2002;105(1): 73-8.

258. Sen-Chowdhry S, Syrris P, Ward D, et al. Clinical and genetic characterization of families with arrhythmogenic right ventricular dysplasia/cardiomyopathy provides novel insights into patterns of disease expression. Circulation. [Comparative Study Research Support, Non-U.S. Gov't]. 2007;115(13):1710-20.
259. Bender V, Vauthier M, Mabo P, et al. Characteristics and outcome in arrhythmogenic right ventricular dysplasia. Am J Cardiol. 1995 ;75(5):411-4.
260. Towbin JA, Bowles NE. The failing heart. Nature. [Review]. 2002;415(6868): 227-33.
261. Thiene G, Basso C, Calabrese F, Angelini A, Valente M. Pathology and pathogenesis of arrhythmogenic right ventricular cardiomyopathy. Herz. [Research Support, Non-U.S. Gov't Review]. 2000;25(3):210-5.
262. Nava A, Canciani B, Buja G, et al. Electrovectorcardiographic study of negative T waves on precordial leads in arrhythmogenic right ventricular dysplasia: relationship with right ventricular volumes. J Electrocardiol. [Research Support, Non-U.S. Gov't]. 1988;21(3):239-45.
263. Metzger JT, de Chillou C, Cheriex E, et al. Value of the 12-lead electrocardiogram in arrhythmogenic right ventricular dysplasia, and absence of correlation with echocardiographic findings. Am J Cardiol. [Research Support, Non-U.S. Gov't]. 1993;72(12):964-7.
264. Nasir K, Bomma C, Tandri H, et al. Electrocardiographic features of arrhythmogenic right ventricular dysplasia/cardiomyopathy according to disease severity: a need to broaden diagnostic criteria. Circulation. [Evaluation Studies Research Support, Non-U.S. Gov't]. 2004;110(12):1527-34.
265. Daliento L, Turrini P, Nava A, et al. Arrhythmogenic right ventricular cardiomyopathy in young versus adult patients: similarities and differences. J Am Coll Cardiol. [Comparative Study Research Support, Non-U.S. Gov't]. 1995;25(3): 655-64.
266. Trevino A, Razi B, Beller BM. The characteristic electrocardiogram of accidental hypothermia. Arch Intern Med. 1971;127(3):470-3.
267. Covino BG, Hegnauer AH. Ventricular excitability cycle: its modification by pH and hypothermia. Am J Physiol. 1955;181(3):553-8.
268. Navarro-Lopez F, Cinca J, Sanz G, et al. Isolated T wave alternans. Am Heart J. [Case Reports]. 1978;95(3):369-74.
269. Joubert PH, Muller FO, Pansegrouw DF, et al. A correlative study of serum digoxin levels and electrocardiographic measurements. S Afr Med J. 1975;49(29): 1177-81.
270. Ostrander LD, Jr, Weinstein BJ. Electrocardiographic changes after glucose ingestion. Circulation. 1964;30:67-76.
271. Friedberg CK, Zager A. "Non-specific" ST and T-wave changes. Circulation. 1961;23:655-61.
272. Wilson FN and Finch R. The effect of drinking iced-water upon the form of the T deflection of the electrocardiogram. Heart. 1923;10:275.
273. Biberman L, Sarma RN, Surawicz B. T-wave abnormalities during hyperventilation and isoproterenol infusion. Am Heart J. 1971;81(2):166-74.
274. Wasserburger RH, Lorenz TH. The effect of hyperventilation and probanthine on isolated RS-T segment and T-wave abnormalities. Am Heart J. 1956;51(5): 666-83.
275. Wendkos MH. The effects of a potassium mixture on abnormal cardiac repolarization in hospitalized psychiatric patients. Am J Med Sci. 1965;249:412-9.
276. Wasserburger RH. Observations on the juvenile pattern of adult negro males. Am J Med. 1955;18(3):428-37.

277. Tzivoni D, Stern Z, Keren A, Stern S. Electrocardiographic characteristics of neurocirculatory asthenia during everyday activities. Br Heart J. 1980; 44(4): 426–32.
278. Daoud FS, Surawicz B, Gettes LS. Effect of isoproterenol on the abnormal T wave. Am J Cardiol.30((8)):810-9.
279. Abinader EG. Adrenergic beta blockade and ECG changes in the systolic click murmur syndrome. Am Heart J. 1976;91(3):297-302.
280. Lichtman J, O'Rourke RA, Klein A, et al Electrocardiogram of the athlete. Alterations simulating those of organic heart disease. Arch Intern Med. 1973; 132(5):763-70.
281. Seta K, Kleiger R, Hellerstein EE, et al. Effect of potassium and magnesium deficiency on the electrocardiogram and plasma electrolytes of pure-bred beagles. Am J Cardiol. 1966;17(4):516-9.
282. VanderArk CR, Ballantyne F, 3rd, Reynolds EW, Jr. Electrolytes and the electrocardiogram. Cardiovasc Clin. [Review]. 1973;5(3):269-94.
283. Luomanmaki K, Heikkila J, Hartikainen M. T-wave alternans associated with heart failure and hypomagnesemia in alcoholic cardiomyopathy. Eur J Cardiol. [Case Reports]. 1975;3(3):167-70.
284. Ricketts HH, Denison EK, Haywood LJ. Unusual T-wave abnormality. Repolarization alternans associated with hypomagnesemia, acute alcoholism, and cardiomyopathy. JAMA. [Case Reports]. 1969;207(2):365-6.
285. Bronsky D, Dubin A, Waldstein S. Calcium and the electrocardiogram II. The electrocardiographic manifestations of hyperparathyroidism and marked hypercalcemia of various etiologies. Am J Cardiol. 1961;7 833.
286. Patel A, Getsos JP, Moussa G, et al. The Osborn wave of hypothermia in normothermic patients. Clin Cardiol. 1994;17(5):273-6.

Chapter

13 Integration of ECG into Cardiac Diagnosis

Snapshot

- Diagnostic ECG Features and Associated Conditions
- Acute Clinical States
- Sudden Death, Cardiac Arrest/Syncope/Ventricular Tachyarrhythmias
- Valvular Disease
- Myocardial Diseases
- Congenital Heart Defects
- Cardiac Involvement in Systemic Disorders
- Other Miscellaneous Conditions

INTRODUCTION

In this Chapter, we will discuss how electrocardiogram (ECG), an invaluable tool in cardiac diagnosis, can be integrated with the traditional bedside cardiac assessment. In fact, the so-called Five Finger Approach to Cardiac Assessment can be listed as follows: History, Inspection, Palpation, Auscultation and ECG. The ECG is often like one of the pieces of the puzzle that a clinician is called upon to solve in cardiac diagnosis. The role it can take may be quite crucial in certain situations, and in others, it may be ancillary to other clinical data.

The encounter with any patient for assessment of the suspected cardiac problem may involve one or more of the following clinical contexts:

1. Patient may be asymptomatic and may be referred for evaluation because of an abnormal ECG.
2. Patient may be asymptomatic and may be referred for evaluation because of planned entry into competitive sports, high-risk occupation such as the pilot of a commercial jet.
3. Patient could be symptomatic and the symptoms could be quite serious such as syncope, witnessed or unwitnessed cardiac arrest or documented ventricular tachyarrhythmias. The symptoms might be in the form of acute pulmonary edema, acute coronary syndromes, acute dyspnea or collapse, presyncope at rest, atypical chest pain, documented atrial or

other supraventricular arrhythmias with or without palpitations, exertional ischemic chest pains, and exertional presyncope and/or exertional dyspnea.

4. Patient could be referred for other reasons such as the presence of a heart murmur, cardiac enlargement and/or left ventricular dysfunction detected on imaging by other modalities, ischemia detected on imaging, heart failure symptoms and/or signs, family history of heart disease, or family history of sudden death or death during sleep.
5. Patient could be referred to rule out a suspected congenital or acquired heart disease such as atrial septal defect, ventricular septal defect (VSD), cardiomyopathies: hypertrophic and others, critical aortic stenosis, mitral valve prolapse, and other valvular lesions
6. Patient may be referred to rule out cardiac involvement because of the presence of some systemic disorders.

The ECG can be diagnostic in some of the above clinical situations. It may be useful in assessing severity in others and therefore of value in clinical follow up of the patients. The ECG findings can be quite striking and diagnostic by themselves and also suggest consideration of the associated conditions. As to when we actually integrate it for the evaluation of the patient may vary depending on the clinical situation as well. We discuss below the diagnostic value of ECG in relation to a number of different clinical contexts.

DIAGNOSTIC ECG FEATURES AND ASSOCIATED CONDITIONS

Certain ECG features are diagnostic by themselves such as the presence of typical WPW pattern, abnormal Q waves of old infarct or scar, classic left ventricular hypertrophy (LVH) with strain pattern of ST-T waves or right ventricular hypertrophy (RVH) with strain pattern and abnormally long QT intervals. Obviously, the significance of any one of these findings needs to be interpreted in the clinical context. In addition, some of these findings may in fact suggest consideration of associated lesions. For instance, WPW pattern will raise the question of certain associated lesions such as possible hypertrophic cardiomyopathy (HCM) and Ebstein's anomaly. Abnormal Q waves might raise the question of coronary artery disease (CAD), anomalous origin of the left coronary artery (LCA) from the pulmonary artery as well as septal hypertrophy in HCM. In anomalous origin of the LCA from the pulmonary trunk, as a result of decreased perfusion pressure and hypoxemic blood flow through the LCA, anterolateral myocardial infarction (MI) usually tends to occur before clinical recognition. The ECG often will show abnormal deep Q waves in leads I, aVL, V5 and V6.[1] The LVH strain pattern might suggest uncontrolled severe hypertension, significant aortic stenosis, as well as HCM. Marked RVH stain pattern will raise the question of significant pulmonary hypertension (primary or secondary) and severe pulmonary stenosis. Prolonged QT intervals will need consideration of many factors in terms of etiology, which were discussed in the previous chapter.

ACUTE CLINICAL STATES

The ECG may also be diagnostic in certain ***acute clinical states*** such as acute pulmonary edema secondary to acute MI as well as acute dyspnea or collapse such as due to acute pulmonary embolism. It is crucial in acute coronary syndromes (MI and/or pericarditis), not only in diagnosis but also in formulating and planning therapy (STEMI vs. NON-STEMI).

SUDDEN DEATH, CARDIAC ARREST/ SYNCOPE/VENTRICULAR TACHYARRHYTHMIAS

In the assessment of patients with history of survival from sudden death events, cardiac arrest/syncope, family history of sudden death or death during sleep, ECG plays an important part in diagnosis of both the actual patient and in the investigation of the first-degree relatives. Atherosclerotic coronary artery disease is the underlying etiology in the majority of the cases of sudden death in subjects over the age of 40 years. The most frequent structural cardiac diseases in pooled analysis in the general population are premature coronary artery disease (31.3%), myocarditis (9.1%), LVH (7.7%) and HCM (7.5%).[2,3] The inherited causes of sudden cardiac death include the following:

1. The cardiomyopathies, in particular HCM and arrhythmogenic ventricular dysplasia/cardiomyopathy (ARVD/C) and dilated cardiomyopathy (DCM).
2. Premature CAD (from inherited dyslipidemia and other cardiac risk factors).
3. Primary arrhythmia syndromes such as catecholaminergic polymorphic ventricular tachycardia (CPVT)-(usually seen in children and young adults with stress and emotion-induced polymorphic VT with high catecholamine state, believed to result from abnormalities in ryanodine receptors that are responsible for release of calcium from sarcoplasmic reticulum following calcium entry into the cell),[4–6] long-QT syndromes and Brugada syndromes. The Brugada syndrome is considered to account for about one-fifth of all sudden deaths in the adults with structurally normal hearts.[7] All of these have autosomal dominant pattern of inheritance. Most of these patients are usually under the age of 40 years. Because of the inheritance pattern, the first-degree relatives will have a 50% a priori likelihood of being affected. The ECG plays a crucial role in diagnosis. Some of the patients may need exercise testing, ambulatory monitoring and sometimes also pharmacological testing (Brugada

pattern may be unmasked by sodium channel blocking drugs, febrile state or vagotonic agents).

Other inherited syndrome that may be associated with serious ventricular arrhythmias and sudden death is the inherited short QT syndrome. This implies that in this clinical context, attention must also be paid to the QTc interval on the ECG.

In patients with documented ventricular (wide QRS) tachyarrhythmia, one also needs to consider WPW with atrial flutter or fibrillation with rapid accessory pathway conduction in the differential diagnosis.

The common clinical association with ***ventricular tachycardia (VT)***, of course, is *the severity of the structural heart disease and the underlying left ventricular function.* About 50% of deaths in patients with congestive heart failure secondary to ischemic heart disease or dilated cardiomyopathy result from arrhythmias including ventricular fibrillation (VF), VT and VT degenerating into VF.[8] In the summarized studies, the sudden death averaged 14% per year. Besides the causes discussed above including HCM, ARVD/C, VT causing syncope has been reported in rare patients with mitral valve prolapse.[9] In adult patients following repair of tetralogy, sudden cardiac death is the most common cause of death late after repair. This will be discussed further in the later section of this chapter under congenital heart defects.

The QRS morphology during VT may also provide some insight into the site of origin of the VT. More often right bundle branch block (RBBB) morphology of VT is associated with left ventricular origin of VT. The left bundle branch block (LBBB) morphology and inferior axis is usually associated with RV outflow tract as site of origin (Fig. 13.1).[10] But LBBB morphology can also be associated with LV site of origin due to alterations of conduction pathway.[11] Ventricular tachycardia with LBBB morphology is also seen in ARVD/C[12] and after surgical repair of tetralogy of Fallot.

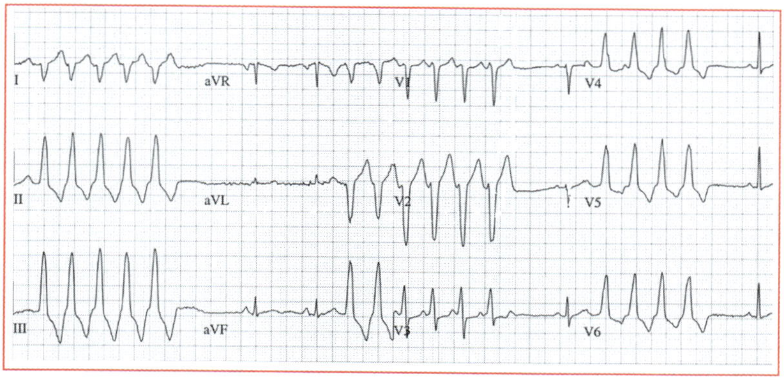

Fig. 13.1: ECG from a patient with suspicious ARVD/C and ventricular tachycardia of possible right ventricular outflow tract origin. The wide QRS complexes of the tachycardia have LBBB morphology with an inferior axis. (LBBB: Left bundle branch block).

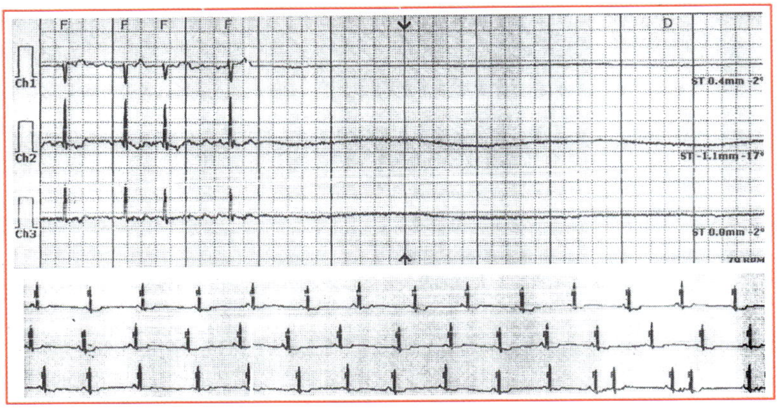

Fig. 13.2: ECG from a patient with sick sinus syndrome with atrial arrhythmias and episodes of syncope. The rhythm shows the patient to be in atrial fibrillation and suddenly develops a long pause in excess of 7 seconds.

In patients presenting with syncope, besides ventricular tachyarrhythmia, one must also consider significant bradyarrhythmias including those caused by sinus node dysfunction, high degrees of atrioventricular (AV) blocks associated with AV nodal and/or distal conduction system disease. The ECG may offer clues to the presence of trifascicular disease as discussed in Chapter 12. Also serious bradycardia may supervene in patients presenting with atrial tachyarrhythmias due to overdrive suppression especially when the underlying disorder is caused by sick sinus syndrome (Fig. 13.2). The sick sinus syndrome may result from a variety of etiologic causes including familial, congenital and acquired origin. The acquired causes include ischemic and hypertensive heart disease, primary as well as secondary cardiomyopathies, rheumatic heart disease, myocarditis, as well as those caused by surgical trauma.[13,14]

VALVULAR DISEASE

In patients with valvular disease, ECG may show signs of chamber hypertrophy or overload depending on the predominant hemodynamic abnormalities, resulting from the specific lesion and its severity. *In mitral stenosis, ECG can be quite diagnostic if typical left atrial overload is noted in combination with right axis deviation or RVH signs* (Fig. 13.3). In mitral regurgitation, no specific clues may be noted. In chronic severe mitralregurgitation, signs of atrial fibrillation with LVH voltage may be seen. Butthis can be quite non-specific. In severe aortic valve disease, signs of LVH may be noted. If the stenosis is dominant, one may see LVH strain pattern. In elderly patients with calcific aortic valve disease, LBBB may be noted. Sometimes however in the elderly, ECG could be even unremarkable despite severe aortic stenosis. The ECG is also useful for the follow-up of patients particularly with mitral stenosis.

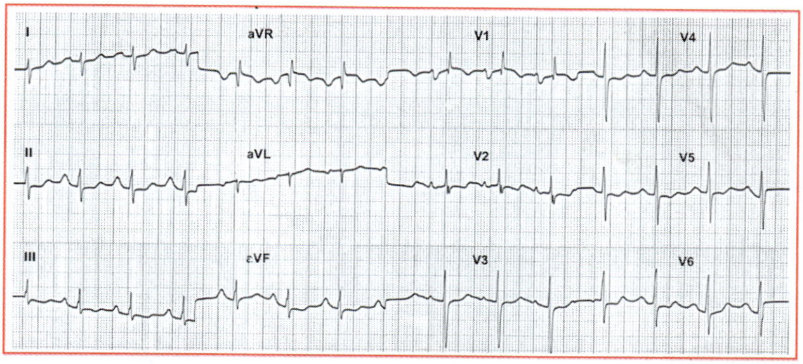

Fig. 13.3: ECG from a 45-year-old woman from India. Shows right axis deviation (RAD) with dominant R waves in V1 and V2 with abnormal T waves suggestive of left ventricular hypertrophy (RVH). Also note the P wave in V1 has typical features of left atrial overload (LAO). The combination of LAO and the signs of RVH immediately suggest mitral stenosis. This patient in fact had significant mitral stenosis with pulmonary hypertension as suggested by the signs of RVH in the ECG.

MYOCARDIAL DISEASES

In dilated cardiomyopathy, ECG may show signs of chamber enlargement, intraventricular conduction defects and sometimes abnormal Q waves of scars unrelated to ischemic disease. The incidence of LBBB appears to be higher in non-ischemic cardiomyopathy compared to the ischemic variety. *In a patient with clinical signs of LV enlargement (with large area displaced and sustained apex with medial retraction) ECG showing LBBB is highly suggestive of non-ischemic dilated cardiomyopathy.* In HCM, the most common findings are signs of LVH and abnormal Q waves. The latter has been shown to be due to increased septal thickness.[15] The WPW pattern is also not an uncommon finding. Marked T wave inversions are noted in apical type of HCM.[16] In Takotsubo cardiomyopathy, patients present with chest pain and have ST segment changes of infarction and show transient left ventricular ballooning. It is seen mostly in post-menopausal women. QT interval is prolonged but not usually associated with ventricular tachyarrhythmia.[17]

In myocardial diseases from granulomatous involvement such as sarcoidosis and other infectious causes, such as viral myocarditis, diphtheria, lyme carditis and Chagas disease, ECG features can be variable. In viral myocarditis and in cardiac involvement with retrovirus as in acquired immune deficiency syndrome, non-specific ST and T wave abnormalities may be noted. Sometimes intraventricular conduction defects may also be noted. AV block and intraventricular conduction defects are often noted in sarcoidosis, diphtheria and lyme carditis. *The ECG is abnormal in symptomatic Chagas disease and the characteristic feature is RBBB with left anterior fascicular block (LAFB).*[18]

CONGENITAL HEART DEFECTS

Some of the congenital heart defects are encountered in adult patients. Also many of the infants born with congenital defects thrive into their adult years.[19] We will discuss briefly some of the more common lesions and the associated ECG features.

Shunt Lesions

Atrial Septal Defect Secundum

This roughly accounts for one-third of all adult patients with congenital heart disease. Rhythm remains sinus although atrial flutter/fibrillation may develop in the later years past age of 50. An incomplete RBBB pattern (***rSr'*** or ***rsR'*** QRS configuration) is typically noted in the right precordial leads, which likely represents right ventricular volume overload.[20] The QRS axis is often vertical and sometimes rightward. Right axis deviation may supervene with development of pulmonary hypertension.[21] Left anterior fascicular block and left axis deviation are rare and may be seen in the elderly and has been described in the hereditary form of ***Holt-Oram syndrome***. (In this syndrome, the thumb is hypoplastic and often lies in the same plane as the other digits.)[19,22]

In addition, a notch in the apex of the R wave in the inferior leads has been correlated with ASD secundum, the pattern is described as ***"crochetage"*** (Fig. 13.4). It has been noted in 73% of adult patients with ASD and has been shown to be 92% specific when noted in all the inferior leads.[23,24]

Atrial Septal Defect Primum

Ostium primum defects are located in the lower part of the atrial septum. Although they can occur as an isolated abnormality, they often tend to occur as part of an ***incomplete endocardial cushion defect*** (also termed

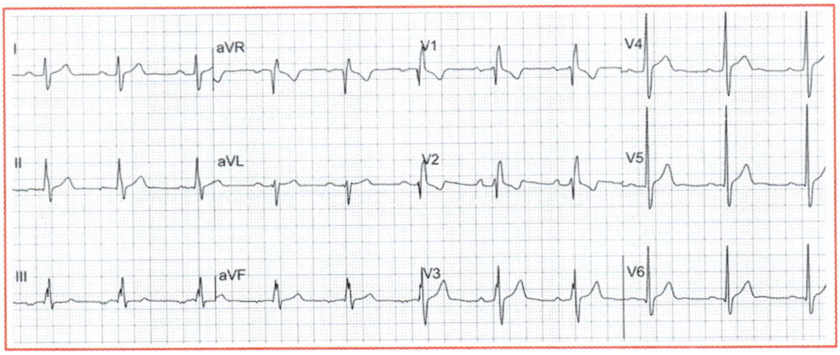

Fig. 13.4: ECG from a 20-year-old woman with clinical and echocardiographic evidence of secundum-type atrial septal defect. ECG shows the "crochetage" pattern in the inferior leads aVF and lead III with an incomplete RBBB pattern. (RBBB: Right bundle branch block).

partial atrioventricular canal defect) with a cleft mitral valve and mitral regurgitation.[25] This defect and the complete forms of the atrioventricular canal defect are associated with abnormal left axis deviation due to a "congenital form" of LAFB. It has been demonstrated to be due to early activation of the posterobasal part of the LV, resulting from the inferior displacement of the His bundle and hypoplastic anterior fascicle of the left bundle.[26,27] The incidence of prolonged PR interval and higher degrees of AV block is also increased in primum type atrial septal defect. The precordial QRS morphology is usually similar to that of secundum type atrial septal defect. The delayed right ventricular activation is considered to be due to a longer than normal right bundle branch arising from the inferiorly displaced His bundle.[28]

Ventricular Septal Defect

Ventricular septal defects encountered in adults are often perimembranous under the aortic valve. The ECG findings relate to hemodynamic abnormalities. Small VSDs usually show no abnormality in ECG. When the defect is large, then the ECG may reflect this by showing left ventricular volume overload. In patients with large defects with developed pulmonary vascular disease, right ventricular pressure overload secondary to the pulmonary hypertension will supervene. Large VSDs may be associated with left atrial overload P waves. QRS axis may shift toward the right and large biphasic QRS complexes may be seen across the precordial leads termed as *"Katz-Wachtel" phenomenon.[29] Deep Q waves in the left precordial leads are often noted with predominant left-to-right shunt* (Fig. 13.5). In Eisenmenger's syndrome, RVH secondary to pulmonary hypertension will dominate.

Persistent Ductus Arteriosus (PDA)

Often when discovered in the adults, the PDA is usually small. When large and not associated with pulmonary vascular disease and Eisenmenger's

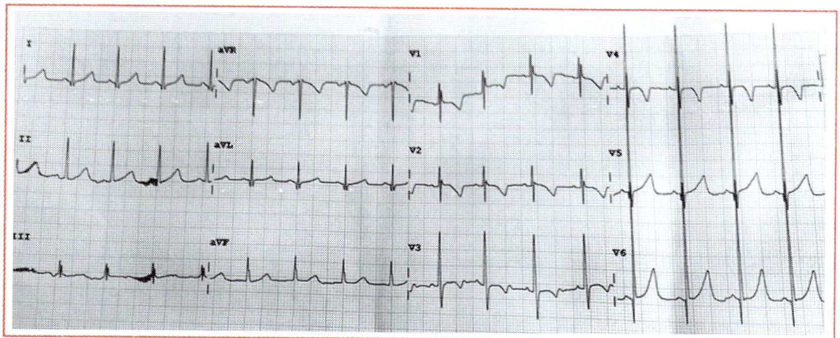

Fig. 13.5: ECG from an infant with a large perimembranous VSD and a significant left-to-right shunt. Shows deep **q** waves in the left precordial leads V5 and V6. (VSD: Ventricular septal defect).

physiology, left ventricular volume overload may be noted with deep S waves in V1 and tall R waves in the V5 and V6 with some non-specific repolarization abnormalities.[30]

Obstructive Lesions

Pulmonary Stenosis

Obstruction of the right ventricular outflow tract can be at the valvular level, below the valve in the infundibulum, or above the valve, in the main pulmonary artery or one of its branches. They may be seen in the adults in unoperated patients or as part of residual defects in operated patients. Congenital pulmonary valvular stenosis accounts for about 10% of all congenital heart defects. Significant pulmonary stenosis will be associated with signs of right atrial overload and RVH. The degree of right axis deviation is correlated with right ventricular pressure.[31] The severity correlates with R/S ratio in leads V1 and V6 and R wave amplitude in V1.[32]

Aortic Stenosis

Discrete sub-valvular aortic stenosis accounts for about one-tenth of all patients with aortic stenosis.[33] This can be due to a fibromuscular ridge or a tunnel-like narrowing of the left ventricular outflow tract. About 20–25% of the patients with discrete sub-aortic stenosis may in fact present with symptoms in their adulthood. Congenital valvular stenosis can occur on a unicuspid valve or a fused bicuspid valve. When significant obstruction is present, patients usually present in their teens or early twenties. Between the ages of 40 and 60 years, a bicuspid aortic valve can become calcific and cause significant stenosis. Rarely, rheumatic valvular involvement may also present in this age group but is most likely to have some mitral involvement as well. In the elderly patients, however, aortic valvular stenosis is often calcific and probably degenerative. Irrespective of the etiology, the hallmark of significant aortic outflow obstruction on the ECG is LVH with or without the strain pattern of the ST-T waves.

Coarctation of Aorta

In adults with isolated coarctation of aorta, P waves of left atrial overload and signs of LVH (especially voltage) are common. Complications in adults (operated or unoperated) with coarctation of aorta include systemic hypertension, heart failure, aortic dissection, premature coronary disease and strokes.[34]

Ebstein's Anomaly, Congenitally Corrected Transposition

Ebstein's Anomaly

Ebstein's anomaly is characterized by downwardly displaced tricuspid valve with partially atrialized right ventricle. The atrialized portion behaves functionally as right atrium but morphologically and electrically as right ventricle.[35] Severity is related to the degree of atrialization of the right ventricle, the tethering of the tricuspid leaflet and the presence or absence of right ventricular outflow obstruction. Associated defects include patent foramen ovale and atrial septal defect secundum. The ECG as pointed out earlier is quite useful and typically shows WPW. In 25% of patients, atrioventricular or atriofascicular pathways are noted.[35] ***P waves*** are often quite tall and broad sometimes described as "***giant***" or "***Himalayan***." The right precordial leads will show low amplitude QRS due to the small size of the right ventricle. In addition, the QRS complexes will show right ventricular conduction delay with atypical features of RBBB (multiphasic QRS complexes).[36] The most common form of presentation in the adult is for the frequent occurrence of supraventricular tachyarrhythmias.[37]

Congenitally Corrected Transposition

Congenitally corrected transposition of the great arteries (TGA) may remain undetected and asymptomatic. The ECG offers clues of which two important features are *atrioventricular conduction disturbances and reversed direction of the initial QRS force.* The sinus node is normally positioned resulting in normal P wave morphology and axis. Abnormal atrioventricular conduction defects are common in three-fourths of the patients and are attributed to the long pathway the His bundle follows in order to reach the base of the ventricular septum.[38] Varying degrees of AV block may be noted.[39] When complete AV block occurs, the QRS remains narrow since the rhythm arises from above the bifurcation of the bundle of His. Since the ventricles are reversed (inverted), the conduction system is also the reverse of the normal. The anatomic left bundle lies on the right side of the interventricular septum.[38] Septal depolarization is "right to left" and therefore the initial QRS force is directed to the left. This leads to the absence of the normal septal ***q*** waves in the left precordial leads. The septal ***q*** waves are instead noted in the right-sided limb and chest leads (Fig. 13.6). *Clinical signs of a large VSD noted together with the absence of normal septal q waves in the left precordial leads in the ECG should lead one to suspect a coexisting corrected TGA.*[40]

The plane of the ventricular septum tends to be perpendicular rather than parallel to the front of the chest with the left side of the septum facing upward. The "right-to-left" septal depolarization makes the initial QRS force to point superior and leftward resulting in the absence of ***q*** in lead I and prominent ***q*** wave in lead III and aVF.[41]

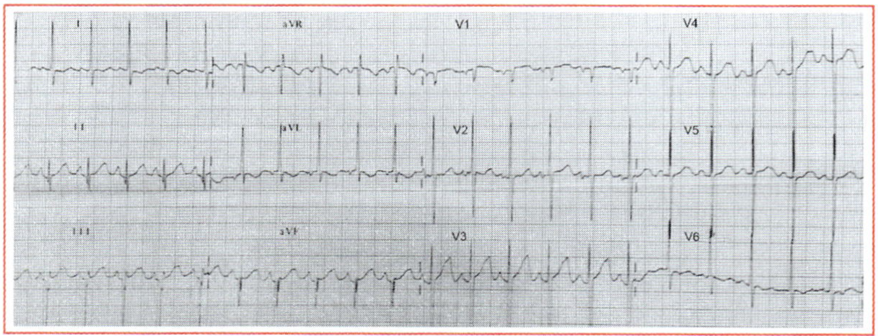

Fig. 13.6: ECG from an infant with congenitally corrected transposition with intact septum, and left-sided AV valve regurgitation presenting with heart failure. Note the absence of normal septal **q** wave in the left precordial leads. The plane of the interventricular septum is parallel to the front of the chest and the left side of the septum faces upward. The right-to-left septal activation is accompanied by deep **q** waves in the inferior leads with superior axis.

The QRS axis is dependent on the dominance of the ventricle. When the *arterial* ventricle is dominant, the axis is leftward and superior. This is also likely to be present if the left atrioventricular valve is incompetent with regurgitation. When the *venous* ventricle is dominant, the QRS axis is directed downward and to the right. This is also likely if there is a coexistent VSD with pulmonary hypertension or significant pulmonary stenosis.[41]

Cardiac Malpositions, Coronary Anomalies, Single Ventricle

Cardiac Malpositions

In the ***situs solitus*** (normally positioned) heart, the aortic arch, the descending aorta, the left atrium, cardiac apex and the stomach are on the left side. In the ***situs inversus*** heart, the arrangement is opposite. It is also referred to as "***the mirror image dextrocardia.***" In this position, the aortic arch, the descending aorta, the left atrium, the cardiac apex and the stomach are on the right side. Two additional terms that are used are ***dextroversion*** and ***levoversion***. Dextroversion exists when the cardiac apex is on the right side, while the aortic arch, the descending aorta, the left atrium and stomach remain in their normal left-sided position (situs solitus). Levoversion exits when the cardiac apex is on the left side while the aortic arch, the descending aorta, the left atrium and the stomach are on the right side (in the situs inversus position)[42] (Fig. 13.7).

In situs inversus, with mirror image dextrocardia, 90–95% of the patients have otherwise normal hearts.[43] The most common associated congenital heart defect is congenitally corrected TGA.

The ECG in mirror image dextrocardia is quite diagnostic. Since the sinus node and the right atrium are on the left side, the P wave axis is oriented

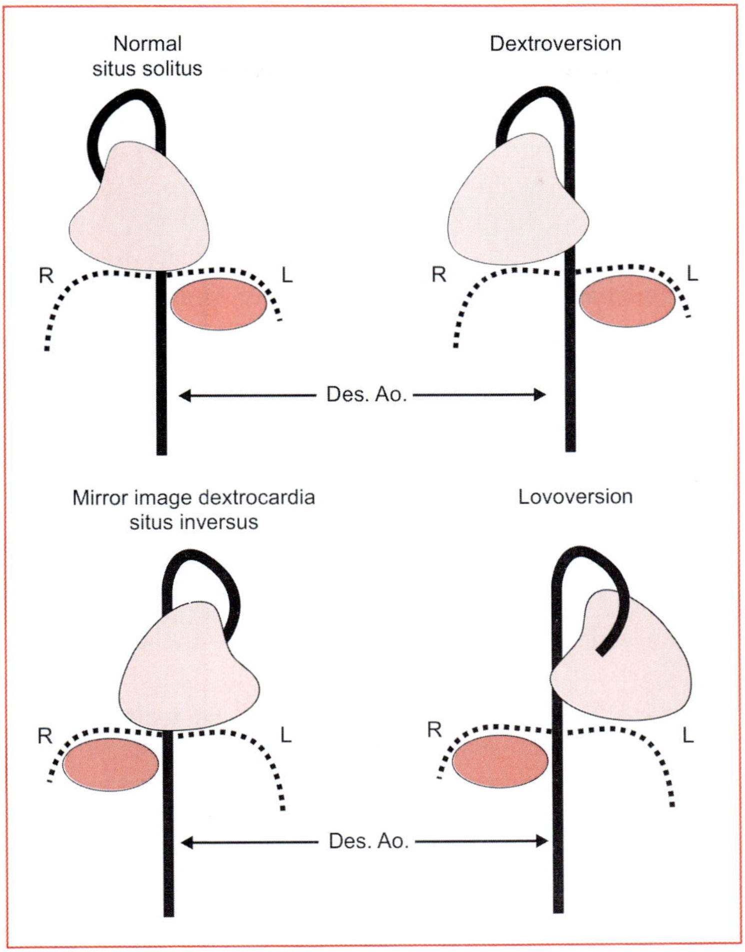

Fig. 13.7: Diagram showing the features of the cardiac malpositions. In situs solitus (the normal position) the aortic arch and the descending aorta, the apex of the heart and the stomach are on the anatomic left side. In dextroversion, the descending aorta and the stomach are on the left side but the apex is on the right side. In situs inversus (mirror image dextrocardia), the descending aorta, the apex and the stomach are on the right side. In levoversion, the descending aorta and the stomach are on the right side but the apex is on the left side.

toward the right and downward. The P wave is, therefore, negative in I and aVL.[44] Ventricular depolarization and repolarization are also inversed. Left-sided leads show negative QRS and T waves, whereas the right-sided leads show upright QRS and T waves. Normal ***R/S*** progression will be seen only when right-sided precordial leads V3R–V6R, are taken that are exact opposite of the left-sided leads, V3 to V6 (*see* Fig.12.29B). The ECG as seen on the limb leads may look like arm lead reversal but the precordial leads become diagnostic.

Coronary Anomalies

Ectopic origins of coronary arteries are encountered roughly in about 1% of patients undergoing coronary angiography. Coronary artery fistulas may result in volume overload due to the shunt. The ECG may show changes of the volume overload of the chamber involved with or without ischemic changes related to coronary steal.[45]

The ECG is useful in the diagnosis of the anomalous origin of the LCA from the pulmonary trunk as mentioned earlier in this chapter. Typically the ECG will show abnormal Q waves in leads I, aVL and V4–V6. In addition, there may be additional secondary changes due to hypertrophy of the posterobasal region of the LV resulting in LVH, left axis deviation as well as nonspecific repolarization abnormalities.[1]

Single Ventricle

Single ventricle implies two atria and one ventricular chamber. Both atrioventricular valves are present, thus excluding tricuspid and mitral atresia. The common variety is a single LV with right ventricular infundibulum. The great vessels are almost always transposed. The defect may or may not be associated with pulmonary stenosis. Survival depends on the relative resistance to flow into the pulmonary artery and the resistance to flow into the aorta. When the pulmonary flow is large, ECG may show signs of left atrial overload. The QRS axis will depend on the location of the infundibular chamber. When the latter is at the right base of the ventricle, then the QRS axis will show left axis deviation. When the infundibular chamber is in the left base, then the QRS axis is downward and right.

Surgically Corrected Congenital Heart Defects with Residual Issues

Surgically Corrected Tetralogy of Fallot

The surgical correction of tetralogy of Fallot often entails atriotomy and/or ventricular incisions and patches. This leads to the late development of arrhythmias.[46] Sudden cardiac death is the most common cause of death late after repair. Right bundle branch block results post-operatively in these patients even in the absence of ventriculotomy incision, due to injury to the right bundle and the myocardium. Late increase in QRS width occurs from RV dilatation.[47] Independent predictors of VT and sudden death in these patients include prolonged QRS > 180 ms,[46] low cardiac index and moderate pulmonary and tricuspid regurgitation.

Complete TGA and Intra-atrial Baffle

The current corrective surgery of choice for complete TGA is the arterial switch operation.[48] Previous procedures included an intra-atrial baffle without prostheses or grafts or using a pericardial patch (Mustard procedure).[49] Late arrhythmic complications include sinus node dysfunction, atrial arrhythmias and even sudden cardiac death.[50]

Post-Fontan Operation

The Fontan procedure involves anastomosis of the right atrium to the pulmonary artery. It was developed as surgical palliation of tricuspid atresia.[51] Intra-atrial re-entrant arrhythmias and atrial fibrillation often occur with significant clinical deterioration.

CARDIAC INVOLVEMENT IN SYSTEMIC DISORDERS

Cardiac involvement in patients with other underlying disorders is not an uncommon problem. The underlying disorder could be significant chronic pulmonary disease. Sometimes the underlying disorder may be systemic and the process can be inflammatory, metabolic and endocrine, infiltrative, neuromuscular or neoplastic in nature. The ECG often can provide clues that can be valuable in assessment of cardiac involvement. The ECG changes of COPD were dealt with in the previous chapter. Typically, the QRS voltage is low in lead I due to attenuation of forces oriented in the X-axis direction due to overinflated lung overlapping the heart. This feature is seen also in mitral stenosis. The QRS axis in mitral stenosis may be vertical or rightward also due to the development of pulmonary hypertension and the consequent RVH. While mitral stenosis will show typical P waves of left atrial overload, the P wave in COPD is often rightward oriented due to dominance of the right atrial forces. This will make the P wave typically negative in aVL. The combination of low voltage in lead I (<5 mm QRS) and a negative P in aVL should make one suspect COPD if the patient is above the age of 45 years since these changes do not occur early on. In addition, young patients who are tall and lean will usually have a mean QRS axis of + 90° (vertical QRS), which will therefore result in low voltage in lead I. That is why the age needs to be taken into account in this analysis. The signs of RVH as well as hypoxemia in COPD have been dealt with before in the previous chapter. Therefore, it will not be discussed here further.

Inflammatory

Many of the connective tissue diseases have associated cardiac involvement. In scleroderma, the heart may be involved by fibrosis of the myocardium. Renal involvement may lead to hypertension and secondarily affect the heart and produce LVH. Pulmonary hypertension may also occur due to vascular disease or pulmonary fibrosis with signs of RVH.[52] Intraventricular conduction defects including complete AV block has been reported.[53] In systemic lupus, the heart may be involved as a result of pericarditis or hypertension and rarely by infarction from coronary vasculitis.[54] In majority of patients with periarteritis nodosa, ECG changes might be noted from hypertension and myocardial ischemia.[55] Dermatomyositis may be associated with myocarditis and conduction system involvement such as LAFB, RBBB and LBBB.[56] Rheumatoid disease may cause pericarditis.[57] In ankylosing spondylitis and Reiter's syndrome, the PR interval is often prolonged and second degree AV block, fascicular and bundle branch block (BBB) and rarely complete AV block have also been noted.[58] In acute rheumatic fever with carditis, the PR interval is often prolonged and second-degree AV block and abnormal T waves may also be noted.[59]

Metabolic and Endocrine

In diabetic patients, ECG abnormalities are fairly common.[60] During therapy of acute ketoacidosis ECG monitoring has been shown to be useful in following the extracellular potassium levels.[61] Abnormal symmetric T wave inversion have also been noted during treatment of diabetic ketoacidosis even when the potassium levels have been restored to normal.[60]

In hyperthyroidism, sinus tachycardia is common and the heart rate reflects the severity of the disorder. Atrial fibrillation may also develop and most commonly so in patients above the age of 55 years.[62] The incidence of atrial fibrillation is higher in T3 thyrotoxicosis.[63] The PR interval tends to be prolonged. The P waves may be tall and the QRS amplitude may be high and suggestive of LVH[64] (Fig. 13.8). Acute ***Thyroid storm*** may lead to VT or fibrillation. It may also show ST segment changes of ischemia or infarct likely secondary to increased myocardial oxygen demand or coronary spasm.

In myxedema heart, the ECG will often show sinus bradycardia, low voltage QRS complexes, and low or inverted T waves.[65] Three types of repolarization abnormalities have been described, flat T waves, ST segment changes of pericarditis and deeply inverted T waves of possible myocardial ischemia.[60] Atrioventricular and intraventricular conduction defects are also not uncommon.

In acromegaly, hypertension and heart failure are often present. The ECG changes are quite common which include signs of LVH, ST-T abnormalities, old infarct patterns (Fig. 13.9) and intraventricular conduction defects.[64]

In pheochromocytoma, ECG changes can occur secondary to hypertension, myocardial ischemia or "catecholamine myocarditis".[64,66] The changes may consist of LVH with sinus tachycardia, ST segment depression and sometimes giant T wave inversion as in sub-archnoid hemorrhage.[60] Tachyarrhythmias including VF have been reported.[67]

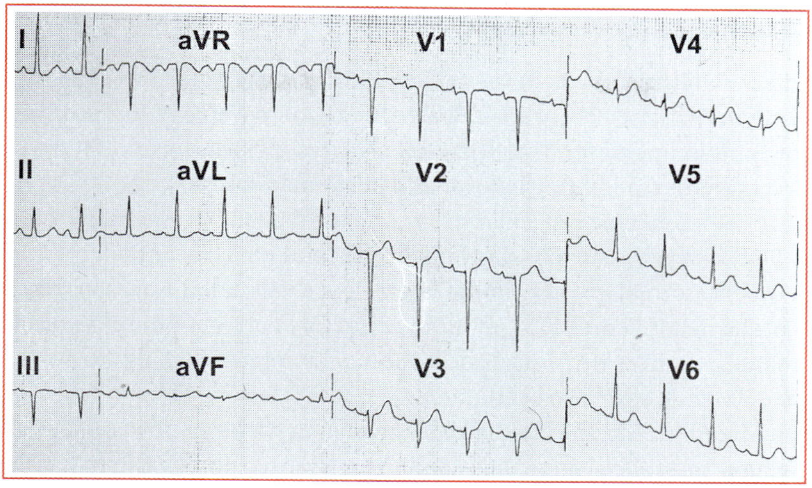

Fig. 13.8: ECG from a patient with hyperthyroidism showing mild sinus tachycardia and voltage for left ventricular hypertrophy.

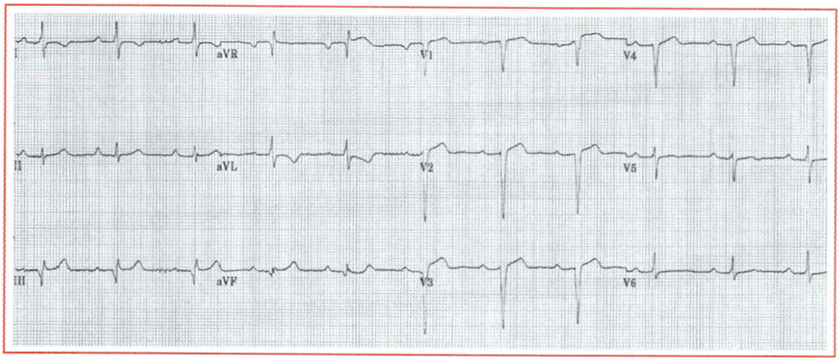

Fig. 13.9: ECG from a patient with acromegaly shows evidence of old inferior and anterior infarct (abnormal **Q** wave in aVF and QS complexes in V1 through V4).

Infiltrative Processes

In hemochromatosis, iron deposits are more pronounced in the working myocardial cells than in the conduction system cells. The ECG manifestations include low voltage, abnormal T waves, conduction defects and atrial arrhythmias secondary to atrial involvement.[68]

In amyloidosis, the ECG abnormalities often reflect the extent of amyloid deposition in the heart.[64] The ECG tends to show low voltage. Other findings include AV and intraventricular conduction defects, old infarct patterns, LVH signs, complex ventricular arrhythmias on ambulatory monitoring.[69]

In lipid storage disease, lipid infiltration will result in conduction defects and chamber enlargement.

Neuromuscular Disorders

Cardiac involvement, as revealed by ECG abnormalities, occurs in the majority of patients with Friedreich's ataxia. The pathology in the myocardium is often one of fibrosis. The ECG changes include axis deviations, old infarct patterns resembling inferior and posterolateral infarction.[70]

In Duchenne type muscular dystrophy, cardiac involvement is common and ECG characteristically shows pattern simulating posterolateral infarction with abnormal Q waves in the lateral leads with tall R waves in the right precordial leads, correlated to fibrosis in the corresponding myocardial segments.[71] Atrial arrhythmias and conduction defects such as the posterior fascicular block have also been noted.

In myotonic dystrophy, cardiac involvement from fibrosis and fatty infiltration may affect the entire conduction system. The ECG abnormalities include prolonged PR interval, LAFB, BBB, abnormal Q waves and ST-T abnormalities.[72,73]

OTHER MISCELLANEOUS CONDITIONS

The ECG is often of value in assessing patients post chest trauma. Tumors both primary and metastatic can involve the heart. Depending on the location and the extent of involvement ECG abnormalities may arise. Atrial myxomas often tend to cause atrial arrhythmias. Metastatic tumor invasion of interventricular septum can produce BBB, AV blocks. In addition, Q waves of old infarct can occur both with primary and secondary tumors.[74] Tumors can also cause pericardial effusions with tamponade showing typical ECG findings of tamponade.

Finally, ECG can become abnormal secondary to myocardial dysfunction caused by certain drugs. Doxorubicin given for chemotherapy can cause cardiomyopathy and myocardial dysfunction. Often non-specific changes may be noted including sinus tachycardia, low voltage, abnormal T waves and prolonged QT intervals.[75]

REFERENCES

1. Burch GE, Depasquale NP. The Anomalous left coronary artery: an experiment of nature. Am J Med. 1964;37:159-61.
2. van der Werf C, van Langen IM, Wilde AA. Sudden death in the young: what do we know about it and how to prevent? Circ Arrhythm Electrophysiol. [Research Support, Non-U.S. Gov't]. 2010;3(1):96-104.
3. Fabre A, Sheppard MN. Sudden adult death syndrome and other non-ischaemic causes of sudden cardiac death. Heart. 2006;92(3):316-20.
4. van der Werf C, Wilde AA. Catecholaminergic polymorphic ventricular tachycardia: important messages from case reports. Europace. [Comment Editorial Research Support, Non-U.S. Gov't]. 2011;13(1):11-3.

5. Leenhardt A, Lucet V, Denjoy I, et al. Catecholaminergic polymorphic ventricular tachycardia in children. A 7-year follow-up of 21 patients. Circulation. 1995; 91(5):1512-9.
6. Francis J, Sankar V, Nair VK, et al. Catecholaminergic polymorphic ventricular tachycardia. Heart Rhythm. [Review]. 2005;2(5):550-54.
7. Antzelevitch C, Brugada P, Borggrefe M, et al. Brugada syndrome: report of the second consensus conference: endorsed by the Heart Rhythm Society and the European Heart Rhythm Association. Circulation. [Consensus Development Conference Research Support, N.I.H., Extramural Research Support, Non-U.S. Gov't Research Support, U.S. Gov't, P.H.S. Review]. 2005;111(5):659-70.
8. Packer M. Sudden unexpected death in patients with congestive heart failure: a second frontier. Circulation. [Research Support, U.S. Gov't, P.H.S.]. 1985;72 (4):681-5.
9. Jeresaty RM. Sudden death in the mitral valve prolapse-click syndrome. Am J Cardiol. [Case Reports Review]. 1976;37(2):317-8.
10. Buxton AE, Waxman HL, Marchlinski FE, et al. Right ventricular tachycardia: clinical and electrophysiologic characteristics. Circulation. [Research Support, Non-U.S. Gov't Research Support, U.S. Gov't, P.H.S.]. 1983;68(5):917-27.
11. Josephson ME, Horowitz LN, Farshidi A, et al. Recurrent sustained ventricular tachycardia. 2. Endocardial mapping. Circulation. 1978;57(3):440-7.
12. Manyari DE, Klein GJ, Gulamhusein S, et al. Arrhythmogenic right ventricular dysplasia: a generalized cardiomyopathy? Circulation. [Research Support, Non-U.S. Gov't]. 1983;68(2):251-7.
13. Ferrer MI. The sick sinus syndrome in atrial disease. JAMA. 1968;206(3):645-6.
14. Sutton R, Kenny RA. The natural history of sick sinus syndrome. Pacing Clin Electrophysiol. [Review]. 1986;9(6 Pt 2):1110-4.
15. Dumont CA, Monserrat L, Soler R, et al. Interpretation of electrocardiographic abnormalities in hypertrophic cardiomyopathy with cardiac magnetic resonance. Eur Heart J. [Research Support, Non-U.S. Gov't]. 2006;27(14):1725-31.
16. Keren G, Belhassen B, Sherez J, et al. Apical hypertrophic cardiomyopathy: evaluation by noninvasive and invasive techniques in 23 patients. Circulation. 1985;71(1):45-56.
17. Bybee KA, Kara T, Prasad A, et al. Systematic review: transient left ventricular apical ballooning: a syndrome that mimics ST-segment elevation myocardial infarction. Ann Intern Med. [Review]. 2004;141(11):858-65.
18. Rosenbaum MB. Chagasic Myocardiopathy. Prog Cardiovasc Dis. [Review]. 1964;7:199-225.
19. Khairy P, Marelli AJ. Clinical use of electrocardiography in adults with congenital heart disease. Circulation. [Research Support, Non-U.S. Gov't Review]. 2007;116(23):2734-46.
20. Sung RJ, Tamer DM, Agha AS, et al. Etiology of the electrocardiographic pattern of "incomplete right bundle branch block" in atrial septal defect: an electrophysiologic study. J Pediatr. 1975;87(6 Pt 2):1182-6.
21. Yamaki S, Horiuchi T, Miura M, et al. Pulmonary vascular disease in secundum atrial septal defect with pulmonary hypertension. Chest. 1986;89(5):694-8.
22. Holt M, Oram S. Familial heart disease with skeletal malformations. Br Heart J. 1960;22:236-42.
23. Rodriguez-Alvarez A, Martinez De Rodriguez G, Goggans AM, et al. The vectorcardiographic equivalent of the "crochetage" of the QRS of the electrocardiogram in atrial septal defect of the ostium secundum type. Preliminary report. Am Heart J. 1959;58:388-94.

24. Heller J, Hagege AA, Besse B, et al. "Crochetage" (notch) on R wave in inferior limb leads: a new independent electrocardiographic sign of atrial septal defect. J Am Coll Cardiol. [Research Support, Non-U.S. Gov't]. 1996;27(4):877-82.
25. Weyn AS, Bartle SH, Nolan TB, et al. Atrial septal defect—primum type. Circulation. 1965;32(6 Suppl):III13-23.
26. Borkon AM, Pieroni DR, Varghese PJ, et al. The superior QRS axis in ostium primum ASD: a proposed mechanism. Am Heart J. 1975;90(2):215-21.
27. Feldt RH, DuShane JW, Titus JL. The atrioventricular conduction system in persistent common atrioventricular canal defect: correlations with electrocardiogram. Circulation. 1970;42(3):437-44.
28. Boineau JP, Moore EN, Patterson DF. Relationship between the ECG, ventricular activation, and the ventricular conduction system in ostium primum ASD. Circulation. 1973;48(3):556-64.
29. Katz LN, Wachtel, H. The diphasic QRS type of electrocardiogram in congenital heart disease. Am Heart J. 1937;13:22-4.
30. Marquis RM, Miller HC, McCormack RJ, et al. Persistence of ductus arteriosus with left to right shunt in the older patient. Br Heart J. 1982;48(5):469-84.
31. Danilowicz D, Hoffman JI, Rudolph AM. Serial studies of pulmonary stenosis in infancy and childhood. Br Heart J. [Research Support, U.S. Gov't, P.H.S.]. 1975;37(8):808-18.
32. Rasmussen K, Sorland SJ. Prediction of right ventricular systolic pressure in pulmonary stenosis from combined vectorcardiographic data. Ame Heart J. 1973;86(3):318-28.
33. Sung CS, Price EC, Cooley DA. Discrete subaortic stenosis in adults. Am J Sardiol. 1978;42(2):283-90.
34. Toro-Salazar OH, Steinberger J, Thomas W, et al. Long-term follow-up of patients after coarctation of the aorta repair. Am J Cardiol. [Research Support, Non-U.S. Gov't Research Support, U.S. Gov't, P.H.S.]. 2002;89(5):541-7.
35. Ho SY, Goltz D, McCarthy K, et al. The atrioventricular junctions in Ebstein malformation. Heart. [Research Support, Non-U.S. Gov't]. 2000;83(4):444-9.
36. Hernandez FA, Rochkind R, Cooper HR. The intracavitary electrocardiogram in the diagnosis of Ebstein's anomaly. Am J Cardiol. 1958;1(2):181-90.
37. Celermajer DS, Bull C, Till JA, et al. Ebstein's anomaly: presentation and outcome from fetus to adult. J Am Coll Cardiol. 1994;23(1):170-6.
38. Lev M, Licata RH, May RC. The Conduction System in Mixed Levocardia with Ventricular Inversion (Corrected Transposition). Circulation. 1963;28:232-7.
39. Honey M. The diagnosis of corrected transposition of the great vessels. Br Heart J. 1963;25:313-33.
40. Ruttenberg HD, Elliott LP, Anderson RC, et al. Congenital corrected transposition of the great vessels. Correlation of electrocardiograms and vector cardiograms with associated cardiac malformations and hemodynamic states. Am J Cardiol. 1966;17(3):339-54.
41. Burch GE, Depasquale, NP. Electrocardiography in the Diagnosis of Congenital Heart Disease. Philadelphia, PA: Lea & Febiger; 1967.
42. Elliott LP, Jue KL, Amplatz K. A roentgen classification of cardiac malpositions. Invest Radiol. 1966;1(1):17-28.
43. Hanson JS, Tabakin BS. Primary and secondary dextrocardia. Their differentiation and the role of cineangiocardiography in diagnosing associated congenital cardiac defects. Am J Cardiol. 1961;8:275-81.

44. Campbell M, Deuchar DC. Dextrocardia and isolated laevocardia. II. Situs inversus and isolated dextrocardia. Br Heart J. [Case Reports]. 1966;28(4): 472-87.
45. McNamara JJ, Gross RE. Congenital coronary artery fistula. Surgery. 1969;65(1): 59-69.
46. Gatzoulis MA, Balaji S, Webber SA, et al. Risk factors for arrhythmia and sudden cardiac death late after repair of tetralogy of Fallot: a multicentre study. Lancet. [Clinical Trial Multicenter Study]. 2000;356(9234):975-81.
47. Gatzoulis MA, Till JA, Somerville J, et al. Mechanoelectrical interaction in tetralogy of Fallot. QRS prolongation relates to right ventricular size and predicts malignant ventricular arrhythmias and sudden death. Circulation. 1995;92(2): 231-7.
48. Jatene AD, Fontes VF, Paulista PP, et al. Anatomic correction of transposition of the great vessels. J Thorac Cardiovasc Surg. [Case Reports]. 1976;72(3):364-70.
49. Warnes CA. Transposition of the great arteries. Circulation. [Review]. 2006;114 (24):2699-709.
50. Gelatt M, Hamilton RM, McCrindle BW, et al. Arrhythmia and mortality after the Mustard procedure: a 30-year single-center experience. J Am Coll Cardiol. 1997;29(1):194-201.
51. Khairy P, Poirier N, Mercier LA. Univentricular heart. Circulation. [Research Support, Non-U.S. Gov't]. 2007;115(6):800-12.
52. Escudero J, Mc DE. The electrocardiogram in scleroderma: analysis of 60 cases and review of the literature. Am Heart J. 1958;56(6):846-55.
53. Lev M, Landowne M, Matchar JC, et al. Systemic scleroderma with complete heart block. Report of a case with comprehensive study of the conduction system. Am Heart J. [Case Reports]. 1966;72(1):13-24.
54. Hejtmancik MR, Wright JC, Quint R, et al. The cardiovascular manifestations of systemic Lupus erythematosus. Am Heart J. [Review]. 1964;68:119-30.
55. Holsinger DR, Osmundson PJ, Edwards JE. The heart in periarteritis nodosa. Circulation. 1962;25:610-8.
56. Haupt HM, Hutchins GM. The heart and cardiac conduction system in polymyositis-dermatomyositis: a clinicopathologic study of 16 autopsied patients. Am J Cardiol. [Research Support, U.S. Gov't, P.H.S.]. 1982;50(5):998-1006.
57. Bonfiglio T, Atwater EC. Heart disease in patients with seropositive rheumatoid arthritis; a controlled autopsy study and review. Arch Intern Med. [Review]. 1969;124(6):714-9.
58. Ruppert GB, Lindsay J, Barth WF. Cardiac conduction abnormalities in Reiter's syndrome. Am J Med. [Case Reports Research Support, Non-U.S. Gov't]. 1982;73 (3):335-40.
59. Bates RC. Acute rheumatic fever: a study of 132 cases in young adults. Ann Intern Med. 1958;48(5):1017-25.
60. Surawicz B, Knilans, T. Chou's Electrocardiography in Clinical Practice, 6th edition Philadelphia, PA: Elsevier Saunders; 2008.
61. Soler NG, Bennett MA, Fitzgerald MG, et al. Electrocardiogram as a guide to potassium replacement in diabetic ketoacidosis. Diabetes. 1974;23(7):610-5.
62. Hoffman I, Lowrey RD. The electrocardiogram in thyrotoxicosis. Am J Cardiol. 1960;6:893-904.
63. Woeber KA. Thyrotoxicosis and the heart. N Engl J Med. [Review]. 1992;327(2): 94-8.

64. Surawicz B, Mangiardi ML. Electrocardiogram in endocrine and metabolic disorders. Cardiovasc Clin. [Review]. 1977;8(3):243-66.
65. Wood P. Diseases of the heart and circulation. London: Eyre & Spottiswoode; 1968.
66. Van Vliet PD, Burchell HB, Titus JL. Focal myocarditis associated with pheochromocytoma. N Engl J Med. 1966;274(20):1102-8.
67. Northfield TC. Cardiac complications of phaeochromocytoma. Br Heart J. 1967; 29(4):588-93.
68. Buja LM, Roberts WC. Iron in the heart. Etiology and clinical significance. Am J Med. 1971;51(2):209-21.
69. Murtagh B, Hammill SC, Gertz MA, et al. Electrocardiographic findings in primary systemic amyloidosis and biopsy-proven cardiac involvement. Am J Cardiol. [Research Support, U.S. Gov't, P.H.S.]. 2005;95(4):535-7.
70. Child JS, Perloff JK, Bach PM, et al. Cardiac involvement in Friedreich's ataxia: a clinical study of 75 patients. J Am Coll Cardiol. [Research Support, Non-U.S. Gov't Research Support, U.S. Gov't, P.H.S.]. 1986;7(6):1370-8.
71. Perloff JK, Roberts WC, de Leon AC, Jr, O'Doherty D. The distinctive electrocardiogram of Duchenne's progressive muscular dystrophy. An electrocardiographic-pathologic correlative study. Am J Med. 1967;42(2):179-88.
72. Olofsson BO, Forsberg H, Andersson S, et al. Electrocardiographic findings in myotonic dystrophy. Br Heart J. 1988;59(1):47-52.
73. Colleran JA, Hawley RJ, Pinnow EE, et al. Value of the electrocardiogram in determining cardiac events and mortality in myotonic dystrophy. Am J Cardiol. [Research Support, Non-U.S. Gov't Research Support, U.S. Gov't, Non-P.H.S.]. 1997;80(11):1494-7.
74. Biran S, Hochman A, Levij IS, et al. Clinical diagnosis of secondary tumors of the heart and pericardium. Dis Chest. 1969;55(3):202-8.
75. Singal PK, Iliskovic N. Doxorubicin-induced cardiomyopathy. N Engl J Med. [Review]. 1998;339(13):900-5.

Chapter

14 Self-Assessment

Snapshot

- Patient 1 to 20
- Questions
- Answers and Discussion

In this final Chapter for the purposes of self-assessment, we present several interesting clinical scenarios using history and/or clinical findings from actual patients seen by us. We believe it will be of help to those who want to test their own clinical and bedside skills and knowledge. It also will stimulate discussion and interchange of ideas when used in clinical teaching and training sessions. The clinical history, the questions as well as the answers with brief explanations will be presented in this chapter. The book has a companion CD, in which we present video recordings of the jugular venous pulsations, and the precordial pulsations as well as audio recordings of heart sounds and murmurs from actual patients. The first part in the CD is the teaching/learning section dealing completely with jugular venous pulsations normal and abnormal, precordial pulsations, heart sounds and murmurs. The CD also has a section for self-assessment with clinical cases together with relevant images, audio and video files.

PATIENT 1

Clinical History

Patient LF is a 51-year-old woman, an ex-smoker admitted with history of progressive increase in dyspnea on exertion over the past year, unable even to climb half a flight of stairs slowly. She also complained of upper left chest tightness precipitated by distress at yelling at her teenage son. The patient had been seen 15 years previously and was told of a "heart murmur". She has been treated in the past few years with digoxin 0.25 mg daily along with furosemide 40 mg for symptoms of dyspnea associated with palpitations. There was no history of rheumatic fever as a child, diabetes or hypertension. The patient has been told to have elevated cholesterol level. Patient's father had angina and suffered a myocardial infarction (MI) at age 77.

Physical Findings

The patient was anxious but in no acute distress. Heart rate (HR) was 80 and regular; blood pressure (BP) was 170/90. There was a slight "malar flush". Jugular venous pulse (JVP) was 10 cm above the sternal angle with double descents (x' and y) which appeared equal. Carotid pulse upstroke was normal with small amplitude. Left ventricular apex was barely palpable in the fifth interspace at the mid-clavicular line. There was a sternal impulse with lateral retraction noted over the precordium. The S2 at the second left interspace was palpable. The S1 was loud. There was a grade I–II early diastolic blowing murmur at the second left interspace. There was an opening snap easily audible at the lower left sternal border that appeared to be close to the S2. There was a grade III long mid-diastolic rumble followed by a presystolic crescendo accentuation at the apex.

The electrocardiogram (ECG) is shown in Figure 14.1.

Question 1: What statement is incorrect with regard to the ECG of this patient?

A. The right axis deviation and the qR in V1 together with ST-T abnormalities in V1 and V2 are highly suggestive of right ventricular hypertrophy (RVH)
B. The P wave in V1 is diagnostic of left atrial overload/abnormality
C. The ST-T waves in the precordial leads V1–V6 are abnormal and anterior ischemia is not excluded
D. The right axis deviation and peaked P wave in Lead II and anterior ST-T abnormalities are suggestive of acute pulmonary embolism

Question 2: At cardiac catheterization and angiography of this patient, what findings are unlikely?

A. Hemodynamics confirming tight mitral stenosis with severe pulmonary hypertension and normal coronary arteries
B. Hemodynamics confirming elevated pulmonary capillary wedge pressures and a full length diastolic gradient in simultaneous LV and wedge pressures

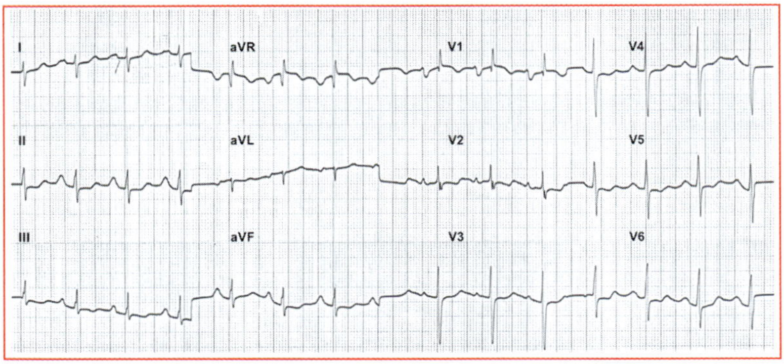

Fig. 14.1: Electrocardiogram.

C. Significant aortic regurgitation and aortic stenosis with normal coronaries

D. Severe mitral regurgitation with pulmonary hypertension

Answer and Discussion

The ECG of this patient shows right axis deviation together with a qR pattern in V1. This is suggestive of RVH. The ST-T abnormalities are probably secondary changes. This together with the clear cut biphasic P wave in V1 with a pronounced terminal negativity indicates strong evidence of left atrial overload/abnormality. The combination of these two alone should raise suspicion of severe mitral stenosis as the underlying cause of the RVH. The absence of tachycardia and the presence of left atrial overload P wave exclude acute pulmonary embolism.

The clinical findings of a dominant right ventricle over the precordium, palpable S2 in the second left interspace and raised jugular venous pressure with double descents all point to significant pulmonary hypertension. When the JVP shows raised levels with equal x' and y descents and if it is due to pulmonary hypertension, then the pulmonary artery systolic pressure is at least 75 mm Hg or more. Palpable S2 in the second left interspace is almost always due to a loud P2 and usually indicates also pulmonary systolic pressure of 75 mm Hg.

In fact, this patient at heart catheterization showed the following findings. The right atrial pressures were elevated to mean of 10 mm Hg and the right ventricular (RV) pressure was 112/12 and the pulmonary artery pressure 107/36 and the pulmonary wedge pressures showed an "a" wave of 30 mm Hg, and "v" wave of 30 mm Hg and a mean of 29 mm Hg. All of these are significantly elevated. The mean mitral diastolic gradient was 14 mm Hg. The findings confirmed severe mitral stenosis and the coronary arteries were normal.

Incidentally, the blowing diastolic murmur heard over the second left interspace on this patient most likely represents pulmonary regurgitation secondary to the severe pulmonary hypertension.

The patient subsequently underwent mitral valve replacement successfully with improvement in her symptoms. The excised mitral valve showed valve orifice of about 0.5 cm^2. At pathology, the valve showed severe fibrosis, commissural fusion and moderate calcification as well. This patient was seen in the 1980s. In the modern era, at least an attempt at possibly balloon valvuloplasty may be considered first before embarking on open-heart surgery and valve replacement. In addition, one of the β-blockers will also be the first choice in attempting to control the rapid ventricular response during atrial fibrillation. Controlling the rapid HR in severe mitral stenosis will help to reduce the mean left atrial pressures as well and improve the symptoms due to the longer diastolic intervals and filling time. Two-dimensional (2D) echocardiographic evaluation is almost always done and a transesophageal echo assessment will probably be required if catheter-based intervention is considered.

PATIENT 2

Clinical History

Patient JS is 46-year-old Caucasian, chronic smoker presented to the emergency department with 1-week history of dyspnea on climbing a flight of stairs, and 4 days in a row of waking up at night with cough and dyspnea, feeling better sitting up. The patient had a dental extraction and filling two and a half weeks prior to this visit. A week prior to this visit, he had been seen in a walk-in-clinic with cough and greenish sputum and was treated for the same with antibiotics. The patient denied history of hypertension, diabetes and dyslipidemia. There was no family history of coronary disease.

Physical Findings

The patient was afebrile. Blood pressure was 170/20 mm Hg. Peripheral pulses were bounding with pistol shot sounds over the femorals. Jugular venous pulse was 12 cm above the sternal angle with a dominant *x′ descent*. Apical impulse was three finger breadths wide and prominent and mildly sustained with an area of retraction medial to it. Right ventricular impulse was palpable in the sub-xiphoid area. S1 was somewhat soft. The S2 was not well split. There was grade II–III decrescendo diastolic murmur over the precordium and the apex. There was also a grade II regurgitant systolic murmur at the apex with a loud S3. Chest was relatively clear. Abdomen showed no organomegaly or tenderness. There were no peripheral signs of endocarditis.

Question 1: Which of the following statements reflect most or all of the physical findings?

A. The patient most likely has developed LV failure secondary to severe aortic regurgitation. Probably also has mild-to-moderate mitral regurgitation.

B. The patient has symptoms and signs consistent with LV failure secondary to severe aortic regurgitation and probably severe mitral regurgitation as well.

C. The patient has biventricular enlargement and the heart failure is probably secondary to a cardiomyopathy.

D. Relatively sudden onset of symptoms with signs of elevated venous pressure and enlarged right ventricle suggest acute pulmonary embolism.

Question 2: Which of the following statements are probably right with regard to the loud S3 and the wide area of the LV apical impulse that was mildly sustained?

A. The loud S3 is suggestive that the mitral regurgitation is probably severe since severe aortic regurgitation alone would be expected to cause functional mitral stenosis and a mid-diastolic rumble (Austin-Flint murmur).

B. The S3 probably reflects underlying myocardial dysfunction and possibly a coexisting cardiomyopathy.
C. The S3 may be secondary to premature closure of the mitral valve and severe elevation of LV diastolic pressures.
D. The S3 is indicative of myocardial damage which is the underlying cause of the heart failure.

Question 3: Likely etiology of this patient's severe aortic regurgitation includes the following *except*:
A. Luetic aortitis
B. Endocarditis on an abnormal aortic valve
C. Dissecting aneurysm of the aorta
D. Rheumatic heart disease

Question 4: Which of the following investigations are probably indicated in this patient?
A. Blood cultures
B. Two-dimensional echocardiography
C. Heart catheterization
D. Serology for syphilis

Question 5: Management of this patient should include which of the following?
A. Medical therapy with Furosemide and angiotensin converting enzyme (ACE) inhibitors
B. Medical therapy of heart failure with ACE inhibitors and β-blockers and nitrates
C. Medical therapy with antibiotics and diuretics
D. Medical therapy with diuretics, ACE inhibitors if tolerated but with prompt referral for valve replacement surgery

Answer and Discussion

This patient presented with clear-cut symptoms of nocturnal dyspnea suggestive of recent onset LV failure. The physical findings of very wide pulse pressure and decrescendo diastolic murmur and enlarged left ventricle suggest significant aortic regurgitation. The presence of systolic regurgitant murmur at the apex is also suggestive of coexisting mitral regurgitation. The abrupt onset of the acute LV failure with significant aortic regurgitation raises the flag that this is probably the most important lesion. Aortic regurgitation when it leads to decompensation characteristically presents with onset of acute LV failure. The etiology of aortic regurgitation usually includes valvular and aortic root causes. The valvular causes include lesions such as the congenital bicuspid aortic valve, aortic valve fenestrations. The acquired causes include rheumatic involvement and endocarditis on an abnormal aortic valve. The aortic root causes include luetic aortitis (not very common these days), aortic root aneurysm such as due to Marfan's syndrome, spondylitis, Paget's disease, osteogenesis imperfecta, hypertensive and atherosclerotic disease as well as secondary to type I aortic dissection.

The absence of pain makes dissection unlikely. But other valvular pathology including endocarditis on a bicuspid or abnormal aortic valve, rheumatic involvement as well as aortic root causes such as luetic involvement need to be excluded. Most other aortic root causes like those associated with Marfan's syndrome, spondylitis and hypertensive/atherosclerotic origin are often suggested by history with clues on general physical examination.

The presence of loud S3 raises the possibility of the coexisting mitral regurgitation to be probably significant and probably moderately severe. Alternative cause could be some associated myocardial dysfunction. The signs of RV enlargement and elevated jugular venous pressure are probably due to secondary pulmonary hypertension associated with the LV failure.

Patients with acute LV failure and severe aortic regurgitation would deteriorate rapidly and therefore would need expedited management that should include medical therapy of congestive failure with loop diuretics and probably ACE inhibitors as tolerated. β-Blockers are not indicated and might actually cause harm. Patients should also be referred to a tertiary care center in an expedited manner to undergo urgent valve replacement surgery. If endocarditis is suspected, blood cultures must be taken followed by appropriate antibiotic therapy adjusted and guided by the causative organism. Referral to surgical centers becomes even more urgent and important in such cases.

This patient received diuretic therapy and got started on some ACE inhibitors. The blood cultures were negative. The echocardiographic studies demonstrated severe aortic regurgitation, moderately severe mitral regurgitation, LV dilatation with grade II-III dysfunction, with no clear-cut vegetations. The aortic root dimension was normal and the left coronary cusp of the aortic valve was somewhat small. He was promptly transferred to a tertiary care center where he underwent aortic valve replacement and annuloplasty of the mitral valve.

Histopathology of the myocardium was relatively normal. But the excised aortic valve showed some myxomatous degeneration. Sections from the aortic wall showed chronic inflammation with lymphocytes and some plasma cells in parts of the media and question of Lues was raised. Actually, serology for syphilis came back positive at a titer of 1:512. The patient received a course of therapy with penicillin. During the early post-operative follow-up period, he still exhibited signs of LV dysfunction suggestive of sustained LV impulse and persistent S3, although it was softer. The ACE inhibitors were continued and he was also placed on carvedilol, uptitrating the dose as tolerated. He is currently doing relatively well seen in follow-up about 10 years post-operatively.

PATIENT 3

Clinical History

Patient RS is a 65-year-old woman from Punjab, India, referred because of a heart murmur. There was no history of rheumatic fever or any symptoms of chest pain, dyspnea, presyncope, syncope or palpitations. The patient appeared to minimize her symptoms, however. She was a non-smoker and a non-drinker. There was a history of hypertension with a previous CVA with full recovery.

Physical Findings

She was about 5'5" in height weighing about 120 lb. Blood pressure 150/70 with HR of 72/min regular. Jugular venous pulse was about 5 cm above the sternal angle with a dominant *x'* descent. Carotid pulse upstroke was normal with normal peripheral pulses. Apical impulse was in the fifth interspace 9 cm from the mid-sternal line. There was a systolic sternal movement together with a palpable sub-xiphoid RV impulse. First heart sound (S1) was loud and somewhat clicky in tone. S2 was diminished in intensity and appeared to be single. There was a grade III ejection murmur audible at the left sternal border maximally loud at the second and the third left interspace and also audible at the left side of the neck (phonocardiogram is shown in Figure 14.2). There was no cyanosis or clubbing. Chest was clear.

Electrocardiogram is shown in Figure 14.3 and the chest X-ray in Figures 14.4A and B.

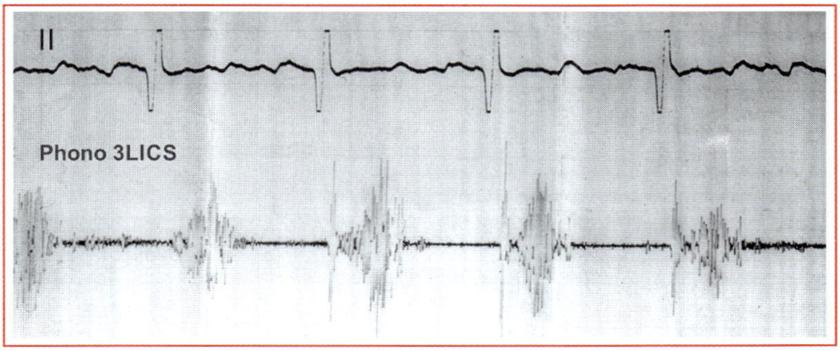

Fig. 14.2: Phono recordings (Phono) taken from the third left interspace.

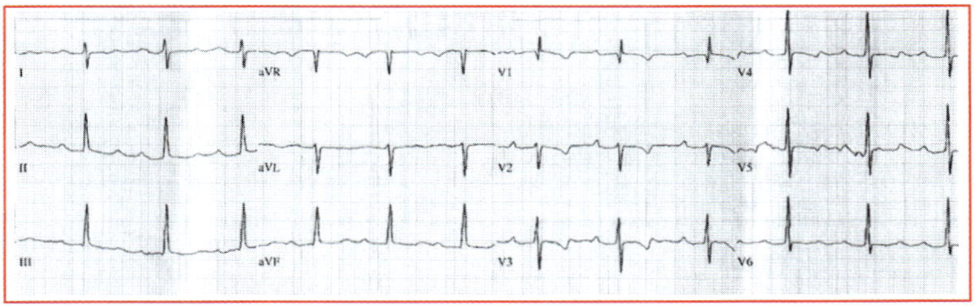

Fig. 14.3: Electrocardiogram.

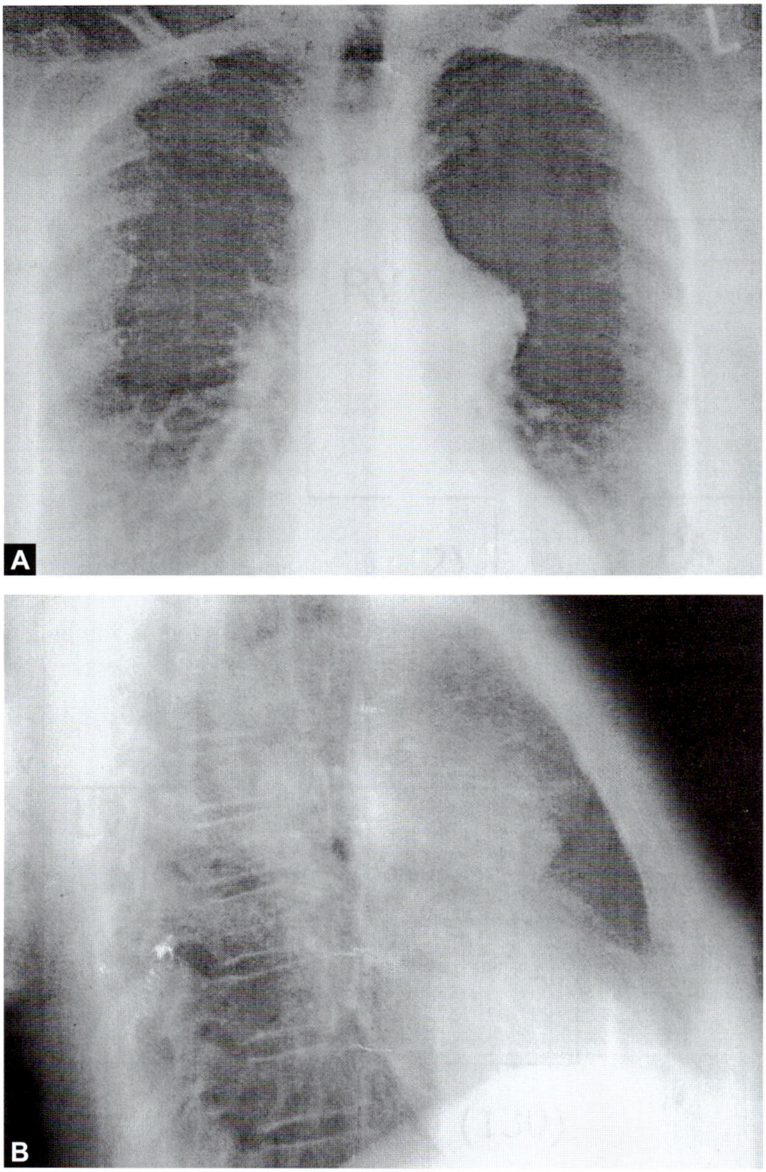

Figs. 14.4A and B: Chest X-ray posterior-anterior and lateral views.

Question 1: Auscultatory findings together with the phonocardiogram are suggestive of:

A. Infundibular pulmonary stenosis
B. Ventricular septal defect (VSD)
C. Aortic stenosis
D. Pulmonary valvular stenosis

Question 2: The chest X-ray shows all of the following *except*:

A. Normal size heart
B. Dilated left atrium
C. No evidence of enlarged left atrium
D. Post-stenotic dilatation of pulmonary artery

Question 3: The ECG is highly suggestive of:

A. Anterior infarction age undetermined
B. Left posterior fascicular block with incomplete right bundle branch block (RBBB) pattern
C. Right ventricular hypertrophy with systolic overload
D. Acute pulmonary embolism

Question 4: The patient underwent cardiac catheterization and coronary angiography. The likely findings are:

A. Moderately elevated pulmonary artery pressures and normal coronaries
B. Severe pulmonary hypertension, normal or mild non-significant coronary artery disease (CAD)
C. Moderate infundibular pulmonary stenosis with CAD
D. Moderate-to-severe pulmonary valvular stenosis with CAD

Answer and Discussion

This patient's physical findings on auscultation are highly suggestive of valvular pulmonary stenosis. The loud clicky S1 is probably a pulmonary ejection click (PEC). It would have been important to know its variation with respiration. Typically, it tends to get softer on inspiration. With milder stenosis, one tends to hear a good separation of the S1 from the PEC. With more severe stenosis, however, the PEC tends to occur earlier and merge with the S1. The murmur was late peaking in the phonocardiogram, also a feature of significant stenosis. The chest X-ray shows post-stenotic dilatation of the main pulmonary artery. There was no left atrial enlargement. The ECG shows right axis deviation with a qR pattern in V1 with negative T waves extending up to V3. This when taken together with the physical findings of systolic sternal movement and palpable sustained sub-xiphoid RV impulse suggests definitely RVH with pressure overload. Obviously because of her age and previous history of hypertension and CVA, one cannot exclude significant CAD.

The cardiac catheterization data did confirm pulmonary valvular systolic gradient of 94 mm Hg indicative of severe pulmonary stenosis. There was a patent foramen ovale with slight arterial desaturation (91%). The cardiac index was somewhat reduced (1.7 L/min/m^2). There was triple vessel CAD. Patient underwent pulmonary valve replacement and four-vessel coronary bypass surgery. She improved post-operatively.

PATIENT 4

Clinical History

Patient SG is a 48-year-old man with history of diabetes treated with oral agents for 5 years and recently also placed on rosuvastatin for slightly elevated cholesterol, was referred with symptoms of exertional dyspnea on climbing two flights of stairs, for about 3 months in duration and one episode of left arm discomfort which woke him up from sleep during the same period. The patient was a chronic smoker who quit smoking 6 months earlier. Both of his parents were in their 70s with history of hypertension and diabetes. The patient denied history of hypertension. The patient was unable to take aspirin due to mild gastric irritation. A recent exercise stress test on the Bruce protocol showed that he exercised 4 minutes and 20 seconds, and achieved a peak HR of 152/min, and a peak BP of 150/70 without symptoms or ST segment changes of ischemia. The nuclear perfusion scans showed a large perfusion defect involving the distal two thirds of the anterior wall, the apex and the septum, with partial reversibility, interpreted as extensive anterior infarct with peri-infarct ischemia. The LV function was reported to be moderately impaired with EF of 40%.

The patient denied symptoms of orthopnea, palpitations, faintness or any central chest discomfort.

Physical Findings

The patient was 5′11″ in height weighing about 230 lb. Blood pressure was 120/80 and HR 89/min regular. Carotid pulse upstroke and amplitude were normal with good peripheral pulses. Jugular venous pulse was normal with *x′ descent*. The apical impulse was not easily felt because of a thick chest. S2 was single. S1 was normal. There was an S3 gallop audible over the precordium without any murmurs. Chest was clear.

Electrocardiogram taken initially at the time of the first visit is shown in Figure 14.5A and a repeat ECG taken a week later shown in Figure 14.5B.

Question 1: The ECG is suggestive of the following:

A. Inferior infarct age undetermined and possible septal infarct
B. Inferior infarct of undetermined age
C. No abnormality noted
D. Inferior infarct old with slightly delayed r/s progression

Question 2: The appropriate management of this patient during this visit will include all of the following *except*:

A. Immediate coronary angiography
B. Assess LV function with 2D echo

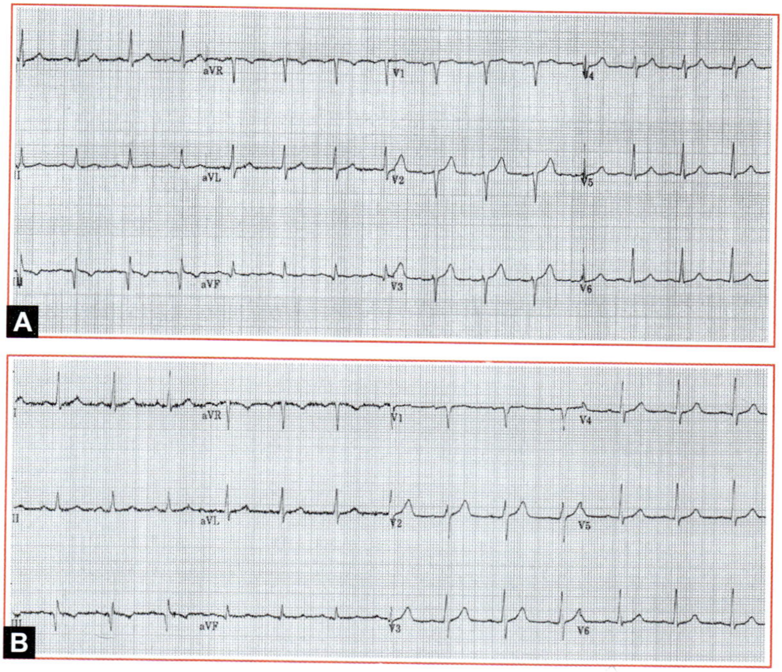

Figs. 14.5A and B: (A). Initial electrocardiogram (ECG).

C. Treat with diuretics for incipient heart failure

D. Start Aspirin (ASA) and β-blocker at low dose with quick follow-up of the response, assess LV function with 2D echo, and follow through with coronary angiography.

The patient was actually started on metoprolol 25 mg twice a day and was told to increase the dose to 50 mg twice a day after 48 hours, if tolerated. He was also placed on 81 mg ASA together with pantoprazole. The patient was seen a few days later at the time of a 2D echocardiographic study. The physical findings at that time showed that the BP was 130/70 with a HR of 80/min. Jugular venous pulse was normal and the S3 was almost inaudible. The initial ECG (Fig. 14.5A) showed old inferior infarct with delayed r/s progression in the precordial leads. The repeat ECG at this time (Fig. 14.5B) showed good r waves in V2 and V3 with better r/s progression and the Q wave in aVF appeared non-significant.

Question 3: The pathophysiologic mechanism for the S3 gallop in this patient is suggestive of the following:

A. High left atrial pressure secondary to significant systolic dysfunction

B. Incipient heart failure

C. Significant silent mitral regurgitation due to papillary muscle dysfunction

D. Ischemic LV diastolic and possibly also some systolic dysfunction

Question 4: The 2D echocardiogram in this patient is likely to show the following:

A. Grade III–IV LV systolic dysfunction
B. Significant silent mitral regurgitation
C. Moderate mitral regurgitation and grade III LV systolic dysfunction
D. Mild LV dysfunction with minimal or no mitral regurgitation

Answer and Discussion

Based on the repeat physical findings and the improvement seen in the ECG, the most likely reason for the S3 was ischemic LV diastolic and perhaps some systolic dysfunction. It was not from heart failure or significant mitral regurgitation. The echocardiogram in fact showed slight left atrial enlargement with mild concentric left ventricular hypertrophy (LVH) and mild LV dysfunction with distal septal and proximal inferior hypokinesis and trivial mitral and trivial aortic regurgitation.

The dose of the metoprolol was increased to 75 mg twice a day. The patient's family physician was told to add an ACE-inhibitor such as ramipril to the regimen starting with a low dose and up titrating the dose during the follow-up. Coronary angiogram showed 100% occlusion of proximal RCA and 99% stenosis of the proximal LAD. The distal right filled through the collaterals. The patient successfully underwent CABG surgery with a LIMA graft to the LAD and saphenous vein graft to the RCA with improvement in symptoms.

PATIENT 5

Clinical History

Patient MC is a 71-year-old lady, from Argentina, non-smoker and non-drinker with history of hypertension going back to her last pregnancy at age 32 years. She was also being treated for type II diabetes and elevated cholesterol for over 10 years. She was being treated with once daily dose of amlodipine 10 mg and candesartan 16 mg and atorvastatin 20 mg in addition to oral medications for diabetes. She was referred because of symptoms of chest pressure with dyspnea of 3-month duration brought on by minimal activity. Typically her discomfort would start in the epigastrium, spread into the mid and left anterior chest region and to the back usually brought on by walking about 400 m. She had no orthopnea. She did have edema of her feet toward the end of the day disappearing by early morning after sleep. She also complained of occasional episodes of dizziness and unsteadiness of short duration. She tended to snore at night and feel sleepy in the afternoons. Her father died from stroke at age 50, mother lived into age 91 years and one brother died of stroke at age 47.

The patient had a stress test with nuclear perfusion studies 2 months prior to this visit. She exercised for a total duration of 3 minutes and 6 seconds with the Bruce protocol. She achieved maximum HR of 146 that was 97% of maximum predicted HR. Resting BP was 180/85 and peak BP was 220/85. The patient had chest pain at peak exercise that resolved after 3 minutes into the recovery phase. Electrocardiogram was uninterpretable for ST segment changes with exercise. The nuclear perfusion scans showed no evidence of ischemia or old infarcts.

Physical Findings

The patient was 5'3" in height and weighed about 72 kg. Blood pressure was 180/85 in the right arm supine position. HR was 71/min, regular. Carotid pulse upstroke was normal with normal peripheral pulses. Jugular venous pulse was normal with an *x' descent*. The apical impulse was not sustained. S2 was well split with the first component becoming soft and inaudible at the apex. The second component was loud. There was a grade I-II short ejection murmur at the apex. There were no extra sounds. Chest was clear.

Question 1: The split S2 in this patient is suggestive of the following:

A. Wide split S2 secondary to possible RBBB
B. Normal splitting of the S2
C. Sequence characteristic of pulmonary hypertension
D. Reversed sequence of left bundle branch block (LBBB)

Question 2: ST segment changes during exercise were not interpretable in this patient for the following reason:

A. Resting ST-T abnormalities secondary to long-standing hypertension
B. Possible LVH with anterior fascicular block on the resting ECG
C. Probable motion artifacts on the ECG during exercise
D. Resting ECG abnormal due to LBBB

Question 3: This patient requires the following:

A. Sleep test to rule out sleep apnea
B. Coronary angiogram to assess the coronary status
C. Better control of BP aided by home monitoring
D. All of the above

Answer and Discussion

The patient's resting ECG most likely showed LBBB and the secondary ST-T abnormalities resulting from the conduction defect must be the reason for the ECG being uninterpretable during exercise. This would typically have reversed sequence of a split S2, with P2 coming before A2. The first component in a reverse sequence being P2 is not normally heard at the apex (LV area) and thus will become soft and inaudible. The second component being A2 is accentuated which is typical of significant hypertension.

This patient most likely has uncontrolled hypertension with increased arterial stiffness that will tend to increase the BP with exercise not only peripherally but also centrally in the aorta. This is to be expected on account of her age as well as the long-standing duration of the hypertension together with the risk factors of diabetes and dyslipidemia. Elevated central aortic pressures on exercise due to central augmentation on minimal exercise will, in turn, produce increased oxygen demands that can produce anginal symptoms even in the absence of significant CAD. Sleep apnea needs to be investigated and treated if present since it is known to aggravate hypertension. Coronary angiography in fact showed normal coronary arteries in this patient. She also had elevated LV end-diastolic pressure at catheterization as a result of diastolic dysfunction probably due to both impaired relaxation as well as secondary to increased stiffness and decreased compliance probably caused by LV hypertrophy. This will also contribute to relative subendocardial ischemia during exercise. This patient would need better control of hypertension that can be aided by home monitoring of BP. Sleep apnea if present is known to aggravate hypertension as well as heart failure.[1-3] Therefore, it needs to be looked for in all patients with hypertension particularly if hypertension is uncontrolled.

PATIENT 6

Clinical History

Patient is a 52-year-old man with history of hypertension of 18 months duration, placed on valsartan that he has not been taking. The patient had mild elevation of cholesterol treated with diet together with family history of hypertension. He had no other risk factors. He denied all cardiac symptoms and has been able to be active doing exercise in a fitness club.

Physical Findings

The patient was 5′7″ in height weighing about 160 lb. Blood pressure was 150/90. Heart rate was 69/min regular. Carotid pulse upstroke was normal with normal peripheral pulses. Jugular venous pulse was normal with an *x′ descent*. Apical impulse was about two finger breadths wide and slightly hyperdynamic. S2 was not split. S1 was not increased in intensity. There was a grade III systolic regurgitation murmur maximally heard at the apex with a soft early S3. The murmur did not appear to diminish significantly on squatting but it did diminish slightly immediately after standing from a squatting position. There were no clicks audible.

Electrocardiogram showed LVH by voltage.

Question 1: The most likely problem in this patient is:

A. Mitral regurgitation secondary to rheumatic disease
B. Mitral regurgitation secondary to papillary muscle dysfunction

C. Prolapsed mitral leaflets and mitral regurgitation
D. Significant mitral regurgitation (non-rheumatic) together with significant uncontrolled hypertension.

A 2D echocardiogram showed moderate-to-severe mitral regurgitation with prolapsed posterior mitral leaflet with enlarged left ventricle and normal LV function. Patient was somewhat irregular in taking his ACE inhibitors at the prescribed doses. Due to symptoms of dry cough, family physician had changed his therapy to an angiotensin receptor blocker. He was referred back about 2.5 years later for symptoms suggestive of progressive increase in exertional dyspnea. Patient had no orthopnea, palpitation or angina.

Physical findings showed BP was 145/85. Heart rate was 75/min, regular. Jugular venous pulse was 6 cm above the sternal angle with an *x′ descent*. Arterial pulses were normal. Apical impulse was about three finger breadths wide and hyperdynamic. S2 was single. There was a grade III mitral regurgitation murmur maximal at the apex with an S3. Electrocardiogram showed vertical axis together with LVH and repolarization abnormalities.

Two-dimensional echocardiogram showed severe mitral regurgitation with prolapsed posterior leaflet, enlarged LV and left atrium with mild global hypokinesis of the LV with grade II dysfunction.

Question 2: Management of this patient at this point requires the following:
A. Better control of hypertension
B. Coronary angiography to rule out CAD
C. Cardiac catheterization, coronary angiography and referral for surgical repair of mitral regurgitation
D. All of the above

Answer and Discussion

This patient had clinical signs (hyperdynamic enlarged LV with loud grade III murmur and S3) of significant isolated mitral regurgitation. Isolated mitral regurgitation is often due to a non-rheumatic cause. The most common among the non-rheumatic causes is mitral regurgitation associated with prolapsed redundant and myxomatous mitral leaflets. The behavior of the murmur despite being due to prolapse of the leaflets was somewhat atypical. It did not diminish in intensity on squatting. It also became softer on standing immediately after squatting. The atypical behavior is attributable to the effect of BP changes on squatting and standing. The former usually raises the BP. That would be expected to increase the degree of mitral regurgitation. The increased venous return on squatting and increase in the heart size should diminish prolapse and should lessen the degree of mitral regurgitation. The murmur did not change significantly probably because of a significant rise in BP. Standing immediately following the squatting will definitely drop the systolic BP due to decreased venous return. This will have a favorable effect on the degree of the mitral regurgitation. This may be opposed by the decrease in heart size which should make the prolapse worse. In this patient the effect of BP change seems to be predominant. The worsening course of his mitral regurgitation over such a short period of follow up of about 30 months, suggests also the significant role played by his hypertension.

Patient had coronary angiogram which showed normal coronaries. He underwent a successful surgical mitral repair with excision of the myxomatous central portion of the posterior leaflet together with a posterior mitral annuloplasty. Seen 13 years following surgery, patient is asymptomatic and more compliant with his medical therapy with better control of his hypertension. The LV size and function are normal, with mild left atrial enlargement and only mild residual mitral regurgitation.

PATIENT 7

Clinical History

Patient FE is a 30-year-old man who is a smoker with history of hypothyroidism treated with thyroid supplement, presented with episodes of left upper chest discomfort radiating to the left shoulder and scapular region lasting for about 2 hours at a time, not always related to activity. Occasionally they were associated with symptoms of feeling strong heart beats at the time. Referring physician found intermittent elevations of BP up to 150/90. Patient denied symptoms of presyncope or syncope and had relatively good exertional tolerance.

His father died of heart attack at age 63, mother at age of 74 of unknown cause. Siblings had no cardiac issues.

Physical Findings

Patient was 5'7" weighing about 210 lb. Blood pressure was 150/85. Carotid pulse upstroke was brisk. Peripheral pulses were symmetrical and normal. Jugular venous pulse was normal with an *x' descent*. Apical impulse was slightly prominent but not sustained. S2 was normally split. S1 was normal. There was an easily audible S4 at the apex without any murmurs in the supine position. Electrocardiogram is shown in Figure 14.6A.

Patient had a perfusion stress test on the Bruce protocol. He exercised for duration of 7 min and 35 sec, and achieved a maximum HR of 135 which was 83% of target HR. The test was terminated because of fatigue with a peak BP of 180/90. The nuclear scan showed reversible perfusion defect involving the inferolateral wall.

Question 1: The following possibilities need to be considered *except*:

A. Uncontrolled hypertension
B. Severe triple vessel CAD
C. Hypertrophic obstructive cardiomyopathy (HOCM)
D. Hypertrophic cardiomyopathy (HCM) without obstruction

Question 2: The cardiac physical examination is incomplete for the following reason:

A. Arterial pulse contour not described
B. Radiofemoral delay not mentioned
C. Auscultation findings in standing position not noted
D. Ankle-brachial BP difference not described

Follow-up Clinical History

Coronary angiogram showed normal coronaries. The LV end-diastolic pressure was elevated to 22 mm Hg. There was no gradient across the LV outflow tract. Patient was treated with metoprolol with improvement in symptoms. Patient quit cigarette smoking. When seen 6 years later, his exertional tolerance was relatively stable and the stress test was similar. He came for follow up again after a lapse of 8 years. His lipid profile showed an LDL of 3.23 mmol, and HDL of 0.79 mmol. The ECG at this time is shown in Figure 14.6B.

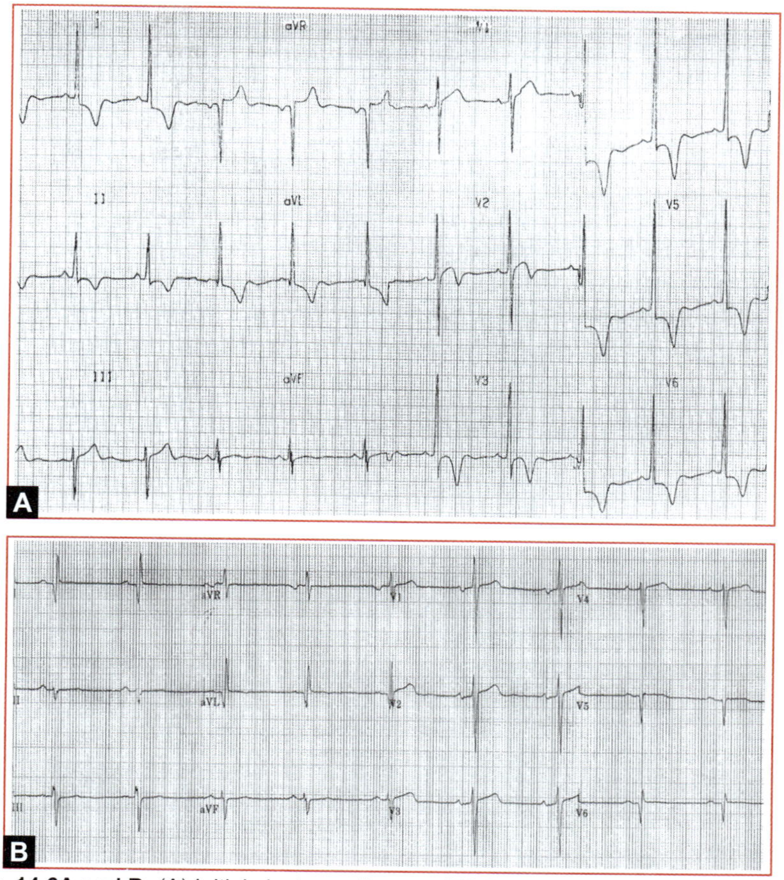

Figs. 14.6A and B: (A) Initial electrocardiogram (ECG). (B) Follow-up, ECG.

Question 1: The current ECG is suspicious of all of the following *except*:

A. Abnormal Q waves suggestive of infarct of the anterolateral wall
B. Abnormal Q waves indicate progression of the underlying hypertrophic cardiomyopathy with fibrosis in the anterolateral wall
C. Pseudoinfarct pattern sometimes seen in HCM
D. Hypertensive heart disease.

Answer and Discussion

This patient essentially presented initially with atypical chest pain and an abnormal ECG showing marked LVH strain pattern with exaggerated T wave inversions seen from V2 to V6. Although he was slightly hypertensive, it was not sufficient to cause such significant ECG changes. As expected, the coronary angiogram was normal. He did have some risk factors including positive family history, mild dyslipidemia and being an ex-smoker. The intervening progression in the ECG without history of any clinical events suggests the likelihood of progression of the underlying HCM with focal fibrosis and scars. He actually had repeat perfusion stress test which showed non-reversible defects corresponding to the Q waves in the anterolateral wall. He currently has no symptoms of angina but does have exertional dyspnea. He probably should have a repeat coronary angiogram to rule out complicating CAD.

PATIENT 8

Clinical History

Patient RK a 26-year-old woman from North India nearing full term with her third pregnancy was first seen a week prior to her due date of delivery. Her previous pregnancies were uncomplicated with normal deliveries. She was asymptomatic. Physical findings showed her to be in no acute distress. Blood pressure was 90/60. Heart rate was 100/min regular. Jugular venous pulse was normal with an *x' descent*. Carotid pulse upstroke was normal with normal peripheral pulses. Apical impulse was slightly hyperdynamic. S2 was not well split. S1 was increased in intensity. There was a grade III diastolic rumble at the apex with presystolic accentuation. No mitral regurgitation murmur was audible. Chest was clear. Abdominal examination showed a gravid uterus. There was no peripheral edema. ECG showed low voltage in lead I with evidence of left atrial overload and sinus tachycardia.

Patient delivered without any cardiac complications. She was followed and remained relatively well for about 10 years except for episodes of atrial tachycardia controlled by atenolol. Two-dimensional echo had shown that her mitral valve area had reduced during this period about 1.5 cm^2 to about 1.2 cm^2. In addition, she had moderate mitral regurgitation and mild aortic regurgitation.

Patient presented to the ER with right upper quadrant pain and was admitted to the surgical service for possible acute cholecystitis. She gave two week history of palpitations and increasing dyspnea and right upper quadrant pain. She also had some cough and was being treated with antibiotics and prednisone by her family physician for possible respiratory infection.

Physical Findings

Blood pressure 110/75 with irregular heart rhythm at rate of 110/min. Arterial pulses were symmetrical with low normal volume. Jugular venous pulse was 12 cm above the sternal angle at 45° with a *v wave* and *y descent*. S1 was accentuated. There was a soft OS and grade III long diastolic rumble. Chest showed bilateral crackles. Liver was enlarged and tender.

Question 1: The clinical history and findings suggest all of the following *except*:

A. At least moderate tricuspid regurgitation
B. Use of prednisone might have contributed to sodium retention and congestion
C. Acute cholecystitis
D. Probable cause of congestive failure is onset of atrial fibrillation in the presence of moderately severe mitral stenosis

Question 2: The reason for the congestive symptoms in this patient as a result of atrial fibrillation is:

A. Excess Oxygen demand placed on the left ventricle from rapid HR
B. Fall in cardiac output due to poor diastolic filling of the left ventricle due to mitral stenosis aggravated by the rapid HR
C. Coronary embolism and resultant myocardial ischemia or infarction
D. Shortened diastolic intervals due to the rapid ventricular rate result in poor emptying of the left atrium due to mitral stenosis leading to increased LA pressures and congestion

Question 3: Management of the patient must include all of the following *except*:

A. Intravenous furosemide followed by daily oral maintenance dose
B. β-Blockers and digoxin to control ventricular rate
C. Anticoagulant therapy with warfarin to maintain INR around 2.5
D. One of the newer antiplatelet and/or oral anticoagulants

Follow-up Clinical History

Patient improved with diuretic therapy and β-blockers and digoxin to control ventricular rate. She was being switched from heparin to warfarin. On the 6th morning following admission, she developed severe acute left upper quadrant abdominal pain which was intermittent but persisted for about 48 hours. This was accompanied by rising serum levels of LDH without rise in serum lactate levels. She appeared to be therapeutically anticoagulated as shown by PT and PTT measurements. A CT scan of abdomen was done.

Question 4: Most likely cause of her abdominal pain is:

A. Mesenteric ischemia
B. Acute gastritis
C. Pulmonary infarct
D. Systemic embolism to the gut, the kidneys or the spleen

Answer and Discussion

This patient had moderately severe mitral stenosis and developed uncontrolled atrial fibrillation with rapid ventricular rate. The rapid ventricular rate during atrial fibrillation results in shortened diastolic intervals. In the presence of moderately severe mitral stenosis, this leads to poor emptying of the LA, resulting in elevated LA pressures which get transmitted to the pulmonary capillary bed causing pulmonary congestion. When significant, it can result in secondary elevation of pulmonary arterial pressure. This acute rise in PA pressure will cause RV decompensation and secondary tricuspid regurgitation. Some of her congestive symptoms might have also been initially aggravated by the use of oral corticosteroids which are known to cause sodium retention.

Atrial fibrillation is a risk for systemic arterial embolism which can affect the brain and cause strokes, affect the coronaries and cause MI or go to the periphery including the abdominal organs.

While she was being adequately treated for the congestive symptoms, and being placed on oral warfarin to prevent systemic embolism which is a serious risk in the presence of atrial fibrillation especially in the presence of mitral stenosis, she actually ended up having systemic embolism to her abdomen. The acute abdominal pain was in fact shown to be secondary to multiple renal infarcts particularly involving the left kidney, as demonstrated by the CT scan of the abdomen.

PATIENT 9

Clinical History

Patient RK a 20-year-old Jamaican had history of heart murmur from the time of his birth. His mother reported that he had some difficulty with breathing during the first year of his life. Subsequently he remained well although his doctors had restricted his activities. He underwent an open heart surgical intervention on his heart about 6 months before this visit. Apparently, two holes were closed with a patch. He was advised to observe endocarditis prophylaxis. He was essentially asymptomatic. Family history was unremarkable.

Physical Findings

Patient was relatively tall and lean. Blood pressure was 100/70 and HR was 75/min regular. Carotid pulse upstroke and all peripheral arterial pulses were normal. Jugular venous pulse was normal with a dominant *x′ descent*. Apical impulse was hyperdynamic and occupied 3 finger breadths in width and was not sustained. There was no palpable RV movement. S2 was normally split on inspiration. There was a grade IV regurgitant systolic murmur audible maximally over the lower left sternal border with an intermittent S3. There was no audible inflow mitral rumble at the apex. Chest was clear.

Electrocardiogram is shown in Figure 14.7.

Question 1: Electrocardiogram shows all of the following *except*:

A. Vertical axis
B. Right ventricular hypertrophy with systolic overload pattern
C. Left ventricular hypertrophy by voltage
D. Incomplete RBBB pattern

Question 2: Based on the physical findings, history and ECG, all of the following are expected to be found on a 2D echo study *except*:

A. Left ventricular enlargement
B. Right ventricular volume overload
C. Dense area in the ventricular septum in the sub-aortic region representing a VSD patch
D. Residual shunt across the ventricular septum by Doppler

Patient when seen in follow-up after 13 years remained well and able to play soccer without symptoms.

The physical findings were as follows: BP was 120/75, HR was 65/min regular and arterial pulses were normal. Jugular venous pulse was normal with *equal x′ and y descents*. Apical impulse was LV, slightly prominent but

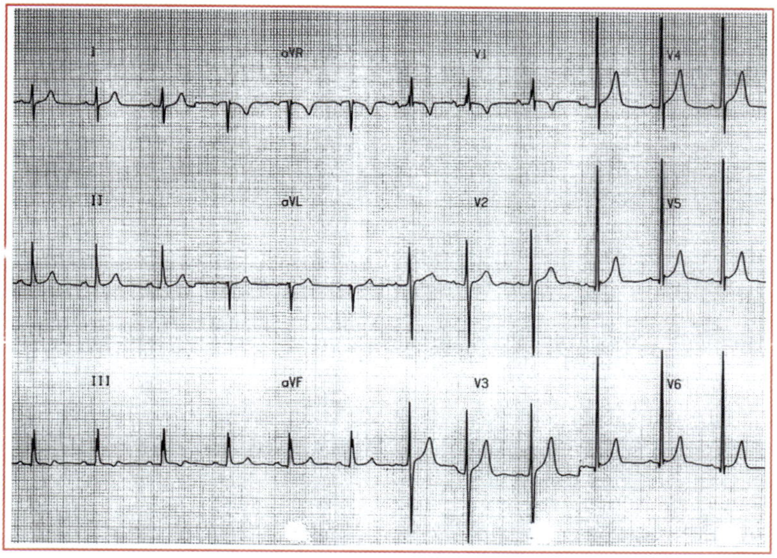

Fig. 14.7: Electrocardiogram.

not sustained. There was a grade III ejection murmur maximal at the second left interspace with normal split S2. There was a grade I regurgitant systolic murmur with predominant high frequency at the lower left sternal border. There were no extra sounds.

Electrocardiogram was not significantly changed.

Question 3: The JVP showing equal *x′ and y descents* is abnormal and in this patient is suggestive of the following:

A. Pulmonary hypertension
B. Post-operative pattern and has no bearing on the RV pressures
C. Need to consider pericardial effusion
D. May sometimes be normal in young adults

Question 4: Based on the current physical findings, all of the following findings are expected on a 2D echo study *except* the following.

A. Left ventricular size and function normal
B. Mild pulmonary regurgitation with mild systolic gradient across the pulmonary valve
C. Dense area in the ventricular septum in the sub-aortic region representing a VSD patch
D. Moderate aortic regurgitation

Answer and Discussion

This patient had repair of two holes on the ventricular septum with a patch. In the early post-operative follow-up, he had a fairly loud VSD murmur audible with a high velocity jet seen on the Doppler across the ventricular septum. The initial ECG showed vertical axis, LVH by voltage and an incomplete RBBB pattern. It did not show any RVH. He also initially had some degree of LV enlargement. But these have improved over the years. The natural history of VSD is such that when large it may cause congestive failure during infancy. If that does not happen and pulmonary hypertension does not develop during teenage years, it may actually remain asymptomatic for the rest of the adult life except for the murmur.

The most common type of VSD is infracristal (i.e. below the level of the crista supraventricularis muscle, a ridge that separates the main body of the RV from the infundibulum or the RV outflow tract). They are in the region of the membranous septum. When viewed from the left side, they are beneath the aortic valve close to the commissure joining the right and the non-coronary cusps. Although they are membranous, they may involve some adjacent portion of the muscular septum. On the right side, they are hidden partially by the septal leaflet of the tricuspid valve. Ventricular septal defects can occasionally be multiple. This patient is reported to have had two defects. Another important feature of VSD is the relatively common occurrence of spontaneous closure. This may account actually for the lesser incidence of VSD in adults compared to the children.[4] While the majority of the defects close during early childhood, delayed closure has also been noted. The closure may involve a variety of mechanisms, including direct apposition of the margins, ingrowth of fibrous tissue, endocardial proliferation, adherence of the septal leaflet of the tricuspid valve or prolapse of the aortic cusp through the defect.[5]

This patient's shunt became less with softer murmur over the left sternal border during follow-up. There could be in fact perhaps partial closure over the years that may account for less shunt and softer murmur. The louder ejection murmur in the second left interspace is probably a pulmonary outflow murmur and is not of much clinical significance.

PATIENT 10

Clinical History

Patient SK is a 39-year-old woman from India referred for evaluation of symptoms of mild dyspnea on rushing. She is a mother of two children between the ages of 8 and 10 years. She has remained well without any prior cardiac issues or risk factors.

Physical Findings

Patient was of average build. Blood pressure was 150/60. Heart rate was 85/min regular and thyroid was somewhat enlarged and nodular. Jugular venous pulse was about 4 cm above the sternal angle with an *x′ descent.* Carotid pulse upstroke was good with peripheral pulses of slapping quality. The apical impulse was hyperdynamic but otherwise normal. S2 was single. S1 was somewhat increased in intensity. There was grade II–III diastolic decrescendo blowing murmur heard over the apex and the left sternal border where it was maximal. At the apex there was grade I regurgitant systolic murmur without any diastolic rumble. Chest was clear.

Electrocardiogram showed voltage for LVH with minor repolarization abnormalities.

Question 1: The increased intensity of the S1 is suggestive of all of the following except:

A. Increased LV contractility due to Starling effect
B. Bicuspid aortic valve with an ejection click fusing with M1
C. Shortened PR interval
D. Thickened mitral leaflets with minimal degree of stenosis

Question 2: The widened pulse pressure in this patient is probably the result of:

A. Mild systolic hypertension with compliant peripheral arteries
B. Possibly associated iron-deficiency anemia
C. Associated hyperthyroidism
D. Moderate to severe aortic regurgitation

Question 3: Based on the current physical findings, all of the following findings are expected on a 2D echo study except the following.

A. Left ventricular size and function—normal
B. Bicuspid aortic valve with aortic regurgitation
C. Non-stenotic rheumatic mitral valve with mild mitral regurgitation
D. Thickened aortic valve cusps with moderate to severe aortic regurgitation

Answer and Discussion

This patient's physical findings are typical for aortic regurgitation of the valvular origin with maximal loudness along the left sternal border. Since she is from India, rheumatic heart disease needs to be considered. Aortic valvular involvement in rheumatic heart disease is usually associated with some mitral involvement. The clinical signs of increased S1 intensity and apical regurgitant systolic murmur are suggestive of associated mitral involvement without significant stenosis. The widened pulse pressure and slightly elevated systolic pressure are suggestive of at least moderate aortic regurgitation. With ECG signs of LVH, the aortic regurgitation is probably long-standing and perhaps more than moderate. She also has mild degree of exertional dyspnea as well that will imply the aortic regurgitation to be significant around moderate-to-severe degree.

PATIENT 11

Clinical History

Patient GK is a 56-year-old man visitor from Greece was well all his life with no history of cardiac murmur, was rushed into the emergency room in a suburban hospital with sudden onset of dyspnea. Patient was dyspneic at rest. Blood pressure was 90/60. Heart rate was 170/min irregular with atrial fibrillation. Coarse crackles were noted over both lung fields. Patient was treated with digoxin and furosemide and transferred to a tertiary care center.

Physical Findings

Patient was well built in no acute distress. Blood pressure was 100/60 and HR was 100/min irregular. Carotid pulse upstroke was normal with normal pulse volume. Jugular venous pulse was upper normal with a *y descent*. Apical impulse was normal. S1 was palpable. S2 was split and audible maximally between the left sternal border and the apex. Grade III long diastolic rumble was heard at the apex.

Electrocardiogram showed atrial fibrillation, low voltage in the limb leads with minor non-specific ST-T abnormalities. Chest X-ray showed clear lung fields with a double density suggestive of left atrial enlargement.

Question 1: Patient's initial symptoms of pulmonary edema were caused by all except:

A. Rapid ventricular rate
B. Myocardial infarction
C. Rapid HR in the presence of significant mitral stenosis
D. Atrial fibrillation

Question 2: Split S2 in this patient is most probably due to the presence of an opening snap. Split A2-P2 can be distinguished from S2-OS by all of the following except:

A. Listening to the split in supine and standing positions
B. By recognizing the presence of a triple sound on inspiration
C. Listening while pressing hard with the diaphragm of the stethoscope
D. By noting the location of the maximal loudness of the split

Answer and Discussion

Mitral stenosis murmur being fairly localized can be easily missed on cursory physical examination. It is not surprising that this patient had no previous history of heart murmur. Even moderately severe mitral stenosis may remain asymptomatic during sinus rhythm. In addition, patients may gradually curtail their usual activities blaming any exertional symptoms to the effect of aging. However when atrial fibrillation sets in secondary to long-standing left atrial enlargement and left atrial pressure elevation secondary to the mitral stenosis, the rapid ventricular rate can hamper significantly diastolic emptying of the left atrium, quite abruptly raising the left atrial pressures to the level of causing acute pulmonary edema.

Pulmonary edema from an acute MI usually implies significant elevations of LV diastolic pressures due to both systolic and diastolic LV dysfunction. It does not require the presence of complicating rapid HR and atrial fibrillation.

The clinical history and the physical findings clearly point to significant mitral stenosis. This patient was seen in 1984 and had hemodynamic investigation with heart catheterization as well as coronary angiography; it confirmed a mean mitral diastolic gradient of 12 mm Hg with a valve area of 0.9 cm^2 suggestive of significant mitral stenosis. The coronary arteries were normal.

The normal A2-P2 split is best heard at the third left interspace where both components are well heard. In the presence of pulmonary hypertension and/or a large right ventricle taking over the precordium, then the P2 may be head over a wide area. The location of maximal loudness of the OS is usually between the lower left sternal border and the apex. OS tends to come later on standing with the decreased left atrial pressure caused by the diminished venous return. Thus, S2-OS gets wider on standing, whereas A2-P2 gets closer. When all three are heard, it causes a trill characteristic of the presence of OS.

PATIENT 12

Clinical History

Patient RS is an 80-year-old lady with no risk factors for CAD presented with dyspnea, cough and orthopnea of 24 hours duration. She gave history of nausea and vomiting 4 days prior to the presenting symptoms. However, patient denied history of chest discomfort.

Physical Findings

Patient was well preserved for age, was in mild distress. BP was 100/70 and HR was 100/min. Jugular venous pulse was about 10 cm above the sternal angle sitting up erect and showed dominant *x′ descent.* Carotid pulse volume was low with a relatively normal upstroke. Apical impulse was slightly sustained. S2 was not well split. There was a grade III regurgitant systolic murmur maximally loud at the apex as well as at the area medial to the apex. In addition, there was a soft S3 audible at the apex. Chest showed crackles bilaterally at the bases. Electrocardiogram is shown in Figure 14.8. Laboratory data: Na 138, K of 4.9, BUN 25, creatinine 362, CPK 346 and LDH 492. Chest X-ray showed pulmonary congestion.

Patient received therapy consisting of intravenous furosemide, topical nitrates, renal dose dopamine infusion and was transferred for surgical intervention.

Question 1: Patient's ECG is suggestive of all of the following except:

A. Sinus tachycardia with RBBB
B. Sinus tachycardia, RBBB, with Q waves and ST elevation of recent anterior and inferior infarction
C. Sinus tachycardia, RBBB with possible LAFB and Q waves and ST elevation of recent anterior and inferior infarction
D. Sinus tachycardia and RBBB suggestive of acute pulmonary embolism

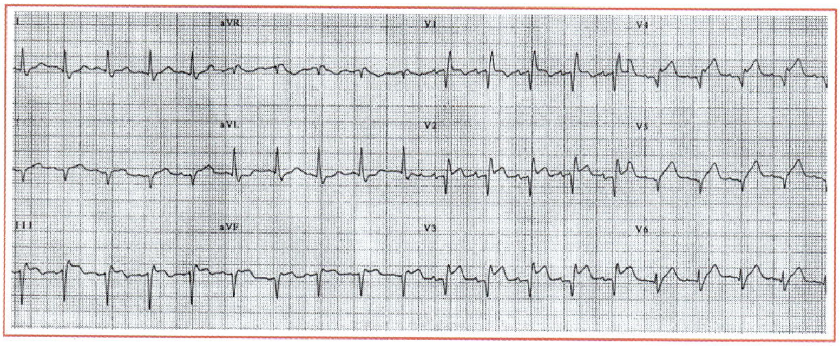

Fig. 14.8: Admission electrocardiogram.

Question 2: The most likely cause of the acute symptoms in this patient is:

A. Severe LV dysfunction due to a large MI
B. Papillary muscle rupture with severe mitral regurgitation
C. Acute ventricular septal rupture
D. RV infarction with tricuspid regurgitation.

Answer and Discussion

This patient quite definitely has had a recent MI. The ECG shows evidence of this in the form of ST segment elevations in the inferior leads and precordial leads V1–V5, suggesting large anterior and inferior infarction probably caused by occlusion of a large LAD that wraps around the apex. In addition, the ECG shows sinus tachycardia probably resulting from increased sympathetic activation secondary to probable decreased cardiac output. In addition, it also shows the evidence of conduction defect in the form of RBBB and possibly also left anterior fascicular block as shown by the superior orientation of the two-thirds of the QRS before the terminal S wave in I. Patient most likely had the onset of the infarction when she had nausea and vomiting 4 days prior to the presentation.

The hemodynamic problem causing the acute congestive symptoms in this patient is most likely due to ventricular septal rupture. If the regurgitant murmur is known to be of new onset in the setting of acute MI, one needs to consider the differential of three causes, namely papillary muscle dysfunction, papillary muscle rupture and septal rupture. The acute hemodynamic deterioration and pulmonary congestion should suggest the possibility of septal rupture versus papillary muscle rupture. Two-dimensional echo study is often quite useful to distinguish between the two. At the bedside, the most useful clinical clue is to locate the area of the maximal loudness of theregurgitant murmur. With mitral regurgitation, it is usually at the apex and is equally loud lateral to the apex. The septal rupture (VSD) murmur is usually loud at the apex as well as over the area medial to the apex. This feature was definitely noted in this patient.

Right ventricular infarction usually occurs in the setting of acute inferior infarction. When RV infarction is large, it can cause severe hypotension and low output state. The clinical picture in this patient is one of pulmonary congestion that does not happen with RV infarction. Furthermore, the dominant *x′ descent* seen in this patient's JVP confirms that the RV contractility is good and unlikely to have any significant tricuspid regurgitation. In fact, good *x′ descent* seen in the JVP in patients admitted with acute inferior infarction should reassure that RV function is normal and therefore the infarction is unlikely to be associated with RV involvement.

Septal rupture has an incidence of about 1% in acute MI and may account for about 5% of all deaths from infarction. It is usually seen in anterior infarction often with the first infarct. Electrocardiogram may show RBBB or complete AV block. Outcome is generally poor if it involves the posterior septum and when associated with cardiogenic shock. Early surgical intervention is often required.

PATIENT 13

Clinical History

Patient JA is a 43-year-old man with history of heart murmur and vague chest pains without any risk factors for CAD, had cardiac arrest at home and was defibrillated six times by the paramedics and subsequently admitted to the intensive care unit of the hospital. He had transient mental cloudiness and confusion but subsequently recovered fully. He was treated with sotalol, topical nitrates and enteric coated aspirin. Patient was referred for cardiac catheterization 4 weeks after the event.

Physical Findings

Patient was relatively tall. Blood pressure was 110/70 mm Hg. Heart rate was 54/min. Carotid pulse upstroke was somewhat brisk. Jugular venous pulse was 5 cm above the sternal angle with dominant *x′ descent.* Apical impulse was LV and clearly had a triple impulse. S2 was normal. There was a grade III ejection murmur at the lower left sternal border and maximal at the apex. There was a loud click at the peak of the murmur. There was a soft S3 audible at the apex.

Electrocardiogram is shown in Figure 14.9.

Question 1: Electrocardiogram shows all of the following except:

A. Marked LVH voltage and left atrial overload
B. ST-T waves changes consistent with LVH strain pattern
C. Left anterior fascicular block
D. Recent anteroseptal infarction.

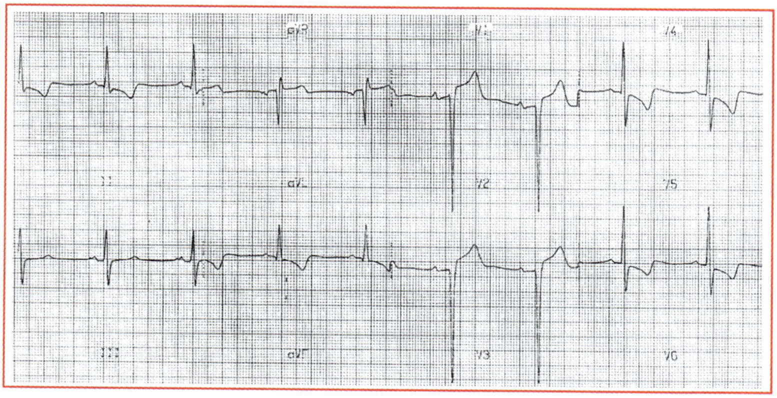

Fig. 14.9: Admission electrocardiogram.

Question 2: The apical impulse described to show triple component is diagnostic of the following:

A. Hypertrophic cardiomyopathy (HCM) non-obstructive
B. Hypertrophic obstructive cardiomyopathy
C. Mitral valve prolapse with severe mitral regurgitation
D. Mitral prolapse with decreased LV compliance due to coexisting CAD.

Question 3: The clinical findings are suggestive of the following:

A. Hypertrophic cardiomyopathy and associated significant CAD
B. Significant CAD and LV dysfunction
C. Hypertrophic obstructive cardiomyopathy with possible prolapsed mitral leaflets
D. Significant CAD and associated aortic stenosis.

At heart catheterization, the pulmonary capillary wedge and the LV end-diastolic pressures were elevated to 30 mm Hg and 23 mm Hg, respectively. There was 110 mm Hg LV outflow tract gradient that was abolished by 100 mg of disopyramide. Left ventricular angiography showed prolapsed posterior mitral leaflet with significant mitral regurgitation. Coronary angiogram showed normal coronary arteries.

Patient underwent sub-aortic myectomy and plication and repair of prolapsed posterior mitral leaflet. Post-operatively, he only had a soft S4. There were no clicks or murmurs noted.

Answer and Discussion

This patient's clinical history is of interest for a variety of reasons. He had suffered the most dreadful complication of the HOCM, namely ventricular fibrillation arrest. Luckily, he did survive this well enough to be able to undergo definite surgical relief of the severe LV outflow tract obstruction. The triple apical LV impulse is diagnostic of HOCM. It indicates the sequential events of an atrial kick (caused by a forceful contraction of the left atrium secondary to decreased LV compliance of hypertrophic LV) followed by a mid-systolic retraction (caused by the mid-systolic obstruction to the outflow with HOCM) (*see* Chapter 5 on Precordial Pulsations). The soft S3 at the apex and the grade III ejection murmur and LVH strain pattern on the ECG go along with this. In addition, ECG also shows possible left atrial overload and left anterior fascicular block.

However, the unusual finding on auscultation was a clearly audible loud click in mid-late systole which in the absence of the ejection murmur would have been considered diagnostic of prolapsed mitral valve. The association of HOCM and the prolapsed mitral leaflets has been observed but the incidence is quite rare. Systolic clicks have been documented on phonocardiography in HOCM before. However, no details about the echocardiographic findings or pathology had been provided.[6] Pseudo-ejection sounds have also been reported in association with HOCM.[7] It was correlated to sudden halting of the systolic anterior movement of the anterior mitral leaflet by echocardiography. It was also found to be associated with significant outflow obstruction. In this patient, however, the systolic click was loud and occurred at the peak of the ejection murmur in mid-late systole. Pathology at surgery confirmed abnormal redundant prolapsed posterior mitral leaflet with significant mitral regurgitation that required repair.

PATIENT 14

Clinical History

Patient JD is a 62-year-old man with chronic renal failure on hemodialysis three times a week and serum creatinine around 300 on dialysis. The patient had an arteriovenous fistula in the left arm for venous access. Patient was in for his routine dialysis. Shortly after going on dialysis, BP was found to fall to 75/50 mm Hg. The nephrologist on call had ordered an urgent echocardiogram. The echocardiogram was reported to have shown pericardial effusion. Cardiac assessment was requested for anticipated therapy of possible cardiac tamponade with pericardiocentesis.

Physical Findings

The patient was slightly anxious but not in severe distress. Denied chest discomfort but admitted to being mildly short of breath. BP was 75/50 mm Hg and HR was 110 min regular. Carotid upstroke was normal. Jugular venous pulse was elevated to the angle of the jaw, with good *x′ and y descents.* The *x′ descent* was slightly dominant. The apical impulse was palpable (11–12 cm from the sternum) despite a thick chest. S1 and S2 were audible but soft. There was a short ejection systolic murmur best heard at the base. Chest showed a few basal crackles. The abdomen was soft. The liver was palpable two finger breadths below the costal margin, and not tender or pulsatile. There was three plus edema around the ankles with mild chronic skin changes.

The ECG showed sinus tachycardia, voltage for LVH, borderline short QT interval with slightly peaked T waves.

Question 1: Does this patient have cardiac tamponade based on the above information or do you need additional information?

A. Not in cardiac tamponade
B. Would like to know about paradoxical pulse as determined by BP cuff
C. Would like to know prior BP and changes from pre to post dialysis
D. Would like to know about the amount of weight gain between each dialysis
E. Need all three mentioned in B, C and D.

Question 2: Of the following statements which one is the most likely:

A. Urgent pericardiocentesis required to alleviate tamponade

B. Urgent pericardiocentesis leaving an in situ drainage tube for prevention
C. Patient in LV pump failure and would require intravenous inotropes
D. No evidence of cardiac tamponade requiring immediate intervention.

Question 3: Description of the ECG findings is consistent with which of the following:
A. Low calcium levels
B. Hyperkalemia
C. Hypercalcemia
D. Moderate hyperkalemia and possibly some hypercalcemia.

Answer and Discussion

Tamponade by definition represents restriction to ventricular filling throughout all three phases of diastole, including the rapid filling phase, the slow filling phase and the atrial contraction end-diastolic phase. It is a major emergency because it severely diminishes the cardiac output and tissue perfusion. No blood can enter the heart throughout diastole because of the external pressure from the tense fluid filled pericardial sac. In diastole, blood is transferred from atria to the ventricles. Since no blood enters the heart during diastole, the patient cannot possibly have a *y descent* in the jugular, which represents diastolic flow into the heart. The presence of a good *y descent* in this patient is a good sign that the patient is not in tamponade. The elevated venous pressure is to be expected in chronic renal failure due to volume overload especially when off dialysis for 2 or 3 days. The *y descent* in fact will be expected to be exaggerated in the presence of elevated *v wave* pressure (and mean pressure in the right atrium) as long as the ventricle is able to expand and drop its pressure to zero as it does in the normal patients during the early rapid filling phase of diastole. This of course is not possible in tamponade.

In cardiac tamponade, the JVP therefore will be elevated but pulsations will be poor. The flow into the heart can occur only during systole corresponding to an *x′ descent*, but this descent will also be poorly visible due to very high venous pressure. The systolic flow can only be recorded by Doppler and that too perhaps only during inspiration.

Pericardial effusions are fairly common in chronic renal failure. The presence of pericardial effusion does not necessarily imply tamponade even in the presence of hypotension. In some patients, when they go on dialysis, initially there can be a sudden drop in BP, which gradually and usually returns back to normal levels after a period of time. This is probably related to changes in the intravascular volume caused by dialysis and the rate of re-expansion of the intravascular volume from redistribution from the extravascular compartment.

With the definite recognition of jugular pulse contour showing good *x′ and y descents,* measurement of pulsus paradoxus becomes less critical. Paradoxical pulse needs to be checked by noting the amount of BP loss on inspiration. It varies from patient to patient. It would be also important to note the baseline measurement when the patient is not hypotensive so that abnormal elevations could be properly recognized. In most clinical situations, this is not generally measured routinely. Thus, paradoxus of at least 15 mm Hg or more would be required to be considered abnormal. For whatever reason, if the contour of the jugular pulsation could not be assessed properly, one should certainly measure pulsus paradoxus.

The patient also was not in cardiogenic shock due to a poor LV function and low cardiac output. The heart sounds were distant and somewhat poorly audible. The thick chest wall and the pericardial effusion together would tend to decrease the intensity of the heart sounds. The S2 being almost inaudible at the base (which is not affected by the pericardial effusion) likely is the function of low BP. The S1 intensity, which would be more affected by the pericardial effusion, if in fact louder than the S2 it will tend to rule out severe pump failure. The fact that in a thick chested person the apex was at all palpable tends to indicate even possibly a hyperdynamic LV that is handling large volume. Patients with chronic renal failure are volume overloaded from sodium and fluid retention. They also tend to be anemic. In addition, this patient had an arteriovenous shunt that would cause a left-to-right shunt and left-sided volume overload. The jugular contour was $x' > y$, which indicated normal RV function that was able to handle the volume overload. A contour showing $x' = y$ or $x' < y$ would indicate some RV dysfunction. If the latter was as a result of a left-sided problem such as hypertensive heart disease, then it would also likely represent some pulmonary hypertension. In fact, the contour of *equal* x' *and* y ($x' = y$) *descents* in the absence of pericardial effusion will raise suspicion of significant pulmonary hypertension.

Within an hour, the patient's BP returned back to normal. The echocardiogram had shown good LV contractility and borderline LV wall thickness. The patient prior to going on dialysis was in fact hypertensive.

Electrocardiogram showed peaked T waves that are commonly seen in hyperkalemia. Since P waves were noted, the hyperkalemia likely is not severe. In addition, patients with chronic renal failure tend to develop resistance to hyperkalemia and do not get into as much trouble as someone who gets an acute rise. The short QT interval in this patient reflects probably hypercalcemia that often coexists with hyperkalemia in chronic renal failure.

PATIENT 15

Clinical History

Patient AR is a 52-year-old mother of four children relatively asymptomatic except for occasional palpitation was sent for evaluation to rule out atrial septal defect.

Physical Findings

The patient was of average build. Blood pressure was 135/80 mm Hg. Heart rate was 75/min. Carotid pulse upstroke was brisk with normal volume and normal peripheral pulses. Jugular venous pulse was 6 cm above the sternal angle with dominant *x′ descent*. Apical impulse was left ventricular, felt over three finger breadths with clear medial retraction and was slightly hyperdynamic. No definite RV impulse was felt by sub-xiphoid palpation. S2 was narrowly split and the split was audible over the left sternal border but not over the apex. There was a grade III regurgitant systolic murmur audible maximally over the apex area. There were no extra sounds heard.

Electrocardiogram showed incomplete RBBB pattern with normal QRS axis in the frontal plane. There were no signs of any chamber hypertrophy, enlargement or overloads.

Question 1: Physical findings are suggestive of the following:
A. Confirmatory of atrial septal defect secundum
B. Unusual to have hyperdynamic apex formed by LV in ASD
C. ASD not excluded. If present it is complicated by left-sided pathology
D. ASD if present must be associated with mitral regurgitation.

Question 2: Which of the following features are not typical of secundum ASD:
A. Apical impulse with medial retraction
B. Loud ejection murmur maximal at the second left interspace
C. Apical impulse with lateral retraction
D. Relatively fixed split S2.

Question 3: Mitral regurgitation if noted in a patient with ASD, the following may be causative:
A. Lutembacher syndrome
B. CAD with papillary muscle dysfunction
C. Atrial septal defect primum with congenital cleft mitral valve
D. Mitral regurgitation with prolapsed mitral leaflets.

Answer and Discussion

This patient's clinical findings are atypical for atrial septal defect as shown by the presence of a hyperdynamic LV apical impulse with somewhat widened area implying an enlarged left ventricle with perhaps a volume overload lesion such as mitral regurgitation. Atrial septal defect with predominant left-to-right shunt at the atrial level would divert the blood away from the left ventricle that in fact will become under filled and therefore will be inconspicuous on palpation.

If atrial septal defect is in fact suspected, a prominent or hyperdynamic LV apex confirmed by the presence of medial retraction should immediately raise the suspicion of an associated LV volume overload lesion. The common conditions based on usual association with ASD are two. First is a possible primum-type defect that is often associated with a cleft mitral valve and the consequent mitral regurgitation. The ECG often will show the presence of left anterior fascicular block with left axis deviation. If this is not the case then one can also consider the presence of associated mitral valve prolapse type lesions associated with a secundum ASD. The characteristic feature of the mitral lesion accompanying secundum atrial septal defect is described as a dislocation of the mitral leaflet toward the left atrial side in the area of coaptation. It gives the appearance similar to mitral valve prolapse caused by the floppy mitral valve, though their causative factors may be different.[8]

ASD is often asymptomatic for years until the patients are in their early forties or fifties. The symptoms of palpitation and mild exertional fatigue may start around that age. Palpitation may result from atrial arrhythmias. Patient may become quite symptomatic once atrial fibrillation develops.

This patient is reported to have had narrowly split S2 which was heard over a wide area of the anterior precordium to the level of the lower left sternal border. This definitely is suspicious of RV enlargement. Patient must be auscultated in the standing position to make sure that the split S2 is still heard and to ensure that there is no significant respiratory variations. This will help in confirming the relatively fixed S2 split. If it is relatively fixed then the diagnosis of ASD becomes more certain on clinical grounds. Ejection murmurs due to increased pulmonary flow may or may not be audible in all patients with ASD.

Lutembacher syndrome implies ASD associated with mitral stenosis (congenital or acquired). The findings vary depending on the size of the atrial septal defect. A large ASD has a beneficial effect on the mitral stenosis. It will help to lower the left atrial pressures. However, the mitral stenosis will end up exaggerating the left-to-right shunt. When the ASD is small, then the clinical picture is that of mitral stenosis.[9,10]

A proper 2D echo study will be of help to confirm the lesions.

PATIENT 16

Clinical History

Patient AN is a 25-year-old woman with history of anorexia nervosa was brought to the emergency room having taken orally 60 tablets of astemizole (histamine-1 receptor antagonist—10 mg tablets). Shortly after arrival around 18.45 hours, patient lost consciousness for about 1 minute.

Physical Findings

The patient was somewhat asthenic, slightly drowsy but arousable. Blood pressure was 100/70. Heart rate was 90/min regular. Carotid pulse upstroke was normal. Peripheral pulses were normal. Jugular venous pulse was low normal with *x′ descent*. Apical impulse was normal and left ventricular. S2 was closely split on inspiration. S1 was slightly split and moderate in intensity. There were no extra sounds. Chest was clear. Extremities were normal and warm. There was no focal neurological deficit.

Cardiologist on call placed a transvenous pacing catheter in the right heart and the patient's rhythm and BP remained stable subsequently. Admission electrocardiogram is shown in Figure 14.10.

Question 1: Patient's monitor showed wide complex tachycardia (not shown). What is the most likely rhythm?

A. Sinus tachycardia rate 140 with LBBB-type conduction
B. Wide QRS tachycardia, probably ventricular tachycardia
C. Supraventricular tachycardia with aberrant conduction
D. Ventricular paced rhythm at a rate of 140/min.

Question 2: What would be the reason for this patient's transient loss of consciousness and why was transvenous pacing wire placed in the right heart?

A. Rapid atrioventricular re-entrant tachycardia with hypotension and the pacing wire was meant for overdrive suppression therapy
B. Tachy-Brady syndrome with asystolic pauses and pacemaker was prophylactic
C. Complete AV block with severe bradycardia requiring temporary pacemaker
D. Torsade de pointe—polymorphic ventricular tachyarrhythmia. Rapid ventricular pacing to prevent recurrences while waiting for the drug levels to fall.

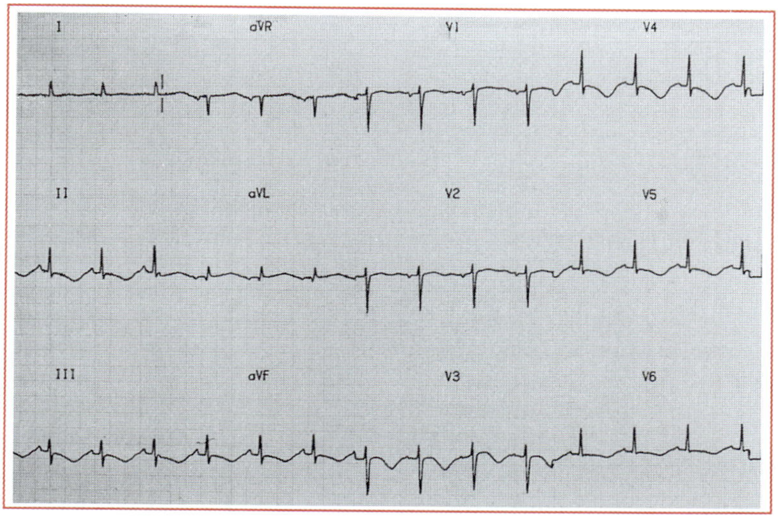

Fig. 14.10: Admission electrocardiogram.

Answer and Discussion

This patient overdosed herself with an antihistaminic agent that has been noted to cause significant QT interval prolongation. The latter implies that the repolarization is prolonged. The duration of repolarization in the cells of the His-Purkinje system is actually the time taken to recover the resting membrane potential after each wave of excitation causing depolarization. In other words, this refractory period of the His-Purkinje system cells is essentially the same as the duration of the action potential. The latter varies according to the frequency of the excitation, namely with the HR, in the intact heart. It is shorter with rapid rates and longer with slower HRs. In this patient, the marked prolongation of the QTc intervals actually caused Torsade type polymorphic ventricular tachycardia and transient loss of consciousness while being monitored in the ER. The QT interval will remain prolonged as long as the drug effects last in the body and predispose to further recurrences of the ventricular arrhythmia. In fact, she was noted to have several short recurrences while being monitored. Fortunately, they were not prolonged. The drug effect was expected to last for at least 24 hours or more depending on the hepatic and renal function.

Since QT interval can be shortened by increasing the ventricular rate, a transvenous pacer wire was placed in the right heart in an attempt to pace her to a faster HR. That should improve the repolarization by shortening the action potential duration and thereby prevent recurrences of the Torsade type tachyarrhythmia while waiting for the drug effects to wear off. That was the purpose of transvenous ventricular pacing at a rate of 140/min in this patient. Since the patient was young and her cardiac function was normal, she was able to tolerate the slightly increased HR. In fact, patient remained stable without further tachyarrhythmia recurrences and was able to be discharged in stable condition after 24 hours.

PATIENT 17

Clinical History

Patient VG is a 51-year-old man with chronic renal failure of 6 years duration secondary to chronic glomerulonephritis on hemodialysis presented with 6-month history of recurrent ascites, ankle swelling and increasing dyspnea unable to walk >30 feet on the level. He had no orthopnea, nocturnal dyspnea, chest discomfort or palpitations. His BP has been on the low side for about 2 months.

Physical Findings

The patient was in no acute distress, somewhat pale and pigmented with some muscle wasting. Blood pressure was 70/50 with no paradoxus. Heart rate was 70/min regular. Carotid upstroke was relatively normal. Peripheral pulses were normal except for low volume. Jugular venous pulse was elevated to the angle of the jaw sitting up with *equal x′ and y descents*. The apical impulse was not palpable. S1 and S2 were soft. There was an early diastolic sound heard along the left sternal border and at the apex area. Chest showed expiratory rhonchi with decreased air entry at the right base. Abdominal examination showed tense ascites with a liver span of 16 cm.

Electrocardiogram showed sinus rhythm, low voltage and widespread non-specific T wave abnormalities. Chest X-ray is shown in Figures 14.11A and B.

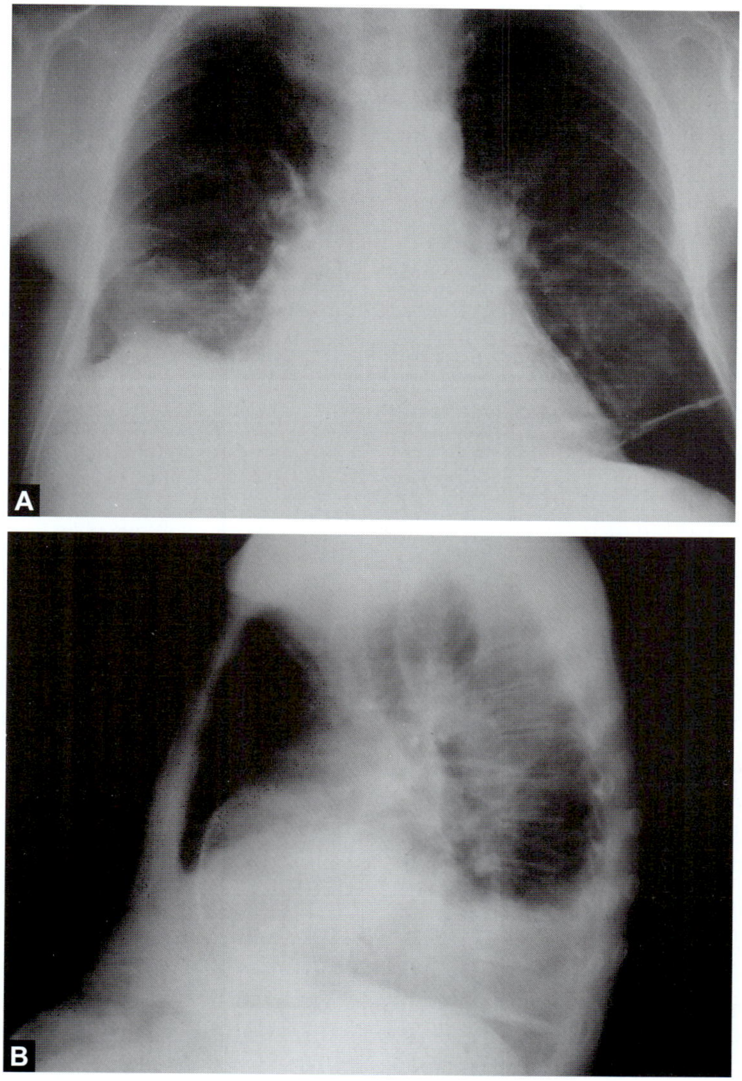

Figs. 14.11A and B: Chest X-ray posterior-anterior and lateral views.

Question 1: Cardiac catheterization will be expected to show all of the following except:

A. Elevated right atrial mean pressures, elevated RV end-diastolic pressures
B. Elevated diastolic pressures in both RV and LV with RV diastolic pressures higher than the LV diastolic pressures
C. Elevated and equal diastolic pressures in the RV and the LV
D. Right atrial pressure wave contour will show equal x′ and y descents. RV diastolic pressure contour will show classic dip and plateau (square root) shape.

Question 2: The extra sound in diastole that was heard is suggestive of the following:

A. Soft opening snap
B. S3 gallop in a patient with heart failure symptoms secondary to cardiomyopathy
C. Possibly a wide split S2 due to pulmonary hypertension and RV failure
D. Probably a loud S3 known as pericardial knock.

Question 3: Chest X-ray is reported to have shown some pericardial calcification and some right pleural effusion. The presence of pleural effusion is:

A. Suggestive of LV failure associated with a cardiomyopathy
B. Not uncommon in chronic constrictive pericarditis and may be due to impaired thoracic lymphatic drainage secondary to elevated venous pressures
C. Unrelated to the underlying process and will need investigation to rule out other causes
D. Needs to be confirmed by CT scan that will also help in identifying pericardial calcification.

Answer and Discussion

This patient has classical signs of chronic constrictive pericarditis. Patients with chronic renal failure can develop pericarditis as well as effusion. The calcific pericardium that was picked up on the chest X-ray in this patient is perhaps a result of this. The causes of chronic constrictive pericarditis are generally listed as follows: idiopathic, remote trauma, post-radiation, uremia and tuberculosis.

The constrictive process being in the pericardium restricts filling of both ventricles in diastole abruptly after the initial expansion during the rapid filing phase. The initial fall in the ventricular pressures to zero during relaxation and the onset of the diastolic phase is followed by a sharp rise to a plateau giving the classic square root appearance of the ventricular pressures (can be termed as "restrictive hemodynamics") (Fig. 14.12). Since the diastolic pressures are elevated, the atrial pressures in turn become elevated. The *y descent* becomes prominent due to elevated right atrial *v wave* pressure head without restriction to filling in the rapid filling phase. As long as the early rapid filling

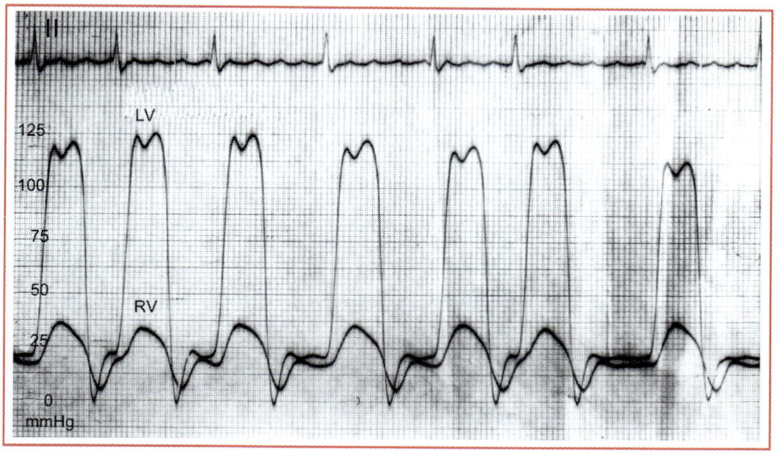

Fig. 14.12: Simultaneous left (LV) and right (RV) ventricular pressures recorded at the time of cardiac catheterization.

is not restricted the *y descent* will be prominent. The *x′ descent* will be well preserved as long as the ventricular function is normal and may become partially diminished when atrial fibrillation sets in the late stage that will result in loss of the atrial contribution to ventricular contractility. The JVP is invariably elevated and will be expected to show good *x′* and *y descents* that will often be equal.

The diastolic pressures are in general equal in both ventricles in constrictive pericarditis. Sometimes in certain patients with pericardial effusion with cardiac tamponade, when the pericardial fluid is drained, the right atrial pressure may still remain elevated. The condition is termed as "effusive constrictive". This is generally encountered in patients with underlying inflammatory process including collagen vascular disease, tuberculosis, and post-radiation pericarditis with effusion.[11]

In restrictive cardiomyopathy, the pressure tracings as well as the clinical features may be similar. However, the LV diastolic pressures will often be higher than that of the RV at rest. If they are nearly equal, mild supine exercise will raise the left-sided diastolic pressures more than that of the RV that can be demonstrated during cardiac catheterization. One study also had shown that mitral annular velocity (E′) measurement by tissue Doppler echocardiography may also be useful. As expected the myocardial function being better in constrictive pericarditis, this measurement is faster in constriction and is usually ≥ 8 cm/s, whereas in restrictive cardiomyopathy such as due to amyloidosis, it is usually reduced.[12]

Most patients with chronic constrictive pericarditis show an early diastolic sound that usually sounds like an S3 and sometimes can be loud and can be termed as pericardial knock. It is caused by the sudden deceleration of the moving column of blood entering the ventricles when the ventricular diastolic expansion and filling comes to abrupt slowing and cessation at the end of the rapid filling phase. This S3 is slightly earlier than the usual S3, but sounds similar in cadence and usually heard at the lower left sternal border and the apex area. It does not vary with respiration. This is the sound that this patient also had. CT or MRI scan will help identify the thickness of the pericardium and show calcification if any.

Pleural effusion is not uncommon in chronic constrictive pericarditis.[13] It may be uni- or bilateral and is probably related to decreased thoracic lymphatic drainage secondary to the elevated venous pressures.

PATIENT 18

Clinical History

Patient JB is a 49-year-old man with history of a heart murmur for some years, essentially remained asymptomatic until about a year ago when he started noticing increasing shortness of breath that he attributed to his asthma. This progressed gradually and approximately 2 months prior to the presentation began to experience paroxysmal nocturnal dyspnea. At around the same time he started feeling rapid pounding of his heart whenever he lay on his left side. For about 4 weeks he was also beginning to experience orthopnea staying up the whole night. He felt comfortable only when he sat up and leaned forward. Patient had no significant risk factors for CAD.

Physical Findings

Patient was in no acute distress. BP was 150/50 and HR was 90/min regular. Carotid upstroke was brisk. Peripheral pulses were bounding and collapsing in nature. Jugular venous pulse was 6 cm above the sternal angle and showed a prominent *a wave* with *dominant x′ descent*. The apical impulse was displaced, was hyperdynamic and occupied about 3 finger breadths in width. (There was a sternal movement felt by the referring physician who thought that it was a RV lift.) There was no impulse felt on sub-xiphoid palpation. The S1 and S2 were not clearly heard. There was a grade III long diastolic murmur of dove-cooing quality audible over both the left and right sternal borders. At the apex there, was a grade II mid-diastolic rumble.

Question 1: The sternal movement described by the referring physician is likely to be due to the following:

A. Right ventricular impulse secondary to pulmonary hypertension
B. Right ventricle pushed forward by expansion of the left atrium during systole
C. Abnormal dyskinetic motion of the anteroseptal wall of the left ventricle
D. Marked sternal retraction secondary to hyperdynamic left ventricle secondary to severe aortic regurgitation.

Question 2: The dove-cooing quality of the murmur is suggestive of all of the following except:

A. Vibrating structures that can be part of the valve cusp and posterior aortic wall
B. Perforation and eversion of the aortic cusp may be contributory
C. Is typically heard in aortic regurgitation of non-rheumatic causes
D. Is related to the LV function.

Question 3: This patient is likely to show other peripheral signs of aortic regurgitation like pistol shot sounds, Duroziez's murmur over the femorals as well as positive Hill's sign. All the following statements are correct about the peripheral signs of aortic regurgitation except:

A. These peripheral signs may be present in other high output states like anemia, thyrotoxicosis, Paget's disease
B. They may also be noted in AV fistulae, persistent ductus, ruptured sinus of Valsalva aneurysm, coronary sinus fistulae
C. They are generally noted only in valvular aortic regurgitation
D. They can be noted in significant aortic regurgitation whether valvular or aortic root in origin.

Answer and Discussion

Aortic regurgitation may result from valvular or aortic root causes. When severe, it will tend to cause marked LV overload and produce a hyperdynamic left ventricle with displaced and enlarged apical impulse. The normal area of medial retraction caused by LV contraction can be quite amplified in severe and isolated aortic regurgitation and can cause marked sternal retraction that this patient actually had (Fig. 14.13). It can be mistaken for RV impulse. But if the sternal movement were to be timed with the arterial pulse, it will be seen to move inward rather than outward during systole, confirming that it is not RV impulse. In fact, marked systolic retraction of the sternum together with bounding peripheral pulses is highly diagnostic of severe aortic regurgitation.

The peripheral signs of aortic regurgitation are noted when the regurgitation is moderate to severe or severe irrespective of etiology of the aortic regurgitation. They can also be noted in other high output states as well as in any conditions that cause early runoff from the arterial system like arteriovenous fistulae, ruptured sinus of Valsalva aneurysm, and coronary sinus fistulae.

The dove cooing quality of the regurgitant murmur is not related to the underlying LV function. It may have three phases of waxing and waning corresponding to the early, mid- and end-diastole. It has been shown to be associated with fluttering of the posterior aortic wall as well as part of the aortic valve cusps. The aortic regurgitant stream appears to produce these vibrations and opening of the anterior mitral leaflet appears to accentuate the resonance of the posterior aortic wall and closing of the anterior mitral leaflet appears to reduce the resonance.[14] Its intensity is shown to be decreased by

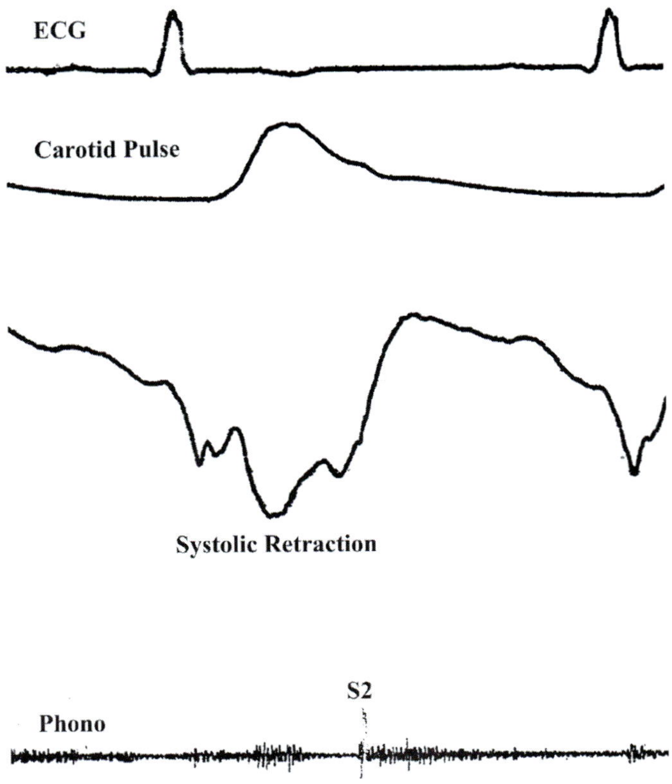

Fig. 14.13: Recording of the movement of the sternum and the left parasternal area with simultaneous carotid pulse and phono recording from the patient. The marked inward movement (retraction) seen to coincide with carotid pulse upstroke during systole.

amyl nitrite inhalation that lessens the degree of aortic regurgitation by arterial dilatation that favors more forward flow.

PATIENT 19

Clinical History

Patient TK a 42-year-old Polish speaking lady, mother of two children, living in Canada for a year, presented with history of chest pain of 2 months duration, described as intermittent throat and chest pressure, usually unprovoked lasting for 5–10 minutes accompanied by dyspnea, relived by sub-lingual nitroglycerine. Patient also felt uncomfortable lying flat. Patient was premenopausal and a chronic smoker had a cholecystectomy in the past and had been treated for hypertension for about 2 months prior to arrival in Canada. Family history is positive for hypertension.

Physical Findings

The patient is slightly obese, anxious with BP 120/80 mm Hg and HR of 90/min regular. Jugular venous pulse was 4 cm above the sternal angle with an *x' descent*. Thyroid was diffusely enlarged. Venous hum grade II was heard over the jugulars. Peripheral pulses were bounding with good carotid pulse upstroke. Pistol shot sounds were heard over the femorals. Apical impulse was barely felt. S1 and S2 were normal. There was a grade II–III ejection murmur audible at the base with a grade I early diastolic decrescendo murmur.

Patient's admission ECG is shown in Figure 14.14.

Question 1: Clinical history and physical findings are suggestive of all of the following except:

A. Unstable angina
B. Hyperkinetic circulatory state suspicious of hyperthyroidism
C. Mild aortic valve disease
D. Aortic valve disease with significant aortic stenosis and aortic regurgitation.

Laboratory data showed normal electrolytes, BUN, blood sugar, creatinine, Ca, P, CPK and LDH levels. Hb was 10.6. ESR was 15. Cholesterol was 3.16, triglyceride 1.17, HDL 1.15 mmol, and LDL of 1.48 mmol. B12, Folate and Ferritin levels were normal.

Thyroid function showed TSH levels of 0.08 (normal range 0.1–3.5). T4 574 (normal range 60–155) and T3 RIA was 10.5 (normal range 0.8–2.7). Antimicrosomal antibody and antithyroglobulin antibody were negative.

Chest X-ray showed pulmonary venous congestion and mild pleural effusions. Patient was placed on IV nitroglycerine, furosemide and propranolol. Patient continued to have recurrence of angina.

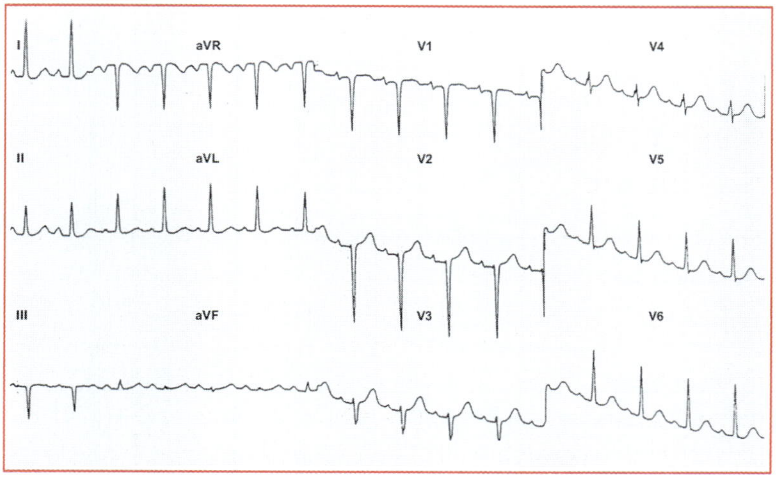

Fig. 14.14: Admission electrocardiogram.

Question 2: Patient would need all of the following except:

A. Urgent coronary angiography
B. Therapy of hyperthyroidism with oral propyl thiouracil (PTU)
C. β-Blockers should be continued
D. Diuretics for pulmonary congestion.

Patient was also begun on therapy with PTU that helped to reduce the symptoms of angina and she was discharged home improved. Repeat T4 was 241 and T3 RIA was 2.5 within 4 weeks of therapy with PTU.
The monitored ECG strips are shown in Figure 14.15.

Question 3: All of the following are the features of angina in thyrotoxicosis except:

A. Angina decubitus is more common
B. Rapid progression but shows significant relief with successful therapy
C. Due to underlying CAD and/or thyroid related coronary spasm
D. Usually indicates significant CAD that would eventually require intervention.

Question 4: All of the following statements are correct in hyperthyroidism except:

A. Congestive heart failure (CHF) does not occur in the absence of underlying LV dysfunction
B. Congestive heart failure rare but can occur in the absence of LV dysfunction
C. Atrial arrhythmias are common
D. AV block is not uncommon.

Answer and Discussion

This patient clearly presented with unstable angina and had classical clinical features of hyperthyroidism. The venous hum is very characteristic and this clinical finding should be looked for in all patients suspected of

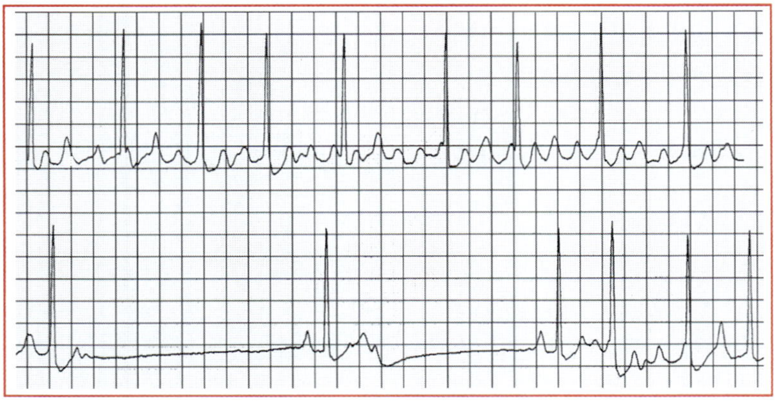

Fig. 14.15: Monitored strips from electrocardiogram.

hyperthyroidism. She also incidentally had clinical findings of mild aortic valve disease without much aortic stenosis and perhaps mild degree of aortic regurgitation. Her peripheral arterial pulses are consistent with the hyperkinetic circulatory state of hyperthyroidism. Thyroid functions and palpably enlarged thyroid go along with the rest of the clinical features.

Her chest X-ray showed findings consistent with pulmonary congestion and her orthopnea got better with furosemide. CHF can occur in the absence of underlying LV dysfunction in hyperthyroidism. However, it is rare. In experimental animals, CHF can be induced by administration of thyroid hormone. Children with prolonged hyperthyroid state without underlying heart disease can develop cardiomegaly and CHF. Abnormal LV function response to exercise not reversed by β-blocker but reversed by antithyroid therapy has also been demonstrated in hyperthyroidism.[15-17]

Characteristics of angina in thyrotoxicosis are such that angina at rest (angina decubitus) is more common, the angina tends to show rapid progression and relief usually occurs with successful antithyroid therapy.[18] Angina in hyperthyroidism can also result from coronary spasm induced by the hyperthyroid state.[19]

Finally, it is well known that hyperthyroidism can cause atrial arrhythmias such as atrial fibrillation and flutter. In fact, it is always a prudent practice to screen for hyperthyroidism in all patients presenting with atrial fibrillation whether or not there is a pre-existent cardiac condition that would predispose to atrial fibrillation. Besides atrial arrhythmias, hyperthyroidism is also known to cause AV blocks.[20,21] This patient exhibited all these cardiac complications, unstable angina, pulmonary congestion, atrial arrhythmias with pauses.

PATIENT 20

Clinical History

Patient JV is a 58-year-old woman with history of hypertension and diabetes for over 10 years, with history of hypothyroidism secondary to I^{131} therapy, as well as a previous history of MI, was admitted with symptoms of exertional dyspnea and angina of 3 years duration and previous episodes of CHF and angina at rest.

Physical Findings

Patient was in no acute distress. BP was 160/80 and HR was 50/min regular. Jugular venous pulse was 8 cm above the sternal angle with a contour showing a prominent *a wave* and $x' > y$ *descents*. Carotid pulse upstroke was normal. Apical impulse was left ventricular, was displaced and was sustained with a palpable atrial kick. An RV impulse was felt by sub-xiphoid palpation.

S2 was closely split. S2 was also loud and palpable at the second left interspace. There was a grade III ejection systolic murmur audible at the base. There was bilateral peripheral edema in the feet. Chest showed relatively clear lung fields.

Electrocardiogram showed slightly prolonged PR interval, suspicious of old inferior scar, T wave inversion in I, aVL and V5 and V6.

Two-dimensional echo study showed concentric LV hypertrophy (15 mm in thickness), normal LV contractility and function, slightly enlarged left atrium that measured 5 cm in width.

The chest X-ray is shown in Figure 14.16.

Question 1: The chest X-ray is suggestive of all of the following except:

A. Cardiomegaly
B. Pulmonary venous redistribution
C. Basal congestion
D. Suspicious of consolidation at the right base.

Question 2: All of the following statements are correct with regard to this patient's symptoms and signs of CHF except:

A. Hypertensive heart disease with significant diastolic dysfunction
B. Congestive heart failure with preserved systolic function
C. Several factors contribute to the marked diastolic dysfunction in this patient including long-standing hypertension and diabetes as well as hypothyroid state with or without significant CAD
D. Possible ischemic cardiomyopathy.

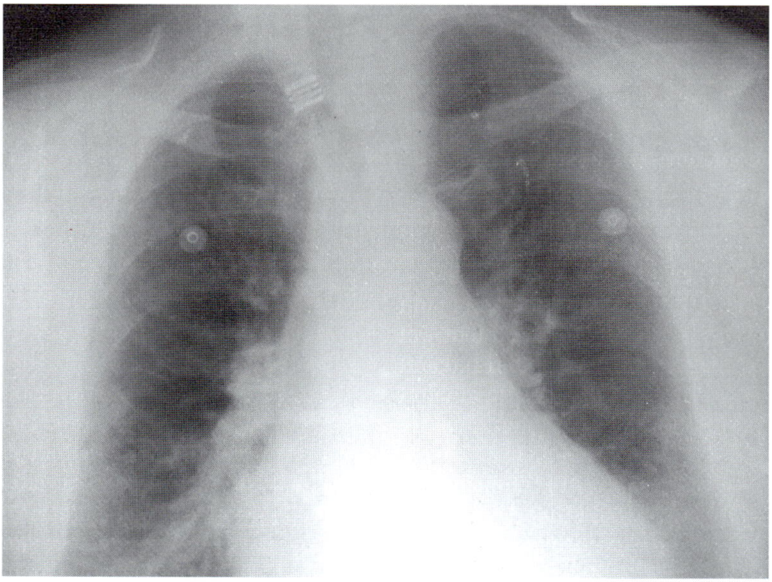

Fig. 14.16: Chest X-ray posterior-anterior view.

Question 3: The palpable S2 in the second left interspace is suggestive of the following:

A. Significant pulmonary hypertension with pulmonary systolic pressures >75 mm Hg
B. Unlikely to be due to pulmonary hypertension since the patient's BP is elevated
C. May be related to the thickness of the chest wall
D. Does not necessarily imply pulmonary hypertension.

Question 4: The cardiac catheterization and coronary angiography in this patient will likely show all of the following except:

A. Normal LV angiogram with normal function
B. Elevated LV diastolic pressures
C. Elevated right-sided pressures and evidence of significant pulmonary hypertension
D. Normal coronaries.

Answer and Discussion

This patient's history and clinical findings are of particular interest. Together with the chest X-ray and echocardiographic findings confirm that the most likely cause of the CHF symptoms and signs in this patient are due to a predominant diastolic dysfunction. The LV systolic function is relatively well preserved. Long-standing history of hypertension is particularly relevant.

Previous history of MI together with suspicious inferior scar in the ECG is suggestive of associated CAD. The elevated JVP with sub-xiphoid RV impulse, *dominant x′ descent* but a visible and good *y descent* together with a palpable S2 in the second left interspace are all suggestive of significant pulmonary hypertension.

In fact, the cardiac catheterization data showed not only normal LV systolic function, significant CAD with 90% LAD and 75% left circumflex coronary disease. The right atrial mean pressure was elevated to 20 mm Hg with an *"a" wave* of 24 mm Hg. The pulmonary capillary wedge pressure measured mean of 32 mm Hg and *v wave* of 25 mm Hg. The pulmonary arterial (PA) pressure was 110/40 mm Hg confirming severe pulmonary hypertension. Left ventricular diastolic pressure was 24 with an *"a" wave* of 32 mm Hg. The hemodynamics clearly reflect significant LV diastolic dysfunction with probable secondary pulmonary hypertension. Underlying CAD is also probably contributory.

These findings clearly demonstrate that a palpable S2 in the second left interspace is highly suggestive of pulmonary hypertension with PA systolic pressures probably in excess of 75 mm Hg. This seems to hold true even in the presence of systemic hypertension as noted in this patient.

Congestive heart failure secondary to predominant LV diastolic dysfunction with preserved systolic function is known to account for more than one-third of all patients with heart failure. The clearest marker of the presence of diastolic dysfunction is the presence of left atrial enlargement in the absence of mitral disease. In fact, impaired left atrial function has been demonstrated in this condition.[22-24] The available therapy at the current time seems to be mainly symptomatic and involve predominantly control of coexisting contributory factors particularly hypertension and relief of ischemia.

REFERENCES

1. Gilat H, Vinker S, Buda I, et al. Obstructive sleep apnea and cardiovascular comorbidities: a large epidemiologic study. Medicine (Baltimore). 2014;93:e45.
2. Somers VK, White DP, Amin R, et al. Sleep apnea and cardiovascular disease: an American Heart Association/american College Of Cardiology Foundation Scientific Statement from the American Heart Association Council for High Blood Pressure Research Professional Education Committee, Council on Clinical Cardiology, Stroke Council, and Council On Cardiovascular Nursing. In collaboration with the National Heart, Lung, and Blood Institute National Center on Sleep Disorders Research (National Institutes of Health). Circulation 2008;118:1080-111.
3. Baguet JP, Narkiewicz K, Mallion JM. Update on Hypertension Management: obstructive sleep apnea and hypertension. J Hypertens. 2006;24:205-8.
4. Simmons RF, Moller JH, Edwards JE. Anatomic evidence for spontaneous closure of ventricular septal defect. Circulation. 1966;34:38.
5. Perloff JK. Clinical recognition of congenital heart disease. Philadelphia, PA: WB Saunders Company; 1970.
6. Luisada AA, Frazin L, Singhal A, et al. Various types of systolic clicks in patients with muscular subaortic stenosis. Jpn Heart J. 1985;26:133-43.
7. Sze KC, Shah PM. Pseudoejection sound in hypertrophic subaortic stenosis: an echocardiographic correlative study. Circulation. 1976;54:504-9.
8. Nagata S, Nimura Y, Sakakibara H, et al. Mitral valve lesion associated with secundum atrial septal defect. Analysis by real time two dimensional echocardiography. Br Heart J. 1983;49:51-8.
9. Craig RJ, Selzer A. Natural history and prognosis of atrial septal defect. Circulation. 1968;37:805-15.
10. Sambhi MP, Zimmerman HA. Pathologic physiology of Lutembacher syndrome. Am J Cardiol. 1958;2:681-6.
11. Syed FF, Ntsekhe M, Mayosi BM, et al. Effusive-constrictive pericarditis. Heart Fail Rev. 2013;18:277-87.
12. Ha JW, Ommen SR, Tajik AJ, et al. Differentiation of constrictive pericarditis from restrictive cardiomyopathy using mitral annular velocity by tissue Doppler echocardiography. Am J Cardiol. 2004;94:316-9.
13. Spodick DH. Chronic and Constrictive Pericarditis: Grune & Stratton; 1964. p. 248.
14. Kohno K, Hiroki T, Arakawa K. Aortic regurgitation with dove-coo murmur with special references to the mechanism of its generation using dual echocardiography. Jpn Heart J. 1981;22:861-9.
15. Skelton CL. The heart and hyperthyroidism. N Engl J Med. 1982;307:1206-8.
16. Foldes J, Istvanffy M, Halmagyi M, et al. Hyperthyroidism and the heart: study of left ventricular function in preclinical hyperthyroidism. Acta Med Hung. 1986;43:23-9.

17. Forfar JC, Muir AL, Sawers SA, et al. Abnormal left ventricular function in hyperthyroidism: evidence for a possible reversible cardiomyopathy. N Engl J Med. 1982;307:1165-70.
18. Somerville W, Levine SA. Angina pectoris and thyrotoxicosis. Br Heart J. 1950; 12:245-57.
19. Featherstone HJ, Stewart DK. Angina in thyrotoxicosis. Thyroid-related coronary artery spasm. Arch Intern Med. 1983;143:554-5.
20. von Olshausen K, Bischoff S, Kahaly G, et al. Cardiac arrhythmias and heart rate in hyperthyroidism. Am J Cardiol. 1989;63:930-3.
21. Sriussadaporn S, Vannasaeng S, Trisukosol D, et al. Complete heart block complicating hyperthyroidism: a case report. J Med Assoc Thai. 1990;73:53-7.
22. Yancy CW, Lopatin M, Stevenson LW, et al. Clinical presentation, management, and in-hospital outcomes of patients admitted with acute decompensated heart failure with preserved systolic function: a report from the Acute Decompensated Heart Failure National Registry (ADHERE) Database. J Am Coll Cardiol. 2006;47:76-84.
23. Fonarow GC, Stough WG, Abraham WT, et al. Characteristics, treatments, and outcomes of patients with preserved systolic function hospitalized for heart failure: a report from the OPTIMIZE-HF Registry. J Am Coll Cardiol. 2007;50: 768-77.
24. Santos AB, Kraigher-Krainer E, Gupta DK, et al. Impaired left atrial function in heart failure with preserved ejection fraction. Eur J Heart Fail. 2014.

Index

Note: Page numbers followed by *f* and *t* indicate for figure and table respectively.

A

B

Buerger's disease, 452, 470

C

D

E

F

K

L

M

N

O

P

Q

R

S

T

Y

ERRATA

Page 123: Table 4.3, Column 2, line 6 from the bottom, "and capacitance" - should be just "capacitance".

Page 398: Table 10.1, Column 1, bullet point 11, "Incresed flow" - should be "Increased flow".

Page 426: Table 10.11, Column 2, Bullet point 6, "Acsites" - should be "Ascites".

Page 453: Paragraph 3, line 2, "Palmerton's sign" - should be "Pemberton sign".

Page 653: Figure 13.7: The diagram in the lower right corner is labelled "Lovoversion" - should be "Levoversion".